MOSBY'S MEDICAL SPELLER

MOSBY'S MEDICAL
SPELLER

The C. V. Mosby Company

ST. LOUIS   TORONTO   1983

Publisher: Thomas A. Manning
Editor: Nancy L. Mullins
Editing supervisor: Judi Wolken
Manuscript editor: Dale Woolery
Design: Gail Morey Hudson
Production: Barbara Merritt

The C.V. Mosby Company
11830 Westline Industrial Drive, St. Louis, Missouri 63146

Library of Congress Cataloging in Publication Data

Main entry under title:

Mosby's medical speller.

    1. Medicine—Terminology.   2.   Spellers.
I. C. V. Mosby Company. [DNLM: 1. Nomenclature.
W 15 M894]
R123.M74 1983   610'.14   83-8262
ISBN 0-8016-3532-2

GW/D/D 9 8 7 6 5 4 3 2 1   02/D/246

CONTRIBUTORS

Contributing editors

KATHLEEN R. COLE and WILLIAM R. COLE

Special consultants

Miriam G. Austrin

Allied Health Careers Consultant;
formerly Coordinator-Director,
Medical Assistant Program,
St. Louis Community College,
St. Louis, Missouri

Kathryn Howard, M.Ed., R.R.A.

Chairperson, Department of Medical Records Administration,
University of Texas School of Allied Health Sciences,
Galveston, Texas

Anne M. Loochtan, B.S., R.R.T.

Clinical Coordinator, Respiratory Therapy,
Pueblo Community College,
Pueblo, Colorado

Helen J. Remboldt, R.N., M.S.

Nursing Instructor,
Grayson County College,
Denison, Texas

Sister Mary Alphonsus Smith, R.S.M.

Chairperson, Medical Secretarial Curriculum,
Mount Aloysius Junior College,
Cresson, Pennsylvania

PRACTICAL GUIDE FOR
THE USER

Language is not only the foundation of general communication but that essential tool by which the concepts and ideas of various professions are transmitted and ultimately measured. *Mosby's Medical Speller* was designed to establish a standard for the accurate and effective communication of the language of the health care professions. Over 60,000 words have been alphabetically listed, correctly spelled, divided into syllables according to recognized phonetic criteria, and pluralized where appropriate.

The selection of words included in the *Speller* was based on those words judged most difficult to spell or most often misspelled. *Mosby's Medical and Nursing Dictionary* and other authoritative and up-to-date medical dictionaries, journals, and references served as our source material to ensure the comprehensive and effective nature of the *Speller*.

To facilitate the user's quick access to information, the following guidelines are offered.

WORD ORDER

All entries are arranged in strict alphabetical order. Multiword phrases are not included in these lists; therefore the user should look up each key element of such word groups. This format eliminates lengthy lists following key word elements.

WORD DIVISION

Each word is divided into syllables by means of a centered dot. For the sake of simplicity, we have used phonetic syllabification exclusively, for example:

an·thro·pol·o·gy
an·thro·pom·e·ter
an·thro·po·met·ric

In typing or typesetting, an important consideration in end-of-line divisions is that a single letter of a word should not end (such as a·bate) or begin (such as ech·o) a line; however, words in which this is possible have been syllabified completely to help clarify pronunciation rather than showing those components as having only one syllable.

Aberrant forms of plurals are presented in the following way:

fis·tu·la
pl fis·tu·las
or fis·tu·lae

SPELLING VARIATIONS

For alternate words or spellings, the format is:

ab·sinthe
or ab·sinth

and, for British spellings:

dac·ry·or·rhoe·a
var of dac·ry·or·rhe·a

We have cross-referenced *or* for alternate word spellings and from British to American English spellings, but not from American English to British spellings.

PREFIXES

We have included many terms with common prefixes such as:

ab·dom·i·no·cen·te·sis
an·te·car·di·um

and within that listing, we have continued to include plurals, word forms, and variants such as:

ab·dom·i·no·cen·te·sis
   pl ab·dom·i·no·cen·te·ses
and
an·te·car·di·um
   pl an·te·car·di·a
   or an·ti·car·di·um
   pl an·ti·car·di·a

The user will also find a complete listing of prefixes and suffixes that are commonly part of medical terminology in the appendix of the *Speller*.

WORD FORMS

In cases where the noun form may be two words but the adjective form is hyphenated, only the adjectival form is given, for example:

test tube (noun)
test-tube (adjective)

We have chosen not to list verb forms where the past tense and participle are formed regularly. The user will find only the irregular forms, for example:

a·cid·i·fy
   a·cid·i·fied
   a·cid·i·fy·ing

PROPER NAMES

Many terms that incorporate the proper name of an individual are included because of the difficulty in spelling often associated with proper names. Examples include:

Teich·mann crys·tals
Tren·de·len·burg po·si·tion

Please note that *'s* is eliminated from all eponyms.

APPENDIXES

The appendixes have been compiled to increase the practical and comprehensive nature of the *Speller* for the user. They provide a quick reference source and contribute to the user's understanding of medical terminology. They include:

- Abbreviations of medical terms and substances
- Weights, measures, conversion tables, and physical element chart
- Prefixes and suffixes commonly used in combining forms
- Pharmaceutical abbreviations

Mosby's Medical Speller may be useful to all those people who are either directly or indirectly associated with the health care professions, such as physicians (all specialty areas), nurses, hospital personnel, medical and legal secretaries, transcriptionists, attorneys, insurance personnel, pharmacists, medical educators, medical record technicians, students, and writers. We think you will find it an invaluable addition to your medical reference library.

CONTENTS

A

ab·a·ca
a·bac·te·ri·al
ab·al·ien·a·tion
a·bar·og·no·sis
a·bar·thro·sis
  pl ab·ar·thro·ses
ab·ar·tic·u·lar
ab·ar·tic·u·la·tion
a·ba·si·a
a·bate
a·bate·ment
ab·ax·i·al
ab·ax·ile
Ab·der·hal·den re·ac·tion
ab·de·rite
ab·do·men
  pl ab·do·mens
  or ab·dom·i·na
ab·dom·i·nal
ab·dom·i·nal·ly
ab·dom·i·no·an·te·ri·or
ab·dom·i·no·cen·te·sis
  pl ab·dom·i·no·cen·te·ses
ab·dom·i·no·cys·tic
ab·dom·i·no·hys·ter·ec·to·
  my
ab·dom·i·no·hys·ter·ot·
  o·my
  pl ab·dom·i·no·hys·ter·ot·o·
    mies
ab·dom·i·no·jug·u·lar
ab·dom·i·no·pel·vic
ab·dom·i·no·per·i·ne·al
ab·dom·i·no·pos·te·ri·or
ab·dom·i·nos·co·py
ab·dom·i·no·tho·rac·ic
ab·dom·i·nous
ab·dom·i·no·vag·i·nal
ab·dom·i·no·ves·i·cal
ab·duce
ab·du·cens
  pl ab·du·cen·tes
ab·du·cent
ab·duct
ab·duc·tion
ab·duc·tor
  pl ab·duc·tors
  or ab·duc·to·res

A·begg rule
ab·em·bry·on·ic
ab·en·ter·ic
ab·er·ran·cy
  pl ab·er·ran·cies
ab·er·rant
ab·er·ra·tion
ab·er·rom·e·ter
a·be·ta·lip·o·pro·te·in·ae·
  mi·a
  var of a·be·ta·lip·o·pro·te·
    in·e·mi·a
a·be·ta·lip·o·pro·te·in·e·
  mi·a
a·bey·ance
ab·i·ent
A·bi·es
a·bi·et·ic
a·bi·o·gen·e·sis
  pl a·bi·o·gen·e·ses
a·bi·o·ge·net·ic
a·bi·on·er·gy
a·bi·o·sis
  pl a·bi·o·ses
a·bi·ot·ic
a·bi·o·troph·ic
a·bi·ot·ro·phy
  pl a·bi·ot·ro·phies
ab·ir·ri·tant
ab·ir·ri·ta·tion
ab·lac·ta·tion
a·blas·te·mic
a·blas·tin
ab·late
ab·la·tion
ab·la·tive
a·ble·phar·i·a
a·blep·si·a
ab·lu·ent
ab·lu·tion
ab·lu·to·ma·ni·a
ab·mor·tal
ab·ner·val
ab·nor·mal
ab·nor·mal·i·ty
  pl ab·nor·mal·i·ties
ab·nor·mi·ty
  pl ab·nor·mi·ties
ABO sys·tem

ab·o·ma·sal
ab·o·ma·si·tis
ab·o·ma·sum
  pl ab·o·ma·sa
ab·o·ma·sus
  pl ab·o·ma·si
ab·o·rad
ab·o·ral
a·bort
a·bort·er
a·bor·ti·fa·cient
a·bor·tion
a·bor·tion·ist
a·bor·tive
a·bor·tus
  pl a·bor·tus·es
abou·li·a
  or a·bu·li·a
a·bra·chi·a
a·bra·chi·o·ce·pha·li·a
a·brade
a·bra·si·o
a·bra·sion
a·bra·sive
ab·re·act
ab·re·ac·tion
ab·rup·ti·o
A·brus
ab·scess
ab·scis·sa
  pl ab·scis·sas
  or ab·scis·sae
ab·scis·sion
ab·sco·pal
ab·sence
ab·sinth
  or ab·sinthe
ab·sinthe
  or ab·sinth
ab·sin·thism
ab·sin·thi·um
ab·sin·thol
ab·so·lute
ab·sorb
ab·sorb·a·ble
ab·sorb·ance
ab·sor·be·fa·cient
ab·sorb·en·cy
  pl ab·sorb·en·cies

1

ab·sorb·ent
ab·sorp·ti·om·e·ter
ab·sorp·tion
ab·sorp·tive
ab·ster·gent
ab·sti·nence
ab·stract
ab·strac·tion
ab·trop·fung
a·bu·li·a
   or a·bou·li·a
a·bu·lic
a·bu·lo·ma·ni·a
a·buse
a·but
a·but·ment
a·ca·cia
a·cal·ci·co·sis
a·cal·cu·li·a
Ac·a·ly·pha
a·camp·si·a
a·can·tha
ac·an·tha·ceous
a·can·tha·me·bi·a·sis
a·can·thaes·the·si·a
   var of a·can·thes·the·si·a
a·can·thes·the·si·a
a·can·thi·on
   or a·kan·thi·on
a·can·tho·ceph·a·la
a·can·tho·ceph·a·lan
a·can·tho·ceph·a·li·a·sis
a·can·tho·ceph·a·lous
A·can·tho·chei·lo·ne·ma
a·can·tho·chei·lo·ne·mi·a·sis
   pl a·can·tho·chei·lo·ne·mi·a·ses
a·can·tho·cyte
a·can·tho·cy·to·sis
a·can·thoid
a·can·tho·ker·a·to·der·mi·a
ac·an·thol·y·sis
   pl ac·an·thol·y·ses
a·can·tho·lyt·ic
ac·an·tho·ma
   pl· ac·an·tho·mas
   or ac·an·tho·ma·ta
ac·an·tho·ma·tous

a·can·thor·rhex·is
ac·an·tho·sis
   pl ac·an·tho·ses
ac·an·thot·ic
a·can·thro·cyte
a·cap·ni·a
a·car·bi·a
a·car·di·a
a·car·di·a·cus
a·car·di·o·tro·phi·a
a·car·di·us
ac·a·ri·a·sis
   pl ac·a·ri·a·ses
a·car·i·cid·al
a·car·i·cide
ac·a·rid
A·car·i·dae
a·car·i·dan
a·car·i·di·a·sis
Ac·a·ri·na
a·car·i·no·sis
   pl a·car·i·no·ses
ac·a·rol·o·gist
ac·a·rol·o·gy
a·ca·ro·pho·bi·a
ac·a·rus
   pl ac·a·ri
a·car·y·ote
   or a·kar·y·ote
a·cat·a·la·si·a
a·cat·a·lep·si·a
a·cat·a·lep·sy
   pl a·cat·a·lep·sies
a·cat·a·lep·tic
a·cat·a·ma·the·si·a
a·cat·a·pha·si·a
ac·a·thex·i·a
ac·a·thex·is
ac·a·this·i·a
   or ak·a·this·i·a
a·cau·dal
a·cau·date
ac·cel·er·ant
ac·cel·er·a·tion
ac·cel·er·a·tor
ac·cel·er·om·e·ter
ac·cen·tu·a·tion
ac·cen·tu·a·tor
ac·cep·tor

ac·ces·sa·ry
   pl ac·ces·sa·ries
   or ac·ces·so·ry
   pl ac·ces·so·ries
ac·ces·sion
ac·ces·sion·al
ac·ces·so·ri·us
   pl ac·ces·so·ri·i
ac·ces·so·ry
   pl ac·ces·so·ries
   or ac·ces·sa·ry
   pl ac·ces·sa·ries
ac·ci·dent
ac·cip·i·ter
ac·cli·mate
ac·cli·ma·tion
ac·cli·ma·ti·za·tion
ac·cli·ma·tize
ac·com·mo·date
ac·com·mo·da·tion
ac·com·mo·da·tive
ac·couche·ment
ac·cou·cheur
ac·cre·men·ti·tion
ac·crete
ac·cre·tion
ac·cu·mu·la·tor
a·ce·cli·dine
ac·e·dap·sone
a·ce·di·a
a·cel·lu·lar
a·ce·lo·mate
a·ce·lous
a·ce·naes·the·si·a
   var of a·ce·nes·the·si·a
a·ce·nes·the·si·a
   or a·coe·nes·the·si·a
a·cen·o·cou·ma·rol
a·cen·tric
a·ce·pha·li·a
a·ceph·a·lo·bra·chi·a
a·ceph·a·lo·car·di·a
a·ceph·a·lo·chi·ri·a
a·ceph·a·lo·cyst
a·ceph·a·lo·gas·ter
a·ceph·a·lo·gas·tri·a
a·ceph·a·lo·po·di·a
a·ceph·a·lo·po·di·us
a·ceph·a·lor·ra·chi·a

a·ceph·a·lo·sto·mi·a
a·ceph·a·lo·tho·ra·ci·a
a·ceph·a·lous
a·ceph·a·lus
  pl a·ceph·a·li
a·ceph·a·ly
a·cer·in
a·ce·ro·la
a·cer·vu·line
a·cer·vu·lus
  pl a·cer·vu·li
a·ces·cent
a·ces·o·dyne
ac·e·tab·u·lar
ac·e·tab·u·lec·to·my
ac·e·tab·u·lo·plas·ty
ac·e·tab·u·lum
  pl ac·e·tab·u·lums
  or ac·e·tab·u·la
ac·e·tal
ac·et·al·de·hyde
a·cet·a·mide
ac·et·a·mi·no·phen
ac·et·an·i·lid
  or ac·et·an·i·lide
ac·et·an·i·lide
  or ac·et·an·i·lid
ac·e·tan·in
ac·et·ar·sol
ac·et·ar·sone
a·ce·tate
a·cet·a·zol·a·mide
a·cet·di·a·mer·sul·fon·a·
  mides
ac·et·e·nyl
A·ce·test
a·ce·tic
a·ce·ti·fy
  a·ce·ti·fied
ac·e·tim·e·ter
  or ac·e·tom·e·ter
ac·e·tin
ac·e·to·ac·e·tate
ac·e·to·a·ce·tic
ac·e·to·a·ce·tyl
ac·e·to·hex·a·mide
a·cet·o·in
ac·e·to·ki·nase
ac·e·tol

ac·e·tol·y·sis
  pl ac·e·tol·y·ses
ac·e·to·me·roc·tol
ac·e·tom·e·ter
  or ac·e·tim·e·ter
a·ce·to·mor·phine
ac·e·to·nae·mi·a
  var of ac·e·to·ne·mi·a
ac·e·to·nae·mic
  var of ac·e·to·ne·mic
a·ce·to·naph·thone
ac·e·tone
ac·e·to·ne·mi·a
ac·e·to·ne·mic
a·ce·to·ni·trile
a·ce·to·nu·ri·a
ac·e·to·or·ce·in
ac·e·to·phen·a·zine
ac·e·to·phe·net·i·din
  or ac·et·phe·net·i·din
a·ce·to·phe·none
a·ce·to·sol·u·ble
a·ce·to·sul·fone
a·ce·to·tol·u·ide
  or a·ce·to·to·lu·i·dide
a·ce·to·to·lu·i·dide
  or a·ce·to·tol·u·ide
a·ce·tous
ac·et·phe·net·i·din
  or a·ce·to·phe·net·i·din
a·ce·tract
a·ce·tum
  pl a·ce·ta
a·ce·tyl
a·ce·tyl·am·i·no·ben·zine
a·ce·tyl·an·i·line
a·cet·y·lase
a·cet·y·la·tion
ac·e·tyl·be·ta·meth·yl·cho·
  line
ac·e·tyl·car·bro·mal
ac·e·tyl·cho·line
ac·e·tyl·cho·lin·es·ter·ase
a·ce·tyl·co A
a·ce·tyl·co·en·zyme A
a·ce·tyl·cys·te·ine
ac·e·tyl·dig·i·tox·in
a·cet·y·lene
ac·e·tyl·meth·yl·car·bi·nol

ac·et·yl-*p*-am·i·no·phe·nol
ac·e·tyl·phen·yl·hy·dra·
  zine
ac·e·tyl·sa·lic·y·late
a·ce·tyl·sal·i·cyl·ic
ac·e·tyl·stro·phan·thi·din
a·ce·tyl sul·fi·sox·a·zole
ac·e·tyl·trans·fer·ase
ach·a·la·si·a
ache
a·chei·li·a
  or a·chi·li·a
a·chei·ri·a
  or a·chi·ri·a
a·chei·ro·po·di·a
Ach·il·le·a
a·chil·le·ine
A·chil·les ten·don
a·chi·li·a
  or a·chei·li·a
a·chil·lo·bur·si·tis
a·chil·lo·dyn·i·a
ach·il·lor·rha·phy
a·chil·lo·te·not·o·my
ach·il·lot·o·my
  pl ach·il·lot·o·mies
a·chi·ri·a
  or a·chei·ri·a
a·chlor·hy·dri·a
a·chlor·hy·dric
a·chlo·rop·si·a
a·cho·li·a
a·chol·ic
  or ach·o·lous
a·chol·u·ric
ach·o·lous
  or a·chol·ic
a·chon·dro·gen·e·sis
a·chon·dro·pla·si·a
a·chon·dro·plas·tic
a·chor·dal
a·chor·date
A·cho·ri·on
a·chres·tic
a·chro·a·cyte
ach·ro·dex·trin
  or ach·ro·ö·dex·trin
a·chroi·o·cy·thoe·mi·a
  var of a·chroi·o·cy·the·mi·a

3

a·chroi·o·cy·the·mi·a
a·chro·ma
　or a·chro·mi·a
a·chro·ma·cyte
ach·ro·ma·si·a
a·chro·mat
a·chro·mat·ic
a·chro·ma·tin
a·chro·ma·tin·ic
a·chro·ma·tism
a·chro·mat·o·cyte
a·chro·ma·tol·y·sis
　pl a·chro·ma·tol·y·ses
a·chro·ma·to·phil
a·chro·ma·to·phil·i·a
a·chro·ma·to·pi·a
a·chro·ma·top·si·a
a·chro·ma·to·sis
　pl a·chro·ma·to·ses
a·chro·ma·tu·ri·a
a·chro·mi·a
　or a·chro·ma
a·chro·mic
a·chro·mo·cyte
a·chro·mo·phil
a·chro·mo·trich·i·a
Ach·ro·my·cin
ach·ro·ö·dex·trin
　or ach·ro·dex·trin
a·chy
　a·chi·er
　a·chi·est
a·chy·li·a
a·chy·li·a gas·tri·ca
a·chy·lous
a·chy·mi·a
a·cic·u·lar
a·cic·u·lum
ac·id
ac·i·dae·mi·a
　var of ac·i·de·mi·a
ac·id·am·i·nu·ri·a
ac·i·de·mi·a
ac·id·fast
a·cid·ic
a·cid·i·fi·a·ble
a·cid·i·fi·ca·tion
a·cid·i·fi·er

a·cid·i·fy
　a·cid·i·fied
　a·cid·i·fy·ing
ac·i·dim·e·ter
ac·i·dim·e·try
　pl ac·i·dim·e·tries
a·cid·i·ty
　pl a·cid·i·ties
ac·i·do·gen·ic
A·ci·dol
ac·i·dol·o·gy
a·cid·o·phil
　or a·cid·o·phile
a·cid·o·phile
　or a·cid·o·phil
a·cid·o·phil·i·a
ac·i·do·phil·ic
ac·i·doph·i·lism
ac·i·doph·i·lus milk
ac·i·do·sis
　pl ac·i·do·ses
ac·i·dot·ic
ac·cid·u·late
a·cid·u·lous
ac·i·dum
ac·i·du·ri·a
ac·i·du·ric
ac·id·yl
ac·i·e·sis
　or ac·y·e·sis
ac·i·nar
ac·i·ne·si·a
a·cin·ic
ac·i·ni·form
ac·i·ni·tis
ac·i·nose
ac·i·nous
ac·i·nus
　pl ac·i·ni
ack·ee
　or ak·ee
a·clad·i·o·sis
a·cla·sis
　pl ac·la·ses
a·clas·tic
a·cleis·to·car·di·a
a·clu·sion
ac·mae·the·sia
　var of ac·mes·the·sia

ac·me
ac·mes·the·si·a
ac·ne
ac·ne ro·sa·ce·a
　pl ac·nae ro·sa·ce·ae
ac·ne vul·gar·is
　pl ac·nae vul·gar·es
ac·ne·form
　or ac·ne·i·form
ac·ne·gen·ic
ac·ne·i·form
　or ac·ne·form
ac·ni·tis
Ac·o·can·the·ra
　or Ac·o·kan·the·ra
a·coe·lo·mate
a·coe·nes·the·si·a
　or a·ce·nes·the·si·a
a·co·in
　or a·co·ine
a·co·ine
　or a·co·in
ac·o·kan·thera
　or ac·o·can·thera
a·con·i·tase
ac·o·nite
ac·o·nit·ic
a·con·i·tine
Ac·o·ni·tum
ac·o·re·a
a·co·ri·a
　or a·ko·ri·a
a·cor·tan
a·cou·es·the·si·a
　or a·cu·es·the·si·a
a·cou·me·ter
a·cous·ma
　pl a·cous·mas
　or a·cous·ma·ta
a·cous·ma·tam·ne·si·a
a·cous·tic
a·cous·ti·co·fa·cial
a·cous·ti·co·mo·tor
a·cous·ti·co·pal·pe·bral
a·cous·ti·co·pho·bia
a·cous·tics
a·cous·to·gram
ac·quire
ac·qui·si·tion

4

ac·ral
a·cra·ni·a
a·cra·ni·al
ac·rid
ac·ri·dine
ac·rid·i·ty
   pl ac·rid·i·ties
ac·ri·fla·vine
ac·ri·mo·ny
   pl ac·ri·mo·nies
ac·ri·sor·cin
a·crit·i·cal
ac·ro·ag·no·sis
ac·ro·an·es·the·si·a
ac·ro·ar·thri·tis
ac·ro·a·tax·i·a
ac·ro·blast
ac·ro·brach·y·ceph·a·ly
ac·ro·cen·tric
ac·ro·ce·pha·li·a
   or ac·ro·ceph·a·ly
ac·ro·ceph·a·lo·pol·y·syn·
   dac·ty·ly
ac·ro·ceph·a·lo·syn·dac·ty·
   ly
ac·ro·ceph·a·ly
   or ac·ro·ceph·a·li·a
   pl ac·ro·ceph·a·lies
ac·ro·chor·don
ac·ro·ci·ne·sis
ac·ro·con·trac·ture
ac·ro·cy·a·no·sis
   pl ac·ro·cy·a·no·ses
ac·ro·cy·a·not·ic
ac·ro·der·ma·ti·tis
   pl ac·ro·der·ma·ti·tes
   or ac·ro·der·ma·ti·ti·des
ac·ro·der·ma·to·sis
ac·ro·dol·i·cho·me·li·a
ac·ro·dont
ac·ro·dyn·i·a
ac·ro·dys·pla·si·a
ac·ro·e·de·ma
ac·ro·es·the·si·a
ac·rog·no·sis
ac·ro·hy·per·hi·dro·sis
ac·ro·hy·po·ther·my
ac·ro·ker·a·to·sis·
   pl ac·ro·ker·a·to·ses

ac·ro·ki·ne·si·a
ac·ro·le·in
ac·ro·mac·ri·a
ac·ro·ma·ni·a
ac·ro·me·ga·li·a
   or ac·ro·meg·a·ly
ac·ro·me·gal·ic
ac·ro·meg·a·loid
ac·ro·meg·a·ly
   pl ac·ro·meg·a·lies
   or ac·ro·me·ga·li·a
ac·ro·me·lal·gi·a
ac·ro·met·a·gen·e·sis
a·cro·mi·al
ac·ro·mic·ri·a
a·cro·mi·o·cla·vic·u·lar
a·cro·mi·o·cor·a·coid
a·cro·mi·o·hu·mer·al
a·cro·mi·on
a·cro·mi·o·nec·to·my
a·cro·mi·o·scap·u·lar
a·cro·mi·o·tho·rac·ic
a·crom·pha·lus
ac·ro·my·o·to·ni·a
ac·ro·nar·cot·ic
ac·ro·neu·rop·a·thy
ac·ro·neu·ro·sis
ac·ro·nine
ac·ro·nyx
ac·roos·te·ol·y·sis
ac·ro·pa·chy
   pl ac·ro·pach·ies
ac·ro·pach·y·der·ma
ac·ro·pa·ral·y·sis
ac·ro·par·es·the·si·a
ac·ro·pa·thol·o·gy
   pl ac·ro·pa·thol·o·gies
a·crop·a·thy
   pl a·crop·a·thies
a·crop·e·tal
ac·ro·pho·bi·a
ac·ro·pig·men·ta·tion
ac·ro·pos·thi·tis
ac·ro·pur·pu·ra
ac·ro·scle·ro·der·ma
ac·ro·scle·ro·sis
   pl ac·ro·scle·ro·ses
ac·rose
ac·ro·so·mal

ac·ro·some
ac·ros·te·al·gi·a
ac·ro·ter·ic
a·crot·ic
ac·ro·tism
ac·ro·tro·pho·neu·ro·sis
ac·ry·late
a·cryl·ic
ac·ry·lo·ni·trile
act
Ac·tae·a
Ac·ti·dil
ac·tin
ac·tin·ic
ac·ti·nism
ac·tin·i·um
ac·ti·no·bac·il·lo·sis
   pl ac·ti·no·bac·il·lo·ses
ac·ti·no·chem·is·try
   pl ac·ti·no·chem·is·tries
ac·ti·no·cu·ti·tis
ac·ti·no·der·ma·ti·tis
ac·tin·o·gen
ac·ti·no·gen·e·sis
ac·ti·no·gen·ic
ac·tin·o·graph
ac·ti·nog·ra·phy
   pl ac·ti·nog·ra·phies
ac·tin·o·lite
   or ac·tin·o·lyte
ac·ti·nol·o·gy
   pl ac·ti·nol·o·gies
ac·tin·o·lyte
   or ac·tin·o·lite
ac·ti·nom·e·ter
ac·ti·nom·e·try
   pl ac·ti·nom·e·tries
Ac·ti·no·my·ces
Ac·ti·no·my·ce·ta·les
ac·ti·no·my·cete
ac·ti·no·my·cin
ac·ti·no·my·co·ma
   pl ac·ti·no·my·co·mas
   or ac·ti·no·my·co·mata
ac·ti·no·my·co·sis
   pl ac·ti·no·my·co·ses
ac·ti·non
ac·ti·no·neu·ri·tis
Ac·ti·no·po·da

ac·ti·no·ther·a·py
ac·ti·no·tox·e·mi·a
ac·ti·no·tox·in
ac·ti·va·tor
ac·tom·e·ter
ac·to·my·o·sin
Ac·u·ar·i·a
a·cu·es·the·si·a
   or a·cou·es·the·si·a
a·cu·i·ty
   pl a·cu·i·ties
a·cu·le·ate
a·cu·me·ter
a·cu·mi·nate
ac·u·pres·sure
ac·u·punc·ture
a·cute
a·cu·ti·cos·tal
ac·u·tor·sion
a·cy·a·no·blep·si·a
a·cy·a·not·ic
a·cy·clic
ac·y·e·sis
   or ac·i·e·sis
Ac·yl·an·id
ac·y·lase
ac·yl·a·tion
ac·yl·mu·tase
ac·yl·phos·pha·tase
ac·yl·trans·fer·ase
a·cys·ti·a
a·cys·ti·ner·vi·a
a·dac·ry·a
a·dac·tyl·i·a
a·dac·tyl·ous
a·dac·ty·ly
ad·a·man·tine
ad·a·man·ti·no·ma
   pl ad·a·man·ti·no·mas
   or ad·a·man·ti·no·ma·ta
ad·a·man·to·blast
ad·a·man·to·blas·to·ma
   pl ad·a·man·to·blas·to·
     mas
   or ad·a·man·to·blas·to·
     ma·ta
ad·a·man·to·ma
   pl ad·a·man·to·mas
   or ad·a·man·to·ma·ta

Ad·am's ap·ple
Ad·an·so·ni·a
a·dapt
ad·ap·ta·tion
a·dapt·er
   or a·dap·tor
a·dap·tive
a·dap·tor
   or a·dap·ter
ad·ax·i·al
ad·der
ad·dict
ad·dic·tion
ad·dic·tive
Ad·di·so·ni·an
ad·di·son·ism
Ad·di·son dis·ease
add·i·tive
ad·du·cent
ad·duct
ad·duc·tion
ad·duc·tor
a·de·lo·mor·phous
ad·e·nal·gi·a
ad·e·nase
ad·en·as·the·ni·a
a·den·drit·ic
ad·e·nec·to·my
   pl ad·e·nec·to·mies
ad·en·ec·to·pi·a
a·de·ni·a
a·den·i·form
ad·e·nine
ad·e·ni·tis
   pl ad·e·ni·ti·des
   or ad·e·nit·is·es
ad·e·ni·za·tion
ad·e·no·ac·an·tho·ma
   pl ad·e·no·ac·an·tho·mas
   or ad·e·no·ac·an·tho·ma·ta
ad·e·no·a·mel·o·blas·to·
   ma
   pl ad·e·no·a·mel·o·blas·
     to·mas
   or ad·e·no·a·mel·o·blas·
     to·ma·ta
ad·e·no·blast

ad·e·no·car·ci·no·ma
   pl ad·e·no·car·ci·no·mas
   or ad·e·no·car·ci·no·ma·ta
ad·e·no·car·ci·no·ma·tous
ad·e·no·cele
ad·e·no·cel·lu·li·tis
ad·e·no·chon·dro·ma
   pl ad·e·no·chon·dro·mas
   or ad·e·no·chon·dro·ma·ta
ad·e·no·cyst
ad·e·no·cys·tic
ad·e·no·cys·to·ma
   pl ad·e·no·cys·to·mas
   or ad·e·no·cys·to·ma·ta
ad·e·no·cyte
ad·e·no·dyn·i·a
ad·e·no·ep·i·the·li·o·ma
ad·e·no·fi·bro·ma
   pl ad·e·no·fi·bro·mas
   or ad·e·no·fi·bro·ma·ta
ad·e·no·fi·bro·sis
ad·e·nog·e·nous
ad·e·nog·ra·phy
ad·e·no·hy·poph·y·se·al
ad·e·no·hy·poph·y·sec·to·
   my
ad·e·no·hy·poph·y·sis
   pl ad·e·no·hy·poph·y·
     ses
ad·e·noid
ad·e·noid·al
ad·e·noid·ec·to·my
   pl ad·e·noid·ec·to·mies
ad·e·noid·ism
ad·e·noid·i·tis
ad·e·no·lei·o·my·o·ma
   pl ad·e·no·lei·o·my·o·mas
   or ad·e·no·lei·o·my·o·ma·ta
ad·e·no·li·po·ma
   pl ad·e·no·li·po·mas
   or ad·e·no·li·po·ma·ta
ad·e·no·lip·o·ma·to·sis
   pl ad·e·no·lym·pho·mas
   or ad·e·no·lym·pho·ma·ta
ad·e·no·lym·phi·tis
ad·e·no·lym·pho·cele
ad·e·no·lym·pho·ma
   pl ad·e·no·lym·pho·mas
   or ad·e·no·lym·pho·ma·ta

ad·e·no·ma
  pl ad·e·no·mas
  or ad·e·no·ma·ta
ad·e·no·ma·la·ci·a
ad·e·nom·a·toid
ad·e·no·ma·to·sis
  pl ad·e·no·ma·to·ses
ad·e·nom·a·tous
ad·e·no·mere
ad·e·no·my·o·fi·bro·ma
ad·e·no·my·o·ma
  pl ad·e·no·my·o·mas
  or ad·e·no·my·o·ma·ta
ad·e·no·my·o·ma·tous
ad·e·no·my·o·me·tri·tis
ad·e·no·my·o·sar·co·ma
ad·e·no·my·o·sis
  pl ad·e·no·my·o·ses
ad·e·no·myx·o·ma
  pl ad·e·no·myx·o·mas
  or ad·e·no·myx·o·ma·ta
ad·e·no·myxo·sar·co·ma
  pl ad·e·no·myx·o·sar·co·mas
  or ad·e·no·myx·o·sar·co·ma·ta
ad·e·non·cus
ad·e·no·neu·ral
ad·e·nop·a·thy
  pl ad·e·nop·a·thies
ad·e·no·phar·yn·gi·tis
  pl ad·e·no·phar·yn·gi·tis·es
  or ad·e·no·phar·yn·gi·ti·des
ad·e·no·phleg·mon
ad·e·no·sar·co·ma
  pl ad·e·no·sar·co·mas
  or ad·e·no·sar·co·ma·ta
ad·e·no·scle·ro·sis
ad·e·nose
a·den·o·sine
ad·e·no·sis
  pl ad·e·no·ses
ad·e·no·tome
ad·e·not·o·my
  pl ad·e·not·o·mies
ad·e·no·ton·sil·lec·to·my
ad·e·nous

ad·e·no·vi·rus
ad·e·nyl
a·den·yl·ate
ad·e·nyl·ic
ad·e·ny·lyl
ad·eps
  pl ad·i·pes
ad·e·qua·cy
a·der·mi·a
a·der·mo·gen·e·sis
ad·her·ence
ad·her·ent
ad·he·sion
ad·he·si·ot·o·my
  pl ad·he·si·ot·o·mies
ad·he·sive
a·di·ac·tin·ic
a·di·ad·o·cho·ki·ne·si·a
Ad·i·an·tum
a·di·a·pho·ret·ic
a·di·a·pho·ri·a
a·di·a·ther·man·cy
  pl a·di·a·ther·man·cies
ad·i·ent
A·din·i·da
ad·i·o·spi·ro·my·co·sis
ad·i·o·spore
ad·i·pec·to·my
ad·i·phen·ine
a·dip·ic
ad·i·po·cele
ad·i·po·cel·lu·lar
ad·i·po·cere
ad·i·po·fi·bro·ma
  pl ad·i·po·fi·bro·mas
  or ad·i·po·fi·bro·ma·ta
ad·i·po·gen·e·sis
  pl ad·i·po·gen·e·ses
ad·i·po·ge·net·ic
  or ad·i·pog·e·nous
  or ad·i·po·gen·ic
ad·i·po·gen·ic
  or ad·i·po·ge·net·ic
  or ad·i·pog·e·nous
ad·i·pog·e·nous
  or ad·i·po·ge·net·ic
  or ad·i·po·gen·ic
ad·i·po·ki·nin
ad·i·pol·y·sis

ad·i·po·ne·cro·sis
ad·i·po·pex·is
ad·i·pose
ad·i·po·sis
  pl ad·i·po·ses
ad·i·po·si·tis
ad·i·pos·i·ty
  pl ad·i·pos·i·ties
ad·i·po·so·gen·i·tal
ad·i·po·su·ri·a
a·dip·si·a
ad·i·tus
  pl ad·i·tus
  or ad·i·tus·es
ad·junct
ad·junc·tive
ad·ju·vant
ad·ju·van·ti·ci·ty
Ad·le·ri·an
ad·max·il·lar·y
ad·me·di·al
ad·me·di·an
ad·min·is·tra·tion
ad·mix·ture
ad·ner·val
  or ad·neu·ral
ad·neu·ral
  or ad·ner·val
ad·nex·a
ad·nex·al
ad·nex·i·tis
ad·nex·o·gen·e·sis
ad·o·les·cence
ad·o·les·cent
A·do·nis
a·don·i·tol
ad·o·ral
a·dre·nal
a·dre·nal·ec·to·mize
a·dre·na·lec·to·my
  pl a·dre·nal·ec·to·mies
A·dren·a·lin
a·dren·a·line
a·dre·nal·ism
a·dre·nal·i·tis
adren·a·lone
a·dre·nal·op·a·thy
ad·re·ner·gen
ad·ren·er·gic

7

a·dre·no·cep·tor
ad·re·no·chrome
a·dre·no·cor·ti·cal
a·dre·no·cor·ti·co·hy·per·
  pla·si·a
a·dre·no·cor·ti·coid
a·dre·no·cor·ti·co·mi·
  met·ic
ad·re·no·cor·ti·co·ste·roid
a·dre·no·cor·ti·co·troph·
  ic
  or a·dre·no·cor·ti·co·tro·
    pic
a·dre·no·cor·ti·co·troph·
  in
  or a·dre·no·cor·ti·co·tro·
    pin
a·dre·no·cor·ti·co·tro·
  pic
  or a·dre·no·cor·ti·co·
    tro·pic
a·dre·no·cor·ti·co·tro·pin
  or a·dre·no·cor·ti·co·troph·
    in
a·dre·no·gen·i·
  tal
a·dre·no·glo·mer·u·lo·
  tro·pin
a·dre·no·lyt·ic
a·dre·no·med·ul·lar·y
a·dre·no·meg·a·ly
ad·ren·op·a·thy
a·dre·no·pri·val
a·dre·no·re·cep·tor
a·dre·no·ste·rone
a·dre·no·tox·in
ad·re·no·tro·phic
  or ad·re·no·trop·ic
ad·re·no·trop·ic
  or ad·re·no·tro·phic
Ad·royd
ad·sorb
ad·sor·bate
ad·sor·bent
ad·sorp·tion
ad·sorp·tive
ad·tor·sion
a·dult
a·dult·hood

a·dul·ter·ant
a·dul·ter·ate
a·dul·ter·a·tion
a·dum·bra·tion
ad·vance·ment
ad·ven·ti·ti·a
ad·ven·ti·tial
ad·ven·ti·tious
ad·verse
ad·ver·sive
a·dy·nam·i·a
a·dy·nam·ic
A·ë·des
ae·goph·o·ny
  var of e·goph·o·ny
ae·lu·ro·pho·bi·a
  var of ai·lu·ro·pho·bi·a
aer·ate
aer·a·tion
aer·if·er·ous
aer·i·form
aer·obe
aer·o·bic
aer·o·bi·ol·o·gy
  pl aer·o·bi·ol·o·gies
aer·o·bi·o·scope
aer·o·bi·o·sis
  pl aer·o·bi·o·ses
aer·o·bi·ot·ic
aer·o·cele
aer·o·col·pos
aer·o·cys·tos·co·py
aer·o·der·mec·ta·si·a
aer·o·don·tal·gi·a
aer·o·don·ti·a
aer·o·don·tics
aer·o·dy·nam·ics
aer·o·em·bo·lism
aer·o·em·phy·se·ma
aer·o·gel
aer·o·gen
aer·o·gen·ic
aer·og·e·nous
aer·o·gram
aer·o·med·i·cine
aer·om·e·ter
aer·o·neu·ro·sis
  pl aer·o·neu·ro·ses
aer·op·a·thy

aer·o·pause
aer·o·pha·gi·a
aer·oph·a·gy
  pl aer·oph·a·gies
aer·o·phil·ic
aer·o·phore
aer·o·phyte
aer·o·pi·e·so·ther·a·py
aer·o·plank·ton
aer·o·ple·thys·mo·graph
aer·o·si·nus·i·tis
aer·o·sol
aer·o·sol·i·za·tion
aer·o·sol·ize
Aer·o·spor·in
aer·o·stat·ics
aer·o·tax·is
  pl aer·o·tax·es
aer·o·ther·a·peu·tics
aer·o·ther·a·py
  pl aer·o·ther·a·pies
aer·o·ti·tis
aer·o·to·nom·e·ter
aer·ot·ro·pism
ae·ru·go
  pl ae·ru·gos
aes·cu·le·tin
  var of es·cu·le·tin
aes·cu·lin
  var of es·cu·lin
aes·the·si·a
  var of es·the·si·a
aes·the·tics
  or es·the·tics
aes·ti·vate
  var of es·ti·vate
ae·ti·ol·o·gy
  var of e·ti·ol·o·gy
ae·tio·por·phy·rin
  var of e·ti·o·por·phy·rin
a·feb·rile
af·fect
af·fec·tion
af·fec·tive
af·fec·tiv·i·ty
  pl af·fec·tiv·i·ties
af·fec·to·mo·tor
af·fer·ent
af·fi·nin

af·fin·i·ty
   pl af·fin·i·ties
af·fir·ma·tion
af·flux
af·flux·ion
af·fri·cate
af·fu·sion
a·fi·brin·o·ge·ne·mi·a
af·la·tox·i·co·sis
af·la·tox·in
af·ter·birth
af·ter·brain
af·ter·care
af·ter·damp
af·ter·dis·charge
af·ter·ef·fect
af·ter·im·age
af·ter·im·pres·sion
af·ter·load
af·ter·nys·tag·mus
af·ter·po·ten·tial
af·ter·taste
af·to·sa
a·ga·lac·ti·a
a·ga·lac·tous
a·gam·ete
a·ga·met·ic
a·gam·ic
a·gam·ma·glob·u·lin·e·mi·a
a·gam·o·gen·e·sis
   pl a·gam·o·gen·e·ses
a·gam·o·ge·net·ic
ag·a·mog·o·ny
   pl ag·a·mog·o·nies
Ag·a·mo·mer·mis
ag·a·mont
ag·a·mous
a·gan·gli·on·ic
a·gan·gli·o·no·sis
a·gar
a·gar·ic
a·gar·i·cin
A·gar·i·cus
a·gas·tric
A·ga·ve
a·gen·cy
a·ge·ne·si·a

a·gen·e·sis
   pl a·gen·e·ses
a·ge·net·ic
a·gen·i·tal·ism
a·gen·o·so·mi·a
a·gent
a·geu·si·a
ag·ger
ag·glom·er·ate
ag·glom·er·a·tion
ag·glu·ti·na·bil·i·ty
   pl ag·glu·ti·na·bil·i·ties
ag·glu·ti·na·ble
ag·glu·ti·nant
ag·glu·ti·nate
ag·glu·ti·na·tion
ag·glu·ti·na·tive
ag·glu·ti·na·tor
ag·glu·ti·nin
ag·glu·tin·o·gen
ag·glu·ti·no·gen·ic
ag·glu·ti·noid
ag·gre·gate
ag·gre·ga·tion
ag·gre·gen
ag·gres·sin
ag·gres·sion
ag·gres·sive
ag·i·tate
ag·i·ta·tion
a·glau·cop·si·a
a·glo·mer·u·lar
a·glos·si·a
a·glu·con
   or a·glu·cone
a·glu·cone
   or a·glu·con
ag·lu·ti·tion
a·gly·ce·mi·a
a·gly·con
   or a·gly·cone
a·gly·cone
   or a·gly·con
a·gly·co·su·ric
ag·ma·tine
ag·mi·nate
ag·mi·nat·ed
ag·nail
ag·na·thi·a

ag·na·thous
ag·na·thus
ag·no·gen·ic
ag·no·si·a
ag·nos·ter·ol
ag·nos·tic
a·gom·phi·a·sis
a·go·nad
a·gon·a·dal
a·go·nad·ism
ag·o·nal
ag·o·nist
ag·o·nis·tic
ag·o·ny
   pl ag·o·nies
ag·o·ra·pho·bi·a
a·gou·ti
   pl a·gou·tis
   or a·gou·ty
   pl a·gou·ties
a·gou·ty
   pl a·gou·ties
   or a·gou·ti
   pl a·gou·tis
a·graffe
a·gram·ma·tism
a·gran·u·lar
a·gran·u·lo·cyte
a·gran·u·lo·cyt·ic
a·gran·u·lo·cy·to·sis
   pl a·gran·u·lo·cy·to·ses
a·graph·es·the·si·a
a·graph·i·a
a·graph·ic
ag·ri·a
ag·ro·ma·ni·a
Ag·ro·py·ron
a·gryp·ni·a
   pl a·gryp·ni·ai
a·gue
a·gy·ri·a
aid·man
   pl aid·men
ai·lan·thus
ai·le·ron
ail·ment
ai·lu·ro·phil·i·a
ai·lu·ro·phobe
ai·lu·ro·pho·bi·a

ain·hum
air·bra·sive
air·sick
air·sick·ness
air·way
aitch·bone
ai·ti·ol·o·gy
    var of e·ti·ol·o·gy
aj·o·wan
    or ai·wain
a·kan·thi·on
    or a·can·thi·on
a·kar·y·o·cyte
a·kar·y·ote
    or a·car·y·ote
a·kat·a·ma·the·si·a
ak·a·this·i·a
    or ac·a·this·i·a
ak·ee
    or ack·ee
ak·i·ne·si·a
ak·i·ne·sis
    pl ak·i·ne·ses
    or ak·y·ne·sis
    pl ak·y·ne·ses
a·kin·es·the·si·a
ak·i·net·ic
A·ki·ne·ton
a·ko·ri·a
    or a·ca·ri·a
ak·y·ne·sis
    pl ak·y·ne·ses
    or ak·i·ne·sis
    pl ak·i·ne·ses
a·la
    pl a·lae
a·lac·ta·si·a
a·la·li·a
al·a·nine
a·lan·tin
al·a·nyl
a·lar
a·las·trim
a·late
    also a·lat·ed
a·la·tion
Al·ba·my·cin
al·be·do
al·bas·pi·din

Al·bers Schön·berg
al·bi·cans
al·bi·du·ri·a
al·bi·nism
al·bi·nis·mus
al·bi·no
al·bi·nism
al·bi·noid·ism
al·bi·not·ic
al·bo·ci·ne·re·ous
al·bu·gin·e·a
al·bu·go
al·bu·men
al·bu·min
al·bu·mi·nate
al·bu·mi·na·tu·ri·a
al·bu·min·glob·u·lin
al·bu·mi·nim·e·ter
al·bu·mi·no·cho·li·a
al·bu·mi·no·cy·to·log·ic
al·bu·mi·noid
al·bu·mi·nol·y·sin
al·bu·mi·nol·y·sis
al·bu·mi·nom·e·ter
al·bu·mi·nop·ty·sis
al·bu·mi·nous
al·bu·min·u·ret·ic
al·bu·min·u·ri·a
al·bu·min·u·ric
Al·bu·mi·sol
al·bu·mo·scope
al·bu·mose
al·bu·mo·su·ri·a
Al·ca·lig·e·nes
al·cap·ton
    or al·kap·ton
al·cap·ton·u·ria
    or al·kap·ton·u·ri·a
Al·cock ca·nal
al·co·gel
al·co·hol
al·co·hol·ate
al·co·hol·ic
al·co·hol·ism
al·co·hol·ist
al·co·hol·i·za·tion
al·co·hol·ize
al·co·hol·om·e·ter
al·co·hol·u·ri·a

al·co·hol·y·sis
    pl al·co·hol·y·ses
Al·dac·ta·zide
Al·dac·tone
al·de·hyde
al·de·hyde ly·ase
al·do·bi·ur·on·ic
al·do·hex·ose
al·dol
al·dol·ase
al·don·ic
al·do·pen·tose
al·dose
al·do·side
al·do·ster·one
al·do·ster·on·ism
al·do·ster·o·no·ma
al·dox·ime
al·drin
a·lec·i·thal
a·lem·bic
a·lem·mal
Al·e·tris
a·leu·ke·mi·a
a·leu·ke·mic
a·leu·ki·a
a·leu·ko·cyt·ic
a·leu·ko·cy·to·sis
al·eu·ron
    or al·eu·rone
al·eu·rone
    or al·eu·ron
a·lex·i·a
a·lex·in
a·lex·i·phar·mac
a·lex·i·phar·mic
a·lex·i·phar·mi·cal
a·ley·dig·ism
Al·flo·rone
al·ga
    pl al·gas
    or al·gae
al·gal
al·ge·don·ic
al·ge·fa·cient
al·ge·si·a
al·ge·sic
al·ge·sim·e·ter
al·ge·sim·e·try

al·ges·the·si·a
al·ges·the·sis
al·get·ic
al·gi·cide
al·gid
al·gin
al·gi·nate
al·gin·ic
al·go·gen·ic
al·go·lag·ni·a
al·gol·o·gy
al·gom·e·ter
al·gom·e·try
pl al·gom·e·tries
al·go·phi·li·a
al·go·pho·bi·a
al·gor
al·i·cy·clic
Al·i·dase
al·ien·a·tion
a·li·e·ni·a
al·ien·ism
al·ien·ist
al·i·es·ter·ase
al·i·form
a·lign·ment
al·i·ment
al·i·men·ta·ry
al·i·men·ta·tion
al·i·men·to·ther·a·py
pl al·i·men·to·ther·a·pies
a·li·na·sal
al·i·phat·ic
al·i·quot
al·i·sphe·noid
or al·i·sphe·noi·dal
al·i·sphe·noi·dal
or al·i·sphe·noid
a·liz·a·rin
or a·liz·a·rine
a·liz·a·rine
or a·liz·a·rin
al·ka·di·ene
al·ka·le·mi·a
al·ka·les·cence
al·ka·les·cent
al·ka·li
pl al·ka·lies
or al·ka·lis

al·ka·lim·e·ter
al·ka·lim·e·try
pl al·ka·lim·e·tries
al·ka·line
al·ka·lin·i·ty
pl al·ka·lin·i·ties
al·ka·lin·i·za·tion
al·ka·lin·ize
al·ka·li·nu·ri·a
al·ka·li·ther·a·py
al·ka·li·za·tion
al·ka·lize
al·ka·liz·er
al·ka·loid
al·ka·lom·e·try
pl al·ka·lom·e·tries
al·ka·lo·sis
pl al·ka·lo·ses
al·ka·lot·ic
al·ka·mine
al·kane
al·ka·net
al·kan·in
or al·kan·nin
al·kan·nin
or al·kan·in
al·kap·ton
or al·cap·ton
al·kap·ton·u·ri·a
or al·cap·ton·u·ri·a
al·ka·ver·vir
al·kene
al·kide
al·kyl
al·kyl·a·mine
al·ky·late
al·kyl·a·tion
al·kyl·o·gen
al·la·ches·the·si·a
al·lan·ti·a·sis
al·lan·to·cho·ri·on
al·lan·to·ic
al·lan·to·i·case
al·lan·toid
al·lan·to·in
al·lan·to·in·ase
al·lan·to·i·nu·ri·a
al·lan·to·is
pl al·lan·to·i·des

al·lele
al·le·lic
al·lel·ism
al·lel·o·ca·tal·y·sis
pl al·lel·o·ca·tal·y·ses
al·lel·o·cat·a·lyt·ic
al·le·lo·chem·ics
al·le·lo·morph
al·le·lo·mor·phic
al·le·lo·mor·phism
al·le·lo·tax·is
al·ler·gen
al·ler·gen·ic
al·ler·gic
al·ler·gid
al·ler·gin
al·ler·gist
al·ler·gi·za·tion
al·ler·gize
al·ler·gol·o·gy
pl al·ler·gol·o·gies
al·ler·gy
pl al·ler·gies
al·les·the·si·a
al·le·thrin
al·le·vi·ate
al·le·vi·a·tion
al·le·vi·a·tive
or al·le·vi·a·to·ry
al·le·vi·a·to·ry
or al·le·vi·a·tive
al·li·cin
al·li·ga·tion
al·li·in
al·lit·er·a·tion
Al·li·um
al·lo·an·ti·gen
al·lo·bar
ai·lo·bar·bi·tal
al·lo·bar·bi·tone
al·lo·chei·ri·a
or al·lo·chi·ri·a
al·lo·chi·ri·a
or al·lo·chei·ri·a
al·lo·chro·ism
al·lo·chro·ma·si·a
al·lo·cor·tex
al·lo·cy·to·phil·ic
al·lo·dip·loid

al·lo·dip·loi·dy
al·lo·e·rot·ic
al·lo·e·rot·i·cism
al·lo·er·o·tism
al·log·a·my
  pl al·log·a·mies
al·lo·ge·ne·ic
al·lo·gen·ic
al·lo·graft
al·lo·im·mune
al·lo·ki·ne·sis
  pl al·lo·ki·ne·ses
al·lo·la·li·a
al·lom·er·ism
al·lo·met·ric
al·lom·e·tron
al·lom·e·try
  pl al·lom·e·tries
al·lo·mor·phism
al·lo·path
al·lo·path·ic
al·lop·a·thy
  pl al·lop·a·thies
al·lo·phan·a·mide
al·lo·phan·ic
al·lo·phore
al·lo·pla·si·a
al·lo·plast
al·lo·plas·tic
al·lo·plas·ty
al·lo·ploid
al·lo·ploi·dy
al·lo·pol·y·ploid
al·lo·pol·y·ploi·dy
al·lo·psy·chic
al·lo·pu·rin·ol
al·lo·rhyth·mi·a
al·lose
al·lo·some
al·lo·ste·ric
al·lo·ste·ri·cal·ly
al·lo·tet·ra·ploid
al·lo·therm
al·lo·tope
al·lo·trans·plant
al·lo·trans·plan·ta·tion
al·lot·ri·o·don·ti·a
al·lot·ri·o·geus·ti·a

al·lot·ri·oph·a·gy
  pl al·lot·ri·oph·a·gies
al·lo·trope
al·lo·troph·ic
al·lo·trop·ic
al·lot·ro·pism
al·lo·typ·ic
al·lo·typ·i·cal·ly
al·lo·ty·py
  pl al·lo·typ·ies
al·lox·an
al·lox·an·tin
al·lox·a·zine
al·lox·u·re·mi·a
al·lox·u·ri·a
all·spice
al·lyl
al·lyl·a·mine
al·lyl·bar·bi·tu·ric
al·lyl·nor·mor·phine
al·mond
al·lo·chi·a
al·oe
al·oe em·o·din
a·lo·gi·a
al·o·in
al·o·pe·ci·a
al·o·pe·cic
a·lox·i·done
al·pha
al·pha-ad·re·ner·gic
al·pha-di·one
Al·pha·drol
al·pha·he·li·cal
al·pha·he·lix
al·pha·lo·be·line
al·pha·mi·met·ic
al·pha·naph·thol
al·pha·pro·dine
al·pha·re·cep·tor
al·ser·ox·y·lon
Al·sto·ni·a
al·sto·nine
al·ter·ant
al·ter·a·tion
al·ter·a·tive
al·ter·nans
Al·ter·nar·i·a
al·ter·na·tion

al·thae·a
  var of al·the·a
al·the·a
Alt·mann gran·ules
al·tric·ial
al·tri·gen·der·ism
al·tro·hep·tu·lose
al·trose
al·um
a·lu·mi·na
a·lu·mi·no·sis
  pl a·lu·mi·no·ses
a·lu·mi·num
a·lu·mi·num phos·phate
al·ve·o·lar
al·ve·o·lar·ly
al·ve·o·late
al·ve·o·la·tion
al·ve·o·lec·to·my
  pl al·ve·o·lec·to·mies
al·ve·o·li·tis
al·ve·o·lo·ba·sal
al·ve·o·lo·cla·si·a
al·ve·o·lo·con·dyl·e·an
al·ve·o·lo·den·tal
al·ve·o·lo·la·bi·al
al·ve·o·lo·lin·gual
al·ve·o·lo·plas·ty
  pl al·ve·o·lo·plas·ties
al·ve·o·lot·o·my
al·ve·o·lus
  pl al·ve·o·li
al·ver·ine
al·ve·us
  pl al·ve·i
Al·vo·dine
a·lym·phi·a
a·lym·pho·cy·to·sis
  pl a·lym·pho·cy·to·ses
al·lym·pho·pla·si·a
Alz·hei·mer dis·ease
a·maas
am·a·crine
a·mal·gam
Am·a·ni·ta
a·mal·ga·mate
a·mal·ga·ma·tion
a·mal·ga·ma·tor
a·man·din

a·man·ta·dine
am·a·ranth
am·a·roid
am·a·roi·dal
a·mas·ti·a
a·mas·ti·gote
am·a·tho·pho·bi·a
am·a·to·ry
am·au·ro·sis
  pl am·au·ro·ses
am·au·rot·ic
a·max·o·pho·bi·a
Am·a·zo·na
am·be·no·ni·um
am·ber·grease
  or am·ber·gris
am·ber·gris
  or am·ber·grease
am·bi·dex·ter
am·bi·dex·ter·i·ty
  pl am·bi·dex·ter·i·ties
am·bi·dex·trous
am·bi·ent
am·big·u·ous
am·bi·lat·er·al
al·bi·le·vous
am·bi·sex·u·al
am·bi·sex·u·al·i·ty
  pl am·bi·sex·u·al·i·ties
am·biv·a·lence
am·biv·a·lent
am·bi·ver·sion
am·bi·vert
am·bly·a·cou·si·a
am·bly·a·phi·a
am·bly·chro·mat·ic
am·bly·geus·ti·a
Am·bly·om·ma
am·bly·ope
am·bly·o·pi·a
am·bly·o·scope
am·bo
  pl am·bos
  or am·bon
am·bo·cep·tor
Am·bo·dryl
am·bo·mal·le·al
am·bon
  pl am·bo·nes

or am·bo
  pl am·bos
am·bo·sex·u·al
am·bro·sin
am·bu·lance
am·bu·lant
am·bu·late
am·bu·la·tion
am·bu·la·to·ry
a·me·ba
  pl a·me·bas
  or a·me·bae
am·e·bi·a·sis
  pl am·e·bi·a·ses
a·me·bic
a·me·bi·ci·dal
a·me·bi·cide
a·me·bo·cyte
a·me·boid
am·e·bo·ma
a·me·bu·la
  pl a·me·bu·las
  or a·me·bu·lae
am·e·bu·ri·a
am·ei·o·sis
  pl am·ei·o·ses
a·mel·i·a
a·mel·i·fi·ca·tion
a·me·lio·ra·tion
am·e·lo·blast
am·e·lo·blas·tic
am·e·lo·blas·to·ma
  pl am·e·lo·blas·to·mas
  or am·e·lo·blas·to·ma·ta
am·e·lo·den·ti·nal
am·e·lo·gen·e·sis
  pl am·e·lo·gen·e·ses
am·e·lo·gen·ic
am·e·lus
  pl am·e·li
a·me·ni·a
a·men·or·rhe·a
a·men·or·rhe·al
a·men·or·rhe·ic
a·men·or·rhoe·a
  var of a·men·or·rhe·a
a·men·sal·ism
a·men·ti·a
am·er·i·ci·um

am·er·ism
am·er·is·tic
a·meth·o·caine
am·e·thop·ter·in
a·me·tri·a
am·e·tro·pi·a
am·e·tro·pic
a·mi·cro·bic
am·i·dase
am·ide
am·i·do li·gase
am·i·do·gen
am·i·done hy·dro·chlo·ride
a·mi·do·py·rine
Am·i·dos·to·mum
am·i·dox·ime
Am·i·gen
a·mim·i·a
a·min·ac·rine
am·i·nate
a·mine
a·mi·no
a·mi·no·a·ce·tic
a·mi·no·a·ce·tic ac·id
a·mi·no·ac·i·de·mi·a
a·mi·no·ac·i·dop·a·thy
a·mi·no·ac·id·uri·a
a·mi·no·ac·y·lase
a·mi·no·ben·zo·ic
a·mi·no·ca·pro·ic ac·id
a·mi·no·glu·teth·i·mide
a·mi·no·hip·pu·rate
a·mi·nol·y·sis
  pl a·mi·nol·y·ses
a·mi·no·met·ra·dine
a·mi·no·met·ra·mide
a·mi·no·pen·ta·mide
a·mi·no·phen·a·zone
am·i·noph·er·ase
a·mi·no·phyl·line
a·mi·no·pol·y·pep·ti·dase
am·in·op·ter·in
a·mi·no·py·rine
a·mi·no·sa·lic·y·late
a·mi·no·sal·i·cyl·ic ac·id
A·mi·no·sol
am·i·no·trate
am·i·nu·ri·a
am·i·phen·a·zole

13

am·i·so·met·ra·dine
am·i·thi·o·zone
am·i·to·sis
am·i·trip·ty·line
am·me·ter
am·mo·a·ci·du·ri·a
am·mo·ne·mi·a
am·mo·ni·a
am·mo·ni·at·ed mer·cu·ry
am·mo·ni·um
am·mo·ni·u·ri·a
am·mo·nol·y·sis
   pl am·mo·nol·y·ses
am·nal·ge·si·a
am·ne·si·a
am·ni·o·cen·te·sis
   pl am·ni·o·cen·te·ses
am·ni·o·cho·ri·al
am·ni·og·ra·phy
   pl am·ni·og·ra·phies
am·ni·on
   pl am·ni·ons
   or am·ni·a
am·ni·o·ni·tis
am·ni·o·rrhe·a
am·ni·o·rrhex·is
am·ni·o·scope
am·ni·os·co·py
   pl am·ni·os·co·pies
Am·ni·o·ta
am·ni·ot·ic
am·ni·o·ti·tis
am·ni·o·tome
am·ni·ot·o·my
am·o·bar·bi·tal
am·o·di·a·quin
   or am·o·di·a·quine
am·o·di·a·quine
   or am·o·di·a·quin
amoe·ba
   pl a·moe·bas
   or a·moe·bae
   or a·me·ba
   pl a·me·bas
   or a·me·bae
am·oe·bi·a·sis
   or am·e·bi·a·sis
a·moe·bic
   or a·me·bic

a·moe·bo·cyte
   or a·me·bo·cyte
a·moe·boid
   or a·me·boid
A·moe·bo·tae·ni·a
a·moe·bous
a·mok
   or a·muck
a·mo·la·none
a·morph
a·mor·phi·a
a·mor·phic
a·mor·phin·ism
a·mor·phism
a·mor·phous
a·mor·phus
   pl a·mor·phus·es
   or a·mor·phi
a·mo·tio
a·mox·i·cil·lin
am·per·age
am·pere
am·pere·me·ter
Am·phe·dro·xyn
am·phet·a·mine
am·phi·ar·ky·o·chrome
am·phi·ar·thro·di·al
am·phi·ar·thro·sis
   pl am·phi·ar·thro·ses
am·phi·as·ter
am·phi·blas·tic
am·phi·blas·tu·la
   pl am·phi·blas·tu·las
   or am·phi·blas·tu·lae
am·phi·bol·ic
am·phi·ce·lous
am·phi·cen·tric
am·phi·chro·ic
am·phi·chrome
am·phi·cra·ni·a
am·phi·cyt·u·la
am·phi·di·ar·thro·sis
am·phi·dip·loid
am·phi·dip·loi·dy
   pl am·phi·dip·loi·dies
am·phi·er·o·tism
am·phi·gas·tru·la
   pl am·phi·gas·tru·las
   or am·phi·gas·tru·lae

am·phi·gen·e·sis
am·phi·ge·net·ic
am·phi·gon·a·dism
am·phi·kar·y·on
am·phi·mic·tic
am·phi·mic·ti·cal·ly
am·phi·mix·is
   pl am·phi·mix·es
am·phi·mor·u·la
   pl am·phi·mor·u·lae
am·phi·ox·us
   pl am·phi·oxus·es
   or am·phi·ox·i
am·phi·ploid
am·phi·ploi·dy
   pl am·phi·ploi·dies
am·phi·tene
am·phi·the·a·ter
am·phit·ri·chous
am·pho·cyte
am·pho·lyte
am·pho·my·cin
am·pho·phil
am·pho·phil·ic
am·pho·phi·lous
am·pho·ric
am·pho·ric·i·ty
   pl am·pho·ric·i·ties
am·pho·ter·ic
am·pho·ter·i·cin·B
am·pho·ter·ism
am·phot·o·ny
am·pi·cil·lin
am·plex·us
   pl am·plex·us
am·pli·fi·ca·tion
am·pli·fi·er
am·pli·tude
am·pro·tro·pine
am·pul
   or am·pule
am·pule
   or am·pul
am·pul·la
   pl am·pul·lae
am·pul·lar
am·pul·lary
am·pul·lu·la
   pl am·pul·lu·lae

am·pu·tate
am·pu·ta·tion
am·pu·tee
Am·sus·tain
a·muck
  or a·mok
a·mu·si·a
am·y·dri·a·sis
am·y·e·li·a
a·my·e·lin·ic
a·my·e·lon·ic
a·my·e·lot·ro·phy
a·my·e·lus
a·myg·da·la
  pl a·myg·da·lae
a·myg·da·lin
a·myg·da·line
a·myg·da·loid
a·myg·da·loi·dec·to·my
a·myg·da·lo·lith
am·yl
am·y·la·ceous
am·y·lase
am·y·lene
am·yl·ni·trite
am·y·lo·bar·bi·tone
am·y·lo·clas·tic
am·y·lo·dex·trin
am·y·lo·dys·pep·si·a
am·y·lo·gen·e·sis
am·y·loid
am·y·loi·do·sis
  pl am·y·loi·do·ses
am·y·lol·y·sis
  pl am·y·lol·y·ses
am·y·lo·lyt·ic
am·y·lo·pec·tin
am·y·lo·pec·ti·no·sis
am·y·lo·plast
am·y·lop·sin
am·y·lor·rhe·a
am·y·lor·rhex·is
am·y·lose
am·y·lo·su·ri·a
am·y·lum
am·y·lu·ri·a
a·my·o·es·the·si·a
a·my·o·pla·si·a
a·my·o·sta·si·a

a·my·os·the·ni·a
a·my·os·then·ic
a·my·o·tax·ia
a·my·o·ta·xy
a·my·o·to·ni·a
a·my·o·ton·ic
a·my·o·tro·phi·a
a·my·o·troph·ic
am·y·ot·ro·phy
  pl am·y·ot·ro·phies
Am·y·tal
a·myx·i·a
an·a
an·a·bae·na
a·nab·a·sine
a·nab·a·sis
  pl a·nab·a·ses
an·a·bat·ic
an·a·bi·o·sis
  pl an·a·bi·o·ses
an·a·bi·ot·ic
an·a·bol·er·gy
an·a·bo·lic
a·nab·o·lin
a·nab·o·lism
a·nab·o·lite
an·a·cat·a·did·y·mus
  or an·a·kat·a·did·y·mus
an·a·cho·re·sis
an·a·cid·i·ty
a·nac·la·sis
  pl a·nac·la·ses
a·nac·li·sis
an·a·clit·ic
an·a·cou·si·a
  var of an·a·cu·si·a
an·a·crot·ic
a·nac·ro·tism
an·a·cul·ture
an·a·cu·sis
an·a·dip·si·a
an·a·dre·nal·ism
An·a·drol
a·nae·mi·a
  var of a·ne·mi·a
a·nae·mic
  var of a·ne·mic
an·aer·obe
an·aer·o·bic

an·aer·o·bi·cal·ly
an·aer·o·bi·o·sis
  pl an·aer·o·bi·o·ses
an·aer·o·gen·ic
an·aer·o·sis
an·aes·the·si·a
  var of an·es·the·si·a
an·aes·thet·ic
  var of an·es·thet·ic
an·aes·the·tist
  var of an·es·the·tist
an·aes·the·ti·za·tion
  var of an·es·the·ti·za·tion
an·aes·the·tize
  var of an·es·the·tize
an·a·gen
an·a·gen·e·sis
  pl an·a·gen·e·ses
an·a·gen·et·ic
an·a·gog·ic
an·a·kat·a·did·y·mus
  or an·a·cat·a·did·y·mus
an·a·ku·sis
a·nal
an·al·bu·mi·ne·mi·a
an·a·lep·tic
An·a·lex·in
an·al·ge·si·a
an·al·ge·sic
An·al·ge·sine
an·al·get·ic
a·nal·i·ty
  pl a·nal·i·ties
an·al·ler·gic
an·a·log
  or an·alogue
a·nal·o·gous
an·a·logue
  or an·a·log
a·nal·o·gy
a·nal·y·sand
a·nal·y·sis
  pl a·nal·y·ses
an·a·lyst
an·a·lyt·ic
  or an·a·lyt·i·cal
an·a·lyt·i·cal
  or an·a·lyt·ic
an·a·lyze

an·a·lyz·er
an·am·ne·sis
   pl an·am·ne·ses
an·am·nes·tic
an·am·ni·on·ic
an·am·ni·ote
an·am·ni·ot·ic
an·a·mor·pho·sis
   pl an·a·mor·pho·ses
an·a·pau·sis
   pl an·a·pau·ses
an·a·phase
an·a·phi·a
an·a·pho·ri·a
an·aph·ro·dis·i·a
an·aph·ro·dis·i·ac
an·a·phy·lac·tic
an·a·phy·lac·tin
an·a·phy·lac·to·gen
an·a·phy·lac·to·gen·ic
an·a·phy·lac·to·gen·e·sis
an·a·phy·lac·toid
an·a·phy·la·to·xin
an·a·phy·la·xis
   pl an·a·phy·lax·es
an·a·pla·si·a
An·a·plas·ma
   pl An·a·plas·mas
   or An·a·plas·ma·ta
an·a·plas·mo·sis
   pl an·a·plas·mo·ses
an·a·plas·tic
an·a·poph·y·sis
   pl an·a·poph·y·ses
an·a·pro·tas·pis
   pl an·a·pro·tas·pes
an·ap·tic
an·a·rith·mi·a
an·ar·thri·a
an·a·sar·ca
an·a·sar·cous
an·a·stal·sis
an·a·stal·tic
an·a·state
an·as·tig·mat·ic
a·nas·to·le
a·nas·to·mose
a·nas·to·mo·sis
   pl a·nas·to·mo·ses

a·nas·to·mot·ic
an·as·tral
an·a·tom·ic
   or an·a·tom·i·cal
an·a·tom·i·cal
   or an·a·tom·ic
an·a·tom·i·cal·ly
an·a·tom·i·co·path·o·log·ic
a·nat·o·mist
a·nat·o·mize
a·nat·o·my
   pl a·nat·o·mies
an·a·tox·in
an·a·trip·tic
an·a·troph·ic
an·a·tro·pi·a
an·au·di·a
an·chor·age
an·chy·lose
   or an·ky·lose
   or an·cy·lose
an·chy·lo·sis
   pl an·chy·lo·ses
   or an·ky·lose
   pl an·ky·lo·ses
   or an·cy·lose
   pl an·cy·lo·ses
an·chy·lot·ic
   or an·cy·lot·ic
   or an·ky·lot·ic
an·cip·i·tal
an·cip·i·tous
an·co·nad
an·co·nag·ra
an·co·nal
an·co·ne·al
an·co·ne·us
   pl an·co·ne·i
an·co·noid
an·cy·lose
   or an·chy·lose
   or an·ky·lose
an·cy·lo·sis
   pl an·cy·lo·ses
   or an·chy·lose
   pl an·chy·lo·ses
   or an·ky·lose
   pl an·ky·lo·ses
An·cy·los·to·ma

an·cy·lo·sto·mi·a·sis
   pl an·cy·lo·sto·mi·a·ses
an·cy·lot·ic
   or an·chy·lot·ic
   or an·ky·lot·ic
an·cy·roid
   or an·ky·roid
An·di·ra
an·dro·blas·to·ma
   pl an·dro·blas·to·mas
   or an·dro·blas·to·ma·ta
an·dro·cyte
an·dro·gam·one
an·dro·gen
an·dro·gen·e·sis
   pl an·dro·gen·e·ses
an·dro·gen·ic
an·dro·ge·nic·i·ty
an·drog·e·nous
an·dro·gyne
an·drog·y·nism
an·drog·y·nous
an·drog·y·ny
   pl an·drog·y·nies
an·droid
an·drom·e·da
an·drom·e·do·tox·in
an·dro·mer·o·gon
an·dro·mer·og·o·ny
an·dro·mi·met·ic
an·dro·phil·ic
an·dro·pho·bi·a
an·dro·stane
an·dro·stane·di·ol
an·dro·stane·di·one
an·dro·stene
an·dro·stene·di·ol
an·dros·ter·one
an·e·cho·ic
an·ec·ta·sis
An·ec·tine
an·e·lec·tro·ton·ic
an·e·lec·trot·o·nus
a·ne·mi·a
a·ne·mic
an·e·mom·e·ter
an·em·oph·i·lous
an·e·mo·pho·bi·a

16

an·en·ceph·a·li·a
  pl an·en·ceph·a·li·as
  or an·en·ceph·a·ly
  pl an·en·ceph·a·lies
an·en·ceph·al·ic
an·en·ceph·a·lous
an·en·ceph·a·lus
  pl an·en·ceph·a·li
an·en·ceph·a·ly
  pl an·en·ceph·a·lies
  or an·en·ceph·a·li·a
  pl an·en·ceph·a·li·as
an·en·ter·ous
an·en·zy·mi·a
an·er·ga·si·a
an·er·gic
an·er·gy
  pl an·er·gies
an·er·oid
an·e·ryth·ro·pla·si·a
an·e·ryth·ro·poi·e·sis
an·er·y·throp·si·a
an·es·the·ci·ne·si·a
an·es·the·sia
an·es·the·sim·e·ter
A·nes·the·sin
an·es·the·si·ol·o·gist
an·es·the·si·ol·o·gy
  pl an·es·the·si·ol·o·gies
an·es·thet·ic
a·nes·the·tist
a·nes·the·ti·za·tion
a·nes·the·tize
an·es·tric
an·es·trous
  var of an·es·trus
an·es·trum
  pl an·es·tra
an·es·trus
  pl an·es·tri
an·e·thole
an·e·to·der·ma
an·eu·ploid
  pl an·eu·ploi·dies
an·eu·ri·lem·mic
an·eu·rin
  or an·eu·rine
an·eu·rine
  or an·eu·rin

an·eu·rism
  or an·eu·rysm
an·eu·ris·mal
  or an·eu·rys·mal
an·eu·rysm
  or an·eu·rism
an·eu·rys·mal
  or an·eu·ris·mal
an·eu·rys·mec·to·my
an·eu·rys·mo·plas·ty
an·eu·rys·mor·rha·phy
an·eu·rys·mot·o·my
an·frac·tu·os·i·ty
  pl an·frac·tu·os·i·ties
an·frac·tu·ous
an·gel·i·ca
an·gi·as·the·ni·a
an·gi·ec·ta·sis
  pl an·gi·ec·ta·ses
an·gi·ec·to·my
  pl an·gi·ec·to·mies
an·gi·ec·to·pi·a
an·gi·i·tis
  pl an·gi·i·ti·des
an·gi·na
an·gi·nal
an·gi·noid
an·gi·no·pho·bi·a
an·gi·nose
an·gi·nous
an·gi·o·blast
an·gi·o·blas·tic
an·gi·o·blas·to·ma
  pl an·gi·o·blas·to·mas
  or an·gi·o·blas·to·ma·ta
an·gi·o·car·di·o·gram
an·gi·o·car·dio·graph·ic
an·gi·o·car·di·og·ra·phy
  pl an·gio·car·di·og·ra·phies
an·gi·o·car·di·o·ki·net·ic
an·gi·o·car·di·op·a·thy
an·gi·o·car·di·tis
an·gi·o·cho·li·tis
an·gi·o·chon·dro·ma
  pl an·gi·o·chon·dro·mas
  or an·gi·o·chon·dro·ma·ta
an·gi·o·cyst
an·gi·o·di·a·ther·my
an·gi·o·ec·ta·sia

an·gi·o·e·de·ma
  pl an·gi·o·e·de·mas
  or an·gi·o·ed·e·ma·ta
an·gi·o·en·do·the·li·o·ma
  pl an·gi·o·en·do·the·li·
    o·mas
  or an·gi·o·en·do·the·li·o·
    ma·ta
an·gi·o·fi·bro·ma
  pl an·gi·o·fi·bro·mas
  or an·gi·o·fi·bro·ma·ta
an·gi·o·gen·e·sis
  pl an·gi·o·gen·e·ses
an·gi·o·gen·ic
an·gi·o·gli·o·ma
  pl an·gi·o·gli·o·mas
  or an·gi·o·gli·o·ma·ta
an·gi·o·gram
an·gi·og·ra·phy
  pl an·gi·og·ra·phies
an·gi·o·he·mo·phil·i·a
an·gi·o·hy·a·li·no·sis
an·gi·oid
an·gi·o·ker·a·to·ma
  pl an·gi·o·ker·a·to·ma
  or an·gi·o·ker·a·to·ma·ta
an·gi·o·ki·net·ic
an·gi·o·li·po·ma
  pl an·gi·o·li·po·mas
  or an·gi·o·li·po·ma·ta
an·gi·o·lith
an·gi·ol·o·gy
  pl an·gi·ol·o·gies
an·gi·o·lu·poid
an·gi·ol·y·sis
an·gi·o·ma
  pl an·gi·o·mas
  or an·gi·o·ma·ta
an·gi·o·ma·to·sis
  pl an·gi·o·ma·to·ses
an·gi·om·a·tous
an·gi·o·meg·a·ly
an·gi·o·my·o·li·po·ma
  pl an·gi·o·my·o·li·po·mas
  or an·gi·o·my·o·li·po·ma·ta
an·gi·o·my·o·ma
  pl an·gi·o·my·o·mas
  or an·gi·o·my·o·ma·ta

an·gi·o·my·o·neu·ro·ma
   pl an·gi·o·my·o·neu·ro·mas
   or an·gi·o·my·o·neu·ro·
     ma·ta
an·gi·o·my·o·sar·co·ma
   pl an·gi·o·my·o·sar·co·mas
   or an·gi·o·my·o·sar·co·
     ma·ta
an·gi·o·neu·rec·to·my
an·gi·o·neu·ro·ma
   pl an·gi·o·neu·ro·mas
   or an·gi·o·neu·ro·ma·ta
an·gi·o·neu·ro·my·o·ma
   pl an·gi·o·neu·ro·my·o·mes
   or an·gi·o·neu·ro·my·o·
     ma·ta
an·gi·o·neu·rop·a·thy
an·gi·o·neu·rot·ic
an·gi·o·no·ma
an·gi·o·pa·ral·y·sis
an·gi·o·pa·re·sis
an·gi·op·a·thy
   pl an·gi·op·a·thies
an·gi·o·plas·ty
an·gi·o·poi·e·sis
   pl an·gi·o·poi·e·ses
an·gi·o·pres·sure
an·gi·o·rhi·go·sis
an·gi·or·rha·phy
an·gi·o·sar·co·ma
   pl an·gi·o·sar·co·mas
   or an·gi·o·sar·co·ma·ta
an·gi·o·scle·ro·sis
   pl an·gi·o·scle·ro·ses
an·gi·o·scope
an·gi·o·sco·to·ma
   pl an·gi·o·sco·to·mas
   or an·gi·o·sco·to·ma·ta
an·gi·o·sco·tom·e·try
   pl an·gi·o·sco·tom·e·tries
an·gi·o·spasm
an·gi·o·spas·tic
an·gi·o·stax·is
an·gi·o·ste·no·sis
an·gi·os·to·my
   pl an·gi·os·to·mies
an·gi·os·tron·gy·li·a·sis
an·gi·os·tro·phe
an·gi·os·tro·phy

an·gi·o·tel·ec·ta·sis
an·gi·o·ten·sin
an·gi·o·ten·si·nase
an·gi·o·ten·sin·o·gen
an·gi·o·ti·tis
an·gi·o·tome
an·gi·o·to·nase
an·gi·o·ton·ic
an·gi·o·to·nin
an·gi·o·tribe
an·gi·o·troph·ic
an·gos·tu·ra
ang·strom
an·gu·lar
an·gu·la·tion
an·gu·lus
   pl an·gu·li
an·ha·lo·ni·um
an·he·do·ni·a
an·hi·dro·sis
   pl an·hi·dro·ses
   or an·hy·dro·sis
   pl an·hy·dro·ses
   or an·i·dro·sis
   pl an·i·dro·ses
an·hi·drot·ic
   or an·hy·drot·ic
   or an·i·drot·ic
an·his·tic
an·his·tous
an·hy·drae·mi·a
   var of an·hy·dre·mi·a
an·hy·drase
an·hy·dra·tion
an·hy·dre·mi·a
an·hy·dride
an·hy·dro·sis
   pl an·hy·dro·ses
   or an·hi·dro·sis
   pl an·hi·dro·ses
   or an·i·dro·sis
   pl an·i·dro·ses
an·hy·drot·ic
   or an·hi·drot·ic
   or an·i·drot·ic
an·hy·drous
an·i·an·thi·nop·sy
an·ic·ter·ic
a·nid·e·us

an·i·dro·sis
   pl an·i·dro·ses
   or an·hi·dro·sis
   pl an·hi·dro·ses
   or an·hy·dro·sis
   pl an·hy·dro·ses
an·i·drot·ic
   or an·hy·drot·ic
   or an·hi·drot·ic
a·nile
an·i·ler·i·dine
an·i·lide
a·ni·linc·tus
   or a·ni·lin·gus
an·i·line
a·ni·lin·gus
   or a·ni·linc·tus
an·il·in·ism
a·nil·i·ty
   pl a·nil·i·ties
an·i·ma
an·i·mal
an·i·mal·cule
an·i·mal·i·ty
   pl an·i·mal·i·ties
an·i·ma·tion
an·i·mism
an·i·mus
an·i·on
an·i·on·ic
an·i·on·i·cal·ly
an·i·on·ot·ro·py
   pl an·i·on·ot·ro·pies
an·i·rid·i·a
an·is·ate
an·ise
an·is·ei·ko·ni·a
a·nis·ic
an·i·sin·di·one
an·i·so·co·ri·a
an·i·so·cy·to·sis
   pl an·i·so·cy·to·ses
an·i·so·dac·ty·ly
an·i·so·dont
an·i·so·gam·ic
   or an·i·sog·a·mous
an·i·sog·a·mous
   or an·i·so·gam·ic

an·i·sog·a·my
   pl an·i·sog·a·mies
an·i·sog·na·thous
an·is·ole
an·i·so·mas·ti·a
an·i·so·me·li·a
an·i·so·me·tro·pi·a
an·i·so·me·trop·ic
an·i·so·mor·phic
an·i·so·nu·cle·o·sis
an·i·so·pi·e·sis
an·i·so·poi·ki·lo·cy·to·sis
an·i·so·sthen·ic
an·i·so·ton·ic
an·i·so·trop·ic
an·i·so·tro·pine
  meth·yl·bro·mide
an·i·so·tro·pous
an·i·su·ri·a
A·nitsch·kow cell
an·kle
an·kle·bone
an·ky·lo·bleph·a·ron
an·ky·lo·chei·li·a
  or an·ky·lo·chi·li·a
an·ky·lo·chi·li·a
  or an·ky·lo·chei·li·a
an·ky·lo·col·pos
  or an·ky·lo·kol·pos
an·ky·lo·dac·tyl·i·a
an·ky·lo·glos·si·a
an·ky·lo·kol·pos
  or an·ky·lo·col·pos
an·ky·lose
  or an·chy·lose
  or an·cy·lose
an·ky·lo·sis
  pl an·ky·lo·ses
  or an·chy·lo·sis
  pl an·chy·lo·ses
  or an·cy·lo·sis
  pl an·cy·lo·ses
An·ky·los·to·ma
an·ky·lo·sto·mi·a·sis
  pl an·ky·lo·sto·mi·a·ses
an·ky·lo·ti·a
an·ky·lot·ic
  or an·chy·lot·ic
  or an·cy·lot·ic

an·ky·roid
  or an·cy·roid
an·la·ge
  pl an·la·gen
  or an·la·ges
an·neal
an·nec·tant
  or an·nec·tent
an·nec·tent
  or an·nec·tant
an·ne·lid
an·nex·a
an·not·to
an·nu·lar
an·nu·lor·rha·phy
an·nu·lot·o·my
an·nu·lus
  pl an·nu·lus·es
  or an·nu·li
a·no·coc·cyg·e·al
an·o·dal
an·ode
an·od·ic
an·o·don·ti·a
an·o·dyne
an·o·dyn·i·a
an·o·e·si·a
an·oes·trous
  var of an·es·trous
an·oes·trum
  var of an·es·trum
  pl an·oes·tra
an·oes·trus
  var of an·es·trous
an·o·et·ic
a·no·gen·i·tal
a·noi·a
a·nom·a·lo·pi·a
a·nom·a·lo·scope
a·nom·a·lous
a·nom·a·ly
  pl a·nom·a·lies
an·o·mer
a·no·mi·a
an·o·mie
  pl an·o·mies
  or an·o·my
an·o·my
  or an·o·mie

an·o·nych·i·a
a·non·y·ma
  pl a·non·y·mas
  or a·non·y·mae
an·o·op·si·a
  or an·op·si·a
an·op·si·a
  or an·o·op·si·a
a·no·pel·vic
a·no·per·i·ne·al
A·noph·e·les
a·nophe·line
a·noph·e·lism
an·oph·thal·mus
An·o·pla
a·no·plas·ty
  pl a·no·plas·ties
An·op·lo·ceph·a·la
an·op·si·a
an·op·thal·mi·a
an·or·chi·a
an·or·chism
a·no·rec·tal
an·o·rec·tic
a·no·rec·to·co·lon·ic
a·no·rec·tum
an·o·rex·i·a
an·o·rex·i·ant
an·o·rex·ic
an·o·rex·i·gen·ic
an·or·gan·ic
an·or·thog·ra·phy
an·or·tho·pi·a
an·or·tho·sis
a·no·scope
a·nos·co·py
a·no·sig·moi·dos·co·py
an·os·mat·ic
an·os·mi·a
an·os·mic
an·o·sog·no·si·a
an·os·phra·si·a
  or an·os·phre·si·a
an·os·phre·si·a
  or an·os·phra·si·a
a·no·spi·nal
an·os·te·o·pla·si·a
an·os·to·sis
an·o·ti·a

19

an·o·tro·pi·a
an·o·tus
a·no·vag·i·nal
an·o·var·ism
a·no·ves·i·cal
an·o·vu·lant
an·o·vu·lar
an·o·vu·la·tion
an·o·vu·la·to·ry
an·ox·ae·mi·a
   var of an·ox·e·mi·a
an·ox·ae·mic
   var of an·ox·e·mic
an·ox·e·mi·a
an·ox·e·mic
an·ox·i·a
a·nox·ic
an·sa
   pl an·sae
an·sate
   or an·sat·ed
an·sat·ed
   or an·sate
an·ser·ine
an·si·form
ant·ac·id
an·tag·o·nism
an·tag·o·nist
an·tag·o·nis·tic
ant·aph·ro·dis·i·ac
ant·ar·thrit·ic
an·taz·o·line
an·te·bra·chi·al
an·te·bra·chi·um
   pl an·te·bra·chi·a
   or an·ti·bra·chi·um
   pl an·ti·bra·chi·a
an·te·car·di·um
   pl an·te·car·di·a
   or an·ti·car·di·um
   pl an·ti·car·di·a
an·te·ce·dent
an·te·cor·nu
   pl an·te·cor·nua
an·te·cu·bi·tal
an·te·cur·va·ture
an·te·feb·rile
an·te·flex·ion
an·te·mor·tem

an·te·na·tal
an·ten·na
   pl an·ten·nas
   or an·ten·nae
an·te·par·tal
an·te·par·tum
an·te·phase
an·te·po·si·tion
an·te·py·ret·ic
an·te·ri·or
an·ter·o·clu·sion
an·ter·o·ex·ter·nal
an·ter·o·grade
an·ter·o·in·fe·ri·or
an·ter·o·in·ter·nal
an·ter·o·lat·er·al
an·ter·o·me·di·al
an·ter·o·me·di·an
an·ter·o·pos·te·ri·or
an·ter·o·sep·tal
an·ter·o·su·pe·ri·or
an·te·ver·sion
an·te·vert
ant·he·lix
   pl ant·he·lix·es
   or ant·he·li·ces
   or an·ti·he·lix
   pl an·ti·he·lix·es
   or an·ti·he·li·ces
ant·hel·min·thic
   or ant·hel·min·tic
   or an·ti·hel·min·tic
ant·hel·min·tic
   or ant·hel·min·thic
   or an·ti·hel·min·tic
an·the·lone
an·tho·cy·a·nin
   or an·tho·cy·an
an·tho·cy·an
   or an·tho·cy·a·nin
an·tho·pho·bi·a
an·tho·xan·thin
an·thra·cene
an·thrac·nose
an·thra·coid
an·thra·com·e·ter
an·thra·co·ne·cro·sis
an·thra·co·sil·i·co·sis
   pl an·thra·co·sil·i·co·ses

an·thra·co·sis
   pl an·thra·co·ses
an·thra·co·ther·a·py
an·thra·cot·ic
an·thra·gal·lol
an·thra·lin
an·thra·my·cin
an·thra·ni·late
an·thra·nil·ic
an·thra·qui·none
an·thrax
   pl an·thra·ces
an·throne
an·thro·po·cen·tric
an·thro·po·gen·e·sis
   pl an·thro·po·gen·e·ses
an·thro·po·ge·net·ic
an·thro·po·gen·ic
an·thro·pog·e·ny
   pl an·thro·pog·e·nies
an·thro·pog·o·ny
   pl an·thro·pog·o·nies
an·thro·pog·ra·phy
   pl an·thro·pog·ra·phies
an·thro·poid
an·thro·po·ki·net·ics
an·thro·pol·o·gy
   pl an·thro·pol·o·gies
an·thro·pom·e·ter
an·thro·po·met·ric
an·thro·pom·e·try
   pl an·thro·pom·e·tries
an·thro·po·mor·phic
an·thro·po·mor·phism
an·thro·pop·a·thy
   pl an·thro·pop·a·thies
an·thro·poph·a·gy
   pl an·thro·poph·a·gies
an·thro·po·phil·ic
an·thro·pos·o·phy
   pl an·thro·pos·o·phies
an·thro·po·zo·o·no·sis
ant·hys·ter·ic
an·ti·a·bor·tion
an·ti·a·bor·ti·fa·cient
an·ti·a·bor·tion·ist
an·ti·ac·id
an·ti·ad·re·ner·gic
an·ti·ag·glu·ti·nin

an·ti·al·bu·min
an·ti·a·lex·in
an·ti·al·ler·gen·ic
  or an·ti·al·ler·gic
an·ti·al·ler·gic
  or an·ti·al·ler·gen·ic
an·ti·a·me·bic
an·ti·am·y·lase
an·ti·an·a·phy·lac·tin
an·ti·an·a·phy·lax·is
  pl an·ti·an·a·phy·lax·es
an·ti·an·dro·gen
an·ti·an·ti·bod·y
an·ti·anx·i·e·ty
an·ti·ar·rhyth·mic
an·ti·ar·thrit·ic
an·ti·aux·in
an·ti·bac·te·ri·al
an·ti·bech·ic
an·ti·bi·ont
an·ti·bi·o·sis
  pl an·ti·bi·o·ses
an·ti·bi·ot·ic
an·ti·blen·nor·rhag·ic
an·ti·bod·y
  pl an·ti·bod·ies
an·ti·bra·chi·um
  pl an·ti·bra·chi·a
  or an·te·bra·chi·um
  pl an·te·bra·chi·a
an·ti·cal·cu·lous
an·ti·can·cer
  or an·ti·can·cer·ous
an·ti·can·cer·ous
  or an·ti·can·cer
an·ti·car·di·um
  pl an·ti·car·di·a
  or an·te·car·di·um
  pl an·te·car·di·a
an·ti·car·i·o·gen·ic
an·ti·ca·ri·ous
an·ti·cath·ode
an·ti·chei·rot·o·nus
an·ti·cho·les·ter·e·mic
an·ti·cho·lin·er·gic
an·ti·cho·lin·es·ter·ase
an·ti·cli·nal
an·ti·co·ag·u·lant
an·ti·co·ag·u·late

an·ti·co·ag·u·la·tion
an·ti·co·ag·u·la·tive
an·ti·co·ag·u·lin
an·ti·co·don
an·ti·com·ple·ment
an·ti·com·ple·men·ta·ry
an·ti·con·vul·sant
an·ti·con·vul·sive
an·ti·cus
an·ti·cy·tol·y·sin
an·ti·cy·to·tox·in
an·ti·de·pres·sant
an·ti·de·pres·sive
an·ti·di·a·bet·ic
an·ti·di·ar·rhe·al
an·ti·din·ic
an·ti·di·u·re·sis
an·ti·di·u·ret·ic
an·ti·dot·al
an·ti·dot·al·ly
an·ti·dote
an·ti·drom·ic
an·ti·dys·en·ter·ic
an·ti·ec·ze·mat·ic
an·ti·e·met·ic
an·ti·en·zyme
an·ti·ep·i·lep·tic
an·ti·ep·i·the·li·al
an·ti·es·ter·ase
an·ti·fe·brile
an·ti·fer·til·i·ty
an·ti·fer·ti·li·zin
an·ti·fi·bri·nol·y·sin
an·ti·fi·bri·no·lyt·ic
an·ti·flat·u·lent
an·ti·flu·o·ri·da·tion·ist
an·ti·fun·gal
an·ti·ga·lac·tic
an·ti·gen
an·ti·ge·ne·mi·a
an·ti·gen·ic
an·ti·ge·nic·i·ty
  pl an·ti·ge·nic·i·ties
an·ti·glob·u·lin
an·ti·goi·tro·gen·ic
an·ti·hal·lu·ci·na·to·ry
an·ti·he·lix
  pl an·ti·he·li·ces
  or an·ti·he·lix·es

  or ant·he·lix
  pl ant·he·li·ces
  or ant·he·lix·es
an·ti·hel·min·tic
  or an·te·hel·min·tic
  or ant·hel·min·tic
  or ant·hel·min·thic
an·ti·he·mol·y·sin
an·ti·he·mo·phil·ic
an·ti·hem·or·rhag·ic
an·ti·hi·drot·ic
an·ti·his·ta·mine
an·ti·his·ta·min·ic
an·ti·hor·mone
an·ti·hu·man
an·ti·hy·per·cho·les·ter·ol·
  e·mic
an·ti·hy·per·ten·sive
an·ti·hys·ter·ic
an·ti·ic·ter·ic
an·ti·im·mune
an·ti·in·fec·tive
an·ti·in·flam·ma·to·ry
an·ti·i·sol·y·sin
an·ti·ke·no·tox·in
an·ti·ke·to·gen·e·sis
an·ti·ke·to·gen·ic
an·ti·lac·tase
an·ti·leu·ke·mi·a
an·ti·leu·ke·mic
an·ti·leu·ko·cyt·ic
an·ti·lew·is·ite
an·ti·li·pe·mic
an·ti·lith·ic
an·ti·lo·bi·um
  pl an·ti·lo·bi·a
an·ti·lu·et·ic
an·ti·lym·pho·cyte
  or an·ti·lym·pho·cyt·ic
an·ti·lym·pho·cyt·ic
  or an·ti·lym·pho·cyte
an·ti·ly·sin
an·ti·ly·sis
  pl an·ti·ly·ses
an·ti·lyt·ic
an·ti·ma·lar·i·al
an·ti·mere
an·ti·mes·en·ter·ic
an·ti·me·tab·o·lite

21

an·ti·me·tro·pi·a
an·ti·mi·cro·bi·al
an·ti·mi·cro·bic
an·ti·mi·tot·ic
an·ti·mon·go·loid
an·ti·mo·ni·al
an·ti·mo·nic
an·ti·mo·nide
an·ti·mo·ny
   pl an·ti·mo·nies
an·ti·mo·nyl
an·ti·morph
an·ti·mu·ta·gen·ic
an·ti·my·cin
an·ti·my·cot·ic
an·ti·nar·cot·ic
an·ti·nau·se·ant
an·ti·ne·o·plas·tic
an·ti·ne·phrit·ic
an·ti·neu·ral·gic
an·ti·neu·rit·ic
an·tin·i·al
an·tin·i·on
an·ti·no·ci·cep·tive
an·tin·o·my
   pl an·tin·o·mies
an·ti·o·don·tal·gic
an·ti·op·so·nin
an·ti·ov·u·la·to·ry
an·ti·ox·i·dant
an·ti·ox·i·da·tion
an·ti·par·a·lyt·ic
an·ti·par·a·sit·ic
an·ti·pa·thy
   pl an·ti·pa·thies
an·ti·pe·dic·u·lot·ic
an·ti·pep·sin
an·ti·pe·ri·od·ic
an·ti·per·i·stal·sis
   pl an·ti·per·i·stal·ses
an·ti·per·i·stal·tic
an·ti·per·spi·rant
an·ti·phlo·gis·tic
an·ti·plas·min
an·ti·plas·tic
an·ti·pneu·mo·coc·cic
an·tip·o·dal
an·ti·pode
   pl an·tip·o·des

an·ti·pol·lu·tion
an·ti·pol·lu·tion·ist
an·ti·pos·tate
an·ti·pro·te·ase
an·ti·pro·throm·bin
an·ti·pro·to·zo·al
an·ti·pru·rit·ic
an·ti·pso·ri·at·ic
an·ti·psy·chot·ic
an·ti·py·re·sis
   pl an·ti·py·re·ses
an·ti·py·ret·ic
an·ti·py·rine
an·ti·py·rot·ic
an·ti·rab·ic
an·ti·ra·chit·ic
an·ti·ra·di·a·tion
an·ti·re·flec·tion
an·ti·ric·kett·si·al
an·ti·sca·bi·et·ic
an·ti·scor·bu·tic
an·ti·seb·or·rhe·ic
an·ti·se·cre·to·ry
an·ti·sep·sis
   pl an·ti·sep·ses
an·ti·sep·tic
an·ti·sep·ti·cize
an·ti·se·ro·to·nin
an·ti·se·rum
   pl an·ti·ser·ums
   or an·ti·se·ra
an·ti·si·al·a·gog
an·ti·si·al·a·gogue
   var of an·ti·si·al·a·gog
an·ti·si·al·ic
an·ti·sid·er·ic
an·ti·so·cial
an·ti·spas·mod·ic
an·ti·strep·to·coc·cic
an·ti·strep·tol·y·sin
an·ti·su·do·ral
an·ti·su·do·rif·ic
an·ti·sym·pa·thet·ic
an·ti·syph·i·lit·ic
an·ti·the·nar
an·ti·throm·bin
an·ti·throm·bo·plas·tin
an·ti·thy·roid
an·ti·tox·ic

an·ti·tox·in
an·ti·trag·i·cus
   pl an·ti·trag·i·ci
an·ti·tra·gus
   pl an·ti·tra·gi
an·ti·trich·o·mo·nal
an·ti·trope
an·ti·trop·ic
an·ti·try·pan·o·so·mal
an·ti·tryp·sin
an·ti·tryp·tase
an·ti·tryp·tic
an·ti·tu·ber·cu·lar
   or an·ti·tu·ber·cu·lous
an·ti·tu·ber·cu·lin
an·ti·tu·ber·cu·lot·ic
an·ti·tu·ber·cu·lous
   or an·ti·tu·ber·cu·lar
an·ti·tu·mor
   or an·ti·tu·mor·al
an·ti·tu·mor·al
   or an·ti·tu·mor
an·ti·tus·sive
an·ti·ve·ne·re·al
an·ti·ven·in
an·ti·vi·ral
an·ti·vi·ta·min
an·ti·vi·vi·sec·tion·ist
an·ti·xe·roph·thal·mic
an·ti·xe·rot·ic
an·ti·zy·mot·ic
an·tra·cele
   or an·tro·cele
an·tral
an·trec·to·my
an·tri·tis
an·tro·at·ti·cot·o·my
an·tro·buc·cal
an·tro·cele
   or an·tra·cele
an·tro·na·sal
an·tro·py·lo·ric
an·trorse
an·trorse·ly
an·tro·scope
an·tros·to·my
   pl an·tros·to·mies
an·trot·o·my
   pl an·trot·o·mies

an·tro·tym·pan·ic
an·tro·tym·pa·ni·tis
an·trum
pl an·trums
or an·tra
a·nu·cle·ar
an·u·lus
pl an·u·li
an·u·re·sis
pl an·u·re·ses
an·u·ri·a
a·nus
pl a·nus·es
or a·ni
an·vil
anx·i·e·ty
pl anx·i·e·ties
a·or·ta
pl a·or·tas
or a·or·tae
a·or·tal
a·or·tal·gi·a
a·or·tic
a·or·ti·co·pul·mo·nar·y
a·or·ti·co·pul·mon·ic
a·or·ti·co·re·nal
a·or·ti·tis
a·or·to·gram
a·or·tog·ra·phy
pl a·or·tog·ra·phies
a·or·to·il·i·ac
a·or·top·a·thy
a·or·tor·rha·phy
a·or·to·scle·ro·sis
a·or·tot·o·my
a·pal·les·the·si·a
a·pan·cre·a
a·par·a·lyt·ic
a·path·ic
ap·a·thy
pl ap·a·thies
ap·a·tite
a·pel·lous
a·pe·ri·ent
a·pe·ri·od·ic
a·per·i·stal·sis
pl a·per·i·stal·ses
a·per·i·tive
a·per·tog·na·thi·a

ap·er·tom·e·ter
ap·er·ture
a·pex
pl a·pex·es
or a·pi·ces
Ap·gar
a·pha·ci·a
or a·pha·ki·a
a·pha·gi·a
a·pha·ki·a
also a·pha·ci·a
a·pha·kic
aph·a·lan·gi·a
a·pha·si·a
a·pha·si·ac
a·pha·sic
a·pha·si·ol·o·gy
A·phas·mid·ia
aph·e·li·ot·ro·pism
a·phe·mi·a
a·phe·mic
a·pho·ni·a
a·phon·ic
a·phose
a·phot·ic
a·phra·si·a
a·phre·ni·a
aph·ro·dis·i·a
aph·ro·dis·i·ac
aph·tha
pl aph·thae
aph·thoid
aph·tho·sis
pl aph·tho·ses
aph·thous
a·phy·lax·is
ap·i·cal
ap·i·cec·to·my
ap·i·ci·tis
pl a·pi·ci·tes
a·pi·co·ec·to·my
pl a·pi·co·ec·to·mies
a·pi·co·lo·ca·tor
a·pi·col·y·sis
pl a·pi·col·y·ses
a·pi·cos·to·my
a·pi·gen·in
A·pi·um
a·pla·cen·tal

ap·la·nat·ic
a·plan·a·tism
a·pla·si·a
a·plas·tic
ap·ne·a
ap·ne·ic
ap·neu·mi·a
ap·neu·sis
pl ap·neu·ses
ap·neus·tic
ap·noe·a
var of ap·ne·a
ap·noe·ic
var of ap·ne·ic
ap·o·chro·mat·ic
a·poc·o·pe
ap·o·crine
ap·oc·y·nin
Ap·oc·y·num
ap·o·dal
a·po·di·a
ap·o·en·zyme
ap·o·fer·ri·tin
ap·o·gee
a·po·lar
ap·o·mict
ap·o·mic·tic
ap·o·mic·ti·cal·ly
ap·o·mix·is
pl ap·o·mix·es
ap·o·mor·phine
ap·o·neu·rec·to·my
ap·o·neu·ror·rha·phy
ap·o·neu·ro·sis
pl ap·o·neu·ro·ses
ap·o·neu·ro·si·tis
ap·o·neu·rot·ic
ap·o·neu·rot·o·my
a·poph·y·sa·ry
or a·poph·y·se·al
or ap·o·phys·i·al
a·poph·y·se·al
or ap·o·phys·i·al
or a·poph·y·sa·ry
ap·o·phys·i·al
or a·poph·y·sa·ry
or a·poph·y·se·al
a·poph·y·sis
pl a·poph·y·ses

23

a·poph·y·si·tis
ap·o·plec·tic
ap·o·plec·ti·form
ap·o·plex·y
   pl ap·o·plex·ies
ap·o·re·pres·sor
a·por·i·a
   pl a·por·i·as
   or a·por·i·ae
a·pos·ta·sis
   pl a·pos·ta·ses
a·po·stax·is
   pl a·po·stax·es
ap·os·teme
a·pos·thi·a
a·poth·e·car·y
   pl a·poth·e·car·ies
ap·o·them
ap·o·trip·sis
ap·o·zem
ap·oz·e·ma
ap·o·zy·mase
ap·pa·ra·tus
   pl ap·pa·ra·tus·es
   or ap·pa·ra·tus
ap·pear·ance
ap·pend·age
ap·pen·dec·to·my
   pl ap·pen·dec·to·mies
ap·pen·di·cal
   or ap·pen·dic·e·al
   or ap·pen·di·ci·al
ap·pen·dic·e·al
   or ap·pen·di·cal
   or ap·pen·di·ci·al
ap·pen·di·ci·al
   or ap·pen·di·cal
   or ap·pen·dic·e·al
ap·pen·di·cec·to·my
   pl ap·pen·di·cec·to·mies
ap·pen·di·ces
ap·pen·di·ci·tis
ap·pen·di·co·li·thi·a·sis
ap·pen·di·co·ly·sis
ap·pen·di·cos·to·my
   pl ap·pen·di·cos·to·mies
ap·pen·dic·u·lar

ap·pen·dix
   pl ap·pen·dix·es
   or ap·pen·di·ces
ap·per·ceive
ap·per·cep·tion
ap·per·cep·tive
ap·pe·stat
ap·pe·tite
ap·pe·ti·tion
ap·pe·ti·tive
ap·pla·nate
ap·pla·na·tion
ap·pla·nom·e·ter
ap·pli·ance
ap·pli·ca·tor
ap·pli·qué
ap·pre·hen·sion
ap·pose
ap·proach
ap·prox·i·mate
ap·prox·i·ma·tion
a·prac·tic
a·prax·i·a
a·prax·ic
ap·ri·cot
ap·ro·bar·bi·tal
a·proc·ti·a
ap·ros·ex·i·a
a·pros·o·pi·a
ap·sych·i·a
ap·ty·a·li·a
ap·ty·a·lism
a·pul·mo·nism
a·pus
a·pyk·no·mor·phous
a·py·og·e·nous
ap·y·rase
a·py·ret·ic
a·py·rex·i·a
   pl a·py·rex·i·as
   or a·py·rex·y
   pl a·py·rex·ies
a·py·rex·i·al
a·py·rex·y
   pl a·py·rex·ies
   or a·py·rex·i·a
   pl a·py·rex·i·as
a·py·ro·gen·ic

aq·ua
   pl aq·uas
   or aq·uae
aq·ua·pho·bi·a
aq·uat·ic
aq·ue·duct
aq·ue·duc·tal
aq·ue·ous
aq·uo·cap·su·li·tis
aq·uos·i·ty
   pl aq·uos·i·ties
ar·a·ban
ar·a·bic
a·rab·i·nose
a·ra·bi·no·side
a·rab·i·no·syl·cy·to·sine
a·rab·i·tol
ar·ach·ic
   or ar·a·chid·ic
ar·a·chid·ic
   or a·rach·ic
a·rach·i·don·tic
a·ra·chis
A·rach·ni·da
a·rach·nid·ism
a·rach·ni·tis
a·rach·no·dac·ty·ly
   pl a·rach·no·dac·ty·lies
a·rach·no·gas·tri·a
a·rach·noid
ar·ach·noi·dal
a·rach·noid·ism
a·rach·noid·i·tis
a·rach·no·ly·sin
a·rach·no·pho·bi·a
a·rach·no·pi·a
A·ra·li·a
ar·al·kyl
a·ra·ne·ism
a·ra·ne·ous
a·ra·phi·a
ar·a·ro·ba
ar·bor
ar·bo·res·cent
ar·bo·ri·za·tion
ar·bo·rize
ar·bor·vi·tae
ar·bo·vi·rus
ar·bu·tin

ar·bu·tus
ar·cade
ar·chae·o·cyte
  var of ar·che·o·cyte
ar·cha·ic
arch·am·phi·as·ter
ar·chae·us
  pl ar·chae·i
  or ar·che·us
  pl ar·che·i
ar·che·go·ni·al
ar·che·go·ni·ate
ar·che·go·ni·um
  pl ar·che·go·ni·a
arch·en·ceph·a·lon
  pl arch·en·ceph·a·la
arch·en·ter·on
  pl arch·en·ter·a
arch·e·o·cyte
ar·che·o·ki·net·ic
ar·che·spore
  or ar·che·spo·ri·um
  pl ar·che·spo·ri·a
ar·che·spo·ri·um
  pl ar·che·spo·ri·a
  or ar·che·spore
ar·che·type
ar·che·us
  pl ar·che·i
  or ar·chae·us
  pl ar·chae·i
ar·chi·a·ter
ar·chi·blast
ar·chi·gas·ter
ar·chil
  or or·chil
ar·chi·neph·ron
ar·chi·neu·ron
ar·chi·pal·li·um
ar·chi·plasm
ar·chi·tec·ton·ic
ar·chi·tec·ture
ar·cho·plasm
ar·ci·form
arc·ta·tion
arc·to·staph·y·los
ar·cu·al
ar·cu·a·li·a
ar·cu·ate

ar·cu·a·tion
ar·cus
ar·dor
ar·e·a·tus
A·re·ca
a·re·co·line
a·re·flex·i·a
a·re·gen·er·a·tive
ar·e·na·ceous
ar·e·no·vi·rus
a·re·o·la
  pl a·re·o·las
  or a·re·o·lae
a·re·o·lar
ar·e·om·e·ter
Ar·gas
Ar·gas·i·dae
ar·gen·taf·fin
  or ar·gen·taf·fine
ar·gen·taf·fine
  or ar·gen·taf·fin
ar·gen·taf·fi·no·ma
  pl ar·gen·taf·fi·no·mas
  or ar·gen·taf·fi·no·ma·ta
ar·gen·tic
ar·gen·tine
ar·gen·to·phil
  or ar·gen·to·phile
  or ar·gen·to·phil·ic
ar·gen·to·phile
  or ar·gen·to·phil
  or ar·gen·to·phil·ic
ar·gen·to·phil·ic
  or ar·gen·to·phil
  or ar·gen·to·phile
ar·gen·tous
ar·gen·tum
ar·gi·nase
ar·gi·ni·no·suc·cin·ic·ac·id·
  u·ri·a
ar·gon
Ar·gyll-Rob·ert·son pu·pil
ar·gyr·i·a
ar·gyr·ic
ar·gy·ro·phil
  or ar·gy·ro·phile
  or ar·gy·ro·phil·ic

ar·gy·ro·phile
  or ar·gy·ro·phil
  or ar·gy·ro·phil·ic
ar·gy·ro·phil·ic
  or ar·gy·ro·phil
  or ar·gy·ro·phile
ar·gy·ro·sis
  pl ar·gy·ro·ses
a·rhin·en·ce·pha·li·a
  or ar·rhin·en·ce·pha·li·a
a·rhin·i·a
  or ar·rhin·i·a
a·ri·bo·fla·vin·o·sis
  pl a·ri·bo·fla·vin·o·ses
a·rith·mo·ma·ni·a
ar·ma·men·tar·i·um
  pl ar·ma·men·tar·i·ums
  or ar·ma·men·tar·i·a
ar·mar·i·um
  pl ar·mar·i·ums
  or ar·mar·i·a
arm·pit
ar·ni·ca
Ar·nold-Chi·ar·i
  de·for·mi·ty,
  mal·for·ma·tion,
  syn·drome
ar·o·mat·ic
a·ro·ma·tize
a·rous·al
ar·o·yl
ar·rec·tor
  pl ar·rec·to·rs
  or ar·rec·to·res
ar·rest
ar·rhe·no·blas·to·ma
  pl ar·rhe·no·blas·to·mas
  also ar·rhe·no·blas·to·ma·ta
ar·rhin·en·ce·pha·li·a
  or a·rhin·en·ce·pha·li·a
ar·rhin·i·a
  or a·rhin·i·a
ar·rhyth·mi·a
  or ar·ryth·mi·a
ar·rhyth·mic
  or ar·rhyth·mi·cal
ar·rhyth·mi·cal
  or ar·rhyth·mic
ar·row·root

25

ar·ryth·mi·a
   or ar·rhyth·mi·a
ar·se·nate
ar·se·nic
ar·se·nic tri·ox·ide
ar·sen·i·cal
ar·sen·i·cal·ism
ar·se·nide
ar·se·ni·ous
ar·se·nite
ar·sen·iu·ret·ed
   or ar·sen·iu·ret·ted
ar·sen·iu·ret·ted
   or ar·sen·iu·ret·ed
ar·se·ni·um
ar·sen·o·blast
ar·sen·ol·y·sis
ar·se·no·ther·a·py
   pl ar·se·no·ther·a·pies
ar·se·nous
ar·sen·ox·ide
ar·sine
ar·son·ic
ar·so·ni·um
ars·phen·a·mine
ars·thi·nol
ar·te·fac
   or ar·te·fact
   or ar·ti·fact
ar·te·fact
   or ar·te·fac
   or ar·ti·fact
ar·te·fac·ta
Ar·te·mis·i·a
ar·ter·al·gi·a
ar·te·re·nol
ar·te·ri·a
   pl ar·te·ri·ae
ar·te·ri·al
ar·te·ri·al·i·za·tion
ar·te·ri·al·ize
ar·te·ri·ec·ta·sis
ar·te·ri·o·cap·il·lar·y
ar·te·ri·o·gram
ar·te·ri·o·graph·ic
ar·te·ri·og·ra·phy
   pl ar·te·ri·og·ra·phies
ar·te·ri·o·la
   pl ar·te·ri·o·lae

ar·te·ri·o·lar
ar·te·ri·ole
ar·te·ri·o·lith
ar·te·ri·o·li·tis
ar·te·ri·o·lo·ne·cro·sis
   pl ar·te·ri·o·lo·ne·cro·ses
ar·te·ri·o·lo·scle·ro·sis
   pl ar·te·ri·o·lo·scle·ro·ses
ar·te·ri·o·ma·la·ci·a
ar·te·ri·o·mo·tor
ar·te·ri·o·my·o·ma·to·sis
   pl ar·te·ri·o·my·o·ma·to·ses
ar·te·ri·o·ne·cro·sis
   pl ar·te·ri·o·ne·cro·ses
ar·te·ri·o·path·ic
ar·te·ri·op·a·thy
ar·te·ri·o·plas·ty
   pl ar·te·ri·o·plas·ties
ar·te·ri·o·pres·sor
ar·te·ri·or·rha·phy
   pl ar·te·ri·or·rha·phies
ar·te·ri·or·rhex·is
   pl ar·te·ri·or·rhex·es
ar·te·ri·o·scle·ro·sis
   pl ar·te·ri·o·scle·ro·ses
ar·te·ri·o·scle·rot·ic
ar·te·ri·o·spasm
ar·te·ri·o·ste·no·sis
   pl ar·te·ri·o·ste·no·ses
ar·te·ri·o·sym·pa·thec·to·
my
ar·te·ri·o·tome
ar·te·ri·ot·o·my
   pl ar·te·ri·ot·o·mies
ar·te·ri·o·ve·nous
ar·ter·i·tis
ar·ter·y
   pl ar·ter·ies
ar·thrag·ra
ar·thral
ar·thral·gi·a
ar·threc·to·my
   pl ar·threc·to·mies
ar·thrit·ic
ar·thri·tide
ar·thri·tis
   pl ar·thrit·i·des
ar·thri·tism
ar·throc·a·ce

ar·thro·cele
ar·thro·cen·te·sis
   pl ar·thro·cen·te·ses
ar·thro·chon·dri·tis
ar·thro·cla·si·a
ar·thro·de·sis
   pl ar·thro·de·ses
ar·thro·di·a
   pl ar·thro·di·ae
ar·thro·di·al
ar·thro·dyn·i·a
ar·thro·dys·pla·si·a
ar·thro·em·py·e·sis
ar·thro·en·dos·co·py
ar·throg·e·nous
ar·thro·gram
ar·throg·ra·phy
   pl ar·throg·ra·phies
ar·thro·gry·po·sis
ar·thro·ka·tad·y·sis
   pl ar·thro·ka·tad·y·ses
ar·thro·lith
ar·throl·o·gy
   pl ar·throl·o·gies
ar·throl·y·sis
   pl ar·throl·y·ses
ar·throm·e·ter
ar·thro·neu·ral·gi·a
ar·thro·oph·thal·mop·a·thy
ar·throp·a·thy
   pl ar·throp·a·thies
ar·thro·phy·ma
ar·thro·phyte
ar·thro·plas·ty
   pl ar·thro·plas·ties
ar·thro·pod
Ar·throp·o·da
ar·throp·o·dous
ar·thro·py·o·sis
ar·thro·scle·ro·sis
ar·thros·co·py
ar·thro·sis
   pl ar·thro·ses
ar·thro·spore
ar·thro·spor·ic
   or ar·thro·spo·rous
ar·thro·spo·rous
   or ar·thro·spor·ic

ar·thros·to·my
  pl ar·thros·to·mies
ar·thro·syn·o·vi·tis
ar·throt·o·my
  pl ar·throt·o·mies
ar·throx·es·is
Ar·thus phe·nom·e·non
ar·ti·ad
ar·ti·cle
ar·tic·u·lar
ar·tic·u·lar·e
ar·tic·u·late
ar·tic·u·la·ti·o
  pl ar·tic·u·la·ti·o·nes
ar·tic·u·la·tion
ar·tic·u·la·tor
ar·tic·u·la·tory
ar·tic·u·lo
ar·tic·u·lus
  pl ar·tic·u·li
ar·ti·fact
  or ar·te·fact
  or ar·te·fac
ar·ti·fac·ti·tious
ar·ti·fi·cial
Ar·ti·o·dac·ty·la
ar·y·ep·i·glot·tic
ar·y·ep·i·glot·ti·cus
ar·yl
ar·y·te·no·ep·i·glot·tic
ar·y·te·no·ep·i·glot·tid·e·an
ar·y·te·noid
ar·y·te·noi·dec·to·my
  pl ar·y·te·noi·dec·to·mies
ar·y·te·noi·di·tis
ar·y·te·noi·do·pex·y
as·a·fet·id·a
  or as·sa·fet·i·da
as·a·foet·i·da
  var of as·a·fet·i·da
as·a·rum
as·bes·ti·form
as·bes·tos
as·bes·to·sis
  pl as·bes·to·ses
as·ca·ri·a·sis
  pl as·ca·ri·a·ses
as·car·i·cide

as·ca·rid
  pl as·ca·rids
  or as·car·i·des
As·ca·rid·ia
as·car·i·di·a·sis
  pl as·car·i·di·a·ses
as·ca·ris
  pl as·car·i·des
As·ca·rops
as·cer·tain·ment
Asch·heim-Zon·dek test
Asch·off bod·y, nod·ule
as·ci·tes
  pl as·ci·tes
as·cit·ic
as·cle·pi·ad
as·cle·pi·as
as·co·carp
as·co·car·pous
as·co·go·ni·um
  pl as·co·go·ni·a
As·co·my·ce·tes
as·co·my·ce·tous
as·cor·bate
a·scor·bic
as·co·spore
as·co·spor·ic
  or as·co·spor·ous
as·co·spor·ous
  or as·co·spor·ic
as·cus
  pl as·ci
as·e·ma·si·a
a·se·mi·a
a·sep·sis
  pl a·sep·ses
a·sep·tic
a·sex·u·al
a·sex·u·al·i·za·tion
a·si·a·li·a
a·sid·er·o·sis
a·so·cial
a·so·ni·a
as·par·a·gin·ase
as·par·a·gine
as·par·agi·nyl
as·par·a·gus
as·par·tase

as·par·tate
as·par·tic
as·par·to·ki·nase
as·par·to·yl
  or as·par·tyl
as·par·tyl
  or as·par·to·yl
as·pect
As·per·gil·la·les
as·per·gil·lin
as·per·gil·lo·ma
  pl as·per·gil·lo·mas
  or as·per·gil·lo·ma·ta
as·per·gil·lo·sis
  pl as·per·gil·lo·ses
As·per·gil·lus
  pl as·per·gil·li
as·per·gil·lus·tox·i·co·sis
a·sper·ma·tism
a·sper·ma·to·gen·e·sis
a·sper·mi·a
as·per·sion
as·phal·ge·si·a
a·spher·ic
as·phyx·i·a
as·phyx·i·al
as·phyx·i·ant
as·phyx·i·ate
as·pid·i·nol
as·pid·i·um
  pl as·pid·i·a
as·pi·do·sper·ma
as·pi·do·sper·mine
as·pi·rate
as·pi·ra·tion
as·pi·ra·tor
as·pi·rin
a·sple·ni·a
As·ple·ni·um
a·spo·ro·gen·ic
a·spo·rog·e·nous
a·spo·rous
a·spo·ru·late
as·sa·fet·i·da
  or as·a·fet·i·da
as·sa·foet·i·da
  var of as·sa·fet·i·da
as·say
as·sim·i·la·ble

as·sim·i·late
as·sim·i·la·tion
as·sim·i·la·tive
as·so·ci·a·tion
as·so·ci·a·tive
as·so·nance
a·sta·si·a
a·stat·ic
as·ta·tine
a·ste·a·to·sis
as·ter
a·ster·e·og·no·sis
   pl a·ster·e·og·no·ses
as·te·ri·on
   pl as·te·ri·a
as·ter·ix·is
a·ster·ni·a
as·ter·o·coc·cus
   pl as·ter·o·coc·ci
as·ter·oid
as·the·ni·a
as·then·ic
as·the·no·co·ri·a
as·the·no·nom·e·ter
as·the·no·pi·a
as·the·nop·ic
as·the·no·sper·mi·a
asth·ma
asth·mat·ic
asth·mat·i·form
asth·mo·gen·ic
as·tig·mat·ic
a·stig·ma·tism
a·stig·ma·tom·e·ter
a·stig·mi·a
as·tig·mom·e·try
   pl as·tig·mom·e·tries
a·stig·mo·scope
a·stom·a·tous
a·sto·mi·a
a·sto·mous
a·strag·a·lar
a·strag·a·lec·to·my
   pl a·strag·a·lec·to·mies
a·strag·a·lus
   pl a·strag·a·lus·es
   or a·strag·a·li
as·tral
as·tric·tion

as·tringe
a·strin·gent
as·tro·bi·o·log·i·cal
as·tro·bi·ol·o·gy
   pl as·tro·bi·ol·o·gies
as·tro·blast
as·tro·blas·to·ma
   pl as·tro·blas·to·mas
   or as·tro·blas·to·ma·ta
as·tro·cyte
as·tro·cyt·ic
as·tro·cy·to·ma
   pl as·tro·cy·to·mas
   or as·tro·cy·to·ma·ta
as·tro·cy·to·sis
as·trog·li·a
as·troid
as·tro·sphere
a·syl·la·bia
a·sy·lum
a·sym·bo·li·a
a·sym·met·ri·cal
a·sym·me·try
   pl a·sym·me·tries
a·symp·to·mat·ic
a·syn·ap·sis
   pl a·syn·ap·ses
a·syn·chro·nism
a·syn·chro·ny
a·syn·cli·tism
a·syn·de·sis
   pl a·syn·de·ses
a·sy·nech·i·a
a·sy·ner·gi·a
a·sy·ner·gic
a·syn·er·gy
   pl a·syn·er·gies
a·sy·no·vi·a
a·syn·tax·i·a
a·sys·tem·at·ic
a·sys·to·le
a·sys·tol·ic
a·tac·tic
a·tac·ti·form
at·a·rac·tic
   or at·a·rax·ic
at·ar·al·ge·si·a
at·a·rax·ia

at·a·rax·ic
   or at·a·rac·tic
a·tav·ic
at·a·vism
at·a·vis·tic
a·tax·a·pha·si·a
   or a·tax·i·a·pha·si·a
a·tax·i·a
   pl a·tax·i·as
   or a·tax·y
   pl a·tax·ies
a·tax·i·a·gram
a·tax·i·a·graph
a·tax·i·a·pha·si·a
   or a·tax·a·pha·si·a
a·tax·i·a·tel·an·gi·ec·ta·si·a
a·tax·ic
a·tax·o·phe·mi·a
a·tax·y
   pl a·tax·ies
   or a·tax·i·a
   pl a·tax·i·as
at·e·lec·ta·sis
   pl at·el·ec·ta·ses
at·el·ec·tat·ic
a·te·li·a
a·te·li·o·sis
   pl a·te·li·o·ses
a·tel·i·ot·ic
at·e·lo·car·di·a
at·e·lo·ceph·a·lous
at·e·lo·ceph·a·ly
at·e·lo·chei·li·a
at·e·lo·glos·si·a
at·e·lo·my·e·li·a
at·e·lo·rha·chid·i·a
at·e·lo·sto·mi·a
a·the·li·a
a·ther·mic
a·ther·mo·sys·tal·tic
ath·er·o·gen·e·sis
   pl ath·er·o·gen·e·ses
ath·er·o·gen·ic
ath·er·o·ma
   pl ath·er·o·mas
   or ath·er·o·ma·ta
ath·er·o·ma·to·sis
   or ath·er·o·ma·to·ses
ath·er·om·a·tous

ath·er·o·scle·ro·sis
pl ath·er·o·scle·ro·ses
ath·er·o·scle·rot·ic
ath·e·te·sis
pl ath·e·te·ses
ath·e·toid
ath·e·to·sic
ath·e·to·sis
pl ath·e·to·ses
ath·e·tot·ic
a·threp·si·a
a·threp·tic
ath·ro·cyte
ath·ro·cy·to·sis
pl ath·ro·cy·to·ses
a·thy·mi·a
a·thy·mic
a·thy·re·o·sis
pl a·thy·re·o·ses
or a·thy·ro·sis
pl a·thy·ro·ses
a·thy·ri·a
a·thy·ro·sis
pl a·thy·ro·ses
or a·thy·re·o·sis
pl a·thy·re·o·ses
at·lan·tad
at·lan·tal
at·lan·to·ax·i·al
at·lan·to·oc·cip·i·tal
at·lan·to·did·y·mus
at·lan·to·mas·toid
at·las
at·lo·ax·oid
at·lo·did·y·mus
at·mol·y·sis
pl at·mol·y·ses
at·mom·e·ter
at·mos
at·mo·sphere
a·to·ci·a
at·om
a·tom·ic
at·o·mic·i·ty
pl at·o·mic·i·ties
at·om·ism
at·om·is·tic
at·om·i·za·tion
at·om·ize

at·om·iz·er
a·to·nia
a·ton·ic
a·to·nic·i·ty
pl a·to·nic·i·ties
at·o·ny
pl at·o·nies
at·o·pen
a·top·ic
a·top·og·no·si·a
a·top·og·no·sis
pl a·top·og·no·ses
at·o·py
pl at·o·pies
a·tox·ic
ATPase
a·trans·fer·ri·ne·mi·a
a·trau·mat·ic
a·tre·mi·a
a·tre·si·a
a·tre·sic
a·tret·ic
a·tri·al
a·trich·i·a
at·ri·ch·o·sis
pl at·ri·cho·ses
a·tri·chous
a·tri·o·sep·to·pex·y
pl a·tri·o·sep·to·pex·ies
a·tri·o·sep·to·plas·ty
a·tri·ot·o·my
a·tri·o·ven·tric·u·lar
a·tri·o·ven·tric·u·la·ris
   com·mu·nis
a·tri·um
pl a·tri·a
a·tro·phi·a
a·troph·ic
at·ro·pho·der·ma
at·ro·phy
pl at·ro·phies
at·ro·pine
at·ro·pin·i·za·tion
at·ro·pin·ize
at·ro·scine
at·tach·ment
at·tack
at·tar
at·ten·tion

at·ten·u·ate
at·ten·u·a·tion
at·tic
at·tic·i·tis
at·ti·co·an·trot·o·my
pl at·ti·co·an·trot·o·mies
at·ti·co·mas·toid
at·ti·cot·o·my
pl at·ti·cot·o·mies
at·ti·tude
at·ti·tu·di·nal
at·trac·tion
at·tri·tion
a·typ·i·a
a·typ·i·cal
a·typ·ism
au·dile
au·di·o·an·al·ge·si·a
au·di·o·gen·ic
au·di·o·gram
au·di·ol·o·gist
au·di·ol·o·gy
pl au·di·ol·o·gies
au·di·om·e·ter
au·di·om·e·tri·cian
au·di·om·e·trist
au·di·om·e·try
pl au·di·om·e·tries
au·di·o·sur·ger·y
au·di·o·vis·u·al
au·di·tion
au·di·tive
au·di·to·ry
Au·er·bach gan·gli·on,
   plex·us
aug·ment
aug·men·ta·tion
aug·na·thus
au·la
pl au·las
or au·lae
au·ra
pl au·ras
or au·rae
au·ral
au·ral·ly
au·ran·ti·a·sis
pl au·ran·ti·a·ses
au·ri·a·sis

au·ric
au·ri·cle
au·ric·u·la
  pl au·ric·u·las
  or au·ric·u·lae
au·ric·u·lar
au·ric·u·lar·e
  pl au·ric·u·lar·i·a
au·ric·u·lar·is
  pl au·ric·u·lar·es
au·ric·u·late
au·ric·u·lo·cra·ni·al
au·ric·u·lo·pal·pe·bral
au·ric·u·lo·tem·po·ral
au·ric·u·lo·ven·tric·u·lar
au·ri·form
au·rin
au·ri·na·sal
au·ri·punc·ture
au·ris
  pl au·res
au·ri·scope
au·ro·chro·mo·der·ma
au·ro·ther·a·py
au·ro·thi·o·glu·cose
au·ro·thi·o·gly·ca·nide
au·rum
aus·cul·tate
aus·cul·ta·tion
aus·cul·ta·to·ry
aus·ten·it·ic
au·ta·coid
au·tar·ce·sis
au·te·cic
au·te·cious
au·tism
au·tis·tic
au·to·ag·glu·ti·na·tion
au·to·ag·glu·ti·nin
au·to·am·pu·ta·tion
au·to·a·nal·y·sis
  pl au·to·a·nal·y·ses
au·to·an·ti·bod·y
  pl au·to·an·ti·bod·ies
au·to·an·ti·gen
au·to·an·ti·tox·in
au·to·ca·tal·y·sis
  pl au·to·ca·tal·y·ses

au·to·cat·a·lyt·ic
au·to·ca·thar·sis
au·toch·tho·nous
au·toc·la·sis
  pl au·toc·la·ses
au·to·clav·a·ble
au·to·clave
au·to·cy·tol·y·sin
au·to·cy·tol·y·sis
  pl au·to·cy·tol·y·ses
au·to·di·ges·tion
au·to·dip·loi·dy
au·to·ech·o·prax·i·a
au·to·ec·o·la·li·a
au·toe·cious
  var of au·te·cious
au·to·ec·ze·ma·ti·za·tion
au·to·e·rot·ic
au·to·e·rot·i·cism
au·to·er·o·tism
au·tog·a·mous
au·tog·a·my
  pl au·tog·a·mies
au·to·gen·e·sis
  pl au·to·gen·e·ses
au·to·ge·net·ic
au·to·gen·ic
au·tog·e·nous
au·tog·no·sis
  pl au·tog·no·ses
au·to·graft
au·tog·ra·phism
au·to·hem·ag·glu·ti·nin
au·to·he·mag·glu·ti·na·tion
au·to·he·mol·y·sin
au·to·he·mol·y·sis
  pl au·to·he·mol·y·ses
au·to·he·mo·ther·a·py
  pl au·to·he·mo·ther·a·pies
au·to·hyp·no·sis
au·to·im·mune
au·to·im·mu·ni·ty
  pl au·to·im·mu·ni·ties
au·to·im·mu·ni·za·tion
au·to·im·mu·nize
au·to·in·fec·tion
au·to·in·oc·u·la·ble
au·to·in·oc·u·la·tion

au·to·ker·a·to·plas·ty
au·to·ki·ne·sis
  pl au·to·ki·ne·ses
au·to·ki·net·ic
au·to·le·sion
au·to·leu·ko·ag·glu·ti·nin
au·tol·o·gous
au·tol·y·sate
au·tol·y·sin
au·tol·y·sis
  pl au·tol·y·ses
au·to·lyt·ic
au·to·lyze
au·to·ma·nip·u·la·tion
au·to·ma·nip·u·la·tive
au·tom·a·tism
au·to·ma·to·graph
au·to·mix·is
  pl au·to·mix·es
au·tom·ne·si·a
au·to·my·so·pho·bi·a
au·to·ne·phrec·to·my
au·to·nom·ic
au·to·nom·o·trop·ic
au·ton·o·mous
au·ton·o·my
  pl au·ton·o·mies
au·to ox·i·da·tion
au·top·a·thy
au·to·pha·gi·a
au·to·phag·ic
au·toph·a·gy
  pl au·toph·a·gies
au·to·phil·i·a
au·to·pho·bi·a
au·toph·o·ny
au·to·plas·mo·ther·a·py
au·to·plas·tic
au·to·plas·ty
au·to·ploid
au·to·ploi·dy
  pl au·to·ploi·dies
au·to·pol·y·ploi·dy
  pl au·to·pol·y·ploi·dies
au·to·pre·cip·i·tin
au·to·pro·throm·bin
au·top·sy
  pl au·top·sies

au·to·psy·chic
au·to·ra·di·o·gram
au·to·ra·di·og·ra·phy
   pl au·to·ra·di·og·ra·phies
au·to·reg·u·la·tion
au·to·reg·u·la·tive
au·to·reg·u·la·to·ry
au·to·re·in·fu·sion
au·to·scope
au·to·sen·si·ti·za·tion
au·to·sep·ti·ce·mi·a
au·to·se·ro·di·ag·no·sis
au·to·se·rum
au·to·sex·ing
au·to·site
au·to·so·mal
au·to·so·mal·ly
au·to·some
au·to·sple·nec·to·my
au·to·stim·u·la·tion
au·to·sug·ges·ti·bil·i·ty
   pl au·to·sug·gest·i·bil·i·ties
au·to·sug·ges·tion
au·to·ther·a·py
   pl au·to·ther·a·pies
au·tot·o·mize
au·tot·o·my
   pl au·tot·o·mies
au·to·top·ag·no·si·a
au·to·tox·e·mi·a
au·to·tox·in
au·to·trans·fu·sion
au·to·trans·plant
au·to·trans·plan·ta·tion
au·to·troph
au·to·tro·phic
au·to·vac·ci·na·tion
au·to·vac·cine
au·tox·i·da·tion
au·tum·nal
aux·an·o·gram
aux·an·o·graph·ic
aux·a·nog·ra·phy
   pl aux·a·nog·ra·phies
au·xe·sis
   pl aux·e·ses
aux·et·ic
aux·il·i·ar·y

au·xi·lyt·ic
aux·in
aux·i·om·e·ter
aux·o·chrome
aux·o·cyte
aux·o·drome
aux·om·e·try
aux·o·ther·a·py
aux·o·ton·ic
aux·o·troph
aux·o·troph·ic
aux·ot·ro·phy
   pl aux·ot·ro·phies
a·val·vu·lar
a·vas·cu·lar
a·vas·cu·lar·i·za·tion
A·ve·na
a·ve·nin
   or a·ve·nine
a·ve·nine
   or a·ve·nin
av·er·age
a·ver·sion
a·ver·sive
a·ver·sive·ly
a·vi·an
a·vi·an·ize
av·i·din
a·vir·u·lence
a·vir·u·lent
a·vi·ta·min·o·sis
   pl a·vi·ta·min·o·ses
Avo·ga·dro num·ber,
   con·stant
a·void·ance
a·void·ant
av·oir·du·pois
a·vulse
a·vul·sion
a·xen·ic
ax·i·al
ax·i·a·tion
ax·if·u·gal
ax·il
ax·ile
ax·il·la
   pl ax·il·las
   or ax·il·lae

ax·il·lar
ax·il·lar·y
   pl ax·il·lar·ies
ax·i·o·buc·cal
ax·i·o·buc·co·cer·vi·cal
ax·i·o·buc·co·gin·gi·val
ax·i·o·buc·co·lin·gual
ax·i·o·cer·vi·cal
ax·i·o·dis·tal
ax·i·o·dis·to·cer·vi·cal
ax·i·o·dis·to·gin·gi·val
ax·i·o·la·bi·o·lin·gual
ax·i·o·lin·gual
ax·i·o·ling·uo·cer·vi·cal
ax·i·o·ling·uo·gin·gi·val
ax·i·o·ling·uo oc·clu·sal
ax·i·o·me·si·al
ax·i·o·me·si·o·cer·vi·cal
ax·i·o·me·si·o·dis·tal
ax·i·o·me·si·o·gin·gi·val
ax·i·o·me·si·o·in·ci·sal
ax·i·o·me·si·o oc·clu·sal
ax·i·o oc·clu·sal
ax·i·o·pul·pal
ax·ip·e·tal
a·xis
   pl ax·es
a·xis·cyl·in·der
ax·ite
ax·o·den·drite
ax·o·fu·gal
ax·o·lem·ma
ax·ol·y·sis
ax·om·e·ter
ax·on
ax·o·nal
ax·one
ax·o·neme
ax·o·nom·e·ter
ax·on·ot·me·sis
ax·op·e·tal
ax·o·phage
ax·o·plasm
ax·o·po·di·um
ax·o·spon·gi·um
ax·o·style
A·yer·za dis·ease
az·a·cy·clo·nol

a·za·cy·clo·nol
   hy·dro·chlor·ide
az·a·me·tho·ni·um
   bro·mide
az·ap·e·tine
az·a·ser·ine
az·a·thi·o·prine
az·e·la·ic
a·ze·o·trope
a·ze·ot·ro·py
az·ide
az·o·car·mine
a·zo·ic

az·o·lit·min
a·zo·o·sper·mi·a
az·o·pro·te·in
az·o·sul·fa·mide
az·ote
az·o·te·mi·a
az·o·te·ne·sis
az·oth
a·zot·i·fi·ca·tion
az·o·tize
az·o·tom·e·ter
az·o·tor·rhe·a

az·o·tu·ri·a
az·ure
az·u·res·in
a·zu·ro·phil
az·u·ro·phil·i·a
az·u·ro·phil·ic
az·y·go·gram
az·y·gog·ra·phy
az·y·gos
az·y·gous
a·zy·mi·a
a·zy·mic

B

Baas·trup dis·ease
bab·bitt met·al
Bab·cock test
Bab·cock-Le·vy test
Ba·bès-Ernst bod·ies
Ba·be·si·a
bab·e·si·a·sis
   pl ba·be·si·a·ses
Ba·be·si·i·dae
ba·be·si·o·sis
   pl ba·be·si·o·ses
Ba·bés nod·ules
Ba·bin·ski re·flex, sign
Ba·bin·ski-Froeh·lich
   dis·ease
Ba·bin·ski-Na·geotte
   syn·drome
Ba·bin·ski-Va·quez
   syn·drome
bac·cate
bac·ci·form
Ba·cel·li sign
Bach·man test
Bach·mann bun·dle
Bach·ti·a·row sign
ba·cill

Bac·il·la·ce·ae
bac·il·lae·mi·a
   var of bac·il·le·mi·a
bac·il·lar
bac·il·lar·y
bac·il·le·mi·a
ba·cil·li·form
ba·cil·lin
ba·cil·lo·pho·bi·a
bac·il·lo·sis
   pl bac·il·lo·ses
ba·cil·lo·ther·a·py
bac·il·lu·ri·a
ba·cil·lus
   pl ba·cil·li
bac·i·tra·cin
back·ache
back·bone
back·cross
back·ground ra·di·a·tion
back·scat·ter
bac·te·re·mi·a
bac·te·re·mic
Bac·te·ri·a·ce·ae
bac·te·ri·al

bac·te·ri·ci·dal
   or bac·ter·i·o·ci·dal
bac·ter·i·cid·al·ly
bac·te·ri·cide
bac·te·ri·cid·in
   or bac·te·ri·o·cid·in
bac·ter·id
bac·ter·in
bac·te·ri·o·chlo·ro·phyll
bac·ter·i·o·ci·dal
   or bac·ter·i·ci·dal
bac·te·ri·o·cid·in
bac·te·ri·o·cin
   or bac·te·ri·cid·in
bac·te·ri·oc·la·sis
   pl bac·te·ri·oc·la·ses
bac·te·ri·o·er·y·thrin
bac·te·ri·o·flu·o·res·ce·in
bac·te·ri·o·gen·ic
bac·te·ri·og·e·nous
bac·te·ri·o·hae·mol·y·sin
   var of bac·te·ri·o·he·mol·y·
   sin
bac·te·ri·o·he·mol·y·sin
bac·te·ri·oid
   or bac·ter·oid

32

bac·te·ri·oi·dal
or bac·te·roi·dal
bac·te·ri·o·log·ic
or bac·te·ri·o·log·i·cal
bac·te·ri·o·log·i·cal
or bac·te·ri·o·log·ic
bac·te·ri·ol·o·gist
bac·te·ri·ol·o·gy
pl bac·te·ri·ol·o·gies
bac·te·ri·o·ly·sin
bac·te·ri·ol·y·sis
pl bac·te·ri·ol·y·ses
bac·te·ri·o·lyt·ic
bac·te·ri·o·op·son·ic
bac·te·ri·o·op·so·nin
bac·te·ri·o·pex·y
bac·te·ri·o·phage
bac·te·ri·o·pha·gi·a
bac·te·ri·o·phag·ic
bac·te·ri·oph·a·gy
bac·te·ri·o·pho·bi·a
bac·te·ri·o·pre·cip·i·tin
bac·te·ri·o·pro·te·in
bac·te·ri·op·son·ic
bac·te·ri·op·so·nin
bac·te·ri·o·sis
pl bac·te·ri·o·ses
bac·te·ri·os·ta·sis
pl bac·te·ri·os·ta·ses
bac·te·ri·o·stat
bac·te·ri·o·stat·ic
bac·te·ri·o·ther·a·peu·tic
bac·te·ri·o·ther·a·py
bac·te·ri·o·tox·ic
bac·te·ri·o·tox·in
bac·te·ri·o·trop·ic
bac·te·ri·ot·ro·pin
bac·te·ri·um
pl bac·te·ri·a
bac·te·ri·u·ri·a
bac·te·ri·za·tion
bac·te·rize
bac·ter·oid
or bac·te·ri·oid
Bac·ter·oi·da·ce·ae
bac·te·roi·dal
or bac·te·ri·oi·dal
bac·ter·oi·des
bac·ter·u·ria

bac·u·lum
pl bac·u·lums
or bac·u·la
Baer treat·ment
bag
bag·as·sco·sis
pl bag·as·sco·ses
ba·gasse
bag·as·so·sis
pl bag·as·so·ses
Bagh·dad
Ba·hi·a ul·cer
Bail·lar·ger
Bain·bridge re·flex
Ba·ker cyst
bak·ers' yeast
bal·ance
ba·lan·ic
Bal·a·ni·tes
ba·la·ni·tis
bal·a·no·chlam·y·di·tis
bal·a·no·plas·ty
bal·a·no·pos·thi·tis
bal·a·no·pre·pu·tial
bal·a·nor·rha·gi·a
bal·a·nor·rhe·a
bal·a·nor·rhoe·a
var of bal·a·nor·rhe·a
bal·an·tid·i·al
or bal·an·tid·ic
bal·an·ti·di·a·sis
pl bal·an·ti·di·a·ses
or bal·an·tid·i·o·sis
pl bal·an·tid·i·o·ses
bal·an·tid·ic
or bal·an·tid·i·al
bal·an·tid·i·o·sis
pl bal·an·tid·i·o·ses
or bal·an·ti·di·a·sis
pl bal·an·ti·di·a·ses
Bal·an·tid·i·um
pl Bal·an·tid·ia
bal·an·ti·do·sis
bal·a·nus
Bal·bi·a·ni rings
bald
bald·ness
Bal·duz·zi sign
Bald·win op·er·a·tion

Bal·dy-Web·ster
op·er·a·tion
Bal·four op·er·a·tion
Ba·lint syn·drome
Ball oper·a·tion
ball-and-sock·et
Bal·lance op·er·a·tion
Bal·let sign
Bal·lin·gall dis·ease
ball·ing iron, gun
bal·ling scale
bal·lism
bal·lis·mus
bal·lis·tic
bal·lis·to·car·di·o·gram
bal·lis·to·car·di·o·graph
bal·lis·to·car·di·og·ra·phy
pl bal·lis·to·car·di·og·ra·phies
bal·lonne·ment
bal·loon·ing
bal·lot·ta·ble
bal·lotte·ment
balm
bal·ne·a·tion
bal·ne·ol·o·gy
pl bal·ne·ol·o·gies
bal·ne·o·ther·a·peu·tics
bal·ne·o·ther·a·py
pl bal·ne·o·ther·a·pies
Ba·lo con·cen·tric scle·ro·sis
bal·sam
bal·sam·ic
Bal·ser fat ne·cro·sis
Bal·tha·zar-Fos·ter mur·mur
ba·meth·an
bam·i·fyl·line
ba·nal
Ban·croft fil·a·ri·a·sis
ban·crof·to·sis
band
ban·dage
ban·dy-leg
bane
bang
or bhang
Bang dis·ease

ban·i·ster·ine
ban·ting
ban·ting·ism
Ban·ti dis·ease, syn·drome
bap·ti·tox·ine
bar
bar·aes·the·si·a
  var of bar·es·the·si·a
bar·aes·the·si·om·e·ter
  var of bar·es·the·si·om·e·ter
bar·ag·no·sis
  pl bar·ag·no·ses
Bá·rány test
bar·ba
barb·al·o·in
bar·bei·ro
Bar·be·ri·o test
bar·ber·ry
  pl bar·ber·ries
Bar·ber method
bar·ber's itch
bar·bi·tal
bar·bi·tal·ism
bar·bi·tone
bar·bi·tu·ism
bar·bi·tu·rate
bar·bi·tu·ric
bar·bi·tu·rism
bar·bo·ne
bar·bo·tage
Bar·coo rot
Bar·de·le·ben op·er·a·tion
Bar·den·heu·er op·er·a·tion
Bar·det-Bie·dl syn·drome
bare·foot
Bär·en·sprung dis·ease
bar·es·the·si·a
bar·es·the·si·om·e·ter
Bar·foed test
bar·i·a·tri·cian
bar·i·at·rics
bar·ic
ba·ri·lla
bar·i·to·sis
bar·i·um
bark
Bar·ker op·er·a·tion

Bar·low dis·ease
Barns·dale bac·il·lus
bar·o·cep·tor
  or bar·o·re·cep·tor
bar·o·don·tal·gi·a
bar·og·no·sis
  pl bar·og·no·ses
bar·o·graph
bar·o·graph·ic
bar·o·ma·crom·e·ter
ba·rom·e·ter
bar·o·met·ric
baro·met·ro·graph
ba·rom·e·try
bar·o·o·ti·tis
bar·o·phil·ic
bar·o·pho·bi·a
bar·o·re·cep·tor
  or bar·cep·tor
baro·scope
bar·o·si·nus·i·tis
Ba·ros·ma
ba·ros·min
bar·o·stat
bar·o·tal·gi·a
bar·o·tax·is
  pl bar·o·tax·es
bar·o·ti·tis
bar·o·trau·ma
  pl baro·trau·mas
  or baro·trau·ma·ta
Bar·ra·quer dis·ease
Bar·ra·quer-Si·mons
  dis·ease
Bar·ré-Guil·lain
  syn·drome
bar·ren
Bart he·mo·glo·bin
Barth her·ni·a
Bar·tho·lin gland
bar·tho·lin·i·tis
  pl bar·tho·lin·i·tes
Bar·ton·el·la
Bar·ton·el·la·ce·ae
bar·ton·el·le·mi·a
bar·ton·el·li·a·sis
bar·ton·el·lo·sis
  pl bar·ton·el·lo·ses

Bart·ter syn·drome
bar·ye
bar·y·es·the·si·a
bar·y·glos·si·a
bar·y·la·li·a
bar·y·pho·ni·a
ba·ry·ta
ba·ry·tes
ba·sad
bas·al
ba·sal·i·o·ma
  pl ba·sal·i·o·mas
  or ba·sal·i·o·ma·ta
ba·sal·is
  pl ba·sal·es
ba·sal·oid
bas·cu·la·tion
base
bas·e·doid
Ba·se·dow dis·ease
Ba·sel·la
base·line
base·ment
ba·se·o·sis
  pl ba·se·o·ses
base·plate
bas·fond
Bash·am mix·ture
ba·si·al
ba·si·al·ve·o·lar
ba·si·bran·chi·al
ba·si·breg·mat·ic
ba·sic
ba·si·chro·ma·tin
ba·sic·i·ty
  pl ba·sic·i·ties
ba·si·cra·ni·al
ba·sid·i·al
Ba·sid·i·ob·o·lus
ba·sid·i·o·ge·net·ic
ba·sid·i·o·my·cete
Ba·sid·i·o·my·ce·tes
ba·sid·i·o·my·ce·tous
ba·sid·i·o·phore
ba·sid·i·o·spore
ba·sid·i·um
  pl ba·sid·i·a
ba·si·fa·cial

ba·si·hy·al
ba·si·hy·oid
bas·i·lad
bas·i·lar
ba·si·lat·er·al
ba·si·lem·ma
ba·sil·ic
bas·i·lo·breg·mat·ic
bas·i·lo·ma
bas·i·lo·men·tal
bas·i·lo·pha·ryn·ge·al
bas·i·lo·sub·na·sal
ba·si·na·sal
ba·si·o·al·ve·o·lar
ba·si·o·breg·mat·ic
ba·si·oc·cip·i·tal
ba·si·on
ba·si·o·tribe
ba·si·o·trip·sy
ba·sip·e·tal
ba·si·pha·ryn·ge·al
ba·si·pho·bi·a
ba·si·pre·sphe·noid
ba·si·rhi·nal
    or ba·sir·rhi·nal
ba·sir·rhi·nal
    or ba·si·rhi·nal
ba·sis
    pl ba·ses
ba·si·sphe·noid
ba·si·sphe·noi·dal
ba·si·syl·vi·an
ba·si·tem·po·ral
ba·si·ver·te·bral
bas·ket
ba·so·cyte
ba·so·e·ryth·ro·cyte
ba·so·phil
ba·so·phile
ba·so·phil·i·a
ba·so·phil·ic
ba·so·phil·i·lism
ba·so·phil·o·cyt·ic
ba·soph·i·lous
ba·so·pho·bi·a
ba·so·pho·bi·ac
ba·so·pho·bic
ba·so·plasm

ba·so·squa·mous
Bas·sen-Korn·zweig
    syn·drome
Bas·set op·er·a·tion
Bas·si·ni op·er·a·tion
bas·so·rin
Bas·ti·an-Bruns law
bath
bath·aes·the·si·a
    var of bath·es·the·si·a
bath·es·the·si·a
bath·mo·trop·ic
bath·mot·ro·pism
bath·o·chrome
bath·o·chro·mic
bath·o·chro·my
bath·o·pho·bi·a
bath·ro·ceph·a·ly
bath·y·an·es·the·si·a
bath·y·car·di·a
bath·y·chrome
bath·y·chro·mic
bath·y·es·the·si·a
bath·y·hy·per·es·the·si·a
bath·y·hyp·es·the·si·a
bath·yp·ne·a
bat·o·pho·bi·a
ba·tra·chi·an
ba·trach·o·tox·in
Bat·son plex·us
bat·ta·rism
bat·ta·ris·mus
Bat·ten-May·ou dis·ease
bat·ter
bat·ter·y
Bat·tey op·er·a·tion
bat·tle fa·tigue
Bat·tle sign
bat·tle·dore
bat·yl
Bau·de·loque di·a·me·ter
Bau·er test
Bau·hin valve
Bau·mès scale
Bau·mes sign
Baum·gar·ten syn·drome
Ba·u·ru ulcer
baux·ite

bay·ber·ry
    pl bay·ber·ries
bay·cu·ru
Bayle dis·ease
Baz·ett for·mu·la
Ba·zin dis·ease
BCG vac·cine
bdel·li·um
Bdel·lo·nys·sus
bdel·lo·vi·bri·o
bde·lyg·mi·a
beak·er
beam
bear·ber·ry
    pl bear·ber·ries
Beard dis·ease
beat
Beau·lines
be·bee·rine
be·bee·ru
be·can·thone
bech·ic
Bech·te·rew nu·cle·us
Beck op·er·a·tion
Beck·er dis·ease
Bec·que·rel ray
bed·bug
bed·lam
Bed·nar aph·thae
bed·pan
bed·side
bed·so·ni·a
    pl bed·so·ni·ae
bed·sore
bed·wet·ting
Beer law
bees·wax
beet·u·ri·a
Bee·vor sign
be·hav·ior
be·hav·ior·al
be·hav·ior·ism
be·hav·ior·ist
be·hav·ior·is·tic
be·hav·iour
    var of be·hav·ior
Beh·çet dis·ease
be·hen·ic

Behre test
Bei·gal dis·ease
bej·el
Be·ke·sy au·di·o·me·try
Bekh·te·rev re·flex
Bekh·te·rev-Men·del re·flex
bel
bel·ae fruc·tus
belch
be·lem·noid
Bell dis·ease
bel·la·don·na
bel·la·don·nine
bell-crowned
belle in·dif·fe·rence
Belle·vue
Bel·ling ac·e·to·car·mine stain
Bel·li·ni duct, tu·bule
Bell-Ma·gen·die law
bel·lows
bel·ly
    pl bel·lies
bel·ly·ache
bel·ly but·ton
bel·o·ne·pho·bi·a
bel·o·noid
bem·e·gride
ben·ac·ty·zine
Ben·a·cus
ben·an·ser·in
ben·a·zo·line
Bence-Jones pro·tein
Ben·da test
ben·da·zac
Ben·der ge·stalt test
ben·dro·flu·me·thi·a·zide
bends
be·ne
    or ben·ne
Ben·e·dict and Fran·ke meth·od
Ben·e·dict Hitch·cock re·a·gent
Ben·e·dict and New·ton meth·od
Ben·e·dict and Theis meth·od

Ben·e·dict test
Ben·e·dikt syn·drome
be·nign
be·nig·nant
ben·ne
    or be·ne
Ben·nett cells
Benn·hold test
be·nor·ter·one
ben·ox·i·nate
ben·per·i·dol
ben·sa·lan
ben·ton·ite
benz·al·de·hyde
benz·al·dox·ime
benz·al·ko·ni·um
benz·an·thra·cene
ben·za·thine
benz·az·o·line
benz·cu·rine i·o·dide
ben·zene
ben·zes·trol
ben·ze·tho·ni·um
ben·zet·i·mide
benz·hex·ol
benz·hy·dra·mine
ben·zi·dine
ben·zi·lo·ni·um
benz·im·id·az·ole
ben·zin
    or ben·zine
benz·in·do·py·rine
ben·zine
    or ben·zin
ben·zo·ate
ben·zo·caine
benz·oc·ta·mine
ben·zo·dep·a
ben·zo·di·ox·an
ben·zo·di·ox·ane
ben·zo·ic
ben·zo·in
ben·zo·i·nat·ed
ben·zol
ben·zole
ben·zo·na·tate
    or ben·zo·no·na·tate
ben·zo·ni·trile

ben·zo·no·na·tine
    or ben·zo·na·tate
ben·zo·phe·none
ben·zo·py·rene
    or benz·py·rene
ben·zo·qui·none
ben·zo·qui·no·ni·um
ben·zo·sul·fi·mide
ben·zo·yl
ben·zo·yl·ec·go·nine
ben·zo·yl·gly·cine
ben·zo·yl·guai·a·col
ben·zo·yl·meth·yl·ec·go·nine
benz·phet·a·mine
benz·py·rene
    or ben·zo·py·rene
benz·py·rin·i·um
benz·quin·a·mide
benz·thi·a·zide
benz·tro·pine
benz·zyd·a·mine
ben·zyl
ben·zyl·ic
ben·zyl·i·dene
ben·zyl·pen·i·cil·lin
ber·ba·mine
ber·ber·ine
ber·ber·is
ber·dache
ber·ga·mot
ber·gap·ten
    or ber·gap·tene
ber·gap·tene
    or ber·gap·ten
Ber·ga·ra-War·ten·berg sign
Ber·gen·hem op·er·a·tion
Ber·ger op·er·a·tion
Bergh test
Berg·mann cords
Berg·meis·ter pa·pil·la
Ber·go·nine-Tri·bon·deau law
ber·i·ber·i
Ber·ke·feld fil·ter
berke·li·um
Ber·lin blue
ber·lock

ber·loque
Ber·nard syn·drome
Ber·nard-Hor·ner
  syn·drome
Bern·hardt par·es·the·si·a
Bern·hardt-Roth
  syn·drome
Bern·heim syn·drome
Ber·noul·li prin·ci·ple
Bern·reu·ter per·son·al·i·ty
  in·ven·tor·y
Bern·stein theor·y
ber·serk
Ber·ti·el·la
Ber·til·lon sys·tem
ber·til·lon·age
Ber·tin col·umn
be·ryl·li·o·sis
  pl be·ryl·li·o·ses
  or ber·yl·lo·sis
  pl ber·yl·lo·ses
be·ryl·li·um
ber·yl·lo·sis
  pl ber·yl·lo·ses
  or ber·yl·li·o·sis
  pl ber·yl·li·o·ses
bes·i·clom·e·ter
Bes·nier-Boeck dis·ease
Bes·nier-Boeck-
  Schau·mann dis·ease
Best dis·ease
bes·ti·al·i·ty
  pl bes·ti·al·i·ties
be·syl·ate
be·ta
be·ta-ad·re·ner·gic
beta·cism
be·ta-D-al·lo·py·ra·nose
be·ta·eu·caine
be·ta·glob·u·lin
be·ta-he·mo·lyt·ic
be·ta·his·tine
be·ta-hy·poph·a·mine
be·ta·ine
be·ta·ke·to·hy·drox·y·bu·
  tyr·ic
be·ta·meth·a·sone
be·ta·naph·thol
be·ta·naph·thyl

be·ta·ox·i·da·tion
be·ta·pro·pi·o·lac·tone
be·ta-re·cep·tor
be·ta·to·pic
be·ta·tron
be·ta·zole
be·tel
be·thane·chol
be·than·i·dine
Bet·ten·dorff test
Bet·u·la
bet·u·lin
bet·u·lin·ol
be·tween·brain
Betz cell
Bev·an op·er·a·tion
bev·a·tron
bev·el
be·zoar
Be·zold re·flex
Be·zold-Brü·cke ef·fect
Be·zold-Jar·isch re·flex
bhang
  or bang
Bi·al test
bi·al·am·i·col
Bi·an·chi syn·drome
bi·ar·tic·u·lar
bi·a·stig·ma·tism
bi·au·ric·u·lar
bi·ax·i·al
bi·bal·lism
bib·li·o·clast
bib·li·o·klept
bib·li·o·klep·to·ma·ni·a
bib·li·o·ma·ni·a
bib·li·o·ther·a·peu·tic
bib·li·o·ther·a·pist
bib·li·o·ther·a·py
  pl bib·li·o·ther·a·pies
bib·o
bi·bo·rate
bib·u·lous
bi·cam·er·al
bi·cap·i·tate
bi·cap·su·lar
bi·car·bon·ate
bi·car·di·o·gram
bi·cau·dal

bi·cau·date
bi·cel·lu·lar
be·ceph·a·lous
bi·ceph·a·lus
bi·ceps
  pl bi·ceps·es
bi·chlo·ride
bi·chrom·ate
bi·cil·i·ate
bi·cip·i·tal
bi·con·cave
bi·con·vex
bi·cor·nate
bi·cor·nu·ate
bi·cor·nu·ous
bi·co·ro·ni·al
bi·cor·po·rate
bi·cou·de
bi·cus·pid
bi·dac·ty·ly
Bid·der gan·gli·on
Bid·der or·gan
bi·der·mo·ma
  pl bi·der·mo·mas
  or bi·der·mo·ma·ta
bi·det
bid·u·ous
Bie·brich scar·let
Bie·dl-Bar·det syn·drome
bi·e·lec·trol·y·sis
  pl bi·e·lec·trol·y·ses
Biel·schow·sky dis·ease
Biel·schow·sky-Jan·sky
  dis·ease
Bier method
Bier·mer a·ne·mia,
  dis·ease
Bier·nack·i sign
Bi·ett dis·ease
bi·fid
bi·fla·gel·late
bi·fo·cal
bi·fo·rate
bi·fron·tal
bi·fur·cate
bi·fur·ca·ti·o
  pl bi·fur·ca·ti·o·nes
bi·fur·ca·tion
big toe

Big·e·low method
bi·gem·i·nal
bi·gem·i·ny
 pl bi·gem·i·nies
big·head
bi·go·ni·al
bi·is·chi·al
Bik·e·le sign
bi·labe
bi·lam·i·nar
bi·lat·er·al
bi·lat·er·al·ism
bi·lay·er
bile
Bil·har·zi·a
bil·har·zi·a·sis
 pl bil·har·zi·a·ses
 or bil·har·zi·o·sis
 pl bil·har·zi·o·ses
bil·har·zi·o·sis
 pl bil·har·zi·o·ses
 or bil·har·zi·a·sis
 pl bil·har·zi·a·ses
bil·i·a·ry
bil·i·cy·a·nin
bil·i·fi·ca·tion
bil·i·fla·vin
bil·i·fus·cin
bil·i·gen·e·sis
bi·lig·u·late
bi·lig·u·la·tus
bil·i·hu·min
bil·i·leu·kan
bi·lin
bil·i·neu·rine
bil·ious
bil·ious·ness
bil·i·pra·sin
bil·i·pur·pu·rin
bil·i·ra·chi·a
bil·i·ru·bin
bil·i·rub·i·nae·mi·a
 var of bil·i·rub·i·ne·mi·a
bil·i·ru·bin·ate
bil·i·ru·bi·ne·mi·a
bil·i·ru·bin·glo·bin
bil·i·ru·bi·nu·ri·a
bil·i·u·ri·a
bil·i·ver·din

Bill·roth op·er·a·tion
bi·lo·bate
bi·lobed
bi·lob·u·lar
bi·loc·u·lar
bi·loc·u·late
bi·loph·o·dont
bi·man·u·al
bi·mas·toid
bi·mo·dal
bi·mo·lec·u·lar
bin·an·gle
bi·na·ry
 pl bi·na·ries
bi·na·sal
bi·nau·ral
bin·au·ric·u·lar
bind
bind·er
Bi·net age
Bi·net-Si·mon test
Bing sign
Bing-Neel syn·drome
bin·io·dide
bi·noc·u·lar
bi·no·mi·al
bi·not·ic
bin·ov·u·lar
bin·ox·ide
Bins·wang·er dis·ease
bi·nu·cle·ar
bi·nu·cle·ate
bi·nu·cle·a·tion
bi·nu·cle·o·late
bi·o·a·cou·stics
bi·o·ac·tiv·i·ty
 pl bi·o·ac·tiv·i·ties
bi·o·as·say
bi·o·as·tro·nau·ti·cal
bi·o·as·tro·nau·tics
bi·o·au·to·graph
bi·o·au·to·graph·ic
bi·o·au·tog·ra·phy
 pl bi·o·au·tog·ra·phies
bi·o·a·vail·a·bil·i·ty
bi·ob·jec·tive
bi·o·cat·a·lyst
bi·oc·cip·i·tal

bi·o·ce·no·sis
 pl bi·o·ce·no·ses
bi·o·chem·i·cal
bi·o·chem·is·try
 pl bi·o·chem·is·tries
bi·o·chem·or·phic
bi·o·che·mor·phol·o·gy
 pl bi·o·che·mor·phol·o·gies
bi·o·chrome
bi·o·ci·dal
bi·o·cide
bi·o·clean
bi·o·cli·mat·ics
bi·o·cli·ma·tol·o·gy
 pl bi·o·cli·ma·tol·o·gies
bi·o·coe·no·sis
 var of bi·o·ce·no·sis
 pl bi·o·coe·no·ses
bi·o·col·loid
bi·o·cy·ber·net·ics
bi·o·cy·tin
bi·o·de·grad·a·bil·i·ty
 pl bi·o·de·grad·a·bil·i·ties
bi·o·de·grad·a·ble
bi·o·deg·ra·da·tion
bi·o·de·grade
bi·o·de·tri·tus
bi·o·dy·nam·ic
bi·o·dy·nam·ics
bi·o·e·col·o·gy
 pl bi·o·e·col·o·gies
bi·o·e·lec·tric
 or bi·o·e·lec·tri·cal
bi·o·e·lec·tri·cal
 or bi·o·e·lec·tric
bi·o·e·lec·tric·i·ty
 pl bi·o·e·lec·tric·i·ties
bi·o·e·lec·tro·gen·e·sis
 pl bi·o·e·lec·tro·gen·e·ses
bi·o·e·lec·tron·ics
bi·o·en·er·get·ics
bi·o·en·gi·neer·ing
bi·o·en·vi·ron·men·tal
bi·o·feed·back
bi·o·fla·vo·noid
bi·o·gen
bi·o·gen·e·sis
 pl bi·o·gen·e·ses
bi·o·ge·net·ic

bio·gen·ic
bi·og·e·nous
bi·og·e·ny
bi·o·ge·o·chem·is·try
   pl bi·o·ge·o·chem·is·tries
bi·o·ge·og·ra·phy
bi·o·haz·ard
bi·o·in·stru·men·ta·tion
bi·o·ki·net·ics
bi·o·log·ic
   or bi·o·log·i·cal
bi·o·log·i·cal
   or bi·o·log·ic
bi·ol·o·gist
bi·ol·o·gy
   pl bi·ol·o·gies
bi·o·lu·mi·nes·cence
bi·ol·y·sis
   pl bi·ol·y·ses
bi·o·lyt·ic
bi·o·mass
bi·o·ma·te·ri·al
bi·o·math·e·mat·ics
bi·ome
bi·o·me·chan·ics
bi·o·med·i·cal
bi·o·med·i·cine
bi·o·me·te·or·ol·o·gy
bi·om·e·ter
bi·o·me·tri·cian
bi·o·met·rics
bi·om·e·try
bi·o·mi·cro·scope
bi·o·mi·cro·scop·ic
bi·o·mi·cros·co·py
   pl bi·o·mi·cros·co·pies
bi·on
bi·o·ne·cro·sis
bi·on·er·gy
bi·on·ics
bi·o·nom·ics
bi·on·o·my
   pl bi·on·o·mies
bi·o·nu·cle·on·ics
bi·o·or·gan·ic
bi·oph·a·gous
bi·oph·a·gy
   pl bi·oph·a·gies
bi·o·phore

bi·o·pho·tom·e·ter
bi·o·phys·ics
bi·o·phys·i·og·ra·phy
   pl bi·o·phys·i·og·ra·phies
bi·o·phys·i·ol·o·gy
bi·op·la·sis
bi·o·plasm
bi·o·plas·mic
bi·o·plas·tic
bi·o·pol·y·mer
bi·op·sy
   pl bi·op·sies
bi·o·psy·chic
bi·o·psy·cho·log·i·cal
bi·o·psy·chol·o·gy
   pl bi·o·psy·chol·o·gies
bi·op·ter·in
bi·or·bit·al
bi·o·re·search
bi·o·rhythm
bi·o·rhyth·mic
bi·o·rhyth·mic·i·ty
   pl bi·o·rhyth·mic·i·ties
bi·os
   pl bi·os·es
   or bi·oi
bi·o·sat·el·lite
bi·o·sci·ence
bi·o·sci·en·tist
bi·ose
bi·o·sen·sor
bi·o·set
bi·o·spec·trom·e·try
bi·o·spec·tros·co·py
bi·o·sphere
bi·o·sta·tis·tics
bi·os·ter·ol
bi·o·syn·the·sis
   pl bi·o·syn·the·sis
bi·o·syn·thet·ic
Bi·ot breath·ing
bi·o·ta
bi·o·tax·is
bi·o·tax·y
bi·o·tech·no·log·i·cal
bi·o·tech·nol·o·gy
   pl bi·o·tech·nol·o·gies
bi·o·tel·e·met·ric

bi·o·te·lem·e·try
   pl bio·te·lem·e·tries
bi·ot·ic
bi·o·tin
bi·ot·o·my
bi·o·tox·i·ca·tion
bi·o·tox·i·col·o·gy
bi·o·tox·in
bi·o·trans·for·ma·tion
bi·o·tron
bi·o·type
bi·o·typ·ic
bi·o·ty·pol·o·gy
bi·o·vu·lar
bip·a·ra
   pl bip·a·ras
   or bip·a·rae
bi·pa·ren·tal
bi·pa·ri·e·tal
bip·a·rous
bi·par·tite
bi·ped
bi·ped·al
bi·ped·i·cled
bi·pen·nate
bi·pen·ni·form
bi·per·i·den
bi·phe·nyl
bi·phos·phate
bi·po·lar
bi·po·lar·i·ty
bi·po·ten·ti·al·i·ty
   pl bi·po·ten·ti·al·i·ties
bipp
bi·ra·mose
   or bi·ra·mous
bi·ra·mous
   or bi·ra·mose
birch
Bird dis·ease
bi·re·frac·tive
bi·re·frin·gence
bi·re·frin·gent
bi·ri·mose
bi·ro·ta·tion
birth
birth con·trol
birth·mark
birth pang

bis·a·bol
bis·a·co·dyl
bis·a·cro·mi·al
bis·al·bu·mi·ne·mi·a
Bisch·off test
bis·cuit
bi·sect
bi·sec·tion
bi·sex·ous
bi·sex·u·al
bi·sex·u·al·i·ty
bis·fer·i·ens
bis·fer·i·ous
bish·op
bis·hy·drox·y·cou·ma·rin
bis·il·i·ac
bis in di·e
Bis·kra but·ton
bis·muth
bis·mu·thi·a
bis·muth·o·sis
bis·muth·o·tar·trate
bis·muth·yl
bis·o·brin
bis·ox·a·tin
bi·spi·nous
bis·sa
bis·si·no·sis
    or bys·si·no·sis
bi·ste·phan·ic
bis·tou·ry
    pl bis·tou·ries
bi·stra·tal
bis·tri·min
bi·sul·fate
bi·sul·fide
bi·sul·fite
bi·tar·trate
bite
bi·tem·po·ral
bite·wing
bi·thi·o·nol
Bi·thyn·i·a
Bi·tis
Bi·tot spots
bi·tro·chan·ter·ic
bit·ter·ling
bit·ters
Bitt·ner milk fac·tor

bi·tu·ber·al
bi·tu·men
bi·tu·mi·no·sis
bi·u·rate
bi·u·ret
bi·va·lence
bi·va·len·cy
    pl bi·va·len·cies
bi·va·lent
bi·valve
bi·val·vu·lar
bi·ven·ter
bi·ven·tral
bi·ven·tric·u·lar
bix·in
bi·zy·go·mat·ic
Biz·zo·ze·ro
Bjer·rum
black eye
black lung
Black test
black vom·it
black-and-blue
black·head
black·leg
black·out
black·wa·ter
blad·der
blade
blain
Bla·lock-Taus·sig
    op·er·a·tion
blanch
bland
Blan·din glands
Bland-White-Gar·land
    syn·drome
Blan·for·di·a
blast
blas·te·ma
    pl blas·te·mas
    or blas·te·ma·ta
blas·tem·ic
blas·tic
blas·tin
blas·to·chyle
blas·to·coel
    or blas·to·coele

blas·to·coele
    or blas·to·coel
blas·to·coe·lic
blas·to·cyst
Blas·to·cys·tis hom·i·nis
blas·to·cyte
blas·to·cy·to·ma
blas·to·derm
blas·to·der·mal
blas·to·der·mic
blas·to·disc
    or blas·to·disk
blas·to·disk
    or blas·to·disc
blas·to·gen·e·sis
    pl blas·to·gen·e·ses
blas·to·ge·net·ic
blas·to·gen·ic
blas·tog·e·ny
blas·to·ki·ne·sis
    pl blas·to·ki·ne·ses
blas·to·ki·nin
blas·tol·y·sis
    pl blas·tol·y·ses
blas·to·ma
    pl blas·to·mas
    or blas·to·ma·ta
blas·tom·a·to·gen·ic
blas·tom·a·to·sis
blas·tom·a·tous
blas·to·mere
Blas·to·my·ces
Blas·to·my·ce·tes
blas·to·my·ce·tic
blas·to·my·cin
blas·to·my·co·sis
    pl blas·to·my·co·ses
blas·to·neu·ro·pore
blas·toph·tho·ri·a
    pl blas·toph·tho·ri·as
    or blas·toph·tho·ry
    pl blas·toph·tho·ries
blas·toph·thor·ic
blas·toph·tho·ry
    pl blas·toph·tho·ries
    or blas·toph·tho·ri·a
    pl blas·toph·tho·ri·as

blas·to·por·al
  or blas·to·por·ic
blas·to·pore
blas·to·po·ric
  or blas·to·por·al
blas·to·sphere
blas·to·spher·ic
blas·to·spore
blas·to·spo·ric
blas·tot·o·my
  pl blas·tot·o·mies
blas·tu·la
  pl blas·tu·las
  or blas·tu·lae
blas·tu·lar
blas·tu·la·tion
Blat·ta
Blat·tel·la
Blaud pill
blear-eyed
blear·y
bleb
bleed
bleed·er
blem·ish
blem·ma·trope
blend·ing
blenn·ad·e·ni·tis
blenn·o·gen·ic
blenn·oid
blen·noph·thal·mi·a
blen·nor·rha·gi·a
blen·nor·rhe·a
blen·nor·rhe·al
blen·nor·rhoe·a
  var of blen·nor·rhe·a
blen·nor·rhoe·al
  var of blen·nor·rhe·al
blen·nos·ta·sis
blenn·o·tho·rax
blenn·u·ri·a
bleph·ar·ad·e·ni·tis
bleph·a·ral
bleph·a·rec·to·my
bleph·ar·e·de·ma
bleph·a·re·lo·sis
  pl bleph·a·re·lo·ses
bleph·a·rism

bleph·a·ri·tis
  pl bleph·a·rit·i·des
bleph·a·ro·ad·e·ni·tis
bleph·a·ro·ad·e·no·ma
  pl bleph·a·ro·ad·e·no·mas
  or bleph·a·ro·ad·e·no·ma·ta
bleph·a·ro·ath·er·o·ma
  pl bleph·a·ro·ath·er·o·mas
  or bleph·a·ro·ath·er·o·ma·ta
bleph·a·ro·blen·nor·rhe·a
bleph·a·ro·blen·nor·rhoe·a
  var of
    bleph·a·ro·blen·nor·rhe·a
bleph·a·ro·chal·a·sis
bleph·a·ro·chrom·hi·dro·
  sis
bleph·a·ro·clei·sis
bleph·a·roc·lo·nus
bleph·a·ro·con·junc·ti·vi·tis
bleph·a·ro·di·as·ta·sis
bleph·a·ro·dys·chroi·a
bleph·ar·oe·de·ma
  var of bleph·ar·e·de·ma
bleph·a·ro·me·las·ma
bleph·a·ron
  pl bleph·a·ra
bleph·a·ron·cus
  pl bleph·a·ron·ci
bleph·a·ro·pa·chyn·sis
bleph·a·ro·phi·mo·sis
bleph·a·roph·ry·plas·tic
bleph·a·roph·ry·plas·ty
bleph·a·ro·phy·ma
  pl bleph·a·ro·phy·mas
  or bleph·a·ro·phy·ma·ta
bleph·a·ro·plast
bleph·a·ro·plas·tic
bleph·a·ro·plas·ty
bleph·a·ro·ple·gi·a
bleph·a·rop·to·sis
bleph·a·ro·py·or·rhoe·a
  var of bleph·a·ro·py·o·rhe·a
bleph·a·ror·rha·phy
bleph·a·ro·spasm
bleph·a·ro·sphinc·ter·ec·to·
  my
bleph·a·ro·stat
bleph·a·ro·ste·no·sis

bleph·a·ro·sym·phy·sis
  pl bleph·a·ro·sym·phy·ses
bleph·a·ro·sy·nech·i·a
  pl bleph·a·ro·sy·nech·i·ae
Bles·sig-I·van·ov cys·toid
  de·gen·er·a·tion
blind
blind gut
blind spot
blind·ness
blink
blis·ter
bloat
Bloch method
Bloch-Sulz·ber·ger
  syn·drome
block
block·ade
block·er
Blocq dis·ease
Blond·lot rays
blood
blood bank
blood cell
blood count
blood fluke
blood group
blood heat
blood plate·let
blood poi·son·ing
blood pres·sure
blood se·rum
blood sug·ar
blood test
Blood·good oper·a·tion
blood·less
blood·let·ting
blood·line
blood·mo·bile
blood·root
blood·shot
blood·stream
blood·suck·er
blood type
blood·worm
Bloom syn·drome
blotch
Blount-Bar·ber syn·drome

41

blow·fly
  pl blow·flies
blow·pipe
blue baby
blue mold
blue·tongue
Blum·berg sign
Blu·me·nau nu·cle·us
Blu·mer shelf
Blyth test
Bo·a·ri op·er·a·tion
Bo·as test
Bo·as-Op·pler ba·cil·lus
Bob·ruff op·er·a·tion
Boch·da·lek for·a·men
Bock·hart im·pe·ti·go
Bo·dan·sky unit
Bo·di·an stain·ing meth·od
Bod·i·ly
Bo·do
·body
bod·y louse
bod·y wall
Boeck sar·coid, dis·ease
Boer·haa·ve syn·drome
Boer·ner-Lu·kens test
Boet·ti·ger meth·od
Bo·gros space
Böh·ler splint
Böh·mer he·ma·tox·y·lin
Bohr the·o·ry
boil
Boi·vin an·ti·gen
bo·las·ter·one
bol·de·none
bol·dine
bole
Bo·len test
bol·e·nol
Bo·ley gauge
Bolles splint
Bol·lin·ger bod·y
bol·man·ta·late
bo·lom·e·ter
bo·lo·scope
Bol·ton point
Bolt·worth skate
bo·lus
  pl bo·lus·es

Bom·bay blood
bond
bon·duc
Bon·dy op·er·a·tion
bone
bone·let
bone·set·ter
Bon·jean er·got·in
Bonne·vie-Ull·rich
  syn·drome
Bon·nier syn·drome
Bon·will tri·an·gle
bon·y
Bo·oph·i·lus
boost·er
bo·rac·ic
bo·rate
bo·rax
bor·bo·ryg·mat·ic
  or bor·bo·ryg·mic
bor·bo·ryg·mic
  or bor·bo·ryg·mat·ic
bor·bo·ryg·mus
  pl bor·bo·ryg·mi
bor·bo·ryg·my
  pl bor·bo·ryg·mies
Bor·deaux mix·ture
bor·der
bor·der·line
Bor·det·test
Bor·de·tel·la
Bor·det-Gen·gou
  ba·cil·lus, test
Bord·ley-Rich·ards
  meth·od
bo·ric
bo·rism
bor·nane
bor·ne·ol
Born·holm dis·ease
bor·nyl
bo·ro·cit·ric
bo·ro·glyc·er·ide
bo·ro·glyc·er·in
bo·ron
bo·ro·sal·i·cyl·ic
Bor·rel bod·y
Bor·rel·i·a
bor·rel·i·din

boss
bos·se·lat·ed
bos·se·la·tion
boss·ing
Bos·ton sign
bot
Bo·tal·lo duct
bo·tan·ic
  or bo·tan·i·cal
bo·tan·i·cal
  or bo·tan·ic
bot·a·nist
bot·a·ny
botch
bot·fly
  pl bot·flies
bo·thrid·i·um
  pl bo·thrid·i·ums
  or bo·thrid·i·a
Both·ri·o·ceph·a·lus
both·ri·oid
both·ri·on
both·ri·um
  pl both·ri·ums
  or both·ri·i
bo·throp·ic
Bo·throps
bo·tog·e·nin
bot·ry·oid
bot·ry·o·my·co·sis
  pl bot·ry·o·my·co·ses
bot·ry·o·my·cot·ic
Bo·try·tis
bots
Bött·cher cells
bot·tle
bot·u·li·form
bot·u·lin
bot·u·li·nal
bot·u·li·num
  or bot·u·li·nus
bot·u·li·nus
  or bot·u·li·num
bot·u·lism
bou·ba
Bou·chard nodes
Bou·gain·ville
  rheu·ma·tism
bou·gie

42

bou·gie·nage
 or bou·gi·nage
bou·gi·nage
 or bou·gie·nage
Bouil·laud dis·ease
bouil·lon
Bouin flu·id, so·lu·tion
Bou·len·ge·ri·na
bou·lim·i·a
 var of bu·lim·i·a
Boul·ton so·lu·tion
bound
bound·a·ry
bou·quet
bour·donne·ment
Bourne meth·od
Bourne·ville dis·ease
Bour·quin-Sher·man u·nit
bou·stro·phe·don·ic
bou·ton ter·mi·nal
 pl bou·tons ter·mi·nal
bou·ton·neuse fe·ver
bou·ton·niere
Bou·ve·ret syn·drome
Bo·ve·ri test
Bo·vic·o·la
bo·vine
Bow·ditch law
bow·el
Bow·en dis·ease
bow·ing re·flex
bow·leg
Bow·man cap·sule
Bow·man glands
Bow·man mem·brane
box·i·dine
Boy·den sphinc·ter
Boyle law
Boz·zo·lo dis·ease
brace
brace·let
bra·chi·al
bra·chi·al·gi·a
bra·chi·a·lis
bra·chi·ate
bra·chi·a·tion
bra·chi·form
bra·chi·o·ce·phal·ic
ba·chi·o·cru·ral

bra·chi·o·cu·bi·tal
bra·chi·o·cyl·lo·sis
 pl bra·chi·o·cyl·lo·ses
bra·chi·o·cyr·to·sis
bra·chi·o·ra·di·a·lis
bra·chi·ot·o·my
bra·chi·um
 pl bra·chi·a
Brach·mann-de Lange
 syn·drome
Bracht-Wäch·ter bod·ies
brach·y·ba·si·a
brach·y·car·di·a
brach·y·ce·pha·li·a
brach·y·ce·phal·ic
brach·y·ceph·a·lism
brach·y·ceph·a·lous
brach·y·ceph·a·ly
 pl brach·y·ceph·a·lies
brach·y·chei·li·a
 or brach·y·chi·li·a
brach·y·chei·rous
 or brach·y·chi·rous
brach·y·chi·li·a
 or brach·y·chei·li·a
bra·chych·i·ly
brach·y·chi·rous
 or brach·y·chei·rous
brach·y·cra·ni·al
brach·y·dac·tyl·i·a
 pl brach·y·dac·tyl·i·as
 or brach·y·dac·ty·ly
 pl brach·y·dac·ty·lies
brach·y·dac·tyl·ic
brachy·dac·ty·lous
brach·y·dac·ty·ly
 pl brach·y·dac·ty·lies
 or brach·y·dac·tyl·i·a
 pl brach·y·dac·tyl·i·as
brach·y·dont
 or brach·y·o·dont
brach·y·fa·cial
brach·y·glos·sal
brach·y·glos·si·a
brach·y·gna·thi·a
brach·y·gnath·ous
brach·y·ker·kic
brach·y·mei·o·sis
 pl brach·y·mei·o·ses

brach·y·met·a·car·pi·a
brach·y·met·a·po·dy
brach·y·met·a·tar·si·a
brach·y·me·trop·i·a
brach·y·mor·phic
brach·y·mor·phy
brach·y·o·dont
 or brach·y·dont
brach·y·pel·lic
brach·y·pel·vic
brach·y·pha·lan·gi·a
brach·y·pha·lan·gous
brach·y·pha·lan·gy
brach·y·po·dous
brach·y·pro·sop·ic
brach·y·rhin·i·a
brach·y·rhyn·chus
brach·y·skel·ic
brach·y·sta·sis
brach·y·stat·ic
brach·y·ther·a·py
brach·y·u·ran·ic
brack·et
Brack·ett op·er·a·tion
Brad·ford frame
brad·sot
brad·y·a·cu·si·a
brad·y·ar·rhyth·mi·a
brad·y·ar·thri·a
brad·y·aux·e·sis
brad·y·car·di·a
brad·y·ci·ne·si·a
brad·y·ci·ne·sis
brad·y·crot·ic
brad·y·di·as·to·le
brad·y·di·as·to·li·a
brad·y·e·coi·a
brad·y·es·the·si·a
brad·y·gen·e·sis
brad·y·glos·si·a
brad·y·ki·ne·si·a
brad·y·ki·ne·sis
brad·y·ki·net·ic
brad·y·ki·nin
brady·ki·nin·o·gen
brad·y·la·li·a
brad·y·lex·i·a
brad·y·lo·gi·a
brad·y·pha·gi·a

43

brad·y·pha·si·a
brad·y·phe·mi·a
brad·y·phra·si·a
brad·y·phre·ni·a
brad·y·pne·a
brad·y·pra·gi·a
brad·y·prax·i·a
brad·y·rhyth·mi·a
brad·y·sper·ma·tism
brad·y·sper·mi·a
brad·y·sphyg·mi·a
brad·y·stal·sis
brad·y·tach·y·car·di·a
brad·y·tel·e·o·ki·ne·si·a
brad·y·tel·e·o·ki·ne·sis
brad·y·to·ci·a
brad·y·u·ri·a
Brag·ard sign
braille
Brails·ford-Mor·qui·o
  syn·drome
brain stem
brain·case
brain·ed·ness
brain-pan
brain·sick
brain·wash
bran·cher en·zyme
bran·chi·a
  pl bran·chi·ae
bran·chi·al
bran·chi·o·gen·ic
bran·chi·og·e·nous
bran·chi·o·ma
  pl bran·chi·o·mas
  or bran·chi·o·ma·ta
bran·chi·o·mere
bran·chi·om·er·ism
bran·chi·o·mo·tor
Brandt syn·drome
Bran·ham sign
bran·ny
brash
Bras·si·ca
Brat·ton and Mar·shall
  meth·od
Brauer op·er·a·tion
Braun test

Brau·ne ring
brawn·y
Brax·ton Hicks sign
brax·y
  pl brax·ies
bra·ye·ra
bra·zal·um
braze
braz·i·lin
break
  broke
  bro·ken
  break·ing
break·bone fe·ver
break·down
break·through
breast
breast·bone
breast-fed
breath
breathe
Bre·da dis·ease
breech
breed
  bred
  breed·ing
breed·er
breg·ma
  pl breg·ma·ta
breg·mat·ic
breg·ma·to·dym·i·a
breg·ma·to·lam·doid
Breh and Gae·bler
  meth·od
brei
  pl breis
Brem·er test
bren·ner·o·ma
  pl bren·ner·o·mas
  or bren·ner·o·ma·ta
Bren·ner tumor
breph·o·plas·tic
bre·tyl·i·um tos·y·late
Breu·er re·flex
Breus mole
Breutsch dis·ease
brev·i·col·lis
brev·i·lin·e·al

brev·i·ra·di·ate
Brew·er
bridge
bridge·work
bri·dle
Briggs law
Brights dis·ease
Brill dis·ease
Brill-Sym·mers dis·ease
Brill-Zins·ser dis·ease
brim·stone
brin·ase
brine
Bri·nell hard·ness
Bri·nell num·ber
Brin·ton dis·ease
Bri·quet syn·drome
brise·ment
bris·ket
Bris·saud dis·ease
Bris·saud-Ma·rie
  syn·drome
bris·tle
Brit·ish an·ti·lew·is·ite
broach
Broad·bent law
braod-spec·trum
Bro·ca a·pha·si·a
Bro·ca ar·e·a
Bro·ca con·vo·lu·tion
Bro·ca point
Brock syn·drome
Brocq dis·ease
bro·cre·sine
Bro·der clas·si·fi·ca·tion
Bro·die tu·mor
Brod·mann ar·e·a
broke
bro·ken
brom·ac·e·tone
  or bro·mo·ac·e·tone
bro·mate
bro·ma·to·ther·a·py
bro·ma·to·tox·in
bro·ma·tox·ism
bro·maz·e·pam
bro·ma·zine
brom·chlor·e·none

44

brom·cre·sol
  or bro·mo·cre·sol
bro·me·lain
bro·me·lin
brom·eth·ol
brom·hex·ine
brom·hi·dro·si·pho·bi·a
brom·hi·dro·sis
  pl brom·hi·dro·ses
  or bro·mi·dro·sis
  pl bro·mi·dro·ses
bro·mic
bro·mide
bro·mi·dro·sis
  pl bro·mi·dro·ses
  or brom·hi·dro·sis
  pl brom·hi·dro·ses
bro·min·ate
bro·mi·nat·ed
brom·in·di·one
bro·mine
bro·min·ism
bro·mism
brom·i·so·val·um
bro·mo
  pl bro·mos
bro·mo·ac·et·an·i·lid
bro·mo·ac·e·tone
  or brom·ac·e·tone
bro·mo·ben·zyl
bro·mo·cam·phor
bro·mo·chlo·ro·tri·glu·o·ro·eth·ane
bro·mo·cre·sol
  or brom·cre·sol
bro·mo·de·ox·y·u·ri·dine
bro·mo·der·ma
bro·mo·di·phen·hy·dra·mine
bro·mo·form
bro·mo·hy·per·hi·dro·sis
bro·mo·hy·per·i·dro·sis
bro·mo·ma·ni·a
bro·mo·men·or·rhe·a
bro·mo·men·or·rhoe·a
  var of bro·mo·men·or·rhe·a
bro·mo·phe·nol
  or brom·phe·nol

bro·mop·ne·a
bro·mop·noe·a
  var of bro·mop·ne·a
bro·mo·thy·mol
bro·mo·u·ra·cil
brom·phen·ir·a·mine
brom·phe·nol
  or bro·mo·phe·nol
bronch·ad·e·ni·tis
bron·chi·al
bron·chi·al·ly
bron·chi·arc·ti·a
bron·chi·ec·ta·si·a
bron·chi·ec·ta·sis
  pl bron·chi·ec·ta·ses
bron·chi·ec·tat·ic
bron·chil·o·quy
bron·chi·o·cele
bron·chi·o·cri·sis
bron·chi·o·gen·ic
bron·chi·ol·ar
bron·chi·ole
bron·chi·o·lec·ta·sis
  pl bron·chi·o·lec·ta·ses
bron·chi·o·li·tis
bron·chi·o·lus
  pl bron·chi·o·li
bron·chi·o·spasm
bron·chi·o·ste·no·sis
bron·chit·ic
bron·chi·tis
  pl bron·chit·i·des
bron·chi·um
  pl bron·chi·a
bron·cho·bil·i·ar·y
bron·cho·can·di·di·a·sis
  pl bron·cho·can·di·di·a·ses
bron·cho·cav·ern·ous
bron·cho·cele
bron·cho·col·ic
bron·cho·con·stric·tion
bron·cho·con·stric·tor
bron·cho·dil·a·ta·tion
bron·cho·di·la·tor
bron·cho·e·de·ma
  pl bron·cho·e·de·mas
  or bron·cho·e·de·ma·ta
bron·cho·e·goph·o·ny

bron·cho·e·soph·a·ge·al
bron·cho·e·soph·a·gol·o·gy
bron·cho·e·soph·a·gos·co·py
bron·cho·gen·ic
bron·chog·e·nous
bron·cho·gram
bron·cho·graph·ic
bron·chog·ra·phy
  pl bron·chog·ra·phies
bron·cho·lith
bron·cho·li·thi·a·sis
  pl bron·cho·li·thi·a·ses
bron·chol·o·gy
bron·cho·ma·la·ci·a
bron·cho·me·di·as·ti·nal
bron·cho·mon·i·li·a·sis
  pl bron·cho·mon·i·li·a·ses
bron·cho·mo·tor
bron·cho·my·co·sis
  pl bron·cho·my·co·ses
bron·cho·oe·soph·a·ge·al
  var of bron·cho·e·soph·a·ge·al
bron·cho·oe·soph·a·gol·o·gy
  var of bron·cho·e·soph·a·gol·o·gy
bron·cho·oe·soph·a·gos·co·py
  var of bron·cho·e·soph·a·gos·co·py
bron·chop·a·thy
bron·choph·o·ny
  pl bron·choph·o·nies
bron·cho·plas·ty
bron·cho·ple·gi·a
bron·cho·pleu·ral
bron·cho·pneu·mo·ni·a
bron·cho·pneu·mo·ni·tis
bron·cho·pneu·mop·a·thy
bron·cho·pul·mo·nar·y
bron·chor·rha·gi·a
bron·chor·rha·phy
bron·chor·rhe·a
bron·chor·rhe·al
bron·chor·rhoe·a
  var of bron·chor·rhe·a

bron·chor·rhoe·al
var of bron·chor·rhe·al
bron·cho·scope
bron·cho·scopic
bron·chos·co·py
pl bron·chos·co·pies
bron·cho·spasm
bron·cho·spi·ro·chae·to·sis
var of bron·cho·spi·ro·che·to·sis
bron·cho·spi·ro·che·to·sis
bron·cho·spi·rog·ra·phy
bron·cho·spi·rom·e·ter
bron·cho·spi·rom·e·try
pl bron·cho·spi·rom·e·tries
bron·cho·stax·is
bron·cho·ste·no·sis
pl bron·cho·ste·no·ses
bron·chos·to·my
bron·chot·o·my
pl bron·chot·o·mies
bron·cho·tra·che·al
bron·cho·ve·sic·u·lar
bron·chus
pl bron·chi
Brön·sted and Low·ry sub·stance
Brön·sted the·o·ry
bron·to·pho·bi·a
Brooke tu·mor
broom-tops
Bro·phy op·er·a·tion
broth
brow
Brown test
Browne sign
Brown·i·an mo·tion
Brown-Pearce tu·mor
Brown-Sé·quard syn·drome
bru·cel·la
pl bru·cel·las
or bru·cel·lae
Bru·cel·la·ce·ae
bru·cel·lar
bru·cel·ler·gen
or bru·cel·ler·gen
bru·cel·ler·gin
or bru·cel·ler·gen

bru·cel·li·a·sis
pl bru·cel·li·a·ses
bru·cel·lin
bru·cel·lo·sis
pl bru·cel·lo·ses
Bruch mem·brane
bru·cine
Bruck dis·ease
Brü·cke line
Brud·zin·ski signs
Brug·i·a
Brugsch syn·drome
bruis·a·bil·i·ty
bruise
bruit
Brun sign
Brun·hil·de vi·rus
Brunn mem·brane
Brun·ner gland
Bruns law
Brun·schwig op·er·a·tion
Brun·ton rule
brush bor·der
Brush·field spots
brush·ite
Brushy Creek fe·ver
Bru·ton a·gam·ma·glob·u·li·ne·mi·a
bru·xism
brux·o·ma·ni·a
Bry·ant line
bryg·mus
bry·o·ni·a
bry·on·i·din
bry·o·nin
bry·o·phyte
bry·o·phyt·ic
bu·ak·i
bu·ba
bu·bo
pl bu·boes
bu·bon·ad·e·ni·tis
bu·bon·al·gi·a
bu·bon·ic
bu·bon·o·cele
bu·bon·u·lus
pl bu·bon·u·lus·es
or bu·bon·u·li
bu·car·di·a

buc·ca
pl buc·cae
buc·cal
buc·ci·na·tor
buc·co·ax·i·al
buc·co·cer·vi·cal
buc·co·clu·sal
buc·co·clu·sion
buc·co·dis·tal
buc·co·fa·cial
buc·co·gin·gi·val
buc·co·la·bi·al
buc·co·lin·gual
buc·co·me·si·al
buc·co·na·sal
buc·co·pha·ryn·ge·al
buc·co·pha·ryn·ge·us
buc·co·pul·pal
buc·co·ver·sion
buc·cu·la
pl buc·cu·lae
bu·chu
Buck op·er·a·tion
buck·bean
buck·thorn
buck·tooth
pl buck·teeth
buck·toothed
Buck·y di·a·phragm
bu·cli·zine
buc·ne·mi·a
bud
Budd dis·ease
Budd-Chi·a·ri syn·drome
Bü·din·ger-Lud·loff-Lä·wen dis·ease
Bueng·ner bands
Buer·ger dis·ease
Buer·ger dis·ease
Buer·gi hy·poph·e·sis
bu·fa·gin
bu·fa·lin
buff·er
buff·y coat
Bu·fo
bu·fo·gen·in
Bu·fon·i·dae
bu·for·min
bu·fo·tal·in

bu·fo·ten·i·dine
bu·fo·ten·in
 or bu·fo·ten·ine
bu·fo·ten·ine
 or bu·fo·ten·in
bu·fo·tox·in
bug
bug·ger·y
 pl bug·ger·ies
Bu·ie op·er·a·tion
Buist meth·od
bulb
bul·bar
bul·bi·form
bul·bi·tis
bul·bo·a·tri·al
bul·bo·cap·nine
bul·bo·cav·er·no·sus
 pl bul·bo·cav·er·no·si
bul·bo·mem·bra·nous
bul·bo·nu·cle·ar
bul·bo·spi·nal
bul·bo·spon·gi·o·sus
 pl bul·bo·spon·gi·o·si
bul·bo·u·re·thral
bul·bous
bul·bo·ven·tric·u·lar
bul·bus
 pl bul·bi
bu·le·sis
bu·lim·i·a
bu·lim·ic
Bu·li·nus
bul·la
 pl bul·lae
bul·late
 or bul·lat·ed
bul·lat·ed
 or bul·late
bul·la·tion
bul·lec·to·my
Bul·lis fe·ver
bull neck
bull·necked
bull·nose
bull·ock
bul·lose
 or bul·lous
bul·lo·sis

bul·lous
 or bul·lose
Bum·ke pu·pil
bu·nam·i·dine
bun·dle
Bun·ga·rus
bung·eye
bun·ion
bun·ion·ec·to·my
bun·ion·ette
Bun·nell test
bu·no·dont
Bu·nos·to·mum
Bun·sen burn·er
Bun·sen-Ros·coe law
Bun·yam·ve·ra vi·rus
buph·thal·mi·a
buph·thal·mos
 or buph·thal·mos
buph·thal·mus
 or buph·thal·mus
bu·piv·a·caine
bur
 or burr
bu·ra·mate
bur·bot
Bur·chard test
Bur·dach nu·cle·us
bur·dock
Burd·wan fe·ver
bu·ret
 or bu·rette
bu·rette
 or bu·ret
bu·rim·a·mide
Bur·kitt lym·pho·ma, tu·mor
burr
 or bur
burn
Bur·nett syn·drome
bur·nish·er
burn-out
Bu·row so·lu·tion
bur·sa
 pl bur·sas
 or bur·sae
bur·sal

bur·sec·to·my
 pl bur·sec·to·mies
Bur·ser·a·ce·ae
bur·si·tis
bur·so·lith
bur·sop·a·thy
bur·sot·o·my
bur·su·la
 pl bur·su·lae
Bur·y dis·ease
Busch·ke dis·ease
Bus·quet dis·ease
Bus·se-Busch·ke dis·ease
bu·sul·fan
bu·ta·bar·bi·tal
bu·ta·caine
bu·tac·e·tin
bu·ta·di·ene
bu·tal·bi·tal
bu·tal·ly·o·nal
bu·tam·ben
bu·tane
bu·ta·no·ic
bu·ta·nol
bu·ta·per·a·zine
bu·tene
bu·te·nyl
bu·te·thal
bu·teth·a·mine
bu·thi·a·zide
Bu·thus
But·ler and Tut·hill meth·od
But·ler so·lu·tion
bu·to·py·ro·nox·yl
bu·tox·a·mine
bu·trip·ty·line
butt
but·ter
but·ter·fat
but·ter·fly
 pl but·ter·flies
but·ter·milk
but·ter·nut
but·tock
but·ton
but·ton·hole
but·tress
bu·tyl

bu·tyl·a·mine
bu·tyl·ate
bu·tyl·ene
bu·tyl·i·dene
bu·tyl·par·a·ben
bu·ty·ra·ceous
bu·ty·rate
bu·tyr·ic
bu·ty·rin

bu·ty·rin·ase
bu·ty·roid
bu·ty·rom·e·ter
bu·ty·ro·phe·none
bu·ty·rous
bu·tyr·yl
bux·ine
Buz·zard re·flex
Bwam·ba

By·ler dis·ease
by·pass
bys·si·no·sis
    pl bys·si·no·ses
    or bis·si·no·sis
bys·soid
bys·so·phthi·sis
By·wa·ters syn·drome

C

ca·a·pi
Cab·ot ring
cac·aes·the·si·a
    var of cac·es·the·si·a
cac·aes·the·sic
    var of cac·es·the·sic
cac·an·thrax
cac·er·ga·si·a
cac·es·the·si·a
cac·es·the·sic
ca·chec·tic
ca·chet
ca·che·xi·a
    pl ca·chex·i·as
    or ca·chex·y
    pl ca·chex·ies
ca·chex·y
    pl ca·chex·ies
    or ca·chex·i·a
    pl ca·chex·i·as
cach·in·nate
cach·in·na·tion
ca·chou
cac·o·de·mo·ni·a
    or cac·o·de·mo·no·ma·ni·a
cac·o·de·mo·no·ma·ni·a
    or cac·o·de·mo·ni·a
cac·o·dyl
cac·o·dyl·ate
cac·o·dyl·ic

cac·o·e·thes
cac·o·gen·e·sis
    pl cac·o·gen·e·ses
cac·o·gen·ic
cac·o·gen·ics
cac·o·geu·si·a
cac·o·me·li·a
cac·o·pho·ni·a
cac·o·phon·ic
ca·coph·o·ny
ca·cos·mi·a
cac·ti·no·my·cin
ca·cu·men
    pl ca·cu·mi·na
ca·cu·mi·nal
ca·dav·er
ca·dav·er·ic
ca·dav·er·ine
ca·dav·er·ous
ca·dav·er·ous·ly
cad·mi·o·sis
cad·mi·um
ca·du·ca
ca·du·ce·us
    pl ca·du·ce·i
cae·cal
    var of ce·cal
cae·ci·tas

cae·cum
    var of ce·cum
    pl cae·ca
cae·lo·ther·a·py
cae·no·gen·e·sis
    var of ce·no·gen·e·sis
    pl cae·no·gen·e·ses
cae·no·ge·net·ic
    var of ce·no·ge·net·ic
cae·ru·lo·plas·min
    var of ce·ru·lo·plas·min
Caes·al·pin·i·a
cae·sar·e·an
    or cae·sar·i·an
    var of ce·sar·e·an
cae·sar·i·an
    or cae·sar·e·an
    var of ce·sar·e·an
cae·si·um
    var of ce·si·um
ca·fard
caf·fe·ic
caf·feine
caf·fein·ic
caf·fein·ism
caf·fe·ol
    or caf·fe·one
caf·fe·one
    or caf·fe·ol
Caf·fey dis·ease

48

a·hin·ca
  or ca·in·ca
'aille test
a·in·ca
  or ca·hin·ca
ai·no·pho·bi·a
ais·son dis·ease
Ca·jal
aj·a·put
  or caj·e·put
  or caj·u·put
aj·e·put
  or caj·a·put
  or caj·u·put
aj·e·put·ol
  or caj·u·put·ol
aj·u·put
  or caj·a·put
  or caj·e·put
aj·u·put·ol
  or caj·e·put·ol
Cal·a·bar bean
al·a·mine
al·a·mus
  pl cal·a·mi
al·cae·mi·a
  var of cal·ce·mi·a
cal·ca·ne·al
  or cal·ca·ne·an
cal·ca·ne·an
  or cal·ca·ne·al
cal·ca·ne·o·a·poph·y·si·tis
cal·ca·ne·o·as·trag·a·lar
cal·ca·ne·o·a·strag·a·loid
cal·ca·ne·o·ca·vus
cal·ca·ne·o·cu·boid
cal·ca·ne·o·dyn·i·a
cal·ca·ne·o·na·vic·u·lar
cal·ca·ne·o·tib·i·al
cal·ca·ne·o·val·gus
cal·ca·ne·um
  pl cal·ca·ne·a
cal·ca·ne·us
  pl cal·ca·ne·i
cal·ca·no·dyn·i·a
cal·car
  pl cal·car·i·a
cal·car avis
  pl cal·car·i·a av·i·um

cal·ca·rate
cal·car·e·ous
  or cal·car·i·ous
cal·car·e·ous·ly
cal·car·e·ous·ness
cal·ca·rine
cal·car·i·ous
  or cal·car·e·ous
cal·ce·mi·a
cal·car·i·u·ri·a
cal·ci·bil·i·a
cal·cic
cal·ci·co·sis
  pl cal·ci·co·ses
cal·cif·a·mes
cal·cif·er·ol
cal·cif·er·ous
cal·cif·ic
cal·ci·fi·ca·tion
cal·ci·fy
cal·cig·er·ous
cal·cim·e·ter
cal·ci·na·tion
cal·cine
cal·ci·no·sis
  pl cal·ci·no·ses
cal·ci·pe·ni·a
cal·ci·pex·is
  or cal·ci·pex·y
cal·ci·pex·y
  or cal·ci·pex·is
cal·ci·phil·i·a
cal·ci·phy·lax·is
  pl cal·ci·phy·lax·es
cal·ci·priv·i·a
cal·cis
cal·cite
cal·ci·to·nin
cal·ci·um
cal·ci·u·ri·a
cal·co·glob·u·lin
cal·co·sphae·rite
  var of cal·co·sphe·rite
cal·co·spher·ite
cal·co·spher·ule
cal·cu·lar·y
cal·cu·lif·ra·gous
cal·cu·lo·gen·e·sis

cal·cu·lo·sis
  pl cal·cu·lo·ses
cal·cu·lous
cal·cu·lus
  pl cal·cu·lus·es
  or cal·cu·li
Cald·well-Luc op·er·a·tion
Cald·well pro·jec·tion
cal·e·fa·cient
ca·len·du·la
ca·len·du·lin
cal·en·tu·ra
cal·en·ture
calf
  pl calves
cal·i·ber
cal·i·brate
cal·i·bra·ter
  or cal·i·bra·tor
cal·i·bra·tion
cal·i·bra·tor
  or cal·i·brat·er
cal·i·bre
  var of cal·i·ber
cal·i·ce·al
  or cal·y·ce·al
ca·li·cec·ta·sis
  pl ca·li·cec·ta·ses
  or cal·i·ec·ta·sis
  or ca·ly·cec·ta·sis
ca·li·cec·to·my
  or ca·ly·cec·to·my
ca·lic·i·form
  or ca·lyc·i·form
ca·lic·i·nal
  or ca·li·cine
  or ca·lyc·i·nal
  or ca·ly·cine
ca·li·cine
  or ca·ly·cine
  or ca·lyc·i·nal
  or ca·li·ca·nal
cal·i·ci·vi·rus
ca·lic·u·lus
  pl ca·lic·u·lus
  or ca·lyc·u·lus
  or ca·ly·cle

cal·i·ec·ta·sis
  or ca·li·cec·ta·sis
  or ca·ly·cec·ta·sis
cal·i·for·ni·um
cal·i·per
  or cal·li·per
cal·i·sa·ya bark
cal·is·then·ics
ca·lix
  pl ca·li·ces
  or ca·lyx
Cal·kins meth·od
Cal·lan·der am·pu·ta·tion
Call-Ex·ner bod·ies
cal·li·pe·di·a
cal·li·per
  or cal·i·per
Cal·liph·o·ra
cal·liph·o·rid
Cal·li·phor·i·dae
cal·liph·o·rine
Cal·li·thric·i·dae
  or Cal·li·thrich·i·dae
Cal·li·thrix
Cal·li·thrich·i·dae
  or Cal·li·thric·i·dae
Cal·li·tro·ga
cal·lo·ma·ni·a
cal·lo·sal
cal·lose
cal·los·i·tas
cal·los·i·ty
  pl cal·los·i·ties
cal·lo·so·mar·gi·nal
cal·lo·sum
  pl cal·lo·sa
cal·lous
  pl cal·lous·es
  or cal·lus
  pl cal·lus·es
  or cal·li
cal·lus
  pl cal·lus·es
  or cal·lous
  pl cal·lous·es
  or cal·li
calm·a·tive
Cal·mette test

cal·o·mel
cal·or
cal·o·ra·di·ance
cal·o·res·cence
cal·o·res·cent
cal·o·ric
cal·o·rie
  pl cal·o·ries
  or cal·o·ry
ca·lo·ri·fa·cient
cal·o·rif·ic
ca·lo·ri·gen·ic
cal·o·rim·e·ter
cal·o·ri·met·ric
  or cal·o·ri·met·ri·cal
cal·o·ri·met·ri·cal
  or cal·o·ri·met·ric
cal·o·ri·met·ri·cal·ly
cal·o·rim·e·try
  pl cal·o·rim·e·tries
ca·lor·i·punc·ture
ca·lor·i·trop·ic
cal·o·ry
  or cal·o·rie
Ca·lot tri·an·gle
ca·lum·ba
  or co·lom·bo
cal·va·cin
cal·va·ria
  pl cal·var·i·as
cal·var·i·al
cal·var·i·um
  pl cal·var·i·a
Cal·vé dis·ease
cal·vi·ti·es
  pl cal·vi·ti·es
calx
  pl cal·ces
cal·y·can·thine
cal·y·ce·al
  or cal·i·ce·al
ca·ly·cec·ta·sis
  pl ca·ly·cec·ta·ses
  or ca·li·cec·ta·sis
  or cal·i·ec·ta·sis
ca·ly·cec·to·my
  or ca·li·cec·to·my
ca·ly·ces

ca·lyc·i·form
  or ca·lic·i·form
ca·lyc·i·nal
  or ca·lic·i·nal
  or ca·ly·cine
  or ca·li·cine
ca·ly·cine
  or ca·lyc·i·nal
  or ca·li·cine
  or ca·lic·i·nal
ca·ly·cle
  or ca·lyc·u·lus
  or ca·lic·u·lus
ca·lyc·u·li gus·ta·to·ri·i
ca·lyc·u·lus
  pl ca·lyc·u·li
  or ca·lic·u·lus
  or ca·ly·cle
Ca·lym·ma·to·bac·te·ri·um
ca·lyx
  pl ca·lyx·es
  or ca·ly·ces
  or ca·lix
cam·bi·um
  pl cam·bi·ums
  or cam·bi·a
cam·bo·gia
cam·er·a lu·ci·da
  pl cam·er·a lu·ci·das
cam·er·a ob·scu·ra
  pl cam·er·a ob·scu·ras
cam·i·sole
Cam·midge test
cam·o·mile
  or cham·o·mile
Camp·bell op·er·a·tion
Cam·per line
cam·pes·ter·ol
cam·phane
cam·phene
cam·phor
cam·pho·ra·ceous
cam·pho·rate
cam·pho·ric
cam·phor·ism
cam·phor·o·ma·ni·a
cam·pim·e·ter
cam·pim·e·try

50

camp·to·cor·mi·a
camp·to·dac·ty·ly
camp·to·spasm
cam·syl·ate
Cam·u·ra·ti-En·gle·mann dis·ease
can·a·dine
ca·nal of Cor·ti
ca·na·les al·ve·o·lar·es
can·a·lic·u·lar
can·a·lic·u·la·tion
   or can·a·lic·u·li·za·tion
can·a·lic·u·li·za·tion
   or can·a·lic·u·la·tion
can·a·lic·u·lo·plas·ty
can·a·lic·u·lus
   pl can·a·lic·u·li
can·a·line
ca·na·lis
   pl ca·na·les
ca·nal·i·za·tion
ca·nal·ize
ca·nal·o·plas·ty
ca·nals of Pe·tit
Can·a·val·i·a
can·a·val·in
Can·a·van dis·ease
can·a·van·ine
can·cel·late
   or can·cel·lat·ed
can·cel·lat·ed
   or can·cel·late
can·cel·lous
can·cel·lus
   pl can·cel·li
can·cer
can·cer·ate
can·cer·e·mi·a
can·cer·i·ci·dal
can·cer·i·gen·ic
   or can·cer·o·gen·ic
can·cer·ism
can·cer·i·za·tion
can·cer·o·ci·dal
can·cer·o·gen
can·cer·o·gen·ic
   or can·cer·i·gen·ic
can·cer·ol·o·gist

can·cer·ol·o·gy
   pl can·cer·ol·o·gies
can·cer·o·lyt·ic
can·cer·o·pho·bi·a
   or can·cer·pho·bi·a
can·cer·ous
can·cer·ous·ly
can·cer·pho·bi·a
   or can·cer·o·pho·bi·a
can·cri·form
can·croid
can·crum o·ris
   pl can·cra o·ris
can·de·la
can·di·ci·din
Can·di·da al·bi·cans
can·di·dal
can·di·de·mi·a
can·di·di·a·sis
   pl can·di·di·a·ses
can·di·did
can·di·din
can·di·do·sis
can·di·ru
can·dle
ca·nel·la
ca·nes·cine
ca·nic·o·la fe·ver
Can·i·dae
ca·nine
ca·ni·ni·form
ca·ni·nus
   pl ca·ni·ni
Ca·nis
ca·ni·ties
   pl ca·ni·ties
can·ker
can·ker·ous
can·na·bi·di·ol
can·na·bin
can·nab·i·nol
can·na·bis
can·na·bism
Can·niz·za·ro re·ac·tion
can·non bone
Can·non ring
can·nu·la
   pl can·nu·las
   or can·nu·lae

   or can·u·la
   pl can·u·las
   or can·u·lae
can·nu·lar
can·nu·late
can·nu·la·tion
can·nu·li·za·tion
can·nu·lize
can·re·none
can·thal
can·tha·ri·a·sis
can·thar·i·dal
can·thar·i·date
can·tha·ri·de·an
   or can·tha·ri·di·an
can·thar·i·des
can·tha·rid·i·an
   or can·tha·rid·e·an
can·thar·i·din
can·thar·i·dism
can·thar·i·dize
can·thar·is
   pl can·thar·i·des
can·thec·to·my
can·thi·tis
can·thol·y·sis
   pl can·thol·y·ses
can·tho·plas·ty
can·thor·rha·phy
can·thot·o·my
can·thus
   pl can·thi
can·u·la
   pl can·u·las
   or can·u·lae
   or can·nu·la
   pl can·nu·las
   or can·nu·lae
caou·tchouc
ca·pac·i·tance
ca·pac·i·tate
ca·pac·i·ta·tion
ca·pac·i·ta·tive
   or ca·pac·i·tive
ca·pac·i·tive
   or ca·pac·i·ta·tive
ca·pac·i·tor
ca·pac·i·ty
   pl ca·pac·i·ties

cap·e·let
cap·e·line
Cap·gras syn·drome
cap·il·lar·ec·ta·si·a
cap·il·lar·i·a
cap·il·la·ri·a·sis
  pl cap·il·la·ri·a·ses
  or cap·il·lar·i·o·sis
  pl cap·il·lar·i·o·ses
cap·il·lar·id
cap·il·lar·i·o·mo·tor
cap·il·lar·i·o·sis
  pl cap·il·lar·i·o·ses
  or cap·il·la·ri·a·sis
  pl ca·il·la·ri·a·ses
cap·il·lar·i·tis
cap·il·lar·i·ty
  pl cap·il·lar·i·ties
cap·il·lar·o·scope
cap·il·la·ros·co·py
  pl cap·il·la·ros·co·pies
  or cap·il·lar·i·os·copy
  pl cap·il·lar·i·os·co·pies
cap·il·lar·i·os·copy
  pl cap·il·lar·i·os·co·pies
  or cap·il·la·ros·co·py
  pl cap·il·la·ros·co·pies
cap·il·lar·y
  pl cap·il·lar·ies
ca·pil·li·cul·ture
cap·il·li·ti·um
  pl cap·il·li·ti·a
cap·il·lo·ve·nous
ca·pil·lus
  pl ca·pil·li
cap·i·stra·tion
cap·i·tate
cap·i·ta·tion
cap·i·ta·tum
  pl cap·i·ta·ta
cap·i·tel·lar
cap·i·tel·lum
  pl cap·i·tel·la
cap·i·ton·nage
ca·pit·u·lum
  pl ca·pit·u·la
Ca·pi·vac·ci·us ul·cer
Cap·lan syn·drome
cap·no·hep·a·tog·ra·phy

ca·pon·i·za·tion
ca·pon·ize
ca·pote·ment
Capps pleu·ral re·flex
cap·rate
cap·ric
ca·pril·o·quism
cap·rin
cap·ro·ate
cap·ro·ic
cap·ro·in
cap·ro·yl
cap·ry·late
ca·pryl·ic
cap·sa·i·cin
cap·san·thin
cap·si·cum
cap·sid
cap·sid·al
cap·si·tis
cap·so·mer
  or cap·so·mere
cap·so·mere
  or cap·so·mer
cap·sot·o·my
cap·su·la
  pl cap·su·lae
cap·su·lar
cap·su·late
  or cap·su·lat·ed
cap·su·lat·ed
  or cap·su·late
cap·su·la·tion
cap·sule
cap·su·lec·to·my
cap·su·li·tis
cap·su·lo·len·tic·u·lar
cap·su·lo·ma
cap·su·lo·plas·ty
cap·su·lor·rha·phy
cap·su·lo·tha·lam·ic
cap·su·lo·tome
cap·su·lot·o·my
cap·ta·mine
cap·ta·tion
cap·ti·va·tion
cap·to·di·a·mine
cap·to·dram·in

cap·ture
cap·u·ride
cap·ut
  pl ca·pi·ta
ca·put mor·tu·um
  pl ca·pi·ta mor·tu·a
ca·put suc·ce·da·ne·um
  pl ca·pi·ta suc·ce·da·ne·a
Car·a·bel·li cusp
car·a·geen
  or car·ra·geen
  or car·ra·geen·in
  or car·ra·gheen·in
car·am·i·phen
car·a·pace
car·at
ca·ra·te
car·ba·chol
car·ba·cryl·a·mine
car·ba·cryl·ic
car·ba·dox
car·ba·mate
car·bam·az·e·pine
car·bam·ic
car·bam·ide
car·bam·i·dine
carb·a·mi·no
carb·a·mi·no·he·mo·glo·
  bin
car·bam·o·yl
  or car·bam·yl
car·ba·moyl·trans·fer·ase
car·bam·yl
  or car·bam·o·yl
car·bam·y·la·tion
car·bam·yl·cho·line
car·bam·yl·u·re·a
carb·an·i·on
car·bar·sone
car·ba·ryl
car·ba·sus
car·ba·zide
car·baz·o·chrome
car·ba·zole
carb·a·zot·ic
car·ben·i·cil·lin
car·be·ta·pen·tane
carb·he·mo·glo·bin
  or car·bo·he·mo·glo·bin

car·bide
car·bi·nol
car·bin·ox·a·mine
car·bi·phene
car·bo
car·bo·ben·zox·y
  or car·bo·ben·zy·lox·y
car·bo·ben·zy·lox·y
  or car·bo·ben·zox·y
car·bo·cho·line
car·bo·clo·ral
car·bo·cy·clic
car·bo·he·mi·a
car·bo·he·mo·glo·bin
  or carb·he·mo·glo·bin
car·bo·hy·drase
car·bo·hy·drate
car·bo·hy·dra·tu·ri·a
car·bo·late
car·bol·fuch·sin
car·bol·ic
car·bo·li·gase
car·bo·line
car·bo·lism
car·bo·lize
car·bo·lu·ri·a
car·bol·xy·lene
car·bo·mer
car·bo·my·cin
car·bon
car·bo·na·ceous
car·bo·nate
car·bo·ne·mi·a
car·bon·ic
car·bo·ni·um
car·bon·i·za·tion
car·bon·ize
car·bon·om·e·ter
car·bon·om·e·try
car·bon·u·ri·a
car·bon·yl
car·box·y·es·ter·ase
car·box·y·he·mo·glo·bin
car·box·y·he·mo·glo·bi·ne·
  mi·a
car·box·yl
car·box·yl·ase
car·box·yl·ate
car·box·yl·a·tion

car·box·yl·ic
car·box·yl·trans·fer·ase
car·box·yl·ase
car·box·y·meth·yl
car·box·y·meth·yl·cel·lu·
  lose
car·box·y·my·o·glo·bin
car·box·y·pep·ti·dase
car·box·y·pol·y·pep·ti·dase
car·bro·mal
car·bun·cle
car·bun·cu·lar
car·bun·cu·loid
car·bun·cu·lo·sis
  pl car·bun·cu·lo·ses
car·bu·ret
car·bu·ret·ed
  or car·bu·ret·ted
car·bu·ret·ing
  or car·bu·ret·ting
car·bu·ret·ted
  or car·bu·ret·ed
car·bu·ret·ting
  or car·bu·ret·ing
car·bu·ta·mide
car·byl·a·mine
car·cass
car·ce·ag
car·cin·ec·to·my
car·cin·o·em·bry·on·ic
car·ci·no·gen
car·ci·no·gen·e·sis
  pl car·ci·no·gen·e·ses
car·ci·no·ge·net·ic
car·ci·no·gen·ic
car·ci·no·ge·nic·i·ty
car·ci·noid
car·ci·noi·do·sis
car·ci·nol·y·sis
car·ci·no·lyt·ic
car·ci·no·ma
  pl car·ci·no·mas
  or car·ci·no·ma·ta
car·ci·nom·a·toid
car·ci·no·ma·toi·des
car·ci·no·ma·to·sis
  pl car·ci·no·ma·to·ses
car·ci·nom·a·tous

car·ci·no·phil·i·a
car·ci·no·pho·bi·a
car·ci·no·sar·co·ma
  pl car·ci·no·sar·co·mas
  or car·ci·no·sar·co·ma·ta
car·ci·no·sis
  pl car·ci·no·ses
car·da·mom
  or car·da·mum
  or car·da·mon
car·da·mon
  or car·da·mom
  or car·da·mum
car·da·mum
  or car·da·mom
  or car·da·mon
Car·den am·pu·ta·tion
car·di·a
  pl car·di·as
  or car·di·ae
car·di·ac
car·di·a·co ne·gro
car·di·al
car·di·al·gi·a
car·di·am·e·ter
car·di·a·neu·ri·a
car·di·ant
car·di·asth·ma
car·di·cen·te·sis
  pl car·di·cen·te·ses
car·di·ec·ta·sis
  pl car·di·ec·ta·ses
car·di·ec·to·my
  pl car·di·ec·to·mies
car·di·o·ac·cel·er·a·tion
car·di·o·ac·cel·er·a·tor
car·di·o·ac·tive
car·di·o·an·gi·ol·o·gy
car·di·o·a·or·tic
car·di·o·ar·te·ri·al
car·di·o·asth·ma
car·di·o·au·di·to·ry
car·di·o·cele
car·di·o·cen·te·sis
  pl car·di·o·cen·te·ses
car·di·o·cha·la·si·a
car·di·o·ci·net·ic
car·di·o·cir·rho·sis
car·di·o·cla·si·a

car·di·oc·la·sis
  pl car·di·oc·la·ses
car·di·o·di·a·phrag·mat·ic
car·di·o·di·la·tor
car·di·o·di·o·sis
  pl car·di·o·di·o·ses
car·di·o·dy·nam·ic
car·di·o·dy·nam·ics
car·di·o·dy·na·mom·e·try
car·di·o·dyn·i·a
car·di·o·e·soph·a·ge·al
car·di·o·fa·cial
car·di·o·gen·e·sis
car·di·o·gen·ic
car·di·o·gram
car·di·o·graph
car·di·og·ra·pher
car·di·o·graph·ic
car·di·og·ra·phy
  pl car·di·og·ra·phies
car·di·o·he·pat·ic
car·di·oid
car·di·o·in·hib·i·to·ry
car·di·o·ki·net·ic
car·di·o·ky·mog·ra·phy
car·di·o·lip·in
car·di·o·lith
car·di·ol·o·gist
car·di·ol·o·gy
  pl car·di·ol·o·gies
car·di·ol·y·sin
car·di·ol·y·sis
  pl car·di·ol·y·ses
car·di·o·ma·la·ci·a
car·di·o·me·ga·li·a
car·di·o·meg·a·ly
  pl car·di·o·meg·a·lies
car·di·o·mel·a·no·sis
  pl car·di·o·mel·a·no·ses
car·di·o·men·su·ra·tor
car·di·o·men·to·pex·y
car·di·om·e·ter
car·di·o·met·ric
car·di·om·e·try
  pl car·di·om·e·tries
car·di·o·mo·til·i·ty
car·di·o·my·o·li·po·sis
car·di·o·my·op·a·thy
  pl car·di·o·my·op·a·thies

car·di·o·my·o·pex·y
car·di·o·my·ot·o·my
car·di·o·nec·tor
car·di·o·neph·ric
car·di·o·neu·ral
car·di·o·neu·ro·sis
car·di·o·o·men·to·pex·y
car·di·o·pal·u·dism
car·di·o·path
car·di·o·path·i·a
car·di·o·path·ic
car·di·o·pa·thol·o·gy
car·di·op·a·thy
  pl car·di·op·a·thies
car·di·o·per·i·car·di·o·pex·y
  pl car·di·o·per·i·car·di·o·
    pex·ies
car·di·o·per·i·car·di·tis
car·di·o·pho·bi·a
car·di·o·phone
car·di·o·plas·ty
  pl car·di·o·plas·ties
car·di·o·ple·gi·a
car·di·o·pneu·mat·ic
car·di·o·pneu·mo·graph
car·di·o·pneu·mog·ra·phy
car·di·op·to·si·a
car·di·op·to·sis
  pl car·di·op·to·ses
car·di·o·pul·mo·nar·y
car·di·o·pul·mon·ic
car·di·o·punc·ture
car·di·o·py·lor·ic
car·di·o·ra·di·o·log·ic
car·di·o·ra·di·ol·o·gy
car·di·o·re·nal
car·di·o·res·pi·ra·tory
car·di·or·rha·phy
  pl car·di·or·rha·phies
car·di·or·rhex·is
  pl car·di·or·rhex·es
car·di·os·chi·sis
  pl car·di·os·chi·ses
car·di·o·scle·ro·sis
car·di·o·scope
car·di·o·spasm
car·di·o·spas·tic
car·di·o·sphyg·mo·graph
car·di·o·splen·o·pex·y

car·di·o·ste·no·sis
car·di·o·sym·phy·sis
  pl car·di·o·sym·phy·ses
car·di·o·ta·chom·e·ter
car·di·o·ta·chom·e·try
car·di·o·ther·a·py
  pl car·di·o·ther·a·pies
car·di·ot·o·my
  pl car·di·ot·o·mies
car·di·o·ton·ic
car·di·o·to·pom·e·try
car·di·o·tox·ic
car·di·o·val·vu·lar
car·di·o·val·vu·lo·tome
car·di·o·vas·cu·lar
car·di·o·vec·tog·ra·phy
car·di·o·ver·sion
car·di·o·ver·ter
car·di·tis
car·di·val·vu·li·tis
car·e·bar·i·a
car·ene
Car·i·ca
car·ies
  pl car·ies
ca·ri·na
  pl ca·ri·nas
  or ca·ri·nae
ca·ri·nal
car·i·nate
  or car·i·nat·ed
car·i·nat·ed
  or car·i·nate
car·i·o·gen·e·sis
car·i·o·gen·ic
car·i·o·stat·ic
car·i·ous
car·i·so·pro·dol
Carl Smith dis·ease
Carls·bad salt
car·mal·um
Car·man me·nis·cus sign
car·min·a·tive
car·mine
car·min·ic
car·min·o·phil
car·mus·tine
car·nas·si·al
car·ne·ous

car·ni·fi·ca·tion
car·ni·tine
car·ni·tive
Car·niv·o·ra
car·ni·vore
car·niv·o·rous
car·no·sine
car·no·si·ne·mi·a
car·no·si·nu·ri·a
ca·ro
car·ob
car·o·te·nae·mi·a
  var of car·o·te·ne·mi·a
car·o·tene
  or car·o·tin
car·o·te·ne·mi·a
  or car·o·ti·ne·mi·a
ca·rot·e·no·der·mi·a
ca·rot·e·noid
  or ca·rot·i·noid
car·o·te·no·sis
  pl car·o·te·no·ses
  or car·o·ti·no·sis
ca·rot·ic
ca·rot·i·co·cli·noid
ca·rot·i·co·tym·pan·ic
ca·rot·id
ca·rot·i·do·sym·pa·tho·a·tri·al
ca·rot·i·do·va·go·a·tri·al
ca·rot·i·do·ven·tric·u·lar
car·o·tin
  or car·o·tene
car·ot·i·nase
car·o·ti·ne·mi·a
  or car·o·te·ne·mi·a
ca·rot·i·noid
  or ca·rot·i·noid
car·o·ti·no·sis
  pl caro·ti·no·ses
  or car·o·te·no·sis
ca·rot·is
ca·rot·o·dyn·i·a
carp
car·pa·ine
car·pal
car·pa·le
car·pec·to·my
  pl car·pec·to·mies

Car·pen·ter syn·drome
car·phen·a·zine
car·pho·lo·gi·a
  pl car·pho.lo·gi·as
  or car·phol·o·gy
  pl car·phol·o·gies
car·phol·o·gy
  pl car·phol·o·gies
  or car·pho·lo·gi·a
  pl car·pho.lo·gi·as
car·pi·tis
car·po·met·a·car·pal
car·po·pe·dal
car·po·pha·lan·ge·al
car·pop·to·sis
car·pus
  pl car·pi
car·ra·geen
  or car·ra·geen·in
  or car·ra·gheen·in
  or car·a·geen
car·ra·geen·in
  or car·ra·gheen·in
  or car·ra·geen
  or car·a·geen
car·ra·gheen·in
  or car·ra·geen
  or car·ra·geen·in
  or car·a·geen
Car·rel-Da·kin treat·ment
car·ri·er
Car·ri·on dis·ease
car·ron oil
car·sick
car·sick·ness
Cars·well grapes
Car·ter op·er·a·tion
Car·te·sian
Car·tha·mus
car·ti·lage
car·ti·lag·in·e·ous
  or car·ti·lag·i·nous
car·ti·lag·i·nes la·ryn·gis
car·ti·la·gin·i·fi·ca·tion
car·ti·la·gin·i·form
car·ti·lag·i·noid
car·ti·lag·i·nous
  or car·ti·lag·in·e·ous

car·ti·la·go
  pl car·ti·lag·i·nes
Ca·rum
car·un·cle
ca·run·cu·la
  pl ca·run·cu·lae
ca·run·cu·lar
ca·run·cu·late
  ca·run·cu·lat·ed
car·us
car·va·crol
Car·val·lo sign
carv·er
car·vone
car·y·en·chy·ma
  or kar·y·en·chy·ma
car·y·o·chrome
  or kar·y·o·chrome
car·y·o·phyl·lus
Ca·sal col·lar
ca·san·thra·nol
Ca·sa·res-Gil stain
cas·cade
cas·car·a
cas·car·a a·mar·ga
cas·car·a sa·gra·da
cas·ca·ril·la
cas·ca·ril·lin
cas·ca·rin
case
ca·se·ase
ca·se·ate
ca·se·a·tion
case·book
ca·se·ic
ca·se·i·form
ca·sein
ca·sein·ate
ca·sein·o·gen
ca·se·o·cal·cif·ic
ca·se·ous
case·work
case·worm
Cas·i·mi·ro·a
Ca·so·ni test
casque
cas·sa·va
Cas·ser fon·ta·nel
cas·sette

Cas·sia
cast
Cas·taigne meth·od
Cas·ta·nea
Cas·ta·ne·da vac·cine
Cas·tel meth·od
Cas·tel·la·ni paint
Cas·tile soap
cast·ing
cas·tor
cas·to·re·um
cas·trate
cas·tra·tion
cas·tro·phre·ni·a
cas·u·al·ty
   pl ca·su·al·ties
cas·u·is·tics
cat·a·ba·si·al
ca·tab·a·sis
   pl ca·tab·a·ses
cat·a·bat·ic
cat·a·bi·o·sis
   pl cat·a·bi·o·ses
cata·bi·ot·ic
cat·a·bol·er·gy
cat·a·bol·ic
ca·tab·o·lin
  or ca·tab·o·lite
ca·tab·o·lism
  or ka·tab·o·lism
ca·tab·o·lite
  or ca·tab·o·lin
ca·tab·o·lize
cat·a·caus·tic
cat·a·chro·ma·sis
  or kat·a·chro·ma·sis
cat·a·clei·sis
   pl cat·a·clei·sis
cat·a·clon·ic
cat·a·clo·nus
cat·a·cous·tics
cat·a·crot·ic
ca·tac·ro·tism
cat·a·di·cro·tism
cat·a·did·y·mus
  or kat·a·did·y·mus
cat·a·di·op·tric
  or cat·a·di·op·tri·cal

cat·a·di·op·tri·cal
  or cat·a·di·op·tric
cat·a·gel·o·pho·bi·a
cat·a·gen
cat·a·gen·e·sis
   pl cat·a·gen·e·ses
cat·a·ge·net·ic
cat·a·lase
cat·a·lat·ic
cat·a·lep·sis
cat·a·lep·sy
   pl cat·a·lep·sies
cat·a·lep·tic
cat·a·lep·ti·cal·ly
cat·a·lep·ti·form
cat·a·lep·tize
cat·a·lep·toid
cat·a·lo·gi·a
Ca·tal·pa
ca·tal·y·sis
   pl ca·tal·y·ses
cat·a·lyst
cat·a·lyt·ic
cat·a·lyt·i·cal·ly
cat·a·ly·za·tion
cat·a·lyze
cat·a·lyz·er
cat·a·me·ni·a
cat·a·me·ni·al
cat·a·mite
cat·am·ne·sis
   pl cat·am·ne·ses
cat·am·nes·tic
cat·a·pasm
cat·a·pha·si·a
cat·a·pha·sis
ca·taph·o·ra
cat·a·pho·re·sis
   pl cat·a·pho·re·ses
cat·a·pho·ret·ic
cat·a·pho·ret·i·cal·ly
cat·a·pho·ri·a
cat·a·pho·ric
cat·a·phre·ni·a
cat·a·phy·lac·tic
cat·a·phy·lax·is
cat·a·pla·si·a
  or kat·a·pla·si·a

cat·a·pla·sis
   pl ca·tap·la·ses
cat·a·plasm
cat·a·plas·tic
cat·a·plec·tic
cat·a·plex·y
   pl cat·a·plex·ies
cat·a·ract
cat·a·rac·ta
cat·a·rac·tal
cat·a·rac·to·gen·ic
cat·a·rac·tous
cat·a·rhine
  or cat·ar·rhine
ca·tar·i·a
ca·tarrh
ca·tarrh·al
ca·tarrh·al·ly
Cat·ar·rhi·na
cat·ar·rhine
  or cat·a·rhine
cat·ar·rhin·i·an
cat·a·stal·sis
ca·tas·ta·sis
   pl ca·tas·ta·ses
cat·a·state
cat·a·stat·ic
ca·tas·tro·phe
cat·a·stroph·ic
cat·a·ther·mom·e·ter
  or kat·a·ther·mom·e·ter
cat·a·thy·mi·a
cat·a·thy·mic
cat·a·to·ni·a
   pl cat·a·to·ni·as
  or ca·tat·o·ny
   pl ca·tat·o·nies
  or kat·a·to·ni·a
cat·a·ton·ic
ca·tat·o·ny
   pl ca·tat·o·nies
  or cat·a·to·ni·a
   pl cat·a·to·ni·as
  or kat·a·to·ni·a
cat·a·tri·cro·tism
cat·a·tro·pi·a
cat bite fe·ver
catch·ment ar·e·a
cat·e·chin

cat·e·chol
cat·e·chol·a·mine
cat·e·chu
cat·e·chu·ic
cat·e·lec·tro·ton·ic
cat·e·lec·trot·o·nus
cat·e·nate
cat·e·noid
ca·ten·u·late
cat·gut
Cath·a
ca·thaer·e·sis
   var of ca·ther·e·sis
ca·thar·sis
   pl ca·thar·ses
   or ka·thar·sis
   pl ka·thar·ses
ca·thar·tic
   or ka·thar·tic
ca·thect
ca·thec·tic
ca·thec·ti·cize
ca·thep·sin
ca·ther·e·sis
cath·e·ret·ic
cath·e·ter
cath·e·ter·ism
cath·e·ter·i·za·tion
cath·e·ter·ize
cath·e·ter·o·stat
ca·thex·is
   pl ca·thex·es
cath·i·so·pho·bi·a
cath·ode
   or kath·ode
ca·thod·ic
   or ka·thod·ic
cath·od·i·cal·ly
ca·thol·i·con
cat·i·on
   or kat·i·on
cat·i·on·ic
cat·i·on·i·cal·ly
cat·ling
cat·nep
   or cat·nip
cat·nip
   or cat·nep

ca·top·tric
   or ca·top·tri·cal
   pl ca·top·trics
ca·top·tri·cal
   or ca·top·tric
ca·top·tri·cal·ly
ca·top·tro·scope
cat·ta·lo
   pl cat·ta·los
   or cat·ta·loes
Cat·tell test
cat·ter·y
   pl cat·ter·ies
Cau·ca·sian
cau·da
   pl cau·dae
cau·da e·qui·na
   pl cau·dae e·qui·nae
cau·da he·li·cis
   pl cau·dae he·li·cis
cau·dad
cau·dal
cau·dal·ly
cau·date
   or cau·dat·ed
cau·dat·ed
   or cau·date
cau·da·tion
cau·da·to·len·tic·u·lar
cau·da·tum
   pl cau·da·ta
cau·do·ceph·al·ad
caul
cau·li·flow·er
cau·line
cau·lo·phyl·line
cau·lo·phyl·lum
cau·lo·ple·gi·a
cau·maes·the·si·a
   var of cau·me·the·si·a
cau·mes·the·si·a
caus·al
cau·sal·gi·a
cau·sal·gic
cau·sa·tion
caus·a·tive
cause
caus·tic
cau·ter

cau·ter·ant
cau·ter·i·za·tion
cau·ter·ize
cau·ter·y
ca·va
   pl ca·vae
ca·val
cav·al·ry bone
cav·a·scope
cave of Meck·el
cav·ern
ca·ver·na
   pl ca·ver·nae
cav·er·nil·o·quy
cav·er·ni·tis
cav·er·no·ma
   pl cav·er·no·mas
   or cav·er·no·ma·ta
cav·er·no·si·tis
cav·er·nos·to·my
   pl cav·er·nos·to·mies
cav·er·no·sum
   pl cav·er·no·sa
cav·ern·ous
Ca·vi·a
Ca·vi·i·dae
cav·i·tar·y
cav·i·tas
   pl cav·i·ta·tes
cav·i·tate
cav·i·ta·tion
Ca·vi·te
ca·vi·tis
cav·i·ty
   pl cav·i·ties
ca·vo·gram
ca·vog·ra·phy
ca·vo·sur·face
ca·vo·val·gus
ca·vum
   pl ca·va
ca·vus
ca·vy
   pl ca·vies
Ca·ze·nave dis·ease
ce·as·mic
ceb·a·dil·la
   or sa·ba·dil·la
Ce·bi·dae

ce·bo·ce·pha·li·a
ce·bo·ce·phal·ic
ce·bo·ceph·a·lus
ce·bo·ceph·a·ly
Ce·boi·de·a
Ce·bus
ce·cal
ce·cec·to·my
  pl ce·cec·to·mies
ce·ci·tis
ce·ci·ty
ce·co·cele
ce·co·co·lic
ce·co·co·lo·pex·y
ce·co·co·los·to·my
ce·co·il·e·os·to·my
ce·co·pex·y
  pl ce·co·pex·ies
ce·co·pli·ca·tion
ce·cop·to·sis
  pl ce·cop·to·ses
ce·cor·rha·phy
  pl ce·cor·rha·phies
ce·co·sig·moi·dos·to·my
  pl ce·co·sig·moi·dos·to·
    mies
ce·cos·to·my
  pl ce·cos·to·mies
ce·cot·o·my
  pl ce·cot·o·mies
ce·cum
  pl ce·ca
ce·dar
ce·dar·wood
ce·drene
ce·dron
Ce·las·trus
ce·la·tion
ce·len·ter·on
  pl ce·len·ter·a
cel·er·y
  pl cel·er·ies
ce·li·ac
ce·li·a·del·phus
ce·li·ec·ta·si·a
ce·li·ec·to·my
ce·li·o·cen·te·sis
ce·li·o·col·pot·o·my
  pl ce·lio·col·pot·o·mies

ce·li·o·en·ter·ot·o·my
  pl ce·lio·en·ter·ot·o·mies
ce·li·o·gas·trot·o·my
ce·li·o·ma
  pl ce·li·o·mas
  or ce·li·o·ma·ta
ce·li·o·my·o·mec·to·my
ce·li·o·my·o·si·tis
ce·li·o·par·a·cen·te·sis
  pl ce·li·o·par·a·cen·te·ses
ce·li·op·a·thy
ce·li·or·rha·phy
ce·li·o·scope
ce·li·os·co·py
  pl ce·li·os·co·pies
ce·li·ot·o·my
  pl ce·li·ot·o·mies
ce·li·tis
cell of Betz
cell of Clau·di·us
cell of Cor·ti
cel·la
  pl cel·lae
Cel·la·no blood group
cel·lif·u·gal
  or cel·lu·lif·u·gal
cel·lip·e·tal
  or cel·lu·lip·e·tal
cel·lo·bi·ase
cel·lo·bi·ose
cel·loi·din
cel·lose
cel·lu·la
  pl cel·lu·lae
cel·lu·lar
cel·lu·lar·i·ty
  pl cel·lu·lar·i·ties
cel·lu·lase
cel·lule
cel·lu·li·ci·dal
cel·lu·lif·u·gal
  or cel·lif·u·gal
cel·lu·lin
cel·lu·lip·e·tal
  or cel·lip·e·tal
cel·lu·li·tis
cel·lu·lo·fi·brous
cel·lu·lo·neu·ri·tis

cel·lu·lo·ra·dic·u·lo·neu·ri·
  tis
cel·lu·lo·sa
cel·lu·los·an
cel·lu·lose
cel·lu·los·ic
cel·om
ce·lom·ic
ce·los·chi·sis
ce·lo·scope
ce·lo·so·mi·a
ce·lo·so·mus
  pl ce·lo·so·mus·es
  or ce·lo·so·mi
ce·lo·the·li·o·ma
  pl ce·lo·the·li·o·mas
  or ce·lo·the·li·o·ma·ta
cel·o·vi·rus
cel·o·zo·ic
Cel·si·us
ce·ment
ce·men·ta·tion
ce·men·ti·cle
ce·ment·i·fi·ca·tion
ce·ment·ite
ce·men·to·blast
ce·men·to·blas·to·ma
  pl ce·men·to·blas·to·mas
  or ce·men·to·blas·to·ma·ta
ce·men·to·cla·si·a
ce·men·to·cyte
ce·men·to·den·ti·nal
ce·men·to·e·nam·el
ce·men·to·gen·e·sis
  pl ce·men·to·gen·e·ses
ce·men·to·ma
  pl ce·men·to·mas
  or ce·men·to·ma·ta
ce·men·to·path·i·a
ce·men·to·sis
  pl ce·men·to·ses
ce·men·tum
  pl ce·men·ta
cen·a·del·phus
ce·naes·the·si·a
  var of ce·nes·the·si·a
ce·naes·thet·ic
  var of ce·nes·thet·ic
cen·es·the·si·a

58

ce·nes·thet·ic
ce·nes·thop·a·thy
ce·no·cyte
ce·no·cyt·ic
ce·no·gen·e·sis
    pl ce·no·gen·e·ses
ce·no·ge·net·ic
ce·no·pho·bi·a
ce·no·psy·chic
ce·no·sis
ce·no·site
cen·o·type
cen·sor
cen·sor·ship
cen·tau·ry
cen·ter
cen·te·sis
    pl cen·te·ses
cen·ti·bar
cen·ti·grade
cen·ti·gram
cen·ti·li·ter
cen·ti·me·ter
cen·ti·nor·mal
cen·ti·pede
cen·ti·poise
cen·ti·stoke
cen·trad
cen·trage
cen·tral
cen·tra·phose
cen·tre
    var of cen·ter
cen·tren·ce·phal·ic
cen·tric
cen·tri·cip·i·tal
cen·tric·i·put
cen·trif·u·gal
cen·trif·u·gal·i·za·tion
cen·trif·u·gal·ize
cen·trif·u·gate
cen·trif·u·ga·tion
cen·tri·fuge
cen·tri·lob·u·lar
cen·tri·ole
cen·trip·e·tal
cen·tro·ac·i·nar
cen·tro·cyte
cen·tro·des·mose

cen·tro·don·tous
cen·tro·dor·sal
cen·tro·ki·ne·si·a
cen·tro·lec·i·thal
cen·tro·me·di·an
cen·tro·mere
cen·tro·mer·ic
cen·tro·phose
cen·tro·plasm
cen·tro·scle·ro·sis
cen·tro·some
cen·tro·so·mic
cen·tro·sphere
cen·tro·stal·tic
cen·tro·the·ca
cen·trum
    pl cen·trums
    or cen·tra
Cen·tru·roi·des
ce·pha·e·line
Ceph·a·e·lis
ceph·a·lad
ceph·a·lal·gi·a
ceph·a·lal·gic
ceph·a·lal·gy
Ceph·a·lan·thus
ceph·a·le·a
ceph·a·lex·in
ceph·al·he·ma·to·ma
    pl ceph·al·he·ma·to·mas
    or ceph·al·he·ma·to·ma·ta
ceph·al·hy·dro·cele
ce·phal·ic
ceph·a·lin
    or keph·a·lin
ceph·a·line
ceph·a·li·tis
ceph·a·li·za·tion
ceph·a·lo·cau·dal
ceph·a·lo·cele
ceph·a·lo·cen·te·sis
    pl ceph·a·lo·cen·te·ses
ceph·a·lo·chord
Ceph·a·lo·chor·da
ceph·a·lo·di·pro·so·pus
ceph·a·lo·dym·i·a
ceph·a·lo·dyn·i·a
ceph·a·lo·gas·ter

ceph·a·lo·gen·e·sis
    pl ceph·a·lo·gen·e·ses
ceph·a·lo·gly·cin
ceph·a·lo·gram
ceph·a·lo·graph
ceph·a·log·ra·phy
ceph·a·lo·gy·ric
ceph·a·lo·hem·a·to·cele
ceph·a·lo·he·ma·to·ma
    pl ceph·a·lo·he·ma·to·mas
    or ceph·a·lo·he·ma·to·ma·ta
ceph·a·loid
ceph·a·lom·e·lus
ceph·a·lo·me·ni·a
ceph·a·lo·men·in·gi·tis
ceph·a·lom·e·ter
ceph·a·lo·met·ric
ceph·a·lo·met·rics
    or ceph·a·lom·e·try
ceph·a·lom·e·try
    pl ceph·a·lom·e·tries
    or ceph·a·lo·met·rics
ceph·a·lo·mo·tor
ceph·a·lone
ceph·a·lo·ni·a
ceph·a·lo·oc·u·lo·cu·ta·ne·
    ous
ceph·a·lo·or·bi·tal
ceph·a·lop·a·gus
ceph·a·lop·a·gy
ceph·a·lop·a·thy
    pl ceph·a·lop·a·thies
ceph·a·lo·pel·vic
ceph·a·lo·pha·ryn·ge·us
ceph·a·lo·ple·gi·a
ceph·a·lo·pod
ceph·a·lor·i·dine
ceph·a·los·co·py
ceph·a·lo·spo·rin
ceph·a·lo·spo·ri·o·sis
    pl ceph·a·lo·spo·ri·o·ses
Ceph·a·lo·spo·ri·um
ceph·a·lo·stat
ceph·a·lo·thin
ceph·a·lo·tho·rac·ic
ceph·a·lo·tho·ra·co·il·i·op·
    a·gus
ceph·a·lo·tho·ra·cop·a·gus
ceph·a·lo·tome

ceph·a·lot·o·my
pl ceph·a·lot·o·mies
ceph·a·lo·trac·tor
ceph·a·lo·tribe
ceph·a·lo·trid·y·mus
ceph·a·lo·trip·sy
pl ceph·a·lo·trip·sies
ceph·a·lo·trip·tor
ceph·a·lo·trop·ic
ceph·a·lo·try·pe·sis
pl ceph·a·lo·try·pe·ses
ceph·a·lox·i·a
cep·tor
ce·ra
ce·ra·ceous
cer·am·i·dase
cer·am·ide
cer·a·sin
cer·a·sine
cer·a·si·nose
Cer·a·sus
ce·rate
ce·rat·ed
cer·a·tin
or ker·a·tin
cer·a·ti·tis
or ker·a·ti·tis
cer·a·to·con·junc·ti·vi·tis
or ker·a·to·con·junc·ti·vi·tis
cer·a·to·cri·coid
cer·a·to·hy·al
Cer·a·to·ni·a
cer·a·ton·o·sus
cer·a·to·pha·ryn·ge·us
Cer·a·to·phyl·lus
cer·a·to·po·go·nid
cer·a·to·po·gon·i·dae
cer·a·tose
or ker·a·tose
ce·ra·tum
cer·car·i·a
pl cer·car·i·ae
cer·car·i·al
cer·car·i·an
cer·clage
Cer·co·ce·bus
Cer·co·mo·nas
Cer·co·pi·the·ci·dae
Cer·co·pith·e·coi·de·a

Cer·co·pi·the·cus
cer·cus
pl cer·ci
cere
ce·re·a·flex·i·bil·i·tas
ce·re·al
cer·e·bel·lar
cer·e·bel·lif·u·gal
cer·e·bel·lip·e·tal
cer·e·bel·li·tis
cer·e·bel·lo·bul·bar
cer·e·bel·lo·med·ul·lar·y
cer·e·bel·lo·pon·tine
cer·e·bel·lo·ret·i·nal
cer·e·bel·lo·ru·bral
cer·e·bel·lo·ru·bro·spi·nal
cer·e·bel·lo·spi·nal
cer·e·bel·lo·tha·lam·ic
cer·e·bel·lo·ves·tib·u·lar
cer·e·bel·lum
pl cer·e·bel·lums
or cer·e·bel·la
cer·e·bral
cer·e·bral-pal·sied
cer·e·brate
cer·e·bra·tion
cer·e·bric
ce·re·bri·form
cer·e·brif·u·gal
cer·e·brin·ic
cer·e·brip·e·tal
cer·e·bri·tis
cer·e·bro·cer·e·bel·lar
cer·e·bro·cor·ti·cal
cer·e·bro·cu·pre·in
cer·e·bro·hep·a·to·re·nal
cer·e·broid
cer·e·bro·ma
cer·e·bro·mac·u·lar
cer·e·bro·ma·la·ci·a
cer·e·bro·med·ul·lary
cer·e·bro·men·in·gi·tis
cer·e·bron
cer·e·bron·ic
cer·e·bro·oc·u·lar
cer·e·bro·path·i·a
cer·e·brop·a·thy
cer·e·bro·phys·i·ol·o·gy
cer·e·bro·pon·tile

cer·e·bro·pon·tine
cer·e·bro·ret·i·nal
cer·e·bro·scle·ro·sis
pl ce·re·bro·scle·ro·ses
ce·re·brose
ce·re·bro·side
cer·e·bro·sis
cer·e·bro·spi·nal
cer·e·bro·spi·nant
ce·re·bro·ten·di·nous
ce·re·brot·o·my
ce·re·bro·to·ni·a
ce·re·bro·vas·cu·lar
cer·e·brum
pl ce·re·brums
or ce·re·bra
cere·cloth
cere·ment
Ce·ren·kov ra·di·a·tion
or Che·ren·kov ra·di·a·tion
ce·re·ous
cer·e·sin
or cer·e·sine
cer·e·sine
or cer·e·sin
Ce·re·us
ce·ri·a
ce·ric
ce·ri·met·ric
ce·ri·um
ce·roid
ce·ro·ma
ce·ro·plas·ty
ce·rot·ic
ce·rous
cer·ti·fi·a·ble
cer·ti·fi·ca·tion
cer·ti·fy
ce·ru·le·in
ce·ru·lo·plas·min
ce·ru·men
ce·ru·mi·nal
or ce·ru·mi·nous
ce·ru·mi·nol·y·sis
ce·ru·mi·no·sis
pl ce·ru·mi·no·ses
ce·ru·mi·nous
or ce·ru·mi·nal
ce·ruse

60

cer·vi·cal
cer·vi·ca·lis as·cen·dens
cer·vi·cec·to·my
   pl cer·vi·cec·to·mies
cer·vi·ci·tis
cer·vi·co·au·ral
cer·vi·co·au·ric·u·lar
cer·vi·co·ax·il·lar·y
cer·vi·co·bra·chi·al
cer·vi·co·brach·i·al·gi·a
cer·vi·co·buc·cal
cer·vi·co·col·pi·tis
cer·vi·co·dyn·i·a
cer·vi·co·fa·cial
cer·vi·co·la·bi·al
cer·vi·co·lin·gual
cer·vi·co·pu·bic
cer·vi·co·rec·tal
cer·vi·co·tho·rac·ic
cer·vi·co·u·ter·ine
cer·vi·co·vag·i·nal
cer·vi·co·vag·i·ni·tis
cer·vi·co·ves·i·cal
cer·vix
   pl cer·vix·es
   or cer·vic·es
cer·vix u·ter·i
ce·ryl
ce·sar·e·an
   or ce·sar·i·an
Ce·sar·is-De·mel bod·ies
ce·si·um
Ces·tan syn·drome
Ces·tan-Che·nais
   syn·drome
ces·ti·ci·dal
Ces·to·da
ces·to·dan
ces·tode
ces·to·di·a·sis
   pl ces·to·di·a·ses
ces·toid
Ces·toi·de·a
ces·toid·e·an
ce·ta·ce·um
ce·tal·ko·ni·um
ce·tic
ce·tin
ce·tin·ic

ce·to·phen·i·col
Ce·trar·i·a
ce·tri·mide
ce·tyl
ce·tyl·pyr·i·din·i·um
cev·a·dil·la
cev·a·dine
cev·ine
ce·vi·tam·ic ac·id
Cey·lon sick·ness
ceys·sa·tite
Cha·ber·ti·a
Chad·dock sign
chae·ro·ma·ni·a
   var of che·ro·ma·ni·a
chae·ro·pho·bi·a
   var of che·ro·pho·bi·a
Chae·ro·pith·e·cus
chae·ta
   pl chae·tae
chae·tal
chae·to·min
   var of che·to·min
Chae·to·mi·um
chafe
Cha·gas dis·ease
Cha·gas-Cruz dis·ease
cha·go·ma
   pl cha·go·mas
   or cha·go·ma·ta
Cha·gres fe·ver
cha·la·si·a
cha·la·za
   pl cha·la·zas
   or cha·la·zae
cha·la·zi·on
   pl cha·la·zi·a
cha·la·zo·der·mi·a
chal·ci·tis
chal·cone
   or chal·kone
chal·co·sis
chal·i·co·sis
   pl chal·i·co·ses
chal·ki·tis
chal·kone
   or chal·cone
chalk·stone
chal·lenge

chal·one
cha·lyb·e·ate
cham·ae·ce·phal·ic
   var of cham·e·ce·phal·ic
cham·ae·ceph·a·lous
   var of cham·e·ceph·a·lous
cham·ae·ceph·a·lus
   var of cham·e·ceph·a·lus
   pl cham·ae·ceph·a·li
cham·ae·ceph·a·ly
   var of cham·e·ceph·a·ly
cham·ae·conch
   var of cham·e·conch
cham·ae·con·cha
   var of cham·e·con·cha
cham·ae·con·chous
   var of cham·e·con·chous
cham·ae·cra·ni·al
   var of cham·e·cra·ni·al
cham·ae·pro·so·pic
   var of cham·e·pro·so·pic
cham·aer·rhine
Cham·ber·lain line
Cham·ber·land fil·ter
cham·e·ce·phal·ic
cham·e·ceph·a·lous
cham·e·ceph·a·lus
   pl cham·e·ceph·a·li
cham·e·ceph·a·ly
cham·e·conch
cham·e·con·cha
cham·e·con·chous
cham·e·cra·ni·al
cham·e·pro·so·pic
cham·fer
cham·o·mile
   or cam·o·mile
chan·cre
chan·cri·form
chan·croid
chan·crous
ch'ang shan
chan·nel
Cha·os cha·os
Cha·oul
chap
Chap·man bag
Cha·put meth·od
char·ac·ter

char·ac·ter·i·za·tion
char·ac·ter·o·log·ic
 or char·ac·ter·o·log·i·cal
char·ac·ter·o·log·i·cal
 or char·ac·ter·o·log·ic
char·ac·ter·o·log·i·cal·ly
char·ac·ter·ol·o·gist
char·ac·ter·ol·o·gy
 pl char·ac·ter·ol·o·gies
cha·ras
char·bon
char·coal
Char·cot joint
Char·cot-Ley·den crys·tals
Char·cot-Ma·rie-Tooth
 dis·ease
Char·cot-Wil·brand
 syn·drome
char·la·tan
char·la·tan·ism
Charles law
char·ley·horse
Char·lin syn·drome
Charl·ton blanch·ing test
char·ro·pho·bi·a
 or che·ro·pho·bi·a
char·ta
 pl char·tae
chart·ing
char·treu·sin
char·tu·la
 pl char·tu·lae
Chas·sai·gnac tu·ber·cle
Chas·tek pa·ral·y·sis
chauf·fage
Chauf·fard-Min·kow·ski
 syn·drome
Chauf·fard-Still
 syn·drome
chaul·mau·gra
 or chaul·moo·gra
 or chaul·mu·gra
chaul·moo·gra
 or chaul·mu·gra
 or chaul·mau·gra
chaul·moo·grate
chaul·moo·gric

chul·mu·gra
 or chaul·moo·gra
 or chaul·mau·gra
chav·i·cine
chav·i·col
chay
chay·a
Chea·dle dis·ease
check·bite
check·er·ber·ry
 pl check·er·ber·ries
check·up
Che·di·ak-Hi·ga·shi
 a·nom·a·ly
cheek
cheek·bone
chees·y
chei·lal·gi·a
chei·lec·to·my
 pl chei·lec·to·mies
chei·lec·tro·pi·on
 or chi·lec·tro·pi·on
chei·li·tis
 or chi·li·tis
chei·lo·an·gi·o·scope
chei·lo·gnath·o·pal·a·tos·
 chi·sis
chei·lo·gnath·o·pros·o·pos·
 chi·sis
chei·lo·gnath·o·u·ra·nos·
 chi·sis
chei·lo·plas·ty
 pl chei·lo·plas·ties
chei·lor·rha·phy
chei·los·chi·sis
 pl chei·los·chi·ses
chei·lo·sis
 pl chei·lo·ses
chei·lo·sto·ma·to·plas·ty
chei·lot·o·my
chei·ma·pho·bi·a
chei·rag·ra
 or chi·rag·ra
chei·ral·gi·a
 or chi·ral·gi·a
chei·rap·sy
 or chi·rap·sy
chei·ar·thri·tis
 or chi·ar·thri·tis

chei·rog·no·my
 pl chei·rog·no·mies
 or chi·rog·no·my
 pl chi·rog·no·mies
chei·rog·nos·tic
chei·ro·kin·aes·thet·ic
 var of chei·ro·kin·es·thet·ic
chei·ro·kin·es·the·si·a
chei·ro·kin·es·thet·ic
chei·rol·o·gy
 pl chei·rol·o·gies
 or chi·rol·o·gy
 pl chi·rol·o·gies
chei·ro·meg·a·ly
 pl chei·ro·meg·a·lies
 or chi·ro·meg·a·ly
 pl chi·ro·meg·a·lies
chei·ro·plas·ty
 pl chei·ro·plas·ties
 or chi·ro·plas·ty
 pl chi·ro·plas·ty
chei·ro·po·dal·gi·a
chei·ro·pom·pho·lyx
 or chi·ro·pom·pho·lyx
chei·ro·scope
chei·ro·spasm
 or chi·ro·spasm
chek·en
che·late
che·la·tion
che·la·tor
chel·e·ryth·rine
che·lic·er·a
 pl che·lic·er·ae
chel·i·do·nine
Chel·i·do·ni·um
chel·lin
 or khel·lin
chel·li·nin
 or khel·li·nin
che·li·ped
che·loid
 or ke·loid
che·loi·dal
 or ke·loi·dal
Che·lo·ni·a
che·lo·ni·an
chem·a·bra·sion
chem·i·cal

chem·i·co·cau·ter·y
  or che·mo·cau·ter·y
chem·ex·fo·li·a·tion
chem·i·co·gen·e·sis
chem·i·lu·mi·nes·cence
  or che·mo·lu·mi·nes·cence
chem·i·no·sis
chem·i·o·tax·is
  pl chem·i·o·tax·es
  or che·mo·tax·is
  pl che·mo·tax·es
  or che·mo·tax·y
  pl che·mo·tax·es
che·mise
chem·ist
chem·is·try
  pl chem·is·tries
che·mo·au·to·troph
che·mo·au·to·troph·ic
che·mo·au·to·tro·phi·cal·ly
che·mo·au·tot·ro·phy
  pl che·mo·au·tot·ro·phies
che·mo·bi·ot·ic
che·mo·cau·ter·y
  or chem·i·co·cau·ter·y
chem·o·cep·tor
chem·o·co·ag·u·la·tion
che·mo·dec·to·ma
  pl che·mo·dec·to·mas
  or che·mo·dec·to·ma·ta
che·mo·dif·fer·en·ti·a·tion
che·mo·ki·ne·sis
  pl che·mo·ki·ne·ses
che·mo·ki·net·ic
che·mo·lu·mi·nes·cence
  or chem·i·lu·mi·nes·cence
che·mol·y·sis
che·mo·mor·pho·sis
chem·o·nu·cle·ol·y·sis
che·mo·pal·li·dec·to·my
che·mo·pro·phy·lac·tic
che·mo·pro·phy·lax·is
  pl che·mo·pro·phy·lax·es
che·mo·psy·chi·a·try
che·mo·re·cep·tion
che·mo·re·cep·tive
che·mo·re·cep·tiv·i·ty
  pl che·mo·re·cep·tiv·i·ties
che·mo·re·cep·tor

chem·o·re·flex
che·mo·re·sis·tance
che·mo·sen·si·tive
che·mo·sen·si·tiv·i·ty
  pl chem·o·sen·si·tiv·i·ties
che·mo·sen·so·ry
che·mo·se·ro·ther·a·py
che·mo·sis
  pl che·mo·ses
chem·os·mo·sis
  pl chem·os·mo·ses
chem·os·mot·ic
che·mo·stat
che·mo·ster·i·lant
che·mo·ster·il·i·za·tion
che·mo·ster·il·ize
che·mo·sur·gi·cal
che·mo·sur·ger·y
  pl chem·o·sur·ger·ies
chem·o·syn·the·sis
  pl chem·o·syn·the·ses
chem·o·syn·thet·ic
chem·o·tac·tic
chem·o·tac·ti·cal·ly
chem·o·tax·is
  pl chem·o·tax·es
  or chemo·tax·y
  pl chem·o·tax·ies
  or chem·i·o·tax·is
  pl chem·i·o·tax·es
chem·o·tax·y
  pl chem·o·tax·es
  or chem·o·tax·is
  pl chem·o·tax·es
  or chem·i·o·tax·is
  pl chem·i·o·tax·es
chem·o·thal·a·mot·o·my
chem·o·ther·a·peu·tic
  or chem·o·ther·a·peu·ti·cal
chem·o·ther·a·peu·ti·cal
  or chem·o·ther·a·peu·tic
chem·o·ther·a·peut·i·cal·ly
chem·o·ther·a·peu·tics
chem·o·ther·a·pist
chem·o·ther·a·py
  pl chem·o·ther·a·pies
che·mot·ic
che·mo·troph
che·mo·trop·ic

che·mot·ro·pism
chem·ur·gy
Che·nais syn·drome
che·no·de·ox·y·cho·lic
Che·no·po·di·um
Che·ren·kov ra·di·a·tion
  or Ce·ren·kov ra·di·a·tion
che·ro·ma·ni·a
che·ro·pho·bi·a
  or char·ro·pho·bia
Cher·ry and Cran·dall test
cher·ub·ism
Ches·el·den op·er·a·tion
che·to·min
Chev·a·lier Jack·son op·er·a·tion
chev·on
Chev·re·mont-Com·baire meth·od
Cheyne-Stokes breath·ing, res·pi·ra·tion
Chi·a·ri syn·drome
Chi·a·ri-From·mel syn·drome
chi·ar·thri·tis
  or chei·ar·thri·tis
chi·asm
chi·as·ma
  pl chi·as·mas
  or chi·as·ma·ta
chi·as·mal
chi·as·mat·ic
chick·en·pox
chi·cle·ro ul·cer
chig·ger
chig·o
chig·oe
  var of chig·o
chil·blain
child
child·bear·ing
child·bed
child·birth
child·hood
chi·lec·tro·pi·on
  or chei·lec·tro·pi·on
chi·li·tis
  or chei·li·tis
Chi·lo·mas·tix

Chi·lop·o·da
chi·lop·o·dan
chi·lop·o·dous
chi·mae·ra
var of chi·me·ra
chi·me·ra
chi·mer·ism
chim·pan·zee
chi·myl
chin
chin·a·crin
var of quin·a·crine
chin·a·crine
var of quin·a·crine
chin·bone
chinch
chin·cho·na
var of cin·cho·na
chin·co·na
var of cin·cho·na
chine
Chi·nese res·tau·rant syn·drome
chi·ni·o·fon
chi·noi·dine
chin·o·line
var of quin·o·line
chi·on·a·blep·si·a
chi·o·na·blep·sy
Chi·o·nan·thus
chi·o·no·pho·bi·a
chip·blow·er
chi·rag·ra
or chei·rag·ra
chi·ral·gi·a
or chei·ral·gi·a
chi·rap·si·a
chi·rap·sy
or chei·rap·sy
chi·rog·no·my
pl chi·rog·no·mies
or chei·rog·no·my
pl chei·rog·no·mies
chi·rol·o·gy
pl chi·rol·o·gies
or chei·ro·lo·gy
pl chei·ro·lo·gies
chi·ro·meg·a·ly
pl chi·ro·meg·a·lies

or chei·ro·meg·a·ly
pl chei·ro·meg·a·lies
chi·ro·plas·ty
pl chi·ro·plas·ty
or chei·ro·plas·ty
pl chei·ro·plas·ties
chi·ro·po·di·al
chi·rop·o·dist
chi·rop·o·dy
pl chi·rop·o·dies
chi·ro·pom·pho·lyx
or chei·ro·pom·pho·lyx
chi·ro·prac·tic
chi·ro·prac·tor
chi·ro·prax·is
pl chi·ro·prax·es
chi·ro·spasm
or chei·ro·spasm
chi·tin
chi·tin·ous
chi·to·bi·ose
chi·to·sa·mine
Chi·tral fe·ver
chit·tam
chla·my·de·mi·a
Chla·myd·i·a·ce·ae
chla·myd·i·o·sis
chlam·y·do·spore
chla·myd·o·spor·ic
Chlam·y·do·zo·a·ce·ae
Chlam·y·do·zo·on
chlo·as·ma
pl chlo·as·ma·ta
chlo·phe·di·a·nol
chlor·ac·ne
chlor·ae·mi·a
var of chlor·e·mi·a
chlo·ral
chlo·ral·am·ide
chlo·ral·form·am·ide
chlo·ral·ism
chlo·ral·ize
chlo·ra·lose
chlo·ral·u·re·thane
chlor·am·bu·cil
chlor·a·mine
chlor·am·phen·i·col
chlor·a·nae·mi·a
var of chlor·a·ne·mi·a

chlor·a·ne·mi·a
chlor·a·ne·mic
chlo·rate
chlor·bu·ta·nol
or chlo·ro·bu·ta·nol
chlor·bu·tol
chlor·cy·cli·zine
chlor·dan
or chlor·dane
chlor·dane
or chlor·dan
chlor·dan·to·in
chlor·di·az·ep·ox·ide
chlo·rel·lin
chlor·e·mi·a
chlor·eph·i·dro·sis
chlo·ret·ic
chlor·gua·nide
or chlo·ro·gua·nide
chlor·hex·i·dine
chlor·hy·dri·a
chlo·ric
chlo·ride
chlo·ri·dim·e·ter
chlo·ri·dim·e·try
chlo·ri·du·ri·a
chlo·ri·nat·ed
chlo·ri·na·tion
chlor·in·da·nol
chlo·rine
chlor·i·son·da·mine
chlo·rite
chlor·mad·i·none
chlor·mer·o·drin
chlor·mez·a·none
chlo·ro·ac·e·to·phe·none
chlo·ro·a·nae·mi·a
var of chlo·ro·a·ne·mi·a
chlo·ro·a·ne·mi·a
chlo·ro·az·o·din
chlo·ro·bu·ta·nol
or chlor·bu·ta·nol
chlo·ro·cre·sol
chlo·ro·cru·o·rin
chlo·ro·form
chlo·ro·for·mic
chlo·ro·form·ism
chlo·ro·form·i·za·tion

chlo·ro·gua·nide
  or chlor·gua·nide
chlo·ro·labe
chlo·ro·leu·kae·mi·a
  var of chlo·ro·leu·ke·mi·a
chlo·ro·leu·ke·mi·a
chlo·ro·lym·pho·sar·co·ma
chlo·ro·ma
  pl chlo·ro·mas
  or chlo·ro·ma·ta
chlo·rom·a·tous
chlo·ro·meth·ane
chlo·ro·my·e·lo·ma
  pl chlo·ro·my·e·lo·mas
  or chlo·ro·my·e·lo·ma·ta
chlo·ro·per·cha
chlo·ro·pex·i·a
chlo·ro·phane
chlo·ro·phe·nol
  or chlor·phe·nol
chlo·ro·phen·o·thane
chlo·ro·phyll
chlo·ro·phyl·lase
chlo·ro·pi·a
chlo·ro·pic·rin
  or chlor·pic·rin
Chlo·rop·i·dae
chlo·ro·plast
chlo·ro·plas·tin
chlo·ro·pro·caine
chlo·rop·si·a
chlo·ro·pu·rine
chlo·ro·quine
chlo·ro·sar·co·ma
  pl chlo·ro·sar·co·mas
  or chlo·ro·sar·co·ma·ta
chlo·ro·sis
  pl chlo·ro·ses
chlo·ro·stig·ma
chlo·ro·then
chlo·ro·thi·a·zide
chlo·ro·thy·mol
chlo·rot·ic
chlo·rot·i·cal·ly
chlo·ro·tri·an·i·sene
chlo·rous
chlo·ro·vi·nyl·di·chlo·ro·ar·
  sine
chlo·ro·xy·le·nol

chlor·phen·e·sin
chlor·phen·ir·a·mine
chlor·phe·nol
  or chlo·ro·phe·nol
chlor·phen·ox·a·mine
chlor·phen·ter·mine
chlor·pic·rin
  or chlo·ro·pic·rin
chlor·prom·a·zine
chlor·pro·pa·mide
chlor·pro·phen·py·rid·a·
  mine
chlor·pro·thix·ene
chlor·quin·al·dol
chlor·tet·ra·cy·cline
chlor·thal·i·done
chlor·thy·mol
chlor·u·re·sis
chlor·u·ri·a
chlor·zox·a·zone
cho·a·na
  pl cho·a·nae
cho·a·nal
cho·a·nate
Cho·a·no·tae·ni·a
choke
chokes
cho·lae·mi·a
  var of chol·e·mia
cho·lae·mic
  var of cho·le·mic
chol·a·gog
chol·a·gog·ic
chol·a·gogue
  var of chol·a·gog
cho·lal·ic
chol·a·mine
cho·lane
cho·lan·e·re·sis
cho·lan·ge·i·tis
cho·lan·gi·ec·ta·sis
  pl cho·lan·gi·ec·ta·ses
cho·lan·gi·o·car·ci·no·ma
  pl cho·lan·gi·o·car·ci·no·
  mas
  or cho·lan·gi·o·car·ci·no·
  ma·ta
cho·lan·gi·o·en·ter·os·to·
  my

cho·lan·gi·o·gas·tros·to·my
  pl cho·lan·gi·o·gas·tros·to·
  mies
cho·lan·gi·o·gram
cho·lan·gi·o·graph·ic
cho·lan·gi·og·ra·phy
cho·lan·gi·ole
cho·lan·gi·o·lit·ic
cho·lan·gi·o·li·tis
  pl chol·an·gi·o·lit·i·des
cho·lan·gi·o·ma
  pl cho·lan·gi·o·mas
  or chol·an·gi·o·ma·ta
cho·lan·gi·os·to·my
  pl cho·lan·gi·os·to·mies
cho·lan·gi·ot·o·my
  pl cho·lan·gi·ot·o·mies
chol·an·git·ic
chol·an·gi·tis
  pl chol·an·gi·ti·des
cho·lan·ic
cho·lan·o·poi·e·sis
  pl cho·lan·o·poi·e·sis
cho·lan·o·poi·et·ic
chol·an·threne
cho·late
cho·le·bil·i·ru·bin
cho·le·cal·cif·er·ol
cho·le·chro·me·re·sis
cho·le·chro·mo·poi·e·sis
cho·le·cy·a·nin
cho·le·cyst
  or cho·le·cys·tis
cho·le·cyst·a·gogue
cho·le·cys·tal·gi·a
cho·le·cys·tec·ta·si·a
cho·le·cys·tec·to·my
  pl cho·le·cys·tec·to·mies
cho·le·cyst·en·ter·or·rha·
  phy
cho·le·cyst·en·ter·os·to·my
cho·le·cys·tic
cho·le·cys·tis
  or cho·le·cyst
cho·le·cys·ti·tis
  pl cho·le·cys·ti·ti·des
cho·le·cys·to·co·lon·ic
cho·le·cys·to·co·los·to·my
cho·le·cys·to·cu·ta·ne·ous

65

cho·le·cys·to·du·o·de·nal
cho·le·cys·to·du·od·e·no·co·lic
cho·le·cys·to·du·o·de·nos·to·my
   pl cho·le·cys·to·du·o·de·nos·to·mies
cho·le·cys·to·e·lec·tro·co·ag·u·lec·to·my
cho·le·cys·to·en·ter·os·to·my
cho·le·cys·to·gas·tric
cho·le·cys·to·gas·tros·to·my
   pl cho·le·cys·to·gas·tros·to·mies
cho·le·cys·to·gram
cho·le·cys·to·graph·ic
cho·le·cys·tog·ra·phy
   pl cho·le·cys·tog·ra·phies
cho·le·cys·to·il·e·os·to·my
cho·le·cys·to·je·ju·nos·to·my
cho·le·cys·to·ki·net·ic
cho·le·cys·to·ki·nin
cho·le·cys·to·li·thi·a·sis
cho·le·cys·to·li·thot·o·my
cho·le·cys·to·pex·y
   pl cho·le·cys·to·pex·ies
cho·le·cys·tor·rha·phy
cho·le·cys·tos·to·my
   pl cho·le·cys·tos·to·mies
cho·le·cys·tot·o·my
   pl cho·le·cys·tot·o·mies
cho·le·doch
   or cho·led·o·chal
cho·led·o·chal
   or cho·le·doch
cho·led·o·chec·ta·si·a
cho·led·o·chec·to·my
cho·led·o·chi·tis
cho·led·o·cho·cu·ta·ne·ous
cho·led·o·cho·cys·tos·to·my
cho·led·o·cho·cho·do·chor·rha·phy
cho·led·o·cho·cho·du·o·de·nos·to·my

cho·led·o·cho·en·ter·os·to·my
cho·led·o·cho·gas·tros·to·my
cho·led·o·cho·je·ju·nos·to·my
cho·led·o·cho·li·thi·a·sis
   pl cho·led·o·cho·li·thi·a·ses
cho·led·o·cho·li·thot·o·my
   pl cho·led·o·cho·li·thot·o·mies
cho·led·o·cho·lith·o·trip·sy
cho·led·o·cho·plas·ty
cho·led·o·chor·rha·phy
cho·led·o·chos·to·my
   pl cho·led·o·chos·to·mies
cho·led·o·chot·o·my
cho·led·o·chus
   pl cho·led·o·chi
cho·le·glo·bin
cho·le·haem·a·tin
   var of cho·le·hem·a·tin
cho·le·hem·a·tin
cho·le·ic
cho·le·lith
cho·le·li·thi·a·sis
   pl cho·le·li·thi·a·ses
cho·le·lith·ic
cho·le·li·thot·o·my
cho·le·lith·o·trip·sy
cho·le·li·thot·ri·ty
cho·lem·e·sis
   pl cho·lem·e·ses
cho·le·mi·a
cho·le·mic
cho·le·per·i·to·ne·um
cho·le·poi·e·sis
   pl cho·le·poi·e·ses
cho·le·poi·et·ic
cho·le·pra·sin
cho·le·pyr·rhin
chol·er·a
chol·er·a in·fan·tum
chol·er·a mor·bus
chol·er·a·gen
chol·er·a·ic

cho·le·re·sis
   pl cho·le·re·ses
cho·le·ret·ic
chol·er·ic
chol·er·i·form
chol·er·ine
chol·er·oid
chol·er·o·ma·ni·a
chol·er·o·pho·bi·a
chol·er·rha·gi·a
cho·les·tane
cho·les·ta·nol
cho·le·sta·sis
cho·le·stat·ic
cho·les·te·a·to·ma
   pl cho·les·te·a·to·mas
   or cho·les·te·a·to·ma·ta
cho·les·te·a·tom·a·tous
cho·les·te·a·to·sis
   pl cho·les·te·a·to·ses
cho·les·tene
cho·les·te·nol
cho·les·ter·ae·mi·a
   var of cho·les·ter·e·mi·a
cho·les·ter·ase
cho·les·ter·e·mi·a
   or hy·per·cho·les·ter·o·le·mi·a
cho·les·ter·ic
cho·les·ter·in
cho·les·ter·in·e·mi·a
   or cho·les·ter·o·le·mi·a
cho·les·ter·i·nu·ri·a
cho·les·ter·ol
cho·les·ter·o·lae·mi·a
   var of cho·les·ter·o·le·mi·a
cho·les·ter·ol·e·mi·a
   or cho·les·ter·in·e·mi·a
cho·les·ter·ol·er·e·sis
   pl cho·les·ter·ol·er·e·ses
cho·les·ter·ol·o·poi·e·sis
   pl cho·les·ter·ol·o·poi·e·ses
cho·les·ter·ol·o·sis
   pl cho·les·ter·ol·o·ses
cho·les·ter·ol·u·ri·a
cho·les·ter·o·sis
   pl cho·les·ter·o·ses
cho·les·ter·yl

cho·le·ther·a·py
cho·leu·ri·a
cho·le·ver·din
cho·lic
cho·lin·a·cet·yl·ase
cho·line
cho·lin·er·gic
cho·lin·es·ter·ase
cho·li·no·gen·ic
cho·lin·o·lyt·ic
cho·li·no·mi·met·ic
chol·o·chrome
cho·lo·he·mo·tho·rax
cho·lo·lith
cho·lo·li·thi·a·sis
   pl cho·lo·li·thi·a·ses
chol·o·lith·ic
chol·or·rhe·a
cho·lo·tho·rax
cho·lu·ri·a
Cho·man meth·od
chon·do·den·drine
Chon·do·den·dron
chon·dral
chon·dral·gi·a
chon·drec·to·my
   pl chon·drec·to·mies
chon·dri·fi·ca·tion
chon·dri·fy
chon·dri·gen
chon·drin
chon·dri·o·cont
chon·dri·o·ki·ne·sis
   pl chon·dri·o·ki·ne·ses
chon·dri·o·ma
   pl chon·dri·o·mas
   or chon·dri·o·ma·ta
chon·dri·ome
chon·dri·o·mite
chon·dri·o·so·mal
chon·dri·o·some
chon·dri·tis
chon·dro·ad·e·no·ma
chon·dro·al·bu·mi·noid
chon·dro·an·gi·o·ma
chon·dro·an·gi·o·path·i·a
   cal·car·e·a seu punc·ta·ta
chon·dro·blast
chon·dro·blas·tic

chon·dro·blas·to·ma
   pl chon·dro·blas·to·mas
   or chon·dro·blas·to·ma·ta
chon·dro·cal·ci·no·sis
chon·dro·cal·syn·o·vi·tis
chon·dro·cla·sis
   pl chon·dro·cla·ses
chon·dro·clast
chon·dro·co·ni·a
chon·dro·cos·tal
chon·dro·cra·ni·um
   pl chon·dro·cra·ni·ums
   or chon·dro·cra·ni·a
chon·dro·cyte
chon·dro·cyt·ic
chon·dro·der·ma·ti·tis
chon·dro·dyn·i·a
chon·dro·dys·pla·si·a
chon·dro·dys·tro·phi·a
   pl chon·dro·dys·tro·phi·as
   or chon·dro·dys·tro·phy
   pl chon·dro·dys·tro·phies
chon·dro·dys·tro·phic
chon·dro·dys·tro·phy
   pl chon·dro·dys·tro·phies
   or chon·dro·dys·tro·phi·a
   pl chon·dro·dys·tro·phi·as
chon·dro·ec·to·der·mal
chon·dro·en·do·the·li·o·ma
chon·dro·ep·i·phy·si·tis
chon·dro·ep·i·troch·le·ar·is
chon·dro·fi·bro·ma
   pl chon·dro·fi·bro·mas
   or chon·dro·fi·bro·ma·ta
chon·dro·gen
chon·dro·gen·e·sis
   pl chon·dro·gen·e·ses
chon·dro·ge·net·ic
chon·dro·gen·ic
   or chon·drog·e·nous
chon·drog·e·nous
   or chon·dro·gen·ic
chon·dro·glos·sus
   pl chon·dro·glos·si
chon·dro·hu·mer·a·lis
chon·droid
chon·dro·it·ic
chon·dro·i·tin
chon·dro·i·tin·sul·fu·ric

chon·dro·i·tin·u·ri·a
chon·dro·li·po·ma
chon·dro·lip·o·sar·co·ma
   pl chon·dro·lip·o·sar·co·
     mas
   or chon·dro·lip·o·sar·co·
     ma·ta
chon·drol·o·gy
   pl chon·drol·o·gies
chon·dro·ma
   pl chon·dro·mas
   or chon·dro·ma·ta
chon·dro·ma·la·ci·a
chon·dro·ma·to·sis
chon·drom·a·tous
chon·dro·mere
chon·dro·met·a·pla·si·a
chon·dro·mu·cin
chon·dro·mu·coid
chon·dro·mu·co·pro·te·in
chon·dro·my·o·ma
chon·dro·myx·o·he·man·
   gi·o·en·do·the·li·o·sar·
   co·ma
   pl chon·dro·myx·o·he·man·
     gi·o·en·do·the·li·o·sar·
     co·mas
   or chon·dro·myx·o·he·man·
     gi·o·en·do·the·li·o·sar·
     co·ma·ta
chon·dro·myx·oid
chon·dro·myx·o·ma
   pl chon·dro·myx·o·mas
   or chon·dro·myx·o·ma·ta
chon·dro·myx·o·sar·co·ma
   pl chon·dro·myx·o·sar·co·
     mas
   or chon·dro·myx·o·sar·co·
     ma·ta
chon·dro·os·se·ous
chon·dro·os·te·o·dys·tro·
   phy
   pl chon·dro·os·te·o·dys·tro·
     phies
chon·dro·os·te·o·ma
   pl chon·dro·os·te·o·mas
   or chon·dro·os·te·o·ma·ta
chon·dro·os·te·o·sar·co·ma

pl chon·dro·os·te·o·sar·co·mas

or chon·dro·os·te·o·sar·co·ma·ta

chon·drop·a·thy

pl chon·drop·a·thies

chon·dro·pha·ryn·ge·us

pl chon·dro·pha·ryn·ge·i

chon·dro·phyte

chon·dro·pla·si·a

chon·dro·plast

chon·dro·plas·ty

pl chon·dro·plas·ties

chon·dro·po·ro·sis

pl chon·dro·po·ro·ses

chon·dro·pro·te·in

chon·dro·sa·mine

chon·dro·sar·co·ma

pl chon·dro·sar·co·mas

or chon·dro·sar·co·ma·ta

chon·dro·sar·co·ma·tous

chon·dro·sin

chon·dro·sis

pl chon·dro·ses

chon·dro·skel·e·ton

chon·dros·te·o·ma

chon·dro·ster·nal

chon·dro·ster·no·plas·ty

chon·dro·tome

chon·drot·o·my

pl chon·drot·o·mies

chon·dro·xi·phoid

chon·drus

pl chon·dri

cho·ne·chon·dro·ster·non

Cho·part joint

Cho·pra test

chor·da

pl chor·dae

chor·da·blas·to·pore

chor·dae

chor·dal

chor·da·mes·o·blast

chor·da·mes·o·derm

or chor·do·mes·o·derm

chor·da·mes·o·der·mal

or chor·do·mes·o·der·mal

Chor·da·ta

chor·date

chor·da·ten·di·ne·a

pl chor·dae·ten·din·e·ae

chor·dee

chor·de·ic

chord·en·ceph·a·lon

chor·di·tis

chor·do·blas·to·ma

pl chor·do·blas·to·mas

or chor·do·blas·to·ma·ta

chor·do·car·ci·no·ma

pl chor·do·car·ci·no·mas

or chor·do·car·ci·no·ma·ta

chor·do·ep·i·the·li·o·ma

pl chor·do·ep·i·the·li·o·mas

or chor·do·ep·i·the·li·o·ma·ta

chor·doid

chor·do·ma

pl chor·do·mas

or chor·do·ma·ta

chor·do·mes·o·derm

or chor·da·mes·o·derm

chor·do·mes·o·der·mal

or chor·da·mes·o·der·mal

chor·do·skel·e·ton

chor·dot·o·my

pl chor·dot·o·mies

or cor·dot·o·my

pl cor·dot·o·mies

cho·re·a

cho·re·al

cho·re·at·ic

cho·re·ic

cho·re·i·form

cho·re·o·ath·e·toid

or cho·re·o·ath·e·tot·ic

cho·re·o·ath·e·to·sis

pl cho·reo·ath·e·to·ses

cho·re·o·ath·e·tot·ic

or chor·re·o·ath·e·toid

cho·re·oid

cho·re·o·phra·si·a

cho·ri·al

cho·ri·o·ad·e·no·ma

pl cho·ri·o·ad·e·no·mas

or cho·ri·o·ad·e·no·ma·ta

cho·ri·o·al·lan·to·ic

or cho·ri·o·al·lan·to·id

cho·ri·o·al·lan·toid

or cho·ri·o·al·lan·to·ic

cho·ri·o·al·lan·to·is

pl cho·ri·o·al·lan·to·i·des

cho·ri·o·am·ni·on·ic

cho·ri·o·am·ni·o·ni·tis

cho·ri·o·an·gi·o·ma

pl cho·ri·o·an·gi·o·mas

or cho·ri·o·an·gi·o·ma·ta

cho·ri·o·an·gi·op·a·gus

pl cho·ri·o·an·gi·op·a·gi

cho·ri·o·blas·to·sis

pl cho·ri·o·blas·to·ses

cho·ri·o·cap·il·lar·is

cho·ri·o·car·ci·no·ma

pl cho·ri·o·car·ci·no·mas

or cho·ri·o·car·ci·no·ma·ta

cho·ri·o·cele

cho·ri·o·di·tis

or cho·roid·i·tis

cho·ri·o·ep·i·the·li·o·ma

pl cho·ri·o·ep·i·the·li·o·mas

or cho·ri·o·ep·i·the·li·o·ma·ta

cho·rio·ep·i·the·li·o·ma·tous

cho·ri·o·gen·e·sis

pl cho·ri·o·gen·e·ses

cho·ri·oid

or cho·roid

cho·ri·oi·de·a

cho·ri·o·ma

pl cho·ri·o·mas

or cho·ri·o·ma·ta

cho·ri·o·men·in·gi·tis

pl cho·ri·o·men·in·gi·ti·des

cho·ri·on

cho·ri·on·ep·i·the·li·o·ma

pl cho·ri·on·ep·i·the·li·o·mas

or cho·ri·on·ep·i·the·li·o·ma·ta

cho·ri·on·ic

cho·ri·o·ni·tis

Cho·ri·op·tes

cho·ri·op·tic

cho·ri·o·ret·i·nal

cho·ri·o·ret·i·ni·tis

pl cho·ri·o·ret·i·ni·ti·des

or cho·roi·do·ret·i·ni·tis
pl cho·roi·do·ret·i·ni·ti·des
cho·ri·o·ret·i·nop·a·thy
chor·i·sis
  pl chor·i·ses
cho·ris·ta
cho·ris·to·blas·to·ma
  pl cho·ris·to·blas·to·mas
  or cho·ris·to·blas·to·ma·ta
cho·ris·to·ma
  pl cho·ris·to·mas
  or cho·ris·to·ma·ta
cho·roid
  or cho·ri·oid
cho·roi·dal
cho·roi·de·a
cho·roid·e·re·mi·a
cho·roid·i·tis
  or cho·ri·oi·di·tis
cho·roi·do·cy·cli·tis
cho·roi·do·i·ri·tis
cho·roi·do·ret·i·ni·tis
  pl cho·roi·do·ret·i·ni·ti·des
  or cho·ri·o·ret·i·ni·tis
  pl cho·ri·o·ret·i·ni·ti·des
cho·re·ma·ni·a
chre·ma·to·pho·bi·a
Chris·tel·ler meth·od
Chris·ten·sen-Krab·be
  dis·ease
Chris·tian dis·ease
Christian-Web·er dis·ease
Christ·mas dis·ease
chro·maes·the·si·a
  var of chro·mes·the·si·a
chro·maf·fin
  or chro·maf·fine
chro·maf·fine
  or chro·maf·fin
chro·maf·fin·i·ty
chro·maf·fi·no·blas·to·ma
  pl chro·maf·fi·no·blas·to·
    mas
  or chro·maf·fi·no·blas·to·
    ma·ta
chro·maf·fi·no·ma
  pl chor·maf·fi·no·mas
  or chro·maf·fi·no·ma·ta
chro·maf·fi·nop·a·thy

chro·ma·phil
chro·ma·phobe
chro·ma·si·a
chro·mate
chro·ma·te·lop·si·a
chro·ma·te·lop·sis
chro·mat·ic
chro·mat·i·cal·ly
chro·mat·ic·ness
chro·ma·tid
chro·ma·tin
chro·ma·tin-neg·a·tive
chro·ma·tin-pos·i·tive
chro·ma·tism
chro·ma·to·der·ma·to·sis
  pl chro·ma·to·der·ma·to·ses
chro·ma·to·dys·o·pi·a
chro·ma·tog·e·nous
chro·mat·o·gram
chro·mat·o·graph
chro·mat·o·graph·ic
chro·mat·o·graph·i·cal·ly
chro·ma·tog·ra·phy
  pl chro·ma·tog·ra·phies
chro·ma·toid
chro·ma·to·ki·ne·sis
chro·ma·tol·o·gy
chro·ma·tol·y·sis
  pl chro·ma·tol·y·ses
chro·ma·to·lyt·ic
chro·mat·o·mere
chro·ma·tom·e·ter
chro·ma·tom·e·try
chro·ma·to·path·i·a
chro·ma·top·a·thy
  pl chro·ma·top·a·thies
chro·mat·o·phane
chro·mat·o·phil
  or chro·mat·o·phile
chro·mat·o·phile
  or chro·mat·o·phil
chro·ma·to·phil·i·a
  or chro·moph·i·ly
chro·ma·to·pho·bi·a
chro·mat·o·phore
chro·ma·to·pho·ric
chro·ma·to·phor·o·ma
  pl chro·ma·to·phor·o·mas
  or chro·ma·to·phor·o·ma·ta

chro·ma·to·pho·ro·troph·ic
chro·ma·to·pho·ro·trop·ic
chro·ma·toph·o·rous
chro·mat·o·plasm
chro·mat·o·plast
chro·ma·to·pseu·dop·sis
chro·ma·top·si·a
chro·ma·top·sy
chro·mat·op·tom·e·ter
chro·mat·op·tom·e·try
chro·ma·to·sis
  pl chro·ma·to·ses
chro·ma·tu·ri·a
chrome
chro·mes·the·si·a
chrom·het·er·o·tro·pi·a
chrom·hi·dro·sis
  pl chrom·hi·dro·ses
  or chro·mi·dro·sis
  pl chro·mi·dro·ses
chro·mic
chro·mi·cize
chro·mid·i·al
chro·mid·i·o·sis
chro·mid·i·um
  pl chro·mid·i·a
chro·mi·dro·sis
  pl chro·mi·dro·ses
  or chrom·hi·dro·sis
  pl chrom·hi·dro·ses
chro·mi·um
Chro·mo·bac·te·ri·um
  pl Chro·mo·bac·te·ri·a
chro·mo·blast
chro·mo·blas·to·my·co·sis
  pl chro·mo·blas·to·my·co·
    ses
chro·mo·cen·ter
chro·mo·crin·i·a
chro·mo·cys·tos·co·py
chro·mo·cyte
chro·mo·dac·ry·or·rhe·a
chro·mo·der·ma·to·sis
chro·mo·gen
chro·mo·gen·e·sis
  pl chro·mo·gen·e·ses
chro·mo·gen·ic
chro·mo·lip·id
chro·mo·lip·oid

chro·mol·y·sis
chro·mo·mere
chro·mom·e·try
chro·mo·my·co·sis
  pl chro·mo·my·co·ses
chro·mo·nar
chro·mo·ne·ma
  pl chro·mo·ne·ma·ta
chro·mo·ne·mal
chro·mo·nu·cle·ic
chro·mo·nych·i·a
chro·mo·par·ic
chro·mop·a·rous
chro·mo·pec·tic
chro·mo·pex·ic
chro·mo·pex·y
chro·mo·phage
chro·mo·phane
chro·mo·phil
  or chro·mo·phile
chro·mo·phile
  or chro·mo·phil
chro·mo·phil·ic
chro·moph·i·lous
chro·moph·i·ly
  or chro·ma·to·phil·i·a
chro·mo·phobe
chro·mo·pho·bi·a
chro·mo·pho·bic
chro·mo·phore
chro·mo·pho·ric
chro·moph·o·rous
chro·mo·phose
chro·mo·phy·to·sis
chro·mo·plasm
chro·mo·plast
chro·mo·plas·tid
chro·mo·pro·te·in
chro·mop·si·a
chrom·op·tom·e·ter
chro·mo·scope
chro·mo·scop·ic
chro·mos·co·py
  pl chro·mos·co·pies
chro·mo·so·mal
chro·mo·som·al·ly
chro·mo·some
chro·mo·so·mic
chro·mo·ther·a·py

chro·mo·tox·ic
chro·mo·trich·i·al
chro·mo·trich·o·my·co·sis
  vl chro·mo·trich·o·my·co·ses
chro·mo·trope
chro·mo·trop·ic
chro·mous
chro·nax·i·a
  pl chro·nax·i·as
  or chro·nax·ie
  pl chro·nax·ies
  or chro·nax·y
chro·nax·ie
  pl chro·nax·ies
  or chro·nax·y
  or chro·nax·i·a
  pl chro·nax·i·as
chro·nax·im·e·ter
chro·nax·i·met·ric
chro·nax·im·e·try
  pl chro·nax·im·e·tries
chro·nax·y
  or chro·nax·ie
  pl chro·nax·ies
  or chro·nax·i·a
  pl chro·nax·i·as
chron·ic
chro·nic·i·ty
  pl chro·nic·i·ties
chron·o·bi·ol·o·gy
chron·o·graph
chron·o·log·ic
  or chron·o·log·i·cal
chron·o·log·i·cal
  or chron·o·log·ic
chro·nom·e·try
chron·o·pho·bi·a
chron·o·scope
chron·o·tar·ax·is
chron·o·trop·ic
chro·not·ro·pism
chrys·a·lis
  pl chry·sal·i·des
chrys·a·ro·bin
chrys·a·zin
chry·si·a·sis
  pl chry·si·a·ses

chrys·o·cy·a·no·sis
  pl chrys·o·cy·a·no·ses
chrys·o·der·ma
Chrys·o·my·a
Chrys·o·my·i·a
chrys·o·phan
chrys·o·phan·ic
chry·soph·a·nol
Chry·sops
chrys·o·ther·a·py
  pl chrys·o·ther·a·pies
chton·o·pha·gi·a
chtho·noph·a·gy
Church·ill-Cope re·flex
Chvos·tek sign
chy·lae·mi·a
  var of chy·le·mi·a
chy·lan·gi·o·ma
  pl chy·lan·gi·o·mas
  or chy·lan·gi·o·ma·ta
chyle
chy·lec·ta·si·a
chy·le·mi·a
chy·li·dro·sis
chy·li·fa·cient
chy·li·fac·tion
chy·li·fac·tive
chy·lif·er·ous
chy·li·fi·ca·tion
chy·li·form
chy·lo·cele
chy·lo·cyst
chy·lo·der·ma
chy·loid
chy·lol·o·gy
chy·lo·me·di·as·ti·num
chy·lo·mi·cron
  pl chy·lo·mi·crons
  or chy·lo·mi·cra
chy·lo·mi·cro·ne·mi·a
chy·lo·per·i·car·di·um
chy·lo·per·i·to·ne·um
chy·lo·phor·ic
chy·lo·pneu·mo·tho·rax
chy·lo·po·et·ic
  or chy·lo·poi·et·ic
chy·lo·poi·e·sis
  pl chy·lo·poi·e·ses

chy·lo·poi·et·ic
   or chy·lo·po·et·ic
chy·lor·rhe·a
chy·lo·sis
   pl chy·lo·ses
chy·lo·tho·rax
   pl chy·lo·tho·rax·es
   or chy·lo·tho·ra·ces
chy·lous
chy·lu·ri·a
chy·lus
chy·mase
chyme
chy·mi·fi·ca·tion
chy·mo·pa·pa·in
chy·mo·sin
chy·mo·sin·o·gen
chy·mo·tryp·sin
chy·mo·tryp·sin·o·gen
chy·mous
chy·mus
Ciac·ci·o fix·a·tives
ci·bis·o·tome
ci·bo·pho·bi·a
cic·a·trec·to·my
cic·a·tri·cial
cic·a·tric·u·la
   pl cic·a·tric·u·lae
ci·ca·trix
   pl cic·a·trix·es
   or cic·a·tri·ces
cic·a·tri·zant
cic·a·tri·za·tion
cic·a·trize
cic·er·ism
Ci·cu·ta
cic·u·tism
cic·u·tox·in
Cie·szyn·ski rule
ci·gua·ter·a
ci·gua·tox·in
cil·i·ar·i·scope
cil·i·ar·ot·o·my
cil·i·ar·y
Cil·i·a·ta
cil·i·ate
   or cil·i·at·ed
cil·i·at·ed
   or cil·i·ate

cil·i·ec·to·my
cil·i·o·cy·to·pho·ri·a
Cil·i·oph·o·ra
cil·i·oph·o·ran
cil·i·o·ret·i·nal
cil·i·o·scle·ral
cil·i·o·spi·nal
cil·i·um
   pl cil·i·a
cil·i·um in·ver·sum
cil·lo·sis
cil·lot·ic
cim·bi·a
Ci·mex
   pl Cim·i·ces
Ci·mic·i·dae
cim·i·cif·u·ga
cim·i·cif·u·gin
ci·nan·ser·in
cin·cham·i·dine
cin·cho·caine
cin·cho·na
cin·chon·a·mine
cin·chon·ic
cin·chon·i·dine
cin·cho·nine
cin·cho·nism
cin·chon·i·za·tion
cin·chon·ize
cin·cho·phen
cin·cho·tan·nic
cin·cho·tan·nin
cinc·ture
cin·e·an·gi·o·car·di·o·gram
cin·e·an·gi·o·car·di·o·
   graph·ic
cin·e·an·gi·o·car·di·og·ra·
   phy
   pl cin·e·an·gi·o·car·di·og·ra·
   phies
cin·e·an·gi·o·gram
cin·e·an·gi·o·graph·ic
cin·e·an·gi·og·ra·phy
   pl cin·e·an·gi·og·ra·phies
cin·e·den·sig·ra·phy
cin·e·e·soph·a·go·gram
cin·e·flu·o·ro·graph·ic
cin·e·flu·o·rog·ra·phy
   pl cin·e·flu·o·rog·ra·phies

cin·e·mat·ics
   or kin·e·mat·ics
cin·e·mat·o·graph
   or kin·e·mat·o·graph
cin·e·mat·o·graph·ic
cin·e·mat·o·graph·i·cal·ly
cin·e·ma·tog·ra·phy
   pl cin·e·ma·tog·ra·phies
cin·e·ma·to·ra·di·og·ra·phy
cin·e·mi·crog·ra·phy
cin·e·ol
   or cin·e·ole
cin·e·ole
   or cin·e·ol
cin·e·phle·bog·ra·phy
cin·e·plas·tic
cin·e·plas·ty
   pl cin·e·plas·ties
   or kin·e·plas·ty
   pl kin·e·plas·ties
cin·e·ra·di·og·ra·phy
   pl cin·e·ra·di·og·ra·phies
ci·ne·re·a
ci·ne·re·al
cin·er·in
cin·e·roent·gen·o·flu·or·og·
   ra·phy
cin·e·roent·ge·nog·ra·phy
   pl cin·e·roent·ge·nog·ra·
   phies
ci·ne·sis
   or ki·ne·sis
ci·ne·to·plast
   or ki·ne·to·plast
cin·ges·tol
cin·gu·late
cin·gu·lec·to·my
   pl cin·gu·lec·to·mies
cin·gu·lot·o·my
cin·gu·lo·trac·to·my
cin·gu·lum
   pl cin·gu·la
cin·na·mal·de·hyde
cin·na·med·rine
cin·nam·e·in
cin·na·mene
cin·nam·ic
cin·na·mon
cin·nam·yl

cin·nar·i·zine
cin·per·ene
cin·ta·zone
cin·tri·a·mide
ci·on
  or sci·on
cir·ca·di·an
cir·can·nu·al
cir·ci·nate
cir·cle of Wil·lis
cir·cuit
cir·cu·lar
cir·cu·late
cir·cu·la·tion
cir·cu·la·to·ry
cir·cu·lus
  pl cir·cu·li
cir·cum·a·nal
cir·cum·ar·tic·u·lar
cir·cum·cise
cir·cum·ci·sion
cir·cum·cor·ne·al
cir·cum·duc·tion
cir·cum·fer·en·ti·a
cir·cum·fer·en·tial
cir·cum·flex
cir·cum·in·su·lar
cir·cum·len·tal
cir·cum·lo·cu·tion
cir·cum·loc·u·to·ry
cir·cum·ne·vic
cir·cum·nu·cle·ar
cir·cum·oc·u·lar
cir·cum·o·ral
cir·cum·pen·nate
cir·cum·po·lar·i·za·tion
cir·cum·pul·par
cir·cum·re·nal
cir·cum·scribed
cir·cum·stan·ti·al·i·ty
cir·cum·ton·sil·lar
cir·cum·val·late
cir·cum·vas·cu·lar
cir·cus
ci·ro·le·my·cin
cir·rho·sis
  pl cir·rho·ses
cir·rhot·ic

cir·rus
  pl cir·ri
cir·sec·to·my
  pl cir·sec·to·mies
cir·soid
cir·som·pha·los
  pl cir·som·pha·li
cis·sa
Cis·sam·pe·los
cis·tern
cis·ter·na
  pl cis·ter·nae
cis·ter·na chy·li
  pl cis·ter·nae chy·li
cis·ter·na mag·na
  pl cis·ter·nae mag·nae
cis·ter·nae
cis·ter·nal
cis·ter·nog·ra·phy
cis-trans
cis·tron
cis·ves·ti·tism
ci·ten·a·mide
cit·ra·con·ic
cit·ral
cit·ra·min
cit·rate
cit·ric
cit·rin
cit·rine
cit·ri·nin
cir·to·gen·ase
cit·ron
cit·ro·nel·la
cit·ro·nel·lal
ci·tro·vo·rum
ci·trul·lin
cit·rul·li·nae·mi·a
  var of cit·rul·li·ne·mi·a
cit·rul·line
cit·rul·li·ne·mi·a
cit·rul·li·nu·ri·a
Ci·trul·lu
Cit·rus
cit·to·sis
Ci·vat·te poi·ki·lo·der·ma
Civ·i·ni·ni spine
Cla·do·ni·a
clad·o·spo·ri·o·sis

Clad·o·spo·ri·um
clair·voy·ance
  pl clair·voy·an·ces
  or clair·voy·an·cy
  pl clair·voy·an·cies
clair·voy·an·cy
  pl clair·voy·an·cies
  or clair·voy·ance
  pl clair·voy·an·ces
clam·ox·y·quin
clamp
clap
Clar·a cell
clar·i·fi·a·ble
cla·rif·i·cant
clar·i·fi·ca·tion
clar·i·fi·er
clar·i·fy
Clark sign
Clarke col·umn, nu·cle·us
Clarke-Had·field
  syn·drome
clas·mat·o·cyte
clas·mat·o·cyt·ic
clas·ma·to·sis
  pl clas·ma·to·ses
clas·mo·cy·to·ma
  pl clas·mo·cy·to·mas
  or clas·mo·cy·to·ma·ta
clasp
clas·si·fi·ca·tion
clas·si·fy
clas·tic
clas·to·thrix
clath·rate
clath·ra·tion
Clat·wor·thy sign
Claude syn·drome
clau·di·ca·tion
claus·tral
claus·tro·phil·i·a
claus·tro·phobe
claus·tro·pho·bi·a
claus·tro·pho·bi·ac
  or claus·tro·pho·bic
claus·tro·pho·bic
  or claus·tro·pho·bi·ac
claus·trum
  pl claus·tra

72

clau·su·ra
cla·va
pl cla·vae
clav·a·cin
cla·val
cla·vate
or cla·vat·ed
cla·vat·ed
or cla·vate
cla·vate·ly
cla·va·tion
Clav·i·ceps
clav·i·cle
clav·i·cot·o·my
cla·vic·u·la
pl cla·vic·u·lae
cla·vic·u·lar
cla·vic·u·late
cla·vic·u·lec·to·my
clav·i·for·min
clav·i·pec·to·ral
cla·vus
pl cla·vi
Clay·brook sign
Clay·ton gas
clear·ance
clear·ing
cleav·age
cleft
clei·do·cos·tal
clei·do·cra·ni·al
clei·do·hu·iner·al
clei·do·hy·oid
clei·do·ic
clei·do·mas·toid
clei·do·oc·cip·i·tal
clei·do·scap·u·lar
clei·do·ster·nal
clei·dot·o·my
clei·thro·pho·bi·a
clem·as·tine
clem·i·zole
cle·oid
clep·to·ma·ni·a
or klep·to·ma·ni·a
clep·to·ma·ni·ac
or kelp·to·ma·ni·ac
clep·to·pho·bi·a

Cle·ram·bault-Kan·din·sky
com·plex
click
cli·din·i·um
cli·din·i·um bro·mide
cli·er
or cly·er
cli·ma·co·pho·bi·a
cli·mac·te·ri·al
cli·mac·ter·ic
cli·mac·te·ri·um
pl cli·mac·te·ri·a
cli·mac·tic
cli·mate
cli·mat·ic
cli·ma·tol·o·gy
cli·ma·to·ther·a·py
pl cli·ma·to·ther·a·pies
cli·max
clin·da·my·cin
clin·ic
clin·i·cal
clin·i·cal·ly
cli·ni·cian
clin·i·co·haem·a·to·log·ic
var of clin·i·co·hem·a·to·
log·ic
clin·i·co·hem·a·to·log·ic
clin·i·co·path·o·log·ic
or clin·i·co·path·o·log·i·cal
clin·i·co·path·o·log·i·cal
or clin·i·co·path·o·log·ic
clin·i·co·pa·thol·o·gy
clin·i·co·ra·di·o·log·ic
clin·i·co·roent·gen·o·log·ic
clin·i·my·cin
cli·no·ce·phal·ic
cli·no·ceph·a·ly
cli·no·dac·ty·lism
cli·no·dac·ty·lous
cli·no·dac·ty·ly
cli·noid
cli·nom·e·ter
cli·no·met·ric
or cli·no·met·ri·cal
cli·no·met·ri·cal
or cli·no·met·ric
clin·om·e·try
pl clin·om·e·tries

cli·no·scope
cli·ox·a·nide
clip
clis·e·om·e·ter
or klis·e·om·e·ter
clit·i·on
pl clit·i·a
cli·to·ral
or cli·tor·ic
clit·o·ral·gi·a
cli·tor·ic
or cli·to·ral
clit·o·ri·daux·e
cli·to·rid·e·an
clit·o·ri·dec·to·my
pl cli·to·ri·dec·to·mies
clit·o·ri·di·tis
clit·o·ri·dot·o·my
clit·o·ris
pl clit·o·ris·es
or cli·to·ri·des
clit·o·rism
clit·o·ri·tis
clit·o·ro·ma·ni·a
clit·o·ro·meg·a·ly
clit·o·rot·o·my
clit·or·rha·gi·a
cli·vus
pl cli·vi
clo·a·ca
pl clo·a·cae
clo·a·cal
clo·a·ci·tis
clo·a·co·gen·ic
clo·cor·to·lone
clo·faz·i·mine
clo·fi·brate
clo·ges·tone
clo·ma·cran
clo·meth·er·one
clo·min·o·rex
clo·mi·phene
clo·nal
clo·na·ze·pam
clone
clo·nic
clo·nic·i·ty
pl clo·nic·i·ties
clon·i·co·ton·ic

73

clo·nic-ton·ic
clo·ni·dine
clon·ism
clo·ni·trate
clon·o·graph
clo·nor·chi·a·sis
  pl clo·nor·chi·a·ses
  or clo·nor·chi·o·sis
  pl clo·nor·chi·o·ses
clo·nor·chi·o·sis
  pl clo·nor·chi·o·ses
  or clo·nor·chi·a·sis
  pl clo·nor·chi·a·ses
Clo·nor·chis
clo·no·spasm
clo·nus
clo·pam·ide
clo·pen·thix·ol
clo·per·i·done
Clo·quet ca·nal
clor·a·zep·ic
clor·eth·ate
clor·ex·o·lone
clor·o·phene
clor·pren·a·line
clor·ter·mine
clos·trid·i·al
  or clos·trid·i·an
clos·trid·i·an
  or clos·trid·i·al
Clos·trid·i·um
  pl clos·trid·i·a
clo·sure
clo·sy·late
clot
clo·thi·a·pine
clo·thix·a·mide
clo·trim·a·zole
clove
clove-hitch
clown·ism
clox·a·cil·lin
club·bed
club·bing
club·foot
  pl club·feet
club·foot·ed
club·hand
clump·ing

clu·ne·al
clu·nes
clu·pan·o·don·ic
clu·pe·in
  or clu·pe·ine
clu·pe·ine
  or clu·pe·in
Clu·si·a
clus·ter
Clute in·ci·sion
clut·ter·ing
Clut·ton joints
cly·er
  or cli·er
cly·sis
  pl cly·ses
clys·ma
  pl clys·ma·ta
clys·ter
cne·mi·al
cne·mic
cne·mis
  pl cnem·i·des
cni·dar·i·a
cni·do·blast
co·ac·er·vate
co·ac·er·va·tion
co·ad·ap·ta·tion
co·ag·glu·ti·na·tion
co·ag·glu·ti·nin
co·ag·u·la·bil·i·ty
  pl co·ag·u·la·bil·i·ties
co·ag·u·la·ble
co·ag·u·lant
co·ag·u·lase
co·ag·u·late
co·ag·u·la·tion
co·ag·u·la·tive
co·ag·u·lin
co·ag·u·lom·e·ter
co·ag·u·lop·a·thy
co·ag·u·lum
  pl co·ag·u·la
Coak·ley op·er·a·tion
co·a·lesce
co·a·les·cence
co·a·les·cent
co·apt
co·ap·ta·tion

co·arct
co·arc·tate
co·arc·ta·tion
co·arc·tot·o·my
co·ar·tic·u·la·tion
coat
coat·ing
Coats dis·ease
co·bal·a·min
  or co·bal·a·mine
co·bal·a·mine
  or co·bal·a·min
co·balt
co·bal·ti·ni·trite
co·bal·tous
co·bra·ly·sin
co·ca
co·caine
co·cain·ism
co·cain·i·za·tion
co·cain·ize
co·cain·o·ma·ni·a
co·cain·o·ma·ni·ac
co·car·box·y·lase
co·car·cin·o·gen
co·car·cin·o·gen·e·sis
coc·cal
Coc·cid·i·a
coc·cid·i·al
coc·cid·i·an
coc·cid·i·oi·dal
Coc·cid·i·oi·des
coc·cid·i·oi·din
coc·cid·i·oi·do·ma
coc·cid·i·oi·do·my·co·sis
  pl coc·cid·i·oi·do·my·co·
   ses
  or coc·cid·i·o·my·co·sis
  pl coc·cid·i·o·my·co·ses
coc·cid·i·oi·do·sis
  pl coc·cid·i·oi·do·ses
coc·cid·i·o·my·co·sis
  pl coc·cid·i·o·my·co·ses
  or coc·cid·i·oi·do·my·co·sis
  pl coc·cid·i·oi·do·my·co·ses
coc·cid·i·o·sis
  pl coc·cid·i·o·ses
coc·cid·i·o·stat

coc·cid·i·o·stat·ic
coc·cid·i·um
   pl coc·cid·i·a
coc·ci·gen·ic
   or coc·co·gen·ic
coc·ci·nel·la
coc·co·bac·il·la·ry
coc·co·ba·cil·li·form
coc·co·ba·cil·lus
   pl coc·co·ba·cil·li
coc·co·bac·te·ri·a
coc·co·gen·ic
   or coc·ci·gen·ic
coc·cog·e·nous
coc·coid
   or coc·coi·dal
coc·coi·dal
   or coc·coid
coc·cu·lin
coc·cu·lus
coc·cus
   pl coc·ci
coc·cy·al·gi·a
coc·cy·ceph·a·lus
coc·cy·dyn·i·a
coc·cyg·e·al
coc·cy·gec·to·my
   pl coc·cy·gec·to·mies
coc·cyg·e·o·fem·o·ra·lis
coc·cyg·e·o·pu·bic
coc·cyg·e·us
   pl coc·cyg·e·i
coc·cy·go·dyn·i·a
coc·cy·got·o·my
coc·cyx
   pl coc·cyx·es
   or coc·cy·ges
coch·i·ne·al
coch·le·a
   pl coch·le·as
   or coch·le·ae
coch·le·ar
coch·le·are
coch·le·ar·i·form
coch·le·i·tis
coch·le·o·or·bic·u·lar
coch·le·o·pal·pe·bral
coch·le·o·ves·tib·u·lar

Coch·li·o·my·ia
co·chro·ma·to·graph
co·chro·ma·tog·ra·phy
   pl co·chro·ma·tog·ra·phies
co·cil·la·na
Cock·ayne syn·drome
cock·roach
co·con·scious
co·con·scious·ness
co·con·trac·tion
coc·to·an·ti·gen
coc·to·im·mu·no·gen
coc·to·la·bile
coc·to·pre·cip·i·tin
coc·to·sta·bile
co·de·car·box·y·lase
co·de·hy·dro·gen·ase
co·deine
co·dex
   pl cod·i·ces
cod·liv·er oil
Cod·man tri·an·gle
co·dom·i·nance
co·dom·i·nant
co·don
co·dox·ime
co·ef·fi·cient
Coe·len·ter·a·ta
coe·len·ter·ate
coe·len·ter·on
   var of ce·len·ter·on
   pl coe·len·ter·a
coe·li·ac
   var of cel·i·ac
coe·lo·blas·tu·la
coe·lom
   var of cel·om
   or coe·lome
   pl coe·loms
   or coe·lo·ma·ta
coel·o·mate
coe·lome
   or coe·lom
coe·lom·ic
   var of ce·lom·ic
coe·los·chi·sis
   var of ce·los·chi·sis
   pl coe·los·chi·ses

coe·lo·scope
   var of ce·lo·scope
coe·lo·so·my
coe·nes·the·si·a
   var of ce·nes·the·si·a
coe·no·cyte
   var of ce·no·cyte
coe·no·cyt·ic
   var of ce·no·cyt·ic
coe·no·gen·e·sis
   var of ce·no·gen·e·sis
   pl coe·no·gen·e·ses
coe·no·ge·net·ic
   var of ce·no·ge·net·ic
coe·nu·ri·a·sis
   pl coe·nu·ri·a·ses
coe·nu·ro·sis
   pl coe·nu·ro·ses
coe·nu·rus
   pl coe·nu·ri
co·en·zy·mat·ic
co·en·zy·mat·i·cal·ly
co·en·zyme
coeur
co·fac·tor
co·fer·ment
Cof·fey op·er·a·tion
Co·gan syn·drome
cog·nate
cog·ni·tion
cog·ni·tive
co·hab·i·ta·tion
co·here
co·her·ence
co·her·ent
co·he·sion
co·he·sive
Cohn meth·od
Cohn·heim ar·e·a
co·ho·ba
co·hosh
coil
coi·no·site
co·i·tal
co·i·tion
co·i·to·pho·bi·a
co·i·tus
co·i·tus in·ter·rup·tus
   pl co·i·tus in·ter·rup·ti

co·i·tus re·ser·va·tus
  pl co·i·tus re·ser·va·ti
co·la nut
  or ko·la nut
co·la·mine
co·la·tion
col·a·to·ri·um
  pl col·a·to·ri·a
col·a·ture
col·chi·cine
col·chi·cin·i·za·tion
col·chi·cum
cold
cold-blood·ed
co·lec·to·my
  pl col·ec·to·mies
co·le·i·tis
Cole·man-Shaf·fer diet
co·le·o·cele
co·le·o·cys·ti·tis
Co·le·op·ter·a
co·le·op·ter·ous
co·le·op·to·sis
  pl co·le·op·to·ses
co·le·ot·o·my
co·les
Co·ley tox·in
co·li
co·li·bac·il·le·mi·a
co·li·bac·il·lo·sis
co·li·bac·il·lu·ri·a
co·li·ba·cil·lus
  pl co·li·ba·cil·li
col·ic
col·i·ca
col·i·cin
  or col·i·cine
col·i·cine
  or col·i·cin
col·i·ci·no·ge·nic
col·i·ci·no·ge·nic·i·ty
  pl col·i·ci·no·ge·nic·i·ties
col·i·ci·nog·e·ny
  pl col·i·ci·nog·e·nies
col·ick·y
co·li·co·ple·gi·a
co·li·cys·ti·tis
co·li·cys·to·py·e·li·tis
col·i·form

co·li·gran·u·lo·ma
co·li·ne·phri·tis
col·i·phage
co·li·pli·ca·tion
co·li·punc·ture
co·li·py·e·li·tis
co·li·sep·sis
co·lis·ti·meth·ate
co·lis·tin
co·li·tis
co·li·tox·e·mi·a
co·li·tox·i·co·sis
co·li·tox·in
col·i·u·ri·a
col·la·gen
col·la·gen·ase
col·la·gen·a·tion
col·la·gen·ic
col·la·gen·i·za·tion
col·lag·e·no·blast
col·lag·e·no·cyte
col·lag·e·no·gen·ic
col·la·gen·ol·y·sis
col·la·gen·o·lyt·ic
col·la·gen·o·sis
  pl col·la·gen·o·ses
col·lag·e·nous
col·lapse
col·lar
col·lar·bone
col·lar·ette
col·lat·er·al
col·lec·tor
Col·les frac·ture
Col·let syn·drome
col·lic·u·lec·to·my
col·lic·u·li·tis
col·lic·u·lo·ru·bral
col·lic·u·lus
  pl col·lic·u·li
col·li·dine
col·li·ga·tive
col·li·mate
col·li·ma·tion
col·li·ma·tor
col·lin·e·ar
col·lin·e·ar·i·ty
Col·lin·so·ni·a

Col·lip u·nit
col·li·qua·tion
col·li·qua·tive
col·li·tis
col·lo·di·a·phys·e·al
col·lo·di·on
  or col·lo·di·um
col·lo·di·um
  or col·lo·di·on
col·loid
col·loi·dal
col·loi·dal·ly
col·loi·do·cla·si·a
col·loi·do·cla·sis
  pl col·loi·do·cla·ses
col·loi·do·clas·tic
col·loi·do·pex·y
col·loid·oph·a·gy
col·lo·ne·ma
  pl col·lo·ne·mas
  or col·lo·ne·ma·ta
col·lum
  pl col·la
col·lu·nar·i·um
  pl col·lu·nar·i·a
col·lu·to·ri·um
  pl col·lu·to·ri·a
col·lu·to·ry
col·lyr·i·um
  pl col·lyr·i·ums
  or col·lyr·i·a
Col·o·bi·nae
col·o·bine
col·o·bo·ma
  pl col·o·bo·ma·ta
col·o·bo·ma·tous
Col·o·bus
co·lo·ce·cos·to·my
co·lo·cen·te·sis
co·lo·cho·le·cys·tos·to·my
co·loc·ly·sis
co·lo·clys·ter
co·lo·col·ic
co·lo·co·los·to·my
  pl co·lo·co·los·to·mies
co·lo·cu·ta·ne·ous
col·o·cynth
col·o·cyn·thin

76

co·lo·en·ter·i·tis
co·lo·fix·a·tion
co·lo·hep·a·to·pex·y
co·lo·il·e·al
co·lom·bo
  or ca·lum·ba
co·lon
  pl co·lons
  or co·la
co·lo·ni·al
co·lon·al·gi·a
co·lon·ic
co·lon·i·tis
co·lon·op·a·thy
co·lon·or·rha·gi·a
co·lon·or·rhe·a
co·lon·o·scope
co·lon·os·co·py
col·o·ny
col·o·pex·y
col·o·pho·ny
co·lo·pli·ca·tion
co·lo·proc·tec·to·my
co·lo·proc·ti·tis
co·lo·proc·tos·to·my
  pl co·lo·proc·tos·to·mies
col·op·to·si·a
co·lop·to·sis
co·lo·punc·ture
col·or
col·or·blind
co·lo·rec·ti·tis
co·lo·rec·tos·to·my
co·lo·rec·tum
col·or·im·e·ter
col·or·i·met·ric
col·or·im·e·try
  pl col·or·im·e·tries
col·or·rha·phy
co·lo·sig·moid·os·to·my
  pl co·lo·sig·moid·os·to·
    mies
co·los·to·my
  pl co·los·to·mies
co·los·tral
  or co·lus·tric
  or co·los·trous
col·os·tra·tion

co·los·tror·rhe·a
co·los·trum
co·los·trus
  or co·los·tral
  or co·lus·tric
co·lot·o·my
  pl co·lot·o·mies
co·lo·ty·phoid
col·our
  var of col·or
co·lo·vag·i·nal
co·lo·ves·i·cal
col·pal·gi·a
col·pa·tre·si·a
col·pec·ta·si·a
col·pec·to·my
  pl col·pec·to·mies
col·pe·de·ma
col·peu·ry·sis
col·pi·tis
col·po·cele
col·po·clei·sis
  pl col·po·clei·ses
col·po·cys·ti·tis
col·po·cys·to·cele
col·po·cy·to·gram
col·po·cy·tol·o·gy
col·po·dyn·i·a
col·po·hy·per·pla·si·a
col·po·mi·cro·scope
col·po·mi·cros·co·py
col·po·per·i·ne·o·plas·ty
  pl col·po·per·i·ne·o·plas·
    ties
col·po·per·i·ne·or·rha·phy
col·po·pex·y
  pl col·po·pex·ies
col·po·plas·ty
  pl col·po·plas·ties
col·pop·to·sis
col·por·rha·gi·a
col·por·rha·phy
  pl col·por·rha·phies
col·por·rhex·is
  pl col·por·rhex·es
col·po·scope
col·po·scop·ic
col·pos·co·py
  pl col·pos·co·pies

col·po·spasm
col·po·stat
col·po·ste·no·sis
col·po·ste·not·o·my
col·pot·o·my
  pl col·pot·o·mies
col·po·xe·ro·sis
colts·foot
col·u·brid
Co·lu·bri·dae
Col·um·bacz fly
Co·lum·bi·a-SK vi·rus
co·lum·bin
co·lum·bi·um
col·u·mel·la
  pl col·u·mel·lae
col·u·mel·la au·ris
col·u·mel·lar
col·umn of Ber·tin
co·lum·na
  pl co·lum·nae
co·lum·nae a·na·les
co·lum·nar
co·lum·ning
co·lum·ni·za·tion
co·lumns of Mor·ga·gni
co·lus·tric
  or co·los·tral
  or co·los·trous
co·ly·pep·tic
co·ma
com·a·tose
Com·by sign
com·e·do
  pl com·e·do·nes
com·e·do·car·ci·no·ma
  pl com·e·do·car·ci·no·mas
  or com·e·do·car·ci·no·ma·ta
com·e·do·mas·ti·tis
co·mes
  pl com·i·tes
com·frey
com·men·sal
com·men·sal·ism
com·mi·nute
com·mi·nu·tion
Com·miph·o·ra
com·mis·su·ra
  pl com·mis·su·rae

77

com·mis·su·rae
  su·pra·op·ti·cae
com·mis·sur·al
com·mis·sure of Fo·rel
com·mis·sur·or·rha·phy
com·mis·su·ro·spi·nal
com·mis·sur·ot·o·my
  pl com·mis·sur·ot·o·mies
com·mit·ment
com·mo·ti·o
com·mu·ni·ca·bil·i·ty
  pl com·mu·ni·ca·bil·i·ties
com·mu·ni·ca·ble
com·mu·ni·cans
com·mu·ni·cate
com·mu·ni·ca·tion
com·mu·ta·tor
Co·mo·pi·the·cus
com·pac·ta
com·pac·tion
com·par·a·scope
  or com·par·o·scope
com·par·a·tive
com·pa·ra·tor
com·par·o·scope
  or com·par·a·scope
com·pat·i·bil·i·ty
  pl com·pat·i·bil·i·ties
com·pat·i·ble
com·pen·sate
com·pen·sa·tion
com·pen·sa·to·ry
com·pe·tence
com·pe·ten·cy
  pl com·pe·ten·cies
com·pe·tent
com·pe·ti·tive
com·plaint
com·ple·ment
com·ple·men·tal
com·ple·men·ta·ry
com·ple·men·ta·tion
com·ple·men·toid
com·ple·men·to·phil
com·plex
com·plex·ion
com·plex·ion·al
com·plex·ioned

com·plex·us
  pl com·plex·us
com·pli·ance
  or com·pli·an·cy
  pl com·pli·an·cies
com·pli·an·cy
  pl com·pli·an·cies
  or com·pli·ance
com·pli·cate
com·pli·ca·tion
com·po·nent
com·pos men·tis
com·pos·ite
com·po·si·tion
com·pound
com·press
com·pres·sion
com·pres·sor
Comp·ton ef·fect
com·pul·sion
com·pul·sive
co·mus
con·al·bu·min
co·nar·i·um
  pl co·nar·i·a
co·na·tion
co·na·tion·al
con·a·tive
con·can·a·val·in
Con·ca·to dis·ease
con·cave
con·cav·i·ty
  pl con·cav·i·ties
con·ca·vo·con·cave
con·ca·vo·con·vex
con·ceive
con·cen·trate
con·cen·tra·tion
con·cen·tric
con·cept
con·cep·tion
con·cep·tion·al
con·cep·tive
con·cep·tus
  pl con·cep·tus·es
  or con·cep·ti
con·cha
  pl con·chae

con·chi·tis
con·choid·al
con·choid·al·ly
con·cho·tome
con·chot·o·my
con·cli·na·tion
con·com·i·tant
con·cor·dance
con·cre·ment
con·cres·cence
con·cres·cent
con·cre·ti·o
con·cre·tion
con·cre·tiz·ing
con·cur·rent
con·cuss
con·cus·sion
con·cus·sive
con·cus·sive·ly
con·den·sate
con·den·sa·tion
con·dense
con·dens·er
con·di·tion
con·di·tion·al
con·di·tion·al·ly
con·di·tioned
con·di·tion·ing
con·dom
con·duct
con·duc·tance
con·duc·ti·bil·i·ty
con·duc·tion
con·duc·tiv·i·ty
  pl con·duc·tiv·i·ties
con·duc·to·met·ric
con·duc·tom·e·try
con·duc·tor
con·du·pli·ca·to cor·po·re
con·du·ran·gin
con·du·ran·go
con·dy·lar
con·dy·lar·thro·sis
  pl con·dy·lar·thro·ses
con·dyle
con·dy·lec·to·my
con·dyl·i·on
con·dy·loid

con·dy·lo·ma
   pl con·dy·lo·mas
   or con·dy·lo·ma·ta
con·dy·lom·a·tous
con·dy·lot·o·my
   pl con·dy·lot·o·mies
con·dy·lus
   pl con·dy·li
cone
cone-mon·o·chro·mat
cone·nose
co·nex·us
con·fab·u·la·tion
con·fec·ti·o
   pl con·fec·ti·o·nes
con·fec·tion
con·fer·tus
con·fi·den·ti·al·i·ty
con·fig·u·ra·tion
con·fig·u·ra·tion·al
con·fig·u·ra·tion·al·ly
con·fig·u·ra·tive
con·fine·ment
con·flict
con·flu·ence
con·flu·ens sin·u·um
con·flu·ent
con·fo·cal
con·for·ma·tion
con·for·ma·tion·al
con·for·ma·tion·al·ly
con·for·ma·tor
con·form·er
con·fron·ta·tion
con·fu·sion
con·fu·sion·al
con·geal
con·ge·la·tion
con·ge·ne·ic
con·ge·ner
con·ge·ner·ic
con·gen·er·ous
con·gen·i·tal
con·gen·i·tal·ly
con·ger·ies
con·gest
con·gest·ed
con·ges·tin

con·ges·tion
con·ges·tive
con·gi·us
   pl con·gi·i
con·glo·bate
con·glo·ba·tion
con·glom·er·ate
con·glom·er·a·tion
con·glu·tin
con·glu·ti·nant
con·glu·ti·nate
con·glu·ti·na·tion
con·glu·ti·nin
con·gress
con·gru·ence
con·gru·ent
con·hy·drine
con·i·cal
co·nic·e·ine
co·nid·i·al
co·nid·i·o·phore
co·nid·i·oph·o·rous
co·nid·i·o·spore
co·nid·i·um
   pl co·nid·i·a
co·ni·ine
co·ni·o·fi·bro·sis
co·ni·ol·o·gy
   or ko·ni·ol·o·gy
co·ni·om·e·ter
   or ko·ni·om·e·ter
co·ni·o·sis
   or ko·ni·o·sis
co·ni·o·spo·ri·o·sis
co·ni·o·spo·ro·sis
co·ni·o·tox·i·co·sis
co·ni·um
con·i·za·tion
con·joined
con·joint
con·ju·gal
con·ju·gal·i·ty
   pl con·ju·gal·i·ties
con·ju·gal·ly
con·ju·gant
con·ju·ga·ta
   pl con·ju·ga·tae
con·ju·gate

con·ju·ga·tion
con·junc·ti·va
   pl con·junc·ti·vas
   or con·junc·ti·vae
con·junc·ti·val
con·junc·ti·vi·tis
con·junc·ti·vo·ma
con·junc·ti·vo·plas·ty
con·nec·ter
   or con·nec·tor
con·nec·tive
con·nec·tor
   or con·nect·er
Con·nell su·ture
con·nex·us
co·noid
   or co·noid·al
co·noid·al
   or co·noid
Con·ol·ly sys·tem
Co·no·rhi·nus
con·qui·nine
Con·rad·i dis·ease
con·san·guin·e·ous
con·san·guin·e·ous·ly
con·san·guin·i·ty
   pl con·san·guin·i·ties
con·science
con·scious
con·scious·ly
con·scious·ness
con·sec·u·tive
con·sen·su·al
con·sen·su·al·ly
con·sent
con·ser·va·tive
con·serve
con·sis·tence
con·sis·ten·cy
con·sol·i·dant
con·sol·i·date
con·sol·i·da·tion
con·so·lute
con·so·nat·ing
con·sper·gent
con·stant
con·stel·la·tion
con·sti·pate

con·sti·pa·tion
con·sti·tute
con·sti·tu·tion
con·sti·tu·tion·al
con·sti·tu·tive
con·strict
con·stric·tion
con·stric·tive
con·stric·tor
con·sult
con·sul·tant
con·sul·ta·tion
con·sume
con·sum·ma·to·ry
con·sump·tion
con·sump·tive
con·sump·tive·ly
con·tact
con·tac·tant
con·tac·tile
con·tac·tol·o·gy
con·tac·tu·al
con·ta·gion
con·ta·gious
con·ta·gious·ly
con·ta·gious·ness
con·ta·gi·um
   pl con·ta·gi·a
con·tam·i·nant
con·tam·i·nate
con·tam·i·na·tion
con·tem·pla·ti·o
con·tem·pla·tive
con·tent
con·ti·gu·i·ty
   pl con·ti·gu·i·ties
con·tig·u·ous
con·tig·u·ous·ly
con·tig·u·ous·ness
con·ti·nence
co·ti·nent
con·tin·gen·cy
con·tin·u·ous
con·tcr·tion
con·tour
con·tra-an·gles
con·tra-ap·er·ture
con·tra·cep·tion
con·tra·cep·tive

con·tract
con·tract·i·bil·i·ty
   pl con·tract·i·bil·i·ties
   or con·tract·til·i·ty
   pl con·tract·til·i·ties
con·trac·tile
con·trac·til·i·ty
   pl con·trac·til·i·ties
   or con·tract·i·bil·i·ty
   pl con·tract·i·bil·i·ties
con·trac·tion
con·trac·tor
con·trac·ture
con·tra·fis·su·ra
con·tra·fis·sure
con·tra·in·ci·sion
con·tra·in·di·cant
con·tra·in·di·cate
con·tra·in·di·ca·tion
con·tra·in·dic·a·tive
con·tra·lat·er·al
con·trar·i·ness
con·trast
con·tra·stim·u·lant
con·tra·sug·gest·i·bil·i·ty
con·tra·ver·sion
con·tra·ver·sive
con·tre·coup
con·trec·ta·tion
con·trol
con·tuse
con·tu·sion
co·nus
   pl co·ni
co·nus ar·te·ri·o·sus
   pl co·ni ar·te·ri·o·si
con·va·lesce
con·va·les·cence
con·va·les·cent
con·val·lar·i·a
con·vec·tion
con·vec·tive
con·ver·gence
con·ver·gent
con·ver·sion
con·ver·tin
con·vex
con·vex·i·ty
   pl con·vex·i·ties

con·vex·o-con·cave
con·vex·o-con·vex
con·vo·lute
con·vo·lute·ly
con·vo·lu·tion
con·vo·lu·tion·al
con·vol·vu·lin
con·vol·vu·lus
   pl con·vol·vu·lus·es
   or con·vol·vu·li
con·vul·sant
con·vulse
con·vul·sion
con·vul·si·o par·tic·u·lar·is
con·vul·siv·ant
con·vul·sive
con·vul·sive·ly
Con·way meth·od
Con·way-Byrne
   dif·fu·sion meth·od
Cooke-Pon·der meth·od
Coo·ley a·ne·mi·a, dis·ease
Coo·lidge tube
Coombs test
Coons flu·o·res·cent an·ti·
   bod·y meth·od
Coo·per lig·a·ment
Coo·per meth·od
Coo·pe·ri·a
coo·pe·rid
co·or·di·na·tion
co·os·si·fi·ca·tion
co·os·si·fy
coot·ie
co·pai·ba
co·pal
cope
co·pe·pod
Co·pep·o·da
cop·ing
co·pi·o·pi·a
co·pol·y·mer
co·pol·y·mer·ic
co·po·lym·er·i·za·tion
co·po·lym·er·ize
cop·per
cop·per·as
cop·per·head
co·pre·cip·i·tate

o·pre·cip·i·ta·tion
o·pre·cip·i·tin
op·rem·e·sis
  pl cop·rem·e·ses
op·ro·an·ti·bod·y
op·roc·tic
op·ro·cul·ture
op·ro·lag·ni·a
op·ro·lag·nist
op·ro·la·li·a
op·ro·la·lo·ma·ni·a
op·ro·lith
op·rol·o·gy
  pl cop·rol·o·gies
op·ro·ma
op·ro·pha·gi·a
op·ro·phag·ic
op·roph·a·gist
op·roph·a·gous
op·roph·a·gy
  pl cop·roph·a·gies
op·ro·phe·mi·a
op·ro·phil·i·a
op·ro·phil·i·ac
op·ro·phil·ic
op·roph·i·lous
op·ro·pho·bi·a
op·ro·phra·si·a
op·ro·por·phy·ri·a
op·ro·por·phy·rin
op·ro·por·phy·rin·o·gen
op·ro·por·phy·rin·u·ri·a
op·ro·stane
co·pros·ta·nol
cop·ros·ta·sis
co·pros·ter·ol
cop·ro·zo·a
cop·ro·zo·ic
Cop·tis
cop·u·la
  pl cop·u·las
  or cop·u·lae
cop·u·late
cop·u·la·tion
co·quille
cor
cor·a·cid·i·um
  pl cor·a·cid·i·a
cor·a·co·a·cro·mi·al

cor·a·co·bra·chi·a·lis
  pl cor·a·co·bra·chi·a·les
cor·a·co·cla·vic·u·lar
cor·a·co·hu·mer·al
cor·a·coid
cor·al·li·form
cor·al·lin
  or cor·al·line
cor·al·line
  or cor·al·lin
cord
cor·date
cor·date·ly
cor·dec·to·my
  pl cor·dec·to·mies
cor·dial
cor·di·form
cor·di·tis
cor·do·pex·y
  pl cor·do·pex·ies
cor·dot·o·my
  pl cor·dot·o·mies
  or chor·dot·o·my
  pl chor·dot·o·mies
cor·dy
Cor·dy·lo·bi·a
core
cor·e·cli·sis
  pl cor·e·cli·ses
cor·ec·ta·sis
  pl cor·ec·ta·ses
co·rec·tome
co·rec·to·me·di·al·y·sis
co·rec·to·my
cor·ec·to·pi·a
cor·e·di·al·y·sis
  pl cor·e·di·al·y·ses
cor·e·di·as·ta·sis
co·rel·y·sis
  pl co·rel·y·ses
cor·e·mor·pho·sis
cor·en·cli·sis
cor·e·om·e·ter
cor·e·om·e·try
cor·e·o·plas·ty
cor·e·o·pres·sor
cor·e·ste·no·ma
cor·et·o·my
Co·ri cy·cle

co·ri·a·ceous
co·ri·an·der
co·ri·an·drol
Co·ri·ar·i·a
co·ri·um
  pl co·ri·a
cor·ne·a
cor·ne·al
cor·ne·i·tis
Cor·ne·li·a de Lange syn·
  drome
Cor·nell re·sponse
Cor·nell-Coxe scale
cor·ne·o·bleph·a·ron
cor·ne·o·i·ri·tis
cor·ne·o·man·dib·u·lar
cor·ne·o·oc·u·lo·gy·ric
cor·ne·o·pter·y·goid
cor·ne·o·scle·ra
cor·ne·o·scle·ral
cor·ne·ous
cor·ne·um
  pl cor·nea
cor·nic·u·late
cor·nic·u·lum
  pl cor·nic·u·la
cor·ni·fi·ca·tion
cor·ni·fy
cor·noid
cor·nu
  pl cor·nu·a
cor·nu·a sa·cra·li·a
cor·nu·al
  or cor·nu·ate
cor·nu·ate
  or cor·nu·al
cor·nu·com·mis·sur·al
cor·o·clei·sis
  var of cor·o·cli·sis
cor·o·cli·sis
cor·ol·la
co·rom·e·ter
co·ro·na
  pl co·ro·nae
cor·o·nad
cor·o·nal
cor·o·na·le
cor·o·na·lis

co·ro·na ra·di·a·ta
  pl co·ro·nae ra·di·a·tae
cor·o·nar·i·tis
cor·o·nar·y
  pl cor·o·nar·ies
cor·o·na·vi·rus
cor·o·ner
cor·o·net
co·ro·ni·on
  pl co·ro·ni·a
cor·o·ni·tis
cor·o·no·bas·i·lar
co·ro·no·fa·cial
cor·o·noid
cor·o·noi·dec·to·my
co·ros·co·py
co·rot·o·my
Cor·per and Cohn meth·od
cor·po·ra al·bi·can·tes
cor·po·re·al
cor·po·re·al·ly
corpse
corps·man
  pl corps·men
cor·pu·lence
  or cor·pu·len·cy
cor·pu·len·cy
  pl cor·pu·len·cies
  or cor·pu·lence
cor·pu·lent
cor pul·mo·na·le
  pl cor·di·a pul·mo·na·li·a
cor·pus
  pl cor·po·ra
cor·pus al·bi·cans
  pl cor·po·ra al·bi·can·ti·a
cor·pus cal·lo·sum
  pl cor·po·ra cal·lo·sa
cor·pus ca·ver·no·sum
  pl cor·po·ra ca·ver·no·sa
cor·pus de·lic·ti
  pl cor·po·ra de·lic·ti
cor·pus lu·te·um
  pl cor·po·ra lu·te·a
cor·pus stri·a·tum
  pl cor·po·ra stri·a·ta
cor·pus·cle
cor·pus·cle of Has·sall
cor·pus·cle of Herbst

cor·pus·cle of Va·ter
cor·pus·cu·la
cor·pus·cu·lar
cor·pus·cu·lum
  pl cor·pus·cu·la
cor·rect
cor·rec·tion
cor·rec·tive
cor·re·late
cor·re·la·tion
cor·rel·a·tive
cor·re·spon·dence
cor·re·spond·ing
Cor·ri·gen pulse
cor·rin
cor·rode
cor·ro·sion
cor·ro·sive
cor·ro·sive·ly
cor·ros·ive·ness
cor·ru·ga·tor
cor·tex
  pl cor·tex·es
  or cor·ti·ces
cor·tex·one
Cor·ti gan·gli·on, or·gan, teeth
cor·ti·cal
cor·ti·cal·ly
cor·ti·cate
cor·ti·cec·to·my
cor·ti·cif·u·gal
co·ti·cin
cor·ti·cip·e·tal
cor·ti·co·a·dre·nal
cor·ti·co·af·fer·ent
cor·ti·co·bul·bar
cor·ti·co·col·lic·u·lar
cor·ti·co·ef·fer·ent
cor·ti·co·ge·nic·u·late
cor·ti·co·hy·po·tha·lam·ic
cor·ti·coid
cor·ti·co·ni·gral
cor·ti·co·nu·cle·ar
cor·ti·co·pal·li·dal
cor·ti·co·pon·tile
cor·ti·co·pon·tine
cor·ti·co·pon·to·cer·e·bel·lar

cor·ti·co·ru·bral
cor·ti·co·spi·nal
cor·ti·co·ste·roid
cor·ti·cos·ter·one
cor·ti·co·stri·ate
cor·ti·co·stri·a·to·spi·nal
cor·ti·co·stri·o·ni·gral
cro·ti·co·tha·lam·ic
cor·ti·co·troph·ic
cor·ti·co·troph·in
  or cor·ti·co·tro·pin
cor·ti·co·trop·ic
cor·ti·co·tro·pin
  or cor·ti·co·troph·in
cor·tin
cor·ti·sol
cor·ti·sone
cor·to·dox·one
cor·tol
cor·to·lone
cor·run·dum
cor·us·ca·tion
cor·vus
cor·y·ban·tism
co·ryd·a·lis
co·rym·bi·form
Cor·y·ne·bac·te·ri·a·ce·ae
cor·y·ne·bac·te·ri·al
cor·y·ne·bac·te·ri·um
  pl cor·y·ne·bac·te·ria
co·ryne·form
co·ry·za
co·ry·zal
co·ry·za·vi·rus
cos·met·ic
cos·me·ti·cian
cos·mo·tron
cos·ta
  pl cos·tae
cos·tal
cos·tal·gi·a
cos·ta·lis
cos·tate
cos·tec·to·my
  pl cor·tec·to·mies
Cos·ten syn·drome
cos·ti·car·ti·lage
cos·ti·form
cos·tive

cos·tive·ness
cos·to·ar·tic·u·lar
cos·to·cap·u·la·ris
cos·to·car·ti·lage
cos·to·cen·tral
cos·to·cer·vi·cal
cos·to·cer·vi·ca·lis
cos·to·chon·dral
cos·to·chon·dri·tis
cos·to·cla·vic·u·lar
cos·to·col·ic
cos·to·cor·a·coid
cos·to·di·a·phrag·mat·ic
cos·to·gen·ic
cos·to·lum·bar
cos·to·me·di·as·ti·nal
cos·to·phren·ic
cos·to·scap·u·lar
cos·to·ster·nal
cos·to·ster·no·plas·ty
cos·to·tome
cos·tot·o·my
cos·to·trans·verse
cos·to·trans·ver·sec·to·my
   pl cos·to·trans·ver·sec·to·
    mies
cos·to·ver·te·bral
cos·to·xiph·oid
co·syn·tro·pin
co·tar·nine
co·throm·bo·plas·tin
cot·i·nine
co·to
co·trans·duc·tion
cot·ton
cot·ton frac·ture
co·twin
cot·y·le·don
cot·y·le·do·nar·y
cot·y·loid
couch·ing
cou·de
cough
cou·lomb
cou·ma·phos
cou·ma·rin
   or cu·ma·rin
Coun·cil·man bod·ies
coun·sel

coun·seled
   or coun·selled
coun·sel·ing
   or coun·sel·ling
coun·sel·lor
   or coun·sel·or
coun·sel·or
   or coun·sel·lor
count
coun·ter
coun·ter·act
coun·ter·ac·tion
coun·ter·con·di·tion·ing
coun·ter·cur·rent
coun·ter·die
coun·ter·ex·ten·sion
coun·ter·fis·sure
coun·ter·in·ci·sion
coun·ter·in·di·ca·tion
coun·ter·in·vest·ment
coun·ter·ir·ri·tant
coun·ter·ir·ri·tate
coun·ter·ir·ri·ta·tion
coun·ter·o·pen·ing
coun·ter·pho·bi·a
coun·ter·pho·bic
coun·ter·poi·son
coun·ter·pres·sure
coun·ter·pul·sa·tion
coun·ter·punc·ture
coun·ter·shock
coun·ter·stain
coun·ter·stroke
coun·ter·trac·tion
coun·ter·trans·fer·ence
coun·ter·trend
coup
coup-con·tre-coup
cou·pling
course
court plas·ter
Cour·voi·sier law
cou·vade
Cou·ve·laire u·ter·us
co·va·lence
co·va·lent
co·va·ri·ance
cove·plane
cover glass

cover·slip
Cow hock
cow·age
   or cow·hage
Cow·dri·a
Cow·en sign
cow·hage
   or cow·age
cow·hocked
Cow·ie test
cow·itch
Cow·ling rule
Cow·per cyst, gland
cow·per·i·tis
cow·pox
Cox vac·cine
cox·a
   pl cox·ae
cox·al
cox·al·gi·a
   or cox·al·gy
cox·al·gic
cox·al·gy
   pl cox·al·gies
   or cox·al·gi·a
cox·ar·thri·tis
cox·ar·throc·a·ce
cox·ar·thro·lis·thet·ic
cox·ar·throp·a·thy
Cox·i·el·la
cox·i·tis
   pl cox·i·ti·des
cox·o·dyn·i·a
cox·o·fem·o·ral
Cox·sack·ie dis·ease,
   vi·rus
cox·ot·o·my
cox·o·tu·ber·cu·lo·sis
co·zy·mase
Coz·so·li·no zone
Crab·tree ef·fect
cra·dle
Crä·mer meth·od
cramp
Cran·dall test
cra·ni·ad
cra·ni·al
cra·ni·al·ly
Cra·ni·a·ta

cra·ni·ate
cra·ni·ec·to·my
   pl cra·ni·ec·to·mies
cra·ni·o·buc·cal
cra·ni·o·car·po·tar·sal
cra·ni·o·cele
cra·ni·o·cer·e·bral
cra·ni·o·cer·vi·cal
cra·ni·oc·la·sis
   pl cra·ni·oc·la·ses
cra·ni·o·clast
cra·ni·o·clas·ty
cra·ni·o·clei·do·dys·os·to·
   sis
   pl cra·ni·o·clei·do·dys·os·
     to·ses
cra·ni·o·did·y·mus
   pl cra·ni·o·did·y·mi
cra·ni·o·fa·cial
cra·ni·o·fe·nes·tri·a
cra·ni·o·graph
cra·ni·og·ra·phy
cra·ni·o·la·cu·ni·a
cra·ni·ol·o·gy
   pl cra·ni·ol·o·gies
cra·ni·o·ma·la·ci·a
cra·ni·o·me·taph·y·se·al
cra·ni·om·e·ter
cra·ni·o·met·ric
cra·ni·om·e·try
   pl cra·ni·om·e·tries
cra·ni·op·a·gus
   pl cra·ni·op·a·gi
cra·ni·op·a·thy
   pl cra·ni·op·a·thies
cra·ni·o·pha·ryn·ge·al
cra·ni·o·pha·ryn·gi·o·ma
   pl cra·ni·o·pha·ryn·gi·o·mas
   or cra·ni·o·pha·ryn·gi·o·ma·
     ta
cra·ni·o·phore
cra·ni·o·plas·ty
   pl cra·ni·o·plas·ties
cra·ni·o·ra·chis·chi·sis
   pl cra·ni·o·ra·chis·chi·ses
cra·ni·o·sa·cral
cra·ni·os·chi·sis
   pl cra·ni·os·chi·ses

cra·ni·o·scle·ro·sis
cra·ni·os·co·py
   pl cra·ni·os·co·pies
cra·ni·o·spi·nal
cra·ni·o·stat
cra·ni·o·ste·no·sis
   pl cra·ni·o·ste·no·ses
cra·ni·os·to·sis
   pl cra·ni·os·to·ses
cra·ni·o·syn·os·to·sis
   pl cra·ni·o·syn·os·to·sis·es
   or cra·ni·o·syn·os·to·ses
cra·ni·o·ta·bes
   pl cra·ni·o·ta·bes
cra·ni·o·ta·bet·ic
cra·ni·o·tome
cra·ni·ot·o·my
   pl cra·ni·ot·o·mies
cra·ni·o·trac·tor
cra·ni·o·tym·pan·ic
cra·ni·o·ver·te·bral
cra·ni·um
   pl cra·ni·ums
   or cra·ni·a
crap·u·lence
crap·u·lent
crap·u·lous
craque·le
cra·sis
   pl cra·ses
cra·ter
cra·ter·i·form
cra·ter·i·za·tion
cra·vat
craw-craw
C-re·ac·tive
crease
cre·at·ic
cre·a·ti·nae·mi·a
   var of cre·a·ti·ne·mi·a
cre·at·i·nase
cre·a·tine
cre·a·ti·ne·mi·a
crea·tine·phos·pho·ric
cre·at·i·nine
cre·a·tin·u·ri·a
cre·a·tor·rhe·a
cre·a·tor·rhoe·a
   var of cre·a·tor·rhe·a

crè·che
cre·mains
cre·mas·ter
crem·as·te·ri·al
cre·mas·ter·ic
cre·mate
cre·ma·tion
cre·ma·to·ri·um
   pl crema·to·ri·ums
   or crema·to·ri·a
cre·ma·to·ry
   pl crema·to·ries
crème
crem·no·pho·bi·a
cre·na
   pl cre·nae
cre·nate
   or cre·nat·ed
cre·nat·ed
   or cre·nate
cre·na·tion
cre·no·cyte
cre·no·cy·to·sis
Cren·o·thrix po·lys·po·ra
cre·oph·a·gy
   pl cre·oph·a·gies
cre·o·sol
cre·o·sote
cre·o·tox·in
   or kre·o·tox·in
cre·o·tox·ism
   or kre·o·tox·ism
crep·i·tance
crep·i·tant
crep·i·tate
crep·i·ta·ti·o
crep·i·ta·tion
crep·i·tus
   pl crep·i·tus
cre·pus·cu·lar
cres·cent
cres·cen·tic
cres·co·graph
cre·sol
cre·sot·ic
cres·o·tin·ic
crest
cres·yl
cres·yl·ate

cre·syl·ic
cre·ta
cre·ta·ceous
cre·tin
Cré·tin meth·od
cre·tin·oid
cre·tin·ous
Cré·tin-Pou·yanne
  meth·od
cre·tin·ism
Creutz·feldt-Ja·kob
  dis·ease
cre·vice
cre·vic·u·lar
crib·ber
crib·bing
crib·rate
crib·ra·tion
crib·ri·form
crib·rose
cri·brum
cri·ce·tid
Cri·cet·i·dae
cric·e·tine
Cri·ce·tu·lus
Cri·ce·tus
Crich·ton-Browne sign
crick
cri·co·ar·y·te·noid
cri·co·e·soph·a·ge·al
cri·coid
cri·coi·dec·to·my
cri·co·pha·ryn·ge·al
cri·co·pha·ryn·ge·us
cri·co·thy·re·ot·o·my
cri·co·thy·roid
cri·co·thy·rot·o·my
cri·cot·o·my
cri·co·tra·che·al
cri·co·tra·che·ot·o·my
cri·co·vo·cal
cri du chat syn·drome
Crig·ler-Naj·jar syn·drome
Crile the·o·ry
crim·i·nol·o·gy
  pl crim·i·nol·o·gies
cri·nis
  pl cri·nes
crin·o·gen·ic

cri·nos·i·ty
cri·nous
crip·ple
crise de de·glo·bu·li·sa·tion
cri·sis
  pl cri·ses
Crisp an·eu·rysm
cris·pa·tion
cris·pa·tu·ra
cris·ta
  pl cris·tae
cris·ta a·cous·ti·ca
  pl cris·tae a·cous·ti·ca
cris·tate
crit
crith
Cri·thid·i·a
cri·thid·i·form
crit·i·cal
crit·i·cal·ly
crock
Crock·er tu·mor 180
Crocq dis·ease
cro·cus
  pl cro·cus·es
Crohn dis·ease
cro·mo·lyn
Crooke cells
Crookes tube
cross
cross·bite
cross·breed·ing
cross·eye
cross·eyed
cross·fer·ti·li·za·tion
cross·fir·ing
cross·ing o·ver
cross·link
cross·match·ing
cross·re·ac·tion
cross·re·ac·tive
cross·re·ac·tiv·i·ty
cross·way
cro·ta·lid
Cro·tal·i·dae
crot·a·lin
cro·ta·line
cro·ta·lism
Cro·ta·lus

cro·tam·i·ton
cro·taph·i·on
crotch
crotch·et
cro·tin
Cro·ton
cro·ton·al·de·hyde
cro·ton·ic
cro·ton·ism
cro·to·nyl
cro·tox·in
croup
croup·ine
croup·ous
croup·y
Crou·zon dis·ease
Crou·zon-A·pert dis·ease
Crowe sign
crown
crown·ing
cru·ces
cru·cial
cru·ci·ate
cru·ci·ble
cru·ci·form
crude
cru·fo·mate
crup·per
cru·ra
cru·ral
cru·re·us
crur·or
cru·ro·scro·tal
cru·ro·ves·i·cal
crus
  pl cru·ra
crus·ot·o·my
crust
crus·ta
  pl crus·tae
Crus·ta·ce·a
crus·ta·ce·an
crust·al
crutch
Cru·veil·hier dis·ease
Cru·veil·hier-Baum-
  gar·ten syn·drome

crux
  pl crux·es
  or cru·ces
Cruz dis·ease
cry
  cried
cry·aes·the·si·a
  var of cry·es·the·si·a
cry·al·ge·si·a
cry·an·es·the·si·a
cry·es·the·si·a
cry·mo·an·es·the·si·a
cry·mo·dyn·i·a
cry·mo·phil·ic
cry·o·ther·a·py
  pl cry·mo·ther·a·pies
  or cry·o·ther·a·py
  pl cry·o·ther·a·pies
cry·o·bank
cry·o·bi·o·log·i·cal
cry·o·bi·o·log·i·cal·ly
cry·o·bi·ol·o·gist
cry·o·bi·ol·o·gy
  pl cry·o·bi·ol·o·gies
cry·o·cau·ter·y
cry·o·chem
cry·o·crit
cry·o·ex·trac·tion
cry·o·ex·trac·tor
cry·o·fi·brin·o·gen
cry·o·fi·brin·o·gen·e·mi·a
cry·o·gen
cry·o·gen·ic
cry·o·gen·i·cal·ly
cry·o·gen·ics
cry·og·e·ny
  pl cry·og·e·nies
cry·o·glob·u·lin
cry·o·glob·u·li·ne·mi·a
cry·o·hy·drate
cry·o·hy·poph·y·sec·to·my
cry·om·e·ter
cry·on·ics
cry·op·a·thy
cry·o·phil·ic
cry·o·phy·lac·tic
cry·o·pre·cip·i·tate
cry·o·pre·cip·i·ta·tion
cry·o·probe

cry·o·pro·tec·tive
cry·o·pro·te·in
cry·o·scope
cry·o·scop·ic
  or cry·o·scop·i·cal
cry·o·scop·i·cal
  or cry·o·scop·ic
cry·os·co·py
  pl cry·os·co·pies
cry·o·stat
cry·o·sur·geon
cry·o·sur·gi·cal
cry·o·sur·ger·y
cry·o·thal·a·mec·to·my
cry·o·thal·a·mot·o·my
cry·o·ther·a·py
  pl cry·o·ther·a·pies
  or cry·mo·ther·a·py
  pl cry·mo·ther·a·pies
cry·o·tol·er·ant
cry·o·tome
crypt
crypt of Lie·ber·kühn
crypt of Mor·gag·ni
cryp·ta
  pl cryp·tae
cryp·taes·the·si·a
  var of cryp·tes·the·si·a
crypt·am·ne·si·a
crypt·an·am·ne·si·a
crypt·tec·to·my
crypt·ten·a·mine
crypt·tes·the·si·a
cryp·tic
cryp·ti·cal·ly
cryp·ti·tis
cryp·to·bi·o·sis
  pl cryp·to·bi·o·ses
cryp·to·ceph·a·lus
cryp·to·coc·co·sis
  pl cryp·to·coc·co·ses
Cryp·to·coc·cus
  pl Cryp·to·coc·ci
cryp·to·crys·tal·line
cryp·to·did·y·mus
cryp·to·gam
Cryp·to·gam·i·a
cryp·to·gam·ic
  or cryp·tog·a·mous

cryp·tog·a·mous
  or cryp·to·gam·ic
cryp·to·gen·ic
cryp·to·ge·net·ic
cryp·to·gli·o·ma
cryp·to·in·fec·tion
cryp·to·lith
cryp·to·men·or·rhe·a
cryp·to·mer·o·ra·chis·chi·sis
cryp·tom·ne·si·a
cryp·tom·ne·sic
cryp·toph·thal·mi·a
cryp·toph·thal·mos
cryp·to·pine
cryp·to·po·di·a
cryp·top·o·rous
cryp·to·py·ic
cryp·to·pyr·role
cryp·tor·chid
  or cryp·tor·chis
cryp·tor·chi·dec·to·my
cryp·tor·chid·ism
  or cryp·tor·chism
cryp·tor·chi·do·pe·xy
cryp·tor·chis
  or cryp·tor·chid
cryp·tor·chism
  or cryp·tor·chid·ism
cryp·to·xan·thin
cryp·to·zo·ite
cryp·to·zy·gous
crys·tal
crys·tal·bu·min
crys·tal·fi·brin
crys·tal·lin
crys·tal·line
crys·tal·lite
crys·tal·li·za·tion
crys·tal·lize
crys·tal·lo·gram
crys·tal·lo·graph·ic
  or crys·tal·lo·graph·i·cal
crys·tal·lo·graph·i·cal
  or crys·tal·lo·graph·ic
crys·tal·log·ra·phy
  pl crys·tal·lo·graph·ies
crys·tal·loid
crys·tal·loid·al

crys·tal·lo·mag·net·ism
crys·tal·lo·pho·bi·a
crys·tal·lu·ri·a
Cten·o·ce·phal·i·des
cte·noids
Cten·op·syl·lus seg·nis
cu·beb
cu·beb·ism
cu·bi·form
cu·bi·tal
cu·bi·tus
  pl cu·bi·ti
cu·boid
cu·boi·dal
cu·boi·de·o·na·vic·u·lar
cu·boi·do·dig·i·tal
cu·cum·ber
Cu·cu·mis
Cu·cur·bi·ta
cud·bear
cuff
cuff·ing
cui·rass
cul-de-sac
  pl cul-de-sacs
  or culs-de-sac
cul·do·cen·te·sis
  pl cul·do·cen·te·ses
cul·do·plas·ty
cul·do·scope
cul·do·scop·ic
cul·dos·co·py
  pl cul·dos·co·pies
cul·dot·o·my
Cu·lex
Cu·lic·i·dae
cu·li·cide
cu·lic·i·fuge
Cu·li·ci·nae
cu·li·cine
Cu·li·coi·des
Cul·len sign
cul·men
  pl cul·mens
  or cul·mi·na
cul·ti·vate
cul·ti·va·tion
cul·tur·al
cul·ture

cu·ma·rin
  or cou·ma·rin
cu·mene
cu·mic
cu·min
cu·mol
cu·mu·la·tive
cu·mu·lus
  pl cu·mu·li
cu·mu·lus o·oph·o·rus
cu·ne·ate
  or cu·ne·at·ed
cu·ne·at·ed
  or cu·ne·ate
cu·ne·i·form
cu·ne·o·cu·boid
cu·ne·o·na·vic·u·lar
cu·ne·o·scaph·oid
cu·ne·us
  pl cu·ne·i
cu·nic·u·lus
  pl cu·nic·u·li
cun·ni·linc·tus
  or cun·ni·lin·gus
cun·ni·lin·gu·ism
cun·ni·lin·guist
cun·ni·lin·gus
  or cun·ni·linc·tus
cun·nus
  pl cun·ni
cu·o·rin
cup
cu·po·la
cu·pram·mo·ni·a
cu·pre·a
cu·pre·ine
cu·pric
cu·prous
cu·prum
cu·pru·re·sis
cu·pru·ret·ic
cu·pu·la
  pl cu·pu·lae
cu·pu·lo·gram
cu·pu·lom·e·try
cu·ra·ble
cu·rage
cu·ra·re
  or cu·ra·ri

cu·ra·ri
  or cu·ra·re
cu·ra·ri·form
cu·ra·ri·mi·met·ic
cu·ra·rine
cu·rar·i·za·tion
cu·ra·rize
cu·ra·tive
curb
cur·cu·ma
cur·cu·min
curd
cure
cu·ret
cu·ret·tage
  or cu·rette·ment
cu·rette
  var of cu·ret
cu·rette·ment
  or cu·ret·tage
cu·rie
cu·rie·gram
cu·rie·ther·a·py
cu·rine
cu·ri·os·co·py
cu·ri·um
Cur·ling ul·cer
Cur·rens for·mu·la
cur·rent
Cursch·mann spi·rals
cur·va·tor coc·cyg·e·us
cur·va·tu·ra
  pl cur·va·tu·rae
cur·va·ture
curve
cus·cam·i·dine
cus·cam·in
cus·co·hy·grin
Cush·ing syn·drome
cush·ing·oid
cush·ion
cusp
cus·pate
cus·pid
cud·pi·dal
cus·pi·date
  or cud·pi·dat·ed
cus·pi·dat·ed
  or cus·pi·dat·ed

cus·pi·dat·ed
  or cus·pi·date
cus·pis
  pl cus·pi·des
cu·ta·ne·o·gas·tro·in·tes·ti·
  nal
cu·ta·ne·o·in·tes·ti·nal
cu·ta·ne·o·mu·co·sal
cu·ta·ne·ous
cut·down
Cu·ter·e·bra
Cu·te·re·bri·dae
cu·te·re·brine
cu·ti·cule
cu·ti·col·or
cu·tic·u·la
  pl cu·tic·u·lae
cu·tic·u·lar
cu·tic·u·lar·i·za·tion
cu·ti·dure
cu·tin
cu·tin·i·za·tion
cu·ti·re·ac·tion
cu·tis
  pl cu·tis·es
  or cu·tes
cu·tis an·se·ri·na
  pl cu·tes an·se·ri·nae
cu·ti·sec·tor
cu·ti·za·tion
Cut·ler-Pow·er-Wil·der
  test
Cut·ting col·loid·al mas·tic
  test
cu·vet
  or cu·vette
cu·vette
  or cu·vet
Cu·vier
cy·an·a·mid
  or cy·an·a·mide
cy·an·a·mide
  or cy·an·a·mid
cy·a·nate
cy·a·ne·mi·a
cy·an·eph·i·dro·sis
cy·an·he·mo·glo·bin
cy·an·hi·dro·sis

cy·an·hy·drin
  or cy·a·no·hy·drin
cy·an·ic
cy·a·nide
cy·an·i·dine
cy·an·met·he·mo·glo·bin
  or cy·a·no·met·he·mo·glo·
  bin
cy·an·met·my·o·glo·bin
cy·a·no·a·ce·tic
cy·a·no·ac·ry·late
cy·a·no·chroi·a
cy·a·no·co·bal·a·min
cy·a·no·der·ma
cy·an·o·gen
cy·an·o·gen·ic
  or cy·an·o·ge·net·ic
cy·a·no·gen·e·sis
  pl cy·a·no·gen·e·ses
cy·a·no·ge·net·ic
  or cy·a·no·gen·ic
cy·a·no·hy·drin
  or cy·an·hy·drin
cy·a·nol
cy·a·no·labe
cy·a·no·met·he·mo·glo·bin
  or cy·an·met·he·mo·glo·bin
cy·an·o·phil
  or cy·an·o·phile
cy·an·o·phile
  or cy·an·o·phil
cy·a·no·phil·ic
  or cy·a·noph·i·lous
cy·a·noph·i·lous
  or cy·a·no·phil·ic
cy·a·no·phy·ce·ae
cy·a·no·pi·a
cy·a·nop·si·a
cy·a·nop·sin
cy·a·nosed
cy·a·no·sis
  pl cy·a·no·ses
cy·a·not·ic
cy·a·nur·ic
cy·as·ma
  pl cy·as·ma·ta
cy·ber·cul·tur·al
cy·ber·cul·ture
cy·ber·nat·ed

cy·ber·na·tion
cy·ber·net·ic
  or cy·ber·net·i·cal
cy·ber·net·i·cal
  or cy·ber·net·ic
cy·ber·net·i·cal·ly
cy·ber·ne·ti·cian
cy·ber·net·i·cist
cy·ber·net·ics
cy·borg
cy·ca·sin
cy·cla·mate
cy·clam·ic
cy·cla·min
cy·clan·de·late
cy·clar·thro·sis
  pl cy·clar·thro·ses
cy·clase
cy·claz·o·cine
cy·cle
cy·clec·to·my
cy·clen·ceph·a·lus
cy·clen·ceph·a·ly
cyc·lic AMP
cy·cli·cot·o·my
  pl cy·cli·cot·o·mies
cy·clir·a·mine
cy·clit·ic
cy·cli·tis
cy·cli·tol
cy·cli·za·tion
cy·clize
cy·cli·zine
cy·clo·bar·bi·tal
cy·clo·ceph·a·lus
cy·clo·ceph·a·ly
cy·clo·cho·roi·di·tis
cy·clo·cry·o·ther·a·py
cy·clo·cu·ma·rol
cy·clo·di·al·y·sis
  pl cy·clo·di·al·y·ses
cy·clo·di·a·ther·my
  pl cy·clo·di·a·ther·mies
cy·clog·e·ny
cy·clo·gram
cy·clo·gua·nil
cy·clo·hex·ane
cy·clo·hex·a·nol
cy·clo·hex·i·mide

cy·cloid
cy·clo·i·som·er·ase
cy·clo·ker·a·ti·tis
cy·clol
cy·clo·mas·top·a·thy
cy·clo·meth·y·caine
cy·clo·ni·um
cy·clo·par·af·fin
cy·clo·pen·ta·mine
cy·clo·pen·tane
cy·clo·pen·te·no·phe·nan·threne
cy·clo·pen·thi·a·zide
cy·clo·pen·to·late
cy·clo·phen·a·zine
cy·clo·pho·rase
cy·clo·pho·ri·a
cy·clo·phos·pha·mide
cy·clo·phre·ni·a
cy·clo·phren·ic
Cy·clo·phyl·lid·e·a
cy·clo·phyl·lid·e·an
cy·clo·pi·a
   or cy·clo·py
cy·clo·ple·gi·a
cy·clo·ple·gic
cy·clo·pro·pane
cy·clops
   pl cy·clo·pes
cy·clo·py
   pl cy·clo·pies
   or cy·clo·pi·a
cy·clo·scope
cy·clo·ser·ine
cy·clo·sis
   pl cy·clo·ses
cy·clo·stage
Cy·clo·sto·ma·ta
cy·clos·to·mate
   or cy·clo·sto·ma·tous
cy·clo·sto·ma·tous
   or cy·clos·to·mate
cy·clo·stome
Cy·clos·to·mi
cy·clo·thi·a·zide
cy·clo·thyme
cy·clo·thy·mi·a
cy·clo·thy·mi·ac
cy·clo·thy·mic

cy·clo·ti·a
cy·clo·tome
cy·clot·o·my
   pl cy·clot·o·mies
cy·clo·tron
cy·clo·tro·pi·a
cy·clo·tus
cy·cri·mine
Cy·don·i·a
cy·do·ni·um
cy·e·si·og·no·sis
   pl cy·e·si·óg·no·ses
cy·e·si·ol·o·gy
cy·e·sis
   pl cy·e·ses
cy·hep·ta·mide
cyl·in·der
cy·lin·dric
   or cy·lin·dri·cal
cy·lin·dri·cal
   or cy·lin·dric
cy·lin·dri·form
cyl·in·dro·den·drite
cyl·in·droid
cyl·in·droids
cyl·in·dro·ma
   pl cyl·in·dro·mas
   or cyl·in·dro·ma·ta
cyl·in·dro·sis
   pl cyl·in·dro·ses
cyl·in·dru·ri·a
cyl·lo·so·ma
   pl cyl·lo·so·mas
   or cyl·lo·so·ma·ta
cyl·lo·so·mus
cy·ma·rin
cy·ma·rose
cym·ba
   pl cym·bae
cym·ba con·chae
cym·bi·form
cym·bo·ce·phal·ic
   or cym·bo·ceph·a·lous
cym·bo·ceph·a·lous
   or cym·bo·ce·phal·ic
cym·bo·ceph·a·ly
   pl cym·bo·ceph·a·lies
cy·mene
cy·me·nyl

cy·mo·graph
   or ky·mo·graph
cy·mol
cy·nan·che
cyn·an·thro·pi·a
cyn·an·thro·py
   pl cy·nan·thro·pies
cyn·ic
cyn·o·ceph·a·lous
cyn·o·ceph·a·lus
   pl cyn·o·ceph·a·li
cyn·o·dont
Cyn·o·glos·sum
cyn·o·lys·sa
cyn·o·mol·gus
   pl cyn·o·mol·gi
cyn·o·pho·bi·a
Cyn·o·pi·the·cus
cyn·o·rex·i·a
cyn·u·ren·ic
cyn·u·rin
cy·o·pho·ri·a
cy·oph·o·rin
cy·ot·ro·phy
cy·pen·a·mine
Cy·pe·rus
cy·pi·o·nate
cy·pri·do·pho·bi·a
cyp·ri·pe·di·um
Cy·prin·i·dae
cy·pro·hep·ta·dine
cy·pro·li·dol
cy·pro·quin·ate
cy·pro·ter·one
cy·prox·i·mide
cyr·to·ceph·a·lus
cyr·to·cor·y·phus
cyr·to·graph
cyr·toid
cyr·tom·e·ter
cyr·to·met·o·pus
cyr·tom·e·try
cyr·to·pis·tho·cra·ni·us
cyr·to·sis
   pl cyr·to·ses
cyr·tu·ran·us
cyst

cyst·ad·e·no·car·ci·no·ma
  pl cyst·ad·e·no·car·ci·no·
    mas
  or cyst·ad·e·no·car·ci·no·
    ma·ta
cyst·ad·e·no·fi·bro·ma
  pl cyst·ad·e·no·fi·bro·mas
  or cyst·ad·e·no·fi·bro·ma·ta
cys·tad·e·no·ma
  pl cyst·ad·e·no·mas
  or cyst·ad·e·no·ma·ta
cyst·ad·e·no·sar·co·ma
  pl cyst·ad·e·no·sar·co·mas
  or cyst·ad·e·no·sar·co·ma·ta
cys·tal·gi·a
cys·ta·mine
cys·ta·thi·o·nine
cys·ta·thi·o·nin·u·ri·a
cys·te·amine
cys·tec·ta·si·a
cys·tec·to·my
  pl cys·tec·to·mies
cys·te·ic
cys·te·ine
cys·te·in·yl
cys·ten·ceph·a·lus
cys·tic
cys·ti·cer·coid
cys·ti·cer·co·sis
  pl cys·ti·cer·co·ses
cys·ti·cer·cus
  pl cys·ti·cer·ci
Cys·ti·cer·cus cel·lu·lo·sae
cys·ti·form
cys·tig·er·ous
cys·ti·nae·mi·a
  var of cys·ti·ne·mi·a
cys·tine
cys·tine·ly·si·nu·ri·a
cys·ti·ne·mi·a
cys·ti·no·sis
  pl cys·ti·no·ses
cys·ti·nu·ri·a
cys·ti·stax·is
cys·ti·tis
  pl cys·ti·ti·des
cys·ti·tome
cys·tit·o·my

cys·to·ad·e·no·ma
cys·to·bu·bon·o·cele
cys·to·car·ci·no·ma
  pl cys·to·car·ci·no·mas
  or cys·to·car·ci·no·ma·ta
cys·to·cele
cys·to·co·los·to·my
cys·to·dyn·i·a
cys·to·el·y·thro·plas·ty
cys·to·en·ter·o·cele
cys·to·ep·i·the·li·o·ma
cys·to·fi·bro·ma
  pl cys·to·fi·bro·mas
  or cys·to·fi·bro·ma·ta
cys·to·gas·tros·to·my
cys·to·gen·e·sis
cys·to·gen·i·a
cys·to·gram
cys·to·graph·ic
cys·tog·ra·phy
  pl cys·tog·ra·phies
cys·toid
cys·to·je·ju·nos·to·my
cys·to·lith
cys·to·li·thec·to·my
cys·to·li·thi·a·sis
  pl cys·to·li·thi·a·ses
cys·to·lith·ic
cys·to·li·thot·o·my
cys·to·ma
  pl cys·to·mas
  or cys·to·ma·ta
cys·tom·e·ter
cys·to·met·ro·gram
cys·to·me·trog·ra·phy
cys·tom·e·try
cys·to·mor·phous
cys·to·pa·ral·y·sis
cys·to·pex·y
  pl cys·to·pex·ies
cys·to·pho·tog·ra·phy
cys·to·plas·ty
  pl cys·to·plas·ties
cys·to·ple·gi·a
cys·to·proc·tos·to·my
cys·to·pros·ta·tec·to·my
cys·top·to·sis
cys·to·py·e·li·tis

cys·to·py·e·lo·ne·phri·tis
  pl cys·to·py·e·lo·ne·phri·ti·
    des
cys·to·py·e·log·ra·phy
  pl cys·to·py·e·log·ra·phies
cys·tor·rha·phy
  pl cys·tor·rha·phies
cys·tor·rhe·a
cys·to·sar·co·ma
  pl cys·to·sar·co·mas
  or cys·to·sar·co·ma·ta
cys·to·scope
cys·to·scop·ic
cys·tos·co·pist
cys·tos·co·py
  pl cys·tos·co·pies
cys·to·sphinc·ter·om·e·try
cys·to·ste·a·to·ma
  pl cys·to·ste·a·to·mas
  or cys·to·ste·a·to·ma·ta
cys·tos·to·my
  pl cys·tos·to·mies
cys·to·tome
cys·tot·o·my
  pl cys·tot·o·mies
cys·to·u·re·ter·i·tis
cys·to·u·re·ter·o·cele
cys·to·u·re·ter·o·gram
cys·to·u·re·thri·tis
cys·to·u·re·thro·cele
cys·to·u·re·thro·gram
cys·to·u·re·thro·graph·ic
cys·to·u·re·throg·ra·phy
cys·to·u·re·thro·scope
cys·tyl
cyt·ar·a·bine
cy·tase
cy·tas·ter
cyth·ae·mol·y·sis
  var of cyth·e·mol·y·sis
cyth·e·mol·y·sis
cyth·er·o·ma·ni·a
cyt·i·dine
cyt·i·dyl·ic
cyt·i·sine
cy·to·al·bu·mi·no·log·ic
cy·to·an·a·ly·zer
cy·to·ar·chi·tec·ton·ic

cy·to·ar·chi·tec·tur·al
cy·to·ar·chi·tec·ture
cy·to·bi·ol·o·gy
cy·to·blast
cy·to·blas·te·ma
cy·to·cen·trum
cy·to·chal·a·sin
cy·to·chem·i·cal
cy·to·chem·ism
cy·to·chem·is·try
  pl cy·to·chem·is·tries
cy·to·chrome
cy·to·chy·le·ma
cy·to·ci·dal
cy·to·cide
cu·to·ci·ne·sis
cy·toc·la·sis
cy·to·clas·tic
cy·to·crine
cy·to·crin·i·a
cy·tode
cy·to·den·drite
cy·to·derm
cy·to·di·ag·no·sis
  pl cy·to·di·ag·no·ses
cy·to·di·er·e·sis
  pl cy·to·di·er·e·ses
cy·to·dif·fer·en·ti·a·tion
cy·to·dis·tal
cy·to·gene
cy·to·gen·e·sis
cy·to·ge·net·ic
  or cy·to·ge·net·i·cal
cy·to·ge·net·i·cal
  or cy·to·ge·net·ic
cy·to·ge·net·i·cal·ly
cy·to·ge·net·i·cist
cy·to·ge·net·ics
cy·to·gen·ic
cy·tog·e·nous
cy·tog·e·ny
cy·to·glob·u·lin
cy·to·gly·co·pe·ni·a
cy·to·his·to·gen·e·sis
cy·toid
cy·to·ki·ne·sis
  pl cy·to·ki·ne·ses
cy·to·ki·net·ic

cy·to·ki·nin
cy·tol·er·gy
cy·to·lip·o·chrome
cy·to·log·ic
  or cy·to·log·i·cal
cy·to·log·i·cal
  or cy·to·log·ic
cy·to·log·i·cal·ly
cy·tol·o·gist
cy·tol·o·gy
  pl cy·tol·o·gies
cy·to·lymph
cy·tol·y·sin
cy·tol·y·sis
  pl cy·tol·y·ses
cy·to·lyt·ic
cy·to·me·gal·ic
cy·to·meg·a·lo·vi·rus
cy·to·mem·brane
cy·to·met·a·pla·si·a
cy·tom·e·ter
cy·to·met·ric
cy·tom·e·try
cy·to·mi·tome
cy·to·mor·pho·log·i·cal
cy·to·mor·phol·o·gy
  pl cy·to·mor·phol·o·gies
cy·to·mor·pho·sis
  pl cy·to·mor·pho·ses
cy·to·my·co·sis
  pl cy·to·my·co·ses
cy·ton
cy·to·path·ic
cy·to·path·o·gen·e·sis
cy·to·path·o·gen·ic
cy·to·path·o·ge·nic·i·ty
  pl cy·to·path·o·ge·nic·i·ties
cy·to·pa·thol·o·gy
  pl cy·to·pa·thol·o·gies
cy·top·a·thy
cy·to·pemp·sis
cy·to·pe·ni·a
cy·to·phag·ic
  or cy·toph·a·gous
cy·to·phag·o·cy·to·sis
cy·toph·a·gous
  or cy·to·phag·ic

cy·toph·a·gy
  pl cy·toph·a·gies
cy·to·phil
cy·to·phil·ic
cy·to·pho·tom·e·ter
cy·to·pho·to·met·ric
  or cy·to·pho·to·met·ri·cal
cy·to·pho·to·met·ri·cal
  or cy·to·pho·to·met·ric
cy·to·pho·to·met·ri·cal·ly
cy·to·pho·tom·e·try
  pl cy·to·pho·tom·e·tries
cy·to·phy·lax·is
cy·to·phy·let·ic
cy·to·phys·ics
cy·to·phys·i·ol·o·gy
cy·to·pi·pette
cy·to·plasm
cy·to·plas·mic
cy·to·plas·mi·cal·ly
cy·to·plas·tin
cy·to·poi·e·sis
  pl cy·to·poi·e·ses
cy·to·prox·i·mal
cy·to·pyge
cy·to·re·tic·u·lum
cy·tor·rhyc·tes
  pl cy·tor·rhyc·tes
  or cy·to·ryc·tes
  pl cy·to·ryc·tes
cy·to·ryc·tes
  pl cy·to·ryc·tes
  or cy·tor·rhyc·tes
  pl cy·tor·rhyc·tes
cy·to·scop·ic
cy·tos·co·py
cy·to·sid·er·in
cy·to·sine
cy·to·skel·e·ton
cy·to·sol
cy·to·some
cy·to·spon·gi·um
  pl cy·to·spon·gi·a
cy·tost
cy·to·stat·ic
cy·to·stat·i·cal·ly
cy·to·ste·a·to·ne·cro·sis
cy·to·some

cy·to·tac·tic
cy·to·tax·is
cy·to·tax·on·o·my
   pl cy·to·tax·on·o·mies
cy·to·tech
cy·to·tech·nol·o·gist
cy·to·tech·nol·o·gy
   pl cy·to·tech·nol·o·gies

cy·toth·e·sis
cy·to·tox·ic
cy·to·tox·ic·i·ty
   pl cy·to·tox·ic·i·ties
cy·to·tox·in
cy·to·troph·o·blast
cy·to·tro·pic
cy·tot·ro·pism

cy·to·vi·rin
cy·to·zo·ic
cy·to·zo·on
   pl cy·to·zo·a
cy·to·zyme
cyt·u·la
cy·tu·ri·a

D

Da Cos·ta syn·drome
Da·boi·a
dac·ry·ad·e·ni·tis
dac·ry·ad·e·no·scir·rhus
dac·ry·ag·o·ga·tre·si·a
dac·ry·a·gog·ic
dac·ry·a·gogue
dac·ry·o·ad·e·nal·gi·a
dac·ry·o·ad·e·nec·to·my
dac·yr·o·ad·e·ni·tis
dac·ry·o·ag·o·ga·tre·si·a
dac·ry·o·blen·nor·rhe·a
dac·ry·o·blen·nor·rhoe·a
   var of dac·ry·o·blen·nor·
    rhe·a
dac·ry·o·cele
dac·ry·o·cyst
dac·ry·o·cys·tal·gi·a
dac·ry·o·cys·tec·to·my
   pl dac·ry·o·cys·tec·to·mies
dac·ry·o·cys·ti·tis
dac·ry·o·cys·to·blen·nor·
   rhe·a
dac·ry·o·cys·to·blen·nor·
   rhoe·a
   var of dac·ry·o·cys·to·blen·
    nor·rhe·a
dac·ry·o·cys·to·cele
dac·ry·o·cys·top·to·sis

dac·ry·o·cys·to·rhi·no·ste·
   no·sis
dac·ry·o·cys·to·rhi·nos·to·
   my
   pl dac·ry·o·cys·to·rhi·nos·
    to·mies
dac·ry·o·cys·to·rhi·not·
   o·my
dac·ry·o·cys·to·ste·no·sis
dac·ry·o·cys·tos·to·my
dac·ry·o·cys·to·tome
dac·ry·o·cys·tot·o·my
   pl dac·ry·o·cys·tot·o·mies
dac·ry·o·he·mor·rhe·a
dac·ry·o·lin
dac·ry·o·lith
dac·ry·o·li·thi·a·sis
   pl dac·ry·o·li·thi·a·ses
dac·ry·o·ma
   pl dac·ry·o·mas
   or dac·ry·o·ma·ta
dac·ry·on
   pl dac·ry·a
   or dak·ry·on
   pl dak·ry·a
   pl dac·ry·ops
   or dak·ry·ops
dac·ry·op·to·sis

dac·ry·o·py·or·rhe·a
dac·ry·o·py·o·sis
dac·ry·or·rhe·a
dac·ry·or·rhoe·a
   var of dac·ry·or·rhe·a
dac·ry·o·so·le·ni·tis
dac·ry·o·ste·no·sis
   pl dac·ry·o·ste·no·ses
dac·ry·o·syr·inx
   pl dac·ry·o·sy·rin·ges
   or dac·ry·o·syr·inx·es
dac·ti·no·my·cin
dac·tyl
dac·ty·lar
dac·ty·late
dac·ty·lif·er·ous
dac·tyl·i·on
dac·ty·li·tis
dac·tyl·o·gram
dac·tyl·o·graph
dac·ty·log·ra·pher
dac·ty·log·ra·phic
dac·ty·log·ra·phy
   pl dac·ty·log·ra·phies
dac·ty·lo·gry·po·sis
dac·ty·lol·o·gy
   pl dac·ty·lol·o·gies
dac·ty·lol·y·sis
dac·ty·lo·meg·a·ly

dac·tyl·o·scop·ic
dac·ty·los·co·pist
dac·ty·los·co·py
  pl dac·ty·los·co·pies
dac·ty·lo·sym·phy·sis
  pl dac·ty·lo·sym·phy·ses
dac·ty·lus
  pl dac·ty·li
Da·gni·ni ex·ten·sion-ad·
  duc·tion re·flex
Dahl·ia
dah·lin
dahl·lite
Da·kin so·lu·tion
dak·ry·on
  pl dak·ry·a
  or dac·ry·on
  pl dac·ry·a
dak·ry·ops
  or dac·ry·ops
Dal·i·bour wa·ter
Dall·dorf test
Dal·ton law
dal·ton·ism
dam·mar
Da·moi·seau curve
Da·na op·er·a·tion
Da·na-Put·nam syn·drome
Dan·bolt-Closs syn·drome
Dance sign
dan·der
dan·druff
Dan·dy-Walk·er
  syn·drome
Dan·iell cell
Dan·iels·sen-Boeck
  dis·ease
Dan·los syn·drome
dan·thron
D'An·to·ni stain
dan·tro·lene
Dan·ysz phe·nom·e·non,
  ef·fect
Dan·zer and Hook·er
  meth·od
Daph·ne
dap·pen dish, glass
dap·sone

Dar·i·er dis·ease
dark-field
Dark·sche·witsch
  nu·cle·us
Dar·ling dis·ease
darm·brand
dar·nel
Dar·row so·lu·tion
d'Ar·son·val cur·rent
d'ar·son·val·i·za·tion
dar·tos
dar·trous
Dar·win tu·ber·cle
dar·wi·nism
Das·y·proc·ta
das·y·proc·tid
das·y·proc·tine
Das·y·pus
da·tive
da·tum
  pl da·ta
Da·tu·ra
da·tu·ric
da·tu·rism
Dau·cus
dau·er·schlaf
dau·no·my·cin
Da·vai·ne·a for·mo·sa·na
Dav·en·port al·co·ho·lic
  sil·ver ni·trate meth·od
Da·vid·sohn dif·fer·en·tial
  test
Da·vis graft
Daw·son en·ceph·a·li·tis
Day op·er·a·tion
daz·zle re·flex of Pei·per
de Lange syn·drome
de·Li·ma op·er·a·tion
de Mor·gan spot
de Mus·sy point
de Quer·vain dis·ease
de To·ni-Fan·co·ni syn·
  drome
de To·ni-Fan·co·ni-De·bre
  syn·drome
de·a·cid·i·fi·ca·tion
de·a·cid·i·fy
de·ac·ti·vate

de·ac·ti·va·tion
de·ac·yl·ase
dead·ly night·shade
deaf
de·af·fer·en·ta·tion
deaf-mute
deaf-mut·ism
deaf·ness
de·al·bate
de·al·co·hol·i·za·tion
de·am·i·dase
de·am·i·di·za·tion
de·am·i·nase
de·am·i·nate
de·am·i·na·tion
de·an·aes·the·si·ant
  var of de·an·es·the·si·ant
de·an·es·the·si·ant
de·a·nol
  ac·et·am·i·do·ben·zo·ate
de·a·qua·tion
de·ar·te·ri·al·i·za·tion
death
death rat·tle
de·band·ing
De·bar·y·o·my·ces
  ne·o·for·mans
de·bil·i·tant
de·bil·i·tate
de·bil·i·ty
  pl de·bil·i·ties
De·bove dis·ease
de·branch·er
De·bré-de To·ni-Fan·co·ni
  syn·drome
De·bré-Sé·mé·laigne
  syn·drome
de·bride
de·bride·ment
de·bris
de·bri·so·quin
dec·a·dence
dec·a·gram
de·cal·ci·fi·ca·tion
de·cal·ci·fy
dec·a·li·ter
de·cal·vant
dec·a·me·ter

dec·a·me·tho·ni·um
de·can·cel·la·tion
dec·ane
de·can·nu·la·tion
dec·a·no·ate
dec·a·no·ic
dec·a·nor·mal
de·cant
de·can·ta·tion
dec·a·pep·tide
de·cap·i·tate
de·cap·i·ta·tion
de·cap·i·ta·tor
de·cap·su·late
de·cap·su·la·tion
de·car·bon·i·za·tion
de·car·bon·ize
de·car·box·yl·ase
de·car·box·yl·ate
de·car·box·yl·a·tion
de·ca·thec·tion
dec·a·vi·ta·min
de·cay
de·cen·tered
de·cen·tra·tion
de·cer·e·bel·la·tion
de·cer·e·brate
de·cer·e·bra·tion
de·cer·e·brize
de·chlo·ri·da·tion
de·chlo·ri·nate
de·chlo·ri·na·tion
de·chlor·u·ra·tion
de·cho·les·ter·ol·i·za·tion
dec·i·bel
de·cid·u·a
  pl de·cid·u·ae
de·cid·u·al
de·cid·u·ate
de·cid·u·a·tion
de·cid·u·i·tis
de·cid·u·o·ma
  pl de·cid·u·o·mas
  or de·cid·u·o·ma·ta
de·cid·u·o·sis
  pl de·cid·u·o·sis·es
  or de·cid·u·o·ses
de·cid·u·ous
dec·i·gram

dec·i·li·ter
dec·i·me·ter
dec·i·nor·mal
de·cip·a·ra
  pl de·cip·a·ras
  or de·cip·a·rae
dec·li·na·tion
de·clive
de·coct
de·coc·tion
de·coc·tum
  pl de·coc·ta
de·col·late
de·col·la·tion
de·col·la·tor
de·col·or·ant
de·col·or·a·tion
de·col·or·i·za·tion
de·col·or·ize
de·com·pen·sate
de·com·pen·sa·tion
de·com·pose
de·com·po·si·tion
de·com·press
de·com·pres·sion
de·com·pres·sive
de·con·di·tion
de·con·di·tion·ing
de·con·gest
de·con·ges·tant
de·con·ges·tion
de·con·ges·tive
de·con·tam·i·nate
de·con·tam·i·na·tion
de·cor·ti·cate
de·cor·ti·ca·tion
dec·re·ment
dec·re·men·tal
de·crep·i·ta·tion
de·cre·scen·do
de·cres·cent
de·cru·des·cence
de·cu·ba·tion
de·cu·bi·tal
de·cu·bi·tus
  pl de·cu·bi·ti
de·cur·rent
de·cur·tate
de·cus·sate

de·cus·sa·ti·o
  pl de·cus·sa·ti·o·nes
de·cus·sa·tion
de·den·ti·tion
de·dif·fer·en·ti·ate
de·dif·fer·en·ti·a·tion
de·ep·i·car·di·al·i·za·tion
deer·fly
Dees op·er·a·tion
Deet·jen bod·ies
de·fat
def·e·cate
def·e·ca·tion
de·fect
de·fec·tive
de·fem·i·na·tion
de·fem·i·ni·za·tion
de·fem·i·nize
de·fense
def·er·ens
  or def·er·ent
def·er·ent
  or def·er·ens
de·fer·en·tec·to·my
  pl def·er·en·tec·to·mies
def·er·en·tial
def·er·en·ti·o·ves·i·cal
def·er·en·ti·tis
de·fer·ox·a·mine
de·fer·ves·cence
de·fib·ril·late
de·fib·ril·la·tion
de·fib·ril·la·tive
de·fib·ril·la·tor
de·fib·ril·la·to·ry
de·fi·bri·nate
de·fi·bri·na·tion
de·fi·cien·cy
  pl de·fi·cien·cies
de·fi·cient
def·i·cit
def·la·gra·tion
de·flec·tion
def·lo·ra·tion
de·flo·res·cence
de·flu·vi·um
de·flux·i·o
de·flux·ion
de·form

94

de·form·a·bil·i·ty
de·for·ma·tion
de·for·mi·ty
   pl de·for·mi·ties
de·froth·i·cant
de·func·tion·al·i·za·tion
de·fun·da·tion
de·fu·sion
de·gan·gli·on·ate
de·gas
de·gen·er·a·cy
   pl de·gen·er·a·cies
de·gen·er·ate
de·gen·er·a·tion
de·gen·er·a·tive
de·gen·i·tal·i·ty
de·gen·i·tal·ize
de·germ
de·ger·ma·tion
de·glob·u·li·za·tion
de·glov·ing
de·glu·ti·tion
de·glu·ti·tive
de·glu·ti·to·ry
De·gos dis·ease
De·gos-Delort-Tri·cot
   syn·drome
deg·ra·da·tion
de·grade
de·gran·u·la·tion
de·grease
de·gus·ta·tion
De·hi·o test
de·his·cence
de·hu·mid·i·fi·ca·tion
de·hu·mid·i·fi·er
de·hu·mid·i·fy
de·hy·dra·cet·ic
   or de·hy·dro·a·cet·ic
de·hy·drant
de·hy·drase
de·hy·dra·tase
de·hy·drate
de·hy·dra·tion
de·hy·dro·a·cet·ic
   or de·hy·dra·cet·ic
de·hy·dro·a·scor·bic
de·hy·dro·chlo·ri·nase
de·hy·dro·chlo·ri·nate

de·hy·dro·chlo·ri·na·tion
de·hy·dro·cho·late
de·hy·dro·cho·les·ter·ol
de·hy·dro·cho·lic
de·hy·dro·cor·ti·cos·ter·one
de·hy·dro·ep·i·an·dros·ter·
   one
de·hy·dro·gen·ase
de·hy·dro·gen·ate
de·hy·dro·gen·a·tion
de·hy·dro·gen·ize
de·hy·dro·i·so·an·dros·ter·
   one
de·hy·dro·ret·i·nal
de·hy·dro·ret·i·nol
de·hyp·no·tize
de·i·on·i·za·tion
de·i·on·ize
de·i·on·iz·er
Dei·ters cell
Dei·ters nu·cle·us
dé·jà pen·sé
dé·jà vu
   or dé·jà vue
dé·jà vue
   or dé·jà vu
de·jec·ta
de·jec·tion
De·jer·ine syn·drome
De·jer·ine-Klump·ke
   syn·drome
De·jer·ine-Scot·tas
   dis·ease
De·jer·ine-Thom·as
   at·ro·phy
Del Cas·ti·lo syn·drome
del Ri·o Hor·te·ga sil·ver
   meth·od
de·lac·ri·ma·tion
de·lac·ta·tion
Del·a·field he·ma·tox·y·lin
de·lam·i·na·tion
Del·a·so·a sore
de·lead
del·e·te·ri·ous
de·le·tion
Del·hi boil
de·lim·i·ta·tion
de·lim·it·ed

de·lin·quen·cy
   pl de·lin·quen·cies
de·lin·quent
del·i·qui·da·tion
del·i·quesce
del·i·ques·cence
del·i·ques·cent
de·liq·ui·um
de·lir·i·ant
de·lir·i·fa·cient
de·lir·i·ous
de·lir·i·um
   pl de·lir·i·ums
   or de·lir·i·a
de·lir·i·um tre·mens
del·i·tes·cence
   or del·i·tes·cen·cy
del·i·tes·en·cy
   pl del·i·tes·en·cies
   or del·i·tes·ence
de·liv·er
de·liv·er·y
   pl de·liv·er·ies
del·le
   pl del·len
del·len
de·lo·mor·phic
   or de·lo·mor·phous
de·lo·mor·phous
   or de·lo·mor·phic
de·louse
del·phi·nine
Del·phin·i·um
del·ta
del·toid
   pl del·toids
   or del·toi·de·us
   pl del·toi·de·i
del·toi·de·us
   pl del·toi·de·i
   or del·toid
   pl del·toids
del·to·pec·to·ral
de·lu·sion
de·lu·sion·al
de·lu·sion·ar·y
de·lu·sive
de·lu·so·ry
de·mar·cate

de·mar·ca·tion
de·mas·cu·lin·i·za·tion
de·mas·cu·lin·ize
De·ma·ti·um
dem·e·car·i·um
dem·e·clo·cy·cline
dem·e·cy·cline
de·ment
de·ment·ed
de·men·ti·a
   pl de·men·ti·ae
de·men·ti·a par·a·lyt·i·ca
   pl de·men·ti·ae
   par·a·lyt·i·cae
de·men·ti·a prae·cox
   pl de·men·ti·ae prae·co·ces
   or de·men·tia pre·cox
   pl de·men·ti·ae pre·co·ces
de·men·ti·a pre·cox
   pl de·men·ti·ae pre·co·ces
   or de·men·ti·a prae·cox
   pl de·men·ti·ae prae·co·ces
de·meth·yl·ate
de·meth·yl·a·tion
de·meth·yl·chlor·tet·ra·cy·
   cline
dem·i·fac·et
dem·i·lune of Gian·nuz·zi
dem·i·lune of Hei·den·hain
de·min·er·al·i·za·tion
de·min·er·al·ize
dem·i·mon·stros·i·ty
dem·i·pen·ni·form
dem·o·dec·tic
Dem·o·dex
de·mo·gram
de·mog·ra·phy
   pl de·mog·ra·phies
de·mon·i·ac
   or de·mo·ni·a·cal
de·mo·ni·a·cal
   or de·mon·i·ac
de·mon·ol·a·try
de·mon·o·ma·ni·a
de·mon·o·ma·ni·ac
de·mon·op·a·thy
de·mon·o·pho·bi·a
de·mo·pho·bi·a

de·mor·phin·i·za·tion
de·mu·co·sa·tion
de·mul·cent
de·my·e·lin·ate
de·my·e·lin·a·tion
de·my·e·lin·i·za·tion
de·my·e·lin·ize
de·nar·co·tize
de·na·tur·ant
de·na·tur·a·tion
de·na·ture
de·na·tur·i·za·tion
Den·dras·pis
den·drax·on
den·dri·form
den·drite
den·drit·ic
den·droid
den·dron
   pl den·drons
   or den·dra
den·dro·phag·o·cy·to·sis
den·dro·phil·i·a
de·ner·vate
de·ner·va·tion
den·gue
de·ni·al
den·i·da·tion
den·i·gra·tion
Den·is meth·od
de·ni·tri·fy
de·ni·tro·gen·a·tion
Den·nie-Mar·fan
   syn·drome
Den·on·vil·liers syn·drome
dens
   pl den·tes
den·sim·e·ter
den·si·met·ric
den·si·tom·e·ter
den·si·tom·e·try
   pl den·si·tom·e·tries
den·si·ty
den·sog·ra·phy
den·tal
den·tal·gi·a
den·ta·ry
den·tate
   or den·tat·ed

den·tat·ed
   or den·tate
den·ta·tec·to·my
den·ta·tion
den·ta·to·re·tic·u·lar
den·ta·to·ru·bral
den·ta·to·tha·lam·ic
den·ta·to·thal·a·mo·cor·ti·
   cal
den·ta·tum
den·te·la·tion
den·tes
den·tes a·cus·ti·ci
den·tia
den·tia pre·cox
den·ti·buc·cal
den·ti·cle
den·tic·u·late
   or den·tic·u·lat·ed
den·tic·u·lat·ed
   or den·tic·u·late
den·ti·fi·ca·tion
den·ti·form
den·ti·frice
den·tig·er·ous
den·ti·la·bi·al
den·ti·lin·gual
den·tin
   or den·tine
den·ti·nal
den·tine
   or den·tin
den·tin·i·fi·ca·tion
den·ti·no·blas·to·ma
   pl den·ti·no·blas·to·mas
   or den·ti·no·blas·to·ma·ta
den·ti·no·ce·men·tal
den·ti·no·e·nam·el
den·ti·no·gen·e·sis
   pl den·ti·no·gen·e·ses
den·ti·no·gen·ic
den·ti·noid
den·ti·no·ma
   pl den·ti·no·mas
   or den·ti·no·ma·ta
den·ti·nos·te·oid
den·ti·num
den·tip·a·rous
den·ti·phone

en·tist
en·tis·try
   pl den·tis·tries
en·ti·tion
en·to·al·ve·o·lar
en·to·al·ve·o·li·tis
en·to·fa·cial
en·toid
en·to·trop·ic
en·tu·lous
en·ture
e·nu·cle·at·ed
e·nu·da·tion
e·nude
e·ob·stru·ent
e·o·dor·ant
e·on·tol·o·gy
   pl de·on·tol·o·gies
e·or·sum·duc·tion
e·or·sum·ver·gence
e·or·sum·ver·sion
e·os·si·fi·ca·tion
e·ox·i·da·tion
   or de·ox·i·di·za·tion
e·ox·i·di·za·tion
   or de·ox·i·da·tion
e·ox·i·dize
e·ox·y·a·den·o·sine
e·ox·y·cho·late
e·ox·y·cho·lic
e·ox·y·co·late-cit·rate
   a·gar
e·ox·y·cor·ti·cos·ter·one
e·ox·y·cor·tone
e·ox·y·cos·tone
e·ox·y·cy·ti·dine
e·ox·y·e·phed·rine
e·ox·y·gen·ate
e·ox·y·gen·a·tion
e·ox·y·gua·nine
e·ox·y·pen·tose
e·ox·y·pen·tose·nu·cle·ic
e·ox·y·pyr·i·dox·ine
e·ox·y·ri·bo·nu·cle·ase
e·ox·y·ri·bo·nu·cle·ic
e·ox·y·ri·bo·nu·cle·o·pro·
   te·in
e·ox·y·ri·bo·nu·cle·o·side
e·ox·y·ri·bo·nu·cle·o·tide

de·ox·y·ri·bose
de·ox·y·sug·ar
de·ox·y·u·ri·dine
de·pan·cre·a·tize
de·par·af·fin·ize
de·pend·ence
de·per·son·al·i·za·tion
de·per·son·al·ize
de·phos·phor·y·la·tion
de·pig·ment
de·pig·men·ta·tion
dep·i·late
dep·i·la·tion
de·pil·a·to·ry
   pl de·pil·a·to·ries
dep·i·lous
de·plete
de·ple·tion
de·plu·ma·tion
de·po·lar·i·za·tion
de·po·lar·ize
de·po·lym·er·ase
de·po·lym·er·i·za·tion
de·po·lym·er·ize
de·pos·it
de·pot
de·press
de·pres·sant
de·pressed
de·press·ing
de·pres·sion
de·pres·sive
de·pres·so·mo·tor
de·pres·sor
dep·ri·va·tion
dep·side
de·pu·li·za·tion
dep·u·rant
dep·u·rate
dep·u·ra·tion
der·a·del·phus
de·range·ment
Der·cum dis·ease
de·re·al·i·za·tion
de·re·ism
de·re·is·tic
der·en·ceph·a·lus
   pl der·en·ceph·a·li

der·en·ceph·a·ly
   pl der·en·ceph·a·lies
de·re·press
de·re·pres·sion
der·ic
der·i·va·tion
de·riv·a·tive
der·ma
der·ma·bra·sion
Der·ma·cen·tor
Der·ma·cen·trox·e·nus
der·ma·drome
der·ma·fat
der·ma·hae·mi·a
   var of der·ma·he·mi·a
der·ma·he·mi·a
der·mal
der·ma·my·i·a·sis
der·man·a·plas·ty
Der·ma·nys·sus
der·ma·tag·ra
der·ma·tal·gi·a
der·ma·tan
der·ma·ta·neu·ri·a
der·mat·hae·mi·a
   var of der·mat·he·mi·a
der·mat·he·mi·a
der·ma·therm
der·mat·ic
der·ma·ti·tis
   pl der·ma·ti·ti·ses
   or der·ma·ti·ti·des
der·ma·to·au·to·plas·ty
Der·ma·to·bi·a
der·ma·to·bi·a·sis
der·ma·to·cele
der·ma·to·cel·lu·li·tis
der·ma·to·cha·la·sis
   pl der·ma·to·cha·la·sis·es
   or der·ma·to·chal·la·ses
der·ma·to·co·ni·o·sis
   pl der·ma·to·co·ni·o·sis·es
   or der·ma·to·co·ni·o·ses
der·ma·to·cra·ni·um
   pl der·ma·to·cra·ni·ums
   or der·ma·to·cra·ni·a
der·ma·to·cyst
der·ma·to·dyn·i·a

97

der·ma·to·fi·bro·ma
  pl der·ma·to·fi·bro·mas
  or der·ma·to·fi·bro·ma·ta
der·ma·to·fi·bro·sar·co·ma
  pl der·ma·to·fi·bro·sar·co·
    mas
  or der·ma·to·fi·bro·sar·co·
    ma·ta
der·mat·o·gen
der·ma·to·glyph·ics
der·ma·to·graph
der·ma·to·graph·i·a
der·ma·tog·ra·phism
der·ma·tog·ra·phy
  pl der·ma·tog·ra·phies
der·ma·to·het·er·o·plas·ty
  pl der·ma·to·het·er·o·plas·
    ties
der·ma·to·his·tol·o·gy
  pl der·ma·to·his·tol·o·gies
der·ma·toid
der·ma·to·ko·ni·o·sis
  var of der·ma·to·co·ni·o·sis
der·ma·tol
der·ma·to·log·ic
  or der·ma·to·log·i·cal
der·ma·to·log·i·cal
  or der·ma·to·log·ic
der·ma·tol·o·gist
der·ma·tol·o·gy
  pl der·ma·tol·o·gies
der·ma·tol·y·sis
  pl der·ma·tol·y·ses
der·ma·tome
der·ma·to·meg·a·ly
  pl der·ma·to·meg·a·lies
der·ma·to·mere
der·ma·tom·ic
der·ma·to·mu·co·so·my·o·
  si·tis
  pl der·ma·to·mu·co·so·my·
    o·si·tis·es
  or der·ma·to·mu·co·so·my·
    o·si·ti·des
der·ma·to·my·ces
  pl der·ma·to·my·ce·tes
der·ma·to·my·cete
der·ma·to·my·co·sis
  pl der·ma·to·my·co·ses

der·ma·to·my·o·ma
  pl der·ma·to·my·o·mas
  or der·ma·to·my·o·ma·ta
der·ma·to·my·o·si·tis
  pl der·ma·to·my·o·si·tis·es
  or der·ma·to·my·o·si·ti·des
der·ma·to·neu·rol·o·gy
der·ma·to·neu·ro·sis
  pl der·ma·to·neu·ro·ses
der·ma·to·path·i·a
  or der·ma·top·a·thy
der·ma·to·path·ic
der·ma·to·pa·thol·o·gy
  pl der·ma·to·pa·thol·o·gies
der·ma·to·path·o·pho·bi·a
der·ma·top·a·thy
  pl der·ma·top·a·thies
  or der·ma·to·path·i·a
der·ma·to·phi·li·a·sis
  pl der·ma·to·phi·li·a·ses
der·ma·to·phi·lo·sis
Der·ma·toph·i·lus
  pen·e·trans
der·ma·to·phyte
der·ma·to·phy·tid
der·ma·to·phy·to·sis
  pl der·ma·to·phy·to·ses
der·ma·to·plas·ty
  pl der·ma·to·plas·ties
der·ma·to·pol·y·neu·ri·tis
  pl der·ma·to·pol·y·neur·i·
    tis·es
  or der·ma·to·pol·y·neu·ri·
    ti·des
der·ma·tor·rha·gi·a
der·ma·tor·rhex·is
der·ma·to·scle·ro·sis
  pl der·ma·to·scle·ro·ses
der·ma·tos·co·py
  pl der·ma·tos·co·pies
der·ma·to·si·o·pho·bi·a
der·ma·to·sis
  pl der·ma·to·ses
der·ma·to·some
der·ma·to·sto·ma·ti·tis
der·ma·to·ther·a·py
der·ma·to·thla·si·a
der·ma·tot·o·my

der·ma·to·trop·ic
  or der·mo·trop·ic
der·ma·to·zo·on
  pl der·ma·to·zo·a
der·ma·to·zo·o·no·sis
  pl der·ma·to·zo·o·no·ses
der·ma·tro·phi·a
der·mic
der·mis
der·mi·tis
der·mo·blast
der·mo·cy·ma
der·mo·graph·i·a
der·mo·graph·ic
der·mog·ra·phism
der·mog·ra·phy
  pl der·mog·ra·phies
der·mo·hae·mi·a
  var of der·mo·he·mi·a
der·mo·he·mi·a
der·moid
  or der·moid·al
der·moid·al
  or der·moid
der·moi·dec·to·my
  pl der·moi·dec·to·mies
der·mo·la·bi·al
der·mo·lath·y·rism
der·mo·li·po·ma
  pl der·mo·li·po·mas
  or der·mo·li·po·ma·ta
der·mom·e·ter
der·mom·e·try
der·mo·my·co·sis
der·mo·my·o·tome
der·mo·ne·crot·ic
der·mop·a·thy
  pl der·mop·a·thies
der·mo·phle·bi·tis
der·mo·phyte
der·mo·plas·ty
der·mo·skel·e·ton
der·mo·ste·no·sis
  pl der·mo·ste·no·ses
der·mos·to·sis
  pl der·mos·to·ses
der·mo·syn·o·vi·tis
der·mo·syph·i·lop·a·thy
  pl der·mo·syph·i·lop·a·thies

der·mo·trop·ic
  or der·ma·to·trop·ic
der·mo·vas·cu·lar
der·o·did·y·mus
de·rom·e·lus
der·ren·ga·de·ra
der·rid
des·am·i·dase
des·an·i·ma·ni·a
de·sat·u·ra·tion
Des·ce·met mem·brane
des·ce·me·ti·tis
des·ce·met·o·cele
de·scen·dens cer·vi·cis
de·scen·sus
  pl de·scen·sus
des·cin·o·lone a·cet·o·nide
de·sen·si·ti·za·tion
de·sen·si·tize
de·sen·si·ti·zer
de·ser·pi·dine
de·sex
de·sex·u·al·i·za·tion
de·sex·u·al·ize
des·ic·cant
des·ic·cate
des·ic·ca·tion
des·ic·ca·tive
des·ic·ca·tor
des·ic·ca·to·ry
de·sid·er·ize
de·sip·ra·mine
Des·i·vac
des·lan·o·side
des·mi·o·gnath·us
des·mi·tis
des·mo·cra·ni·um
  pl des·mo·cra·ni·ums
  or des·mo·cra·ni·a
des·mo·cyte
des·mog·e·nous
des·mo·gly·co·gen
des·mog·ra·phy
des·moid
des·mo·lase
des·mol·o·gy
des·mo·ma
des·mone
des·mop·a·thy

des·mo·pla·si·a
des·mo·plas·tic
des·mo·some
des·mos·ter·ol
des·mot·o·my
  pl des·mot·o·mies
Des·nos pneu·mon·i·a
des·o·mor·phine
de·sorp·tion
des·ox·y·cho·late
des·ox·y·cho·lic
des·ox·y·cor·ti·cos·ter·one
des·ox·y·e·phed·rine
des·ox·y·pen·tose
des·ox·y·pen·tose·nu·cle·ic
des·ox·y·pyr·i·dox·ine
des·ox·y·ri·bo·nu·cle·ase
des·ox·y·ri·bo·nu·cle·ic
des·ox·y·ri·bose
des·ox·y·sug·ar
de·spe·ci·at·ed
de·spe·ci·a·tion
d'Es·pine sign
des·qua·mate
des·qua·ma·ti·o
des·qua·ma·tion
des·quam·a·tive
des·qua·ma·to·ry
des·thi·o·bi·o·tin
de·stru·do
de·sul·fi·nase
de·sul·fi·na·tion
de·sul·fu·rase
de·tach·ment
de·tec·tor
de·ter·gent
de·te·ri·o·rate
de·te·ri·o·ra·tion
de·ter·mi·nant
de·ter·mi·na·tion
de·ter·mi·na·tive
de·ter·mine
de·ter·min·ism
de·ter·sive
de·tor·sion
de·tox·i·cant
de·tox·i·cate
de·tox·i·ca·tion
de·tox·i·ca·tor

de·tox·i·fi·ca·tion
de·tox·i·fi·er
de·tox·i·fy
Det·re re·ac·tion
de·tri·tal
de·tri·tion
de·tri·tus
  pl de·tri·tus
de·trun·ca·tion
de·tru·sion
de·tru·sor
de·tru·sor u·ri·nae
de·tu·ba·tion
de·tu·mes·cence
de·tu·mes·cent
deu·tan
deu·ter·a·nom·a·lo·pi·a
  or deu·ter·a·nom·a·lop·si·a
deu·ter·a·nom·a·lop·si·a
  or deu·ter·a·nom·a·lo·pi·a
deu·ter·a·nom·a·lous
deu·ter·a·nom·a·ly
  pl deu·ter·a·nom·a·lies
deu·ter·a·nope
deu·ter·a·nop·i·a
deu·ter·a·nop·ic
deu·ter·a·nop·si·a
deu·ter·ate
deu·ter·a·tion
deu·te·ri·um
deu·ter·o·gen·ic
deu·ter·o·he·mo·phil·i·a
deu·ter·on
deu·ter·o·path·ic
deu·ter·op·a·thy
  pl deu·ter·op·a·thies
deu·ter·o·plasm
deu·ter·o·plas·mol·y·sis
deu·ter·o·pro·te·ose
deu·ter·os·to·ma
  pl deu·ter·os·to·mas
  or deu·ter·os·to·ma·ta
deu·ter·ot·o·ky
  pl deu·ter·ot·o·kies
deu·ter·o·tox·in
deu·tom·er·ite
deu·ton
deu·to·plasm

deu·to·plas·mol·y·sis
   pl deu·to·plas·mol·y·ses
deu·to·sco·lex
Deutsch·län·der dis·ease
de·vas·cu·lar·i·za·tion
de·vel·op·ment
de·vel·op·men·tal
de·vi·ant
de·vi·ate
de·vi·a·tion
Dev·ic dis·ease
de·vice
dev·il's-grip
   pl dev·il's-grips
de·vi·om·e·ter
de·vi·tal·i·za·tion
de·vi·tal·ize
dev·o·lu·tion
dew·claw
dew·lap
de·worm
dex·a·meth·a·sone
dex·brom·phen·ir·a·mine
dex·chlor·phen·ir·a·mine
dex·io·car·di·a
dex·iv·a·caine
dex·ox·a·drol
dex·pan·the·nol
dex·ter
dex·trad
dex·tral
dex·tral·i·ty
   pl dex·tral·i·ties
dex·tral·i·za·tion
dex·tral·ly
dex·tran
dex·tran·ase
dex·trase
dex·trau·ral
dex·tri·fer·ron
dex·trin
   or dex·trine
dex·trine
   or dex·trin
dex·tri·no·gen·ic
dex·tri·no·sis
dex·tri·nu·ri·a
dex·tro·am·phet·a·mine
dex·tro·car·di·a

dex·tro·car·di·al
dex·tro·car·di·o·gram
dex·tro·cer·e·bral
dex·tro·cli·na·tion
dex·tro·con·dy·lism
dex·troc·u·lar
de·troc·u·lar·i·ty
   pl dex·troc·u·lar·i·ties
dex·tro·cy·clo·ver·sion
dex·tro·duc·tion
dex·tro·gas·tri·a
dex·tro·glu·cose
dex·tro·gram
dex·tro·gy·rate
dex·tro·gy·ra·tion
dex·tro·man·u·al
dex·tro·man·u·al·i·ty
dex·tro·meth·or·phan
dex·tro·mor·am·ide
dex·tro·ped·al
dex·tro·pho·bi·a
dex·tro·po·si·tion
dex·tro·pro·pox·y·phene
dex·tro·ro·ta·ry
   or dex·tro·ro·ta·to·ry
dex·tro·ro·ta·tion
dex·tro·ro·ta·to·ry
   or dex·tro·ro·ta·ry
dex·trose
dex·tro·sin·is·tral
dex·tro·su·ri·a
dex·tro·tar·tar·ic
dex·tro·thy·rox·ine
dex·tro·tor·sion
dex·tro·trop·ic
dex·trous
dex·tro·ver·sion
dho·bie
Di George syn·drome
di Gu·gliel·mo syn·drome
di·a·be·tes
   pl di·a·be·tes
di·a·be·tes in·sip·i·dus
di·a·be·tes mel·li·tus
di·a·bet·ic
di·a·be·tid
di·a·be·to·gen·ic
di·a·be·tog·e·nous
di·a·be·tom·e·ter

di·a·be·to·pho·bi·a
di·ab·o·lep·sy
di·a·bo·lep·tic
di·a·brot·ic
di·a·caus·tic
di·ac·e·tae·mi·a
   var of di·ac·e·te·mi·a
di·ac·e·tate
di·ac·e·te·mi·a
di·a·ce·tic
di·ac·e·tin
di·ac·e·tu·ri·a
di·ac·e·tyl
di·ac·e·tyl·mor·phine
di·ac·id
di·a·cla·si·a
   or di·a·cla·sis
di·ac·la·sis
   pl di·ac·la·ses
   or di·a·cla·sia
di·a·clast
di·a·clas·tic
di·a·coele
di·ac·o·la·tion
di·ac·ri·sis
di·a·crit·ic
   or di·a·crit·i·cal
di·a·crit·i·cal
   or di·a·crit·ic
di·ac·tin·ic
di·ad
   or dyad
di·a·derm
di·a·der·mal
   or di·a·der·mat·ic
   or di·a·der·mic
di·a·der·mat·ic
   or di·a·der·mal
   or di·a·der·mic
di·a·der·mic
   or di·a·der·mal
   or di·a·der·mat·ic
di·ad·ic
   or dy·a·dic
di·ad·o·cho·ki·ne·si·a
   or di·ad·o·ko·ki·ne·si·a
di·ad·o·ko·ki·ne·si·a
   or di·ad·o·cho·ki·ne·si·a

di·ad·o·cho·ki·ne·sis
  pl di·ad·o·cho·ki·ne·ses
di·ad·o·cho·ki·net·ic
di·ag·nos·a·ble
di·ag·nose
di·ag·no·sis
  pl di·ag·no·ses
di·ag·nos·tic
di·ag·nos·ti·cal·ly
di·ag·nos·ti·cian
di·ag·o·nal
di·a·ki·ne·sis
  pl di·a·ki·ne·ses
Di·ak·i·o·gi·an·nis sign
Di·a·lis·ter
di·al·kyl·a·mine
di·al·lyl·bar·bi·tu·ric
di·al·y·sance
di·al·y·sate
  or di·al·y·zate
di·al·y·sis
  pl di·al·y·ses
di·a·lyt·ic
di·a·lyz·a·ble
di·al·y·zate
  or di·al·y·sate
di·a·lyze
di·a·lyz·er
di·a·mag·net·ic
di·a·mag·net·ism
di·a·mer·sul·fon·a·mides
di·am·e·ter
di·a·met·ric
  or di·a·met·ri·cal
di·a·met·ri·cal
  or di·a·met·ric
di·am·ide
di·am·i·dine
di·a·mine
di·a·mi·no·di·phen·yl·sul·
  fone
di·a·mi·no·pu·rine
di·a·mi·nu·ri·a
Di·a·mond meth·od
di·a·mor·phine
di·am·tha·zole
di·ap·a·mide
di·a·pa·son
di·a·pause

di·a·pe·de·sis
  pl di·a·pe·de·ses
di·a·pe·det·ic
di·a·per
di·a·phane
di·aph·a·nom·e·ter
di·aph·a·no·met·ric
di·a·pha·nom·e·try
di·aph·a·no·scope
di·aph·a·nos·co·py
  pl di·aph·a·nos·co·pies
di·aph·e·met·ric
di·aph·o·rase
di·a·pho·re·sis
  pl di·a·pho·re·ses
di·a·pho·ret·ic
di·a·phragm
di·a·phrag·ma
  pl di·a·phrag·ma·ta
di·a·phrag·mat·ic
di·a·phrag·ma·ti·tis
di·a·phrag·mat·o·cele
di·a·phrag·mi·tis
di·aph·y·se·al
  or di·a·phys·i·al
di·aph·y·sec·to·my
  pl di·aph·y·sec·to·mies
di·a·phy·si·al
  or di·aph·y·se·al
di·aph·y·sis
  pl di·aph·y·ses
di·a·phy·si·tis
di·ap·la·sis
  pl di·ap·la·ses
di·a·plas·tic
di·a·poph·y·sis
  pl di·a·poph·y·ses
di·a·py·e·sis
di·ar·rhae·mi·a
  var of di·ar·rhe·mi·a
di·ar·rhe·a
di·ar·rhe·al
  or di·ar·rhe·ic
di·ar·rhe·ic
  or di·ar·rhe·al
di·ar·rhe·mi·a
di·ar·rhoe·a
  var of di·ar·rhe·a

di·ar·rhoe·al
  var of di·ar·rhe·al
di·ar·rhoe·ic
  var of di·ar·rhe·ic
di·ar·thric
di·ar·thro·di·al
di·ar·thro·sis
  pl di·ar·thro·ses
di·ar·tic·u·lar
di·as·chi·sis
  pl di·as·chi·ses
di·a·schis·tic
di·a·scope
di·a·scop·ic
di·as·co·py
  pl di·as·co·pies
di·a·stal·sis
  pl di·a·stal·ses
di·a·stase
di·as·ta·sis
  pl di·as·ta·ses
di·a·stat·ic
di·a·ste·ma
  pl di·a·ste·ma·ta
di·a·ste·mat·ic
di·a·stem·a·to·cra·ni·a
di·a·ste·ma·to·my·e·li·a
di·a·ste·ma·to·py·e·li·a
di·as·ter
di·a·ster·e·o·i·so·mer
di·a·ster·e·o·i·so·mer·ic
di·a·ster·e·o·i·som·er·ism
di·as·to·le
di·a·stol·ic
di·a·tax·i·a
di·a·ther·mal
di·a·ther·ma·nous
di·a·ther·mi·a
di·a·ther·mic
di·a·ther·mize
di·a·ther·mo·co·ag·u·la·tion
di·a·ther·mom·e·ter
di·a·ther·my
  pl di·a·ther·mies
di·ath·e·sis
  pl di·ath·e·ses
di·a·thet·ic
di·a·tom
di·a·to·ma·ceous

di·a·tom·ic
di·a·tri·zo·ate
di·a·tri·zo·ic
di·a·ver·i·dine
di·ax·on
   or di·ax·one
di·ax·one
   or di·ax·on
di·ax·on·ic
di·az·e·pam
di·a·zine
di·az·o
di·a·zo·ni·um
di·az·o·re·sor·ci·nol
di·az·o·tiz·a·ble
di·az·o·ti·za·tion
di·az·o·tize
di·az·ox·ide
di·ba·sic
di·benz·an·thra·cene
di·ben·ze·pin
di·ben·zyl·chlor·eth·a·mine
di·both·ri·o·ceph·a·li·a·sis
Di·both·ri·o·ceph·a·lus
di·brom·sa·lan
di·bu·caine
di·bu·to·line
di·cal·ci·um
di·car·box·yl·ic
di·cen·tric
di·ce·pha·li·a
di·ceph·a·lism
di·ceph·a·lous
di·ceph·a·lus
   pl di·ceph·a·li
di·ceph·a·ly
di·chei·lus
   or di·chi·lus
di·chei·rus
   or di·chi·rus
di·chi·lus
   or di·chei·lus
di·chi·rus
   or di·chei·rus
di·chlor·a·mine
di·chlor·eth·yl
   or di·chlo·ro·eth·yl
di·chlor·hy·drin
   or di·chlo·ro·hy·drin

di·chlor·i·sone
di·chlo·ro·a·ce·tic
di·chlo·ro·ben·zene
di·chlo·ro·di·eth·yl sul·fide
di·chlo·ro·di·flu·o·ro·meth·ane
di·chlo·ro·di·phen·yl·tri·chlo·ro·eth·yl·ene
di·chlo·ro·eth·yl
   or di·chlor·eth·yl
di·chlo·ro·hy·drin
   or di·chlor·hy·drin
di·chlo·ro·i·so·pro·ter·e·nol
di·chlo·ro·phen·ar·sine
di·chlo·ro·phe·nol·in·do·phe·nol
di·chlo·ro·phen·ox·y·a·ce·tic
di·chlor·phen·a·mide
di·chog·a·mous
   or di·cho·gam·ic
di·cho·gom·ic
   or di·chog·a·mous
di·chog·a·my
   pl di·chog·a·mies
di·cho·ri·al
di·cho·ri·on·ic
di·chot·ic
di·chot·i·cal·ly
di·chot·o·mize
di·chot·o·my
di·chro·ic
   or di·chro·it·ic
di·chro·ine
di·chro·ism
di·chro·it·ic
   or di·chro·ic
di·chro·ma·si·a
di·chro·ma·sy
di·chro·mat
di·chro·mate
di·chro·mat·ic
di·chro·ma·tism
di·chro·ma·top·si·a
di·chro·mic
di·chro·mism
di·chro·mo·phil
di·chro·moph·i·lism
Dick test

di·cli·dot·o·my
   pl di·cli·dot·o·mies
di·clox·a·cil·lin
di·coe·lous
di·co·phane
di·co·ri·a
di·cot·y·le·do·nous
di·cou·ma·rin
di·cou·ma·rol
Di·cro·coe·li·um
di·crot·al
   or di·crot·ic
   or di·cro·tous
di·crot·ic
   or di·cro·tal
   or di·cro·tous
di·cro·tism
di·cro·tous
   or di·crot·ic
   or di·crot·al
Dic·ty·o·cau·lus
dic·ty·o·ki·ne·sis
dic·ty·o·ma
dic·ty·o·some
dic·ty·o·tene
di·cu·ma·rol
di·cy·clic
di·cy·clo·mine
di·cys·te·ine
di·dac·tic
di·dac·tyl
   or di·dac·tyle
   or di·dac·tyl·ous
di·dac·tyle
   or di·dac·tyle
   or di·dac·tyl·ous
di·dac·ty·lism
di·dac·tyl·ous
   or di·dac·tyl
   or di·dac·tyle
di·del·phi·a
di·del·phic
Di·del·phis
Didot op·er·a·tion
did·y·mal·gi·a
did·y·mi·tis
di·dym·i·um
did·y·mous
did·y·mus

di·e·cious
Di·e·go blood group
di·el·drin
di·e·lec·tric
di·em·bry·o·ny
di·en·ce·phal·ic
di·en·ceph·a·lon
die·ner
di·en·es·trol
di·en·oes·trol
   var of di·en·es·trol
Di·ent·a·moe·ba
di·er·e·sis
   pl di·er·e·ses
di·es·ter
di·es·ter·ase
di·es·trous
   or di·es·tru·al
di·es·tru·al
   or di·es·trous
di·es·trum
   or di·es·trus
di·es·trus
   or di·es·trum
di·et
di·e·tar·y
   pl di·e·tar·ies
di·et·er
di·e·tet·ic
di·e·tet·i·cal·ly
di·e·tet·ics
di·eth·a·nol·a·mine
di·eth·a·zine
Die·thelm meth·od
di·eth·yl
di·eth·yl·a·mide
di·eth·yl·a·mine
di·eth·yl·bar·bi·tu·rate
di·eth·yl·bar·bi·tu·ric
di·eth·yl·car·bam·a·zine
di·eth·yl·ene
di·eth·yl·ene·di·a·mine
di·eth·yl·mal·o·nyl·u·re·a
di·eth·yl·pro·pi·on
di·eth·yl·stil·bes·trol
di·eth·yl·tol·u·a·mide
di·eth·yl·tryp·ta·mine
di·e·ti·cian
   or di·e·ti·tian

di·e·tist
di·e·ti·tian
   or di·e·ti·cian
Die·tl cri·sis
di·e·to·ther·a·py
   pl di·e·to·ther·a·pies
Dieu·la·foy dis·ease
dif·fer·en·tial
dif·fer·en·tial·ly
dif·fer·en·ti·ate
dif·fer·en·ti·a·tion
dif·flu·ence
   or dif·lu·ence
dif·flu·ent
dif·frac·tion
dif·fu·sate
dif·fuse
dif·fus·i·bil·i·ty
dif·fus·i·ble
dif·fu·si·om·e·ter
dif·fu·sion
di·flu·a·nine
di·flu·cor·to·lone
dif·lu·ence
   or dif·flu·ence
di·flu·mi·done
di·gal·lic
di·ga·met·ic
di·gas·tric
Di·ge·ne·a
di·ge·ne·ous
di·gen·e·sis
   pl di·gen·e·ses
di·ge·net·ic
di·gen·ic
di·gest
di·ges·tant
di·gest·er
di·ges·ti·bil·i·ty
di·gest·i·ble
di·ges·tion
di·ges·tive
di·ges·tive·ly
di·ges·tive·ness
Digh·ton syn·drome
dig·i·lan·id
   or dig·i·lan·ide
dig·i·lan·ide
   or dig·i·lan·id

dig·it
dig·i·tal
dig·i·tal·gi·a
dig·i·tal·in
dig·i·tal·is
dig·i·tal·i·za·tion
dig·i·tal·ize
dig·i·tal·ly
dig·i·tal·ose
dig·i·tate
   or dig·i·tat·ed
dig·i·tat·ed
   or dig·i·tate
dig·i·tate·ly
dig·i·ta·tion
dig·i·ti·form
dig·i·ti·grade
dig·i·to·gen·in
dig·i·to·nide
dig·i·to·nin
dig·i·to·plan·tar
dig·i·tox·i·gen·in
dig·i·tox·in
dig·i·tox·ose
dig·i·tox·o·side
dig·i·tus
   pl dig·i·ti
di·glos·si·a
di·glos·sus
di·glu·ta·thi·one
di·glyc·er·ide
di·gnath·us
di·gox·i·gen·in
di·gox·in
di·hex·y·ver·ine
di·hy·brid
di·hy·drate
di·hy·dric
di·hy·dro·cho·les·ter·ol
di·hy·dro·cin·chon·i·dine
di·hy·dro·co·de·i·none
di·hy·dro·co·en·zyme
di·hy·dro·er·go·cor·nine
di·hy·dro·er·got·a·mine
di·hy·drol
di·hy·dro·mor·phi·none
di·hy·dro·quin·ine
di·hy·dro·strep·to·my·cin
di·hy·dro·ta·chys·ter·ol

di·hy·dro·the·e·lin
di·hy·drox·y·a·ce·tic
di·hy·drox·y·ac·e·tone
di·hy·drox·y·a·lu·mi·num
di·hy·drox·y·an·thra·nol
di·hy·drox·y·ben·zene
di·hy·drox·y·cho·le·cal·cif·er·ol
di·hy·drox·y·es·trin
di·hy·drox·y·phen·yl·al·a·nine
di·hy·drox·y·pro·pane
di·i·o·do·hy·drox·y·quin
   or di·i·o·do·hy·drox·y·quin·a·lone
di·i·o·do·hy·drox·y·quin·o·line
   or di·i·o·do·hy·drox·y·quin
di·i·o·do·thy·ro·nine
di·i·o·do·ty·ro·sine
di·i·so·pro·pyl
   flu·o·ro·phos·phate
di·kar·y·on
di·ke·to·pi·per·a·zine
dik·ty·o·ma
   pl dik·ty·o·mas
   or dik·ty·o·ma·ta
dik·wa·kwa·di
di·lac·er·a·tion
di·lat·a·ble
di·la·tan·cy
dil·a·ta·tion
dil·a·ta·tion·al
dil·a·ta·tor
di·late
di·la·tion
dil·a·tom·e·ter
dil·a·to·met·ric
di·la·tor
di·lec·a·nus
Dil·ling rule
dil·u·ent
di·lute
di·lu·tion
di·lu·tion·al
Di·mas·tig·a·moe·ba
di·mef·a·dane
di·me·fline
di·meg·a·ly

di·men·hy·dri·nate
di·men·sion
di·mer
di·mer·cap·rol
dim·er·ous
di·meth·a·di·one
di·meth·i·cone
di·meth·in·dene
di·meth·i·so·quin
di·meth·is·ter·one
di·meth·ox·a·nate
di·meth·yl
di·meth·yl phthal·ate
di·meth·yl sulf·ox·ide
di·meth·yl·am·ine
di·meth·yl·a·mi·no·az·o·ben·zene
di·meth·yl·a·mi·no·benz·al·de·hyde
de·meth·yl·ar·sin·ic
di·meth·yl·ben·zene
di·meth·yl·gly·ox·ime
di·meth·yl·ke·tone
di·meth·yl·ni·tros·a·mine
di·meth·yl·tryp·ta·mine
di·meth·yl·tu·bo·cu·ra·rine
di·meth·yl·xan·thine
di·me·tri·a
Di·mi·tri dis·ease
di·mor·phic
di·mor·phism
di·mor·phous
dim·pling
di·neu·ric
di·neu·tron
din·ic
   or din·i·cal
din·i·cal
   or din·ic
di·ni·tro·or·tho·cre·sol
di·ni·tro·phe·nol
di·ni·tro·phen·yl·hy·dra·zine
di·nu·cle·o·tide
di·nus
di·o·coele
Di·oc·to·phy·ma
Di·oc·to·phy·me
di·oc·tyl

di·oc·tyl cal·ci·um sul·fo·suc·ci·nate
di·oc·tyl so·di·um sul·fo·suc·ci·nate
di·o·done
di·oe·cious
   var of di·ec·ious
di·oes·trous
   var of di·es·trous
di·oes·tru·al
   var of di·es·tru·al
di·oes·trum
   var of di·es·trum
di·oes·trus
   var of di·es·trus
di·ol·a·mine
di·o·nism
di·op·ter
di·op·tom·e·ter
di·op·tom·e·try
di·op·tre
   var of di·op·ter
di·op·tric
di·op·trics
di·op·trom·e·ter
di·op·try
   pl di·op·tries
di·or·tho·sis
   pl di·or·tho·ses
di·or·thot·ic
di·os·co·re·a
di·os·co·rine
di·ose
di·os·gen·in
di·os·min
Di·os·py·ros
di·o·tic
di·ov·u·lar
di·ov·u·la·to·ry
di·ox·ane
di·ox·ide
di·ox·in
di·ox·y·ben·zone
di·ox·y·line
di·pen·tene
di·pep·ti·dase
di·pep·tide
di·per·o·don
Di·pet·a·lo·ne·ma

di·pet·a·lo·ne·mi·a·sis
di·phal·lic
di·phal·lus
di·pha·sic
di·pheb·u·zol
di·phem·a·nil
di·phen·a·di·one
di·phen·an
di·phen·hy·dra·mine
di·phen·i·cil·lin
di·phen·i·dol
di·phen·ox·yl·ate
di·phen·yl·a·mine
di·phen·yl·chlor·ar·sine
  or di·phen·yl·chlo·ro·ar·
  sine
di·phen·yl·chlo·ro·ar·sine
  or di·phen·yl·chlor·ar·sine
di·phen·yl·hy·dan·to·in
di·phen·yl·pyr·a·line
di·pho·ni·a
di·phos·gene
di·phos·phate
di·phos·pho·gly·cer·ic
di·phos·pho·pyr·i·dine
  nu·cle·o·tide
di·phos·pho·thi·a·min
  or di·phos·pho·thi·a·mine
di·phos·pho·thi·a·mine
  or di·phos·pho·thi·a·min
diph·the·ri·a
diph·the·ri·al
  or diph·the·ri·an
diph·the·ri·an
  or diph·the·ri·al
diph·the·ri·a·phor
diph·ther·ic
diph·the·rin
diph·the·rit·ic
diph·the·ri·tis
diph·the·roid
diph·the·ro·tox·in
diph·thon·gi·a
diph·y·gen·ic
di·phyl·lo·both·ri·a·sis
Di·phyl·lo·both·ri·i·dae
Di·phyl·lo·both·ri·um
di·phy·o·dont

dip·la·cu·sis
  pl dip·la·cu·ses
di·plas·mat·ic
di·ple·gi·a
di·ple·gic
dip·lo·al·bu·min·u·ri·a
dip·lo·ba·cil·lus
  pl dip·lo·ba·cil·li
dip·lo·bac·te·ri·um
dip·lo·blas·tic
dip·lo·car·di·a
dip·lo·car·di·ac
dip·lo·ce·pha·li·a
dip·lo·ceph·a·lus
dip·lo·ceph·a·ly
dip·lo·coc·cal
dip·lo·coc·cic
dip·lo·coc·coid
dip·lo·coc·cus
  pl dip·lo·coc·ci
dip·lo·co·ri·a
dip·lo·ë
dip·lo·et·ic
dip·lo·gen·e·sis
  pl dip·lo·gen·e·ses
Dip·lo·go·nop·o·rus
  gran·dis
di·plo·ic
di·plo·i·cin
dip·loid
dip·loi·dy
  pl dip·loi·dies
dip·lo·kar·y·on
dip·lo·mate
dip·lo·mel·li·tu·ri·a
dip·lo·my·e·li·a
dip·lo·ne·ma
  pl dip·lo·ne·mas
  or dip·lo·ne·ma·ta
dip·lo·neu·ral
di·plop·a·gus
di·plo·pi·a
di·plo·pi·om·e·ter
dip·lo·scope
di·plo·sis
  pl di·plo·ses
dip·lo·some
dip·lo·so·mi·a
dip·lo·tene

di·po·lar
di·pole
di·po·tas·si·um
dip·ping
dip·pol·dism
di·pro·so·pi·a
di·pro·so·pus
di·pros·o·py
di·pro·tri·zo·ate
dip·se·sis
dip·set·ic
dip·so·gen
dip·so·gen·ic
dip·so·ma·ni·a
dip·so·ma·ni·ac
dip·so·ma·ni·a·cal
dip·so·pho·bi·a
dip·so·rex·i·a
  or dip·sor·rhex·i·a
dip·sor·rhex·i·a
  or dip·so·rex·i·a
dip·so·sis
dip·so·ther·a·py
Dip·ter·a
dip·ter·an
Dip·ter·o·car·pus
dip·ter·ous
Dip·ter·yx
di·pus
di·py·gus
dip·y·li·di·a·sis
Di·py·lid·i·um
di·pyr·id·am·ole
di·py·rone
di·rec·tor
di·rhin·ic
Di·ro·fi·lar·i·a
di·ro·fil·a·ri·a·sis
dir·rhi·nus
dis·a·bil·i·ty
  pl dis·a·bil·i·ties
dis·able
dis·a·ble·ment
di·sac·cha·ri·dase
di·sac·cha·ride
dis·ag·gre·ga·tion
dis·ar·tic·u·late
dis·ar·tic·u·la·tion
dis·as·sim·i·late

dis·as·sim·i·la·tion
dis·as·sim·i·la·tive
dis·as·so·ci·a·tion
dis·as·sor·ta·tive
disc
   or disk
dis·charge
dis·ci·form
dis·cis·sion
dis·ci·tis
   or dis·ki·tis
dis·cli·na·tion
dis·clos·ing
dis·co·blas·tic
dis·co·blas·tu·la
   pl dis·co·blas·tu·las
   or dis·co·blas·tu·lae
dis·co·gas·tru·la
   pl dis·co·gas·tru·las
   or dis·co·gas·tru·lae
dis·co·gen·ic
dis·co·gram
   or dis·ko·gram
dis·cog·ra·phy
   pl dis·cog·ra·phies
dis·coid
dis·coi·dal
dis·col·or·a·tion
dis·com·po·si·tion
dis·con·nec·tion
dis·con·nex·ion
   var of dis·con·nec·tion
dis·cop·a·thy
   pl dis·cop·a·thies
dis·coph·o·rous
dis·co·pla·cen·ta
   pl dis·co·pla·cen·tas
   or dis·co·pla·cen·tae
dis·co·pla·cen·tal
dis·cor·dance
dis·co·ri·a
   or dys·co·ri·a
dis·crete
dis·crim·i·nate
dis·crim·i·na·tion
dis·cus
   pl dis·cus·es
   or dis·ci
dis·cus pro·lig·er·us

dis·cu·tient
dis·di·a·clast
dis·ease
dis·eased
dis·en·gage·ment
dis·e·qui·lib·ri·um
   pl dis·e·qui·lib·ri·ums
   or dis·e·qui·lib·ri·a
dis·func·tion
   var of dys·func·tion
dis·gen·ic
   var of dys·gen·ic
dis·ger·mi·no·ma
dis·gre·gate
dis·gre·ga·tion
dis·im·pact
dis·in·fect
dis·in·fec·tant
dis·in·fec·tion
dis·in·fest
dis·in·fes·tant
dis·in·fes·ta·tion
dis·in·hi·bi·tion
dis·in·sec·tion
dis·in·sec·ti·za·tion
dis·in·ser·tion
dis·in·te·grant
dis·in·te·grate
dis·in·te·gra·tion
dis·in·te·gra·tive
dis·in·te·gra·tor
dis·in·tox·i·cate
dis·in·tox·i·ca·tion
dis·in·vag·i·na·tion
dis·joint
dis·joint·ed
dis·junc·tion
   var of dys·junc·tion
dis·junc·tive
disk
   or disc
dis·ki·form
dis·ki·tis
   or dis·ci·tis
dis·ko·gram
   or dis·co·gram
dis·kog·ra·phy
dis·lo·cate
dis·lo·ca·tion

dis·mem·ber
dis·mem·ber·ment
dis·mu·ta·tion
dis·oc·clude
di·so·di·um
di·so·ma
di·so·mus
di·so·pyr·a·mide
dis·or·der
dis·or·ga·ni·za·tion
dis·or·ga·nize
dis·o·ri·ent
dis·o·ri·en·ta·tion
dis·par·ate
dys·pa·reu·ni·a
   var of dys·pa·reu·ni·a
dis·par·i·ty
dis·pen·sa·ry
   pl dis·pen·sa·ries
dis·pen·sa·to·ry
   pl dis·pen·sa·to·ries
dis·pense
di·sper·mine
di·sper·my
   pl di·sper·mies
dis·per·sant
dis·per·sate
dis·perse
dis·per·sion
dis·per·sive
dis·per·soid
di·spi·rem
   or di·spi·reme
di·spi·reme
   or di·spi·rem
dis·place
dis·place·ment
dis·po·si·tion
dis·pro·por·tion
dis·rup·tion
dis·rup·tive
dis·sect
dis·sec·tion
dis·sec·tor
dis·sem·i·nate
dis·sep·i·ment
dis·sep·i·men·tal
dis·sim·i·late
dis·sim·i·la·tion

dis·sim·u·la·tion
dis·so·ci·ant
dis·so·ci·ate
dis·so·ci·a·tion
dis·so·ci·a·tive
dis·sog·e·ny
dis·so·lu·tion
dis·solve
dis·sol·vent
dis·sor·ta·tive
dis·so·nance
dis·tad
dis·tal
dis·tem·per
dis·tem·per·oid
dis·ten·si·bil·i·ty
  pl dis·ten·si·bil·i·ties
dis·ten·si·ble
dis·ten·sion
  or dis·ten·tion
dis·ten·tion
  or dis·ten·sion
dis·tich·i·a
dis·ti·chi·a·sis
dis·till
dis·til·land
dis·til·late
dis·til·la·tion
dis·to·buc·cal
dis·to·buc·co·oc·clu·sal
dis·to·buc·co·pul·pal
dis·to·cer·vi·cal
dis·to·clu·sion
dis·to·gin·gi·val
dis·to·in·ci·sal
dis·to·la·bi·al
dis·to·lin·gual
dis·to·lin·guo·oc·clu·sal
Dis·to·ma
Dis·to·ma·ta
dis·to·ma·to·sis
  pl dis·to·ma·to·ses
di·sto·mi·a
dis·to·mi·a·sis
  pl dis·to·mi·a·ses
dis·to·mo·lar
Dis·to·mum
di·sto·mus
dis·to·oc·clu·sal

dis·tor·tion
dis·to·ver·sion
dis·tract·i·bil·i·ty
  pl dis·tract·i·bil·i·ties
dis·trac·tion
dis·trac·tive
dis·tress
dis·tri·bute
dis·tri·bu·tion
dis·tri·chi·a·sis
dis·trix
dis·turb
dis·tur·bance
dis·turbed
di·sul·fate
di·sul·fide
di·sul·fi·ram
di·ta
di·ter·pene
di·thi·az·i·nine i·o·dide
di·thi·zone
dith·ra·nol
di·thy·mol di·i·o·dide
dit·o·cous
  or dit·o·kous
dit·o·kous
  or dit·o·cous
Ditt·rich ste·no·sis
di·u·re·ide
di·u·re·sis
  pl di·u·re·ses
di·u·re·tic
di·ur·nal
di·ur·nule
di·va·ga·tion
di·va·lent
di·var·i·ca·tion
di·ver·gence
di·ver·gent
di·ver·tic·u·lar
di·ver·tic·u·lec·to·my
  pl di·ver·tic·u·lec·to·mies
di·ver·tic·u·li·tis
di·ver·tic·u·lo·gram
di·ver·tic·u·lo·sis
di·ver·tic·u·lum
  pl di·ver·tic·u·la

di·vi·di·vi
  pl di·vi·di·vis
  or di·vi·di·vi
di·vi·nyl
di·vi·sion
Div·ry-van Bo·gaert dis·ease
di·vulse
di·vul·sion
di·vul·sor
di·xen·ic
di·zy·got·ic
diz·zi·ness
diz·zy
djen·kol·ic
Dn·ase
  or DNA·ase
DNA·ase
  or DN·ase
Do·bell so·lu·tion
Do·chez se·rum
doc·i·ma·si·a
  pl doc·i·ma·si·as
  or doc·i·ma·sy
  pl doc·i·ma·sies
doc·i·mas·tic
doc·i·ma·sy
  pl doc·i·ma·sies
  or doc·i·ma·si·a
  pl doc·i·ma·si·as
doc·o·sa·no·ic
doc·tor
doc·trine
do·dec·a·no·ic
do·dec·yl
Dö·der·lein ba·cil·lus
Doeh·le bod·ies
Doer·fler-Stew·art test
Do·giel cells
dog·ma·tist
dog·tooth
doigts en lor·gnette
doi·sy·nol·ic
dol
dol·i·cho·ce·phal·ic
  or dol·i·cho·ceph·a·lous
dol·i·cho·ceph·a·lism
dol·i·cho·ceph·a·lous
  or dol·i·cho·ce·phal·ic

dol·i·cho·ceph·a·lus
  pl dol·i·cho·ceph·a·li
dol·i·cho·ceph·a·ly
  pl dol·i·cho·ceph·a·lies
dol·i·cho·cham·ae·cra·ni·al
dol·i·cho·cne·mic
dol·i·cho·co·lon
dol·i·cho·cra·ni·al
dol·i·cho·cra·ny
  pl dol·i·cho·cra·nies
dol·i·cho·de·rus
dol·i·cho·eu·ro·mes·o·
  ceph·a·lus
dol·i·cho·eu·ro·o·pis·tho·
  ceph·a·lus
dol·i·cho·eu·ro·pro·ceph·
  a·lus
dol·i·cho·fa·cial
dol·i·cho·hi·er·ic
dol·i·cho·ker·kic
dol·i·cho·lep·to·ceph·a·lus
dol·i·cho·mor·phic
dol·i·cho·pel·lic
dol·i·cho·pel·vic
dol·i·cho·plat·y·ceph·a·lus
dol·i·cho·pro·sop·ic
dol·i·chor·rhine
Dol·i·chos
dol·i·cho·sten·o·me·li·a
dol·i·cho·u·ran·ic
Do·lin meth·od
Dol·man test
do·lor
  pl do·lo·res
do·lo·rif·ic
do·lo·rim·e·ter
do·lo·ri·met·ric
do·lo·rim·e·try
  pl do·lo·rim·e·tries
do·lo·ro·gen·ic
do·ma·to·pho·bi·a
dom·i·nance
dom·i·nant
dom·i·na·tor
do·mi·phen
Don·a·hue syn·drome
Do·nath-Land·stei·ner test
don·a·tism

Don·der law
do·nee
Don·nan e·qui·li·bri·um
Don·né cor·pus·cles
do·nor
Don·o·van bod·y
Don·o·va·ni·a
  gran·u·lo·ma·tis
do·pa
do·pa·mine
do·pa·min·er·gic
do·pa·ox·i·dase
do·pase
Dopp·ler ef·fect, shift
do·ra·pho·bi·a
Do·rel·lo ca·nal
dor·mant
dor·nase
Dor·ner spore stain
do·ro·ma·ni·a
Dor·o·thy Reed cell
Dor·rance op·er·a·tion
dor·sad
dor·sal
dor·sal·gi·a
dor·sa·lis
  pl dor·sa·les
Dor·set egg me·di·um
dor·si·duct
dor·si·flex
dor·si·flex·ion
dor·si·flex·or
dor·si·lat·er·al
  or dor·so·lat·er·al
dor·si·lum·bar
  or dor·so·lum·bar
dor·si·spi·nal
dor·so·an·te·ri·or
dor·so·ceph·a·lad
dor·so·cu·boi·dal
dor·so·ep·i·troch·le·ar·is
dor·so·lat·er·al
  or dor·si·lat·er·al
dor·so·lum·bar
  or dor·si·lum·bar
dor·so·me·di·ad
dor·so·me·di·al
dor·so·me·di·an

dor·so·na·sal
dor·so·pos·te·ri·or
dor·so·ra·di·al
dor·so·sa·cral
dor·so·ul·nar
dor·so·ven·trad
dor·so·ven·tral
dor·so·ven·tral·ly
dor·sum
  pl dor·sa
dos·age
dose
do·sem·e·ter
  or do·sim·e·ter
do·sim·e·ter
  or dos·em·e·ter
do·si·met·ric
do·sim·e·try
  pl do·sim·e·tries
dou·ble-blind
dou·ble-joint·ed
dou·blet
douche
Doug·las bag
doug·las·i·tis
dou·rine
dou·rou·cou·li
Do·ver pow·der
dove·tail
dow·el
Down syn·drome
Dow·ney cells
dox·a·pram
dox·e·pin
dox·y·cy·cline
dox·yl·a·mine
Doyne cho·roi·di·tis
drachm
  or dram
drac·on·ti·a·sis
  pl drac·on·ti·a·ses
dra·cun·cu·li·a·sis
  pl dra·cun·cu·li·a·ses
dra·cun·cu·lo·sis
  pl dra·cun·cu·lo·ses
Dra·cun·cu·lus
draft
dra·gée

drag·on blood
Drag·stedt graft
drain
drain·age
dram
  or drachm
dram·a·tism
drape
drap·e·to·ma·ni·a
dras·tic
draught
  var of draft
draw·sheet
dream·work
drench
Dre·pan·i·do·tae·ni·a
drep·a·no·cyte
drep·a·no·cy·thae·mi·a
  var of drep·a·no·cy·the·
    mi·a
drep·a·no·cy·the·mi·a
drep·a·no·cyt·ic
drep·a·no·cy·to·sis
  pl drep·a·no·cy·to·ses
Dres·bach syn·drome
dres·sing
Dress·ler syn·drome
Driesch law of con·
    stant vol·ume
Drink·er res·pi·ra·tor
Drink·er-Col·lins
    re·sus·ci·ta·tion
driv·el·ing
dro·car·bil
drom·o·graph
drom·o·ma·ni·a
drom·o·pho·bi·a
drom·o·stan·o·lone
drom·o·trop·ic
dro·per·i·dol
drop·let
drop·per
drop·si·cal
drop·sy
  pl drop·sies
Dro·soph·i·la
drug
drug·fast

drug·gist
drug·mak·er
drug·store
drum·head
drunk·ard
drunk·en
drunk·en·ly
drunk·en·ness
drunk·om·e·ter
drupe
druse
  pl dru·sen
dru·sen
dry·nurse
Dry·op·ter·is
D-state
DTs
du·al
du·al·ism
du·al·is·tic
Du·ane re·trac·tion
    syn·drome
du·az·o·my·cin
Du·bi·ni cho·re·a
Du·bin-John·son
    syn·drome
Du·bin-Sprinz syn·drome
Du·bois cyst
Du·bois-Rey·mond law,
    prin·ci·ple
Du·boi·si·a
Du·bos-Bra·chet meth·od
Du·boscq col·or·im·e·ter
Du·bo·witz syn·drome
Du·chenne dis·ease
Du·chenne-A·ran dis·ease
Du·chenne-Erb pa·ral·y·sis
Du·chenne-Grie·sin·ger
    dis·ease
duck·er·ing
duck·foot·ed
Du·crey ba·cil·lus
duct
duc·tal
duc·tile
duc·til·i·ty
  pl duc·til·i·ties
duc·tion

duct·less
duc·tu·lar
duct·ule
duc·tu·lus
  pl duc·tu·li
duc·tus
  pl duc·tus
duc·tus ar·te·ri·o·sus
duc·tus cho·led·o·chus
duc·tus de·fer·ens
duc·tus ve·no·sus
Duf·fy an·ti·gen, fac·tor
Duf·fy blood group
Du·gas test
Duhr·ing dis·ease
du·ip·a·ra
Dukes dis·ease
dul·ca·ma·ra
dul·cin
dul·cite
dul·ci·tol
Du·long and Pe·tit law
dum·dum fe·ver
dump·ing syn·drome
du·o·chrome
du·o·crin·in
du·o·de·nal
du·o·de·nec·ta·sis
  pl du·o·de·nec·ta·ses
du·o·de·nec·to·my
  pl du·o·de·nec·to·mies
du·o·de·ni·tis
du·o·de·no·chol·an·gi·tis
du·o·de·no·chol·e·cys·tos·
    to·my
du·o·de·no·cho·led·o·chot·
    o·my
du·o·de·no·col·ic
du·o·de·no·cys·tos·to·my
du·o·de·no·en·ter·os·to·my
  pl du·o·de·no·en·ter·os·to·
    mies
du·o·de·no·gram
du·o·de·nog·ra·phy
du·o·de·no·he·pat·ic
du·o·de·no·il·e·os·to·my
du·o·de·no·je·ju·nal
du·o·de·no·jej·u·nos·to·my

du·o·de·no·mes·o·col·ic
du·o·de·no·pan·cre·a·tec·to·
my
du·o·de·no·plas·ty
du·o·de·no·py·lo·rec·to·my
du·o·de·nor·rha·phy
   pl du·o·de·nor·rha·phies
du·o·de·no·scope
du·o·de·nos·co·py
   pl du·o·de·nos·co·pies
du·o·de·nos·to·my
du·o·de·not·o·my
du·o·de·num
   pl du·o·de·nums
   or du·o·de·na
Du·play op·er·a·tion
du·plex·i·ty
du·pli·ca·ta cru·ci·a·ta
du·pli·ca·tion
du·plic·i·tas
du·plic·i·ty
Du·puys-Du·temps
   phe·nom·en·on
Du·puy·tren con·trac·ture,
   frac·ture
du·ra ma·ter
du·ral
Du·rand dis·ease
Du·rand-Ni·co·las-Favre
   dis·ease
Du·ran-Rey·nals fac·tor
du·ra·plas·ty
   pl du·ra·plas·ties
durch·wan·der·ungs
   per·i·to·ni·tis
Dürck nodes
Du·ret he·mor·rha·ges
du·ri·tis
du·ro·ar·ach·ni·tis
du·ro·sar·co·ma
   pl du·ro·sar·co·mas
   or du·ro·sar·co·ma·ta
Du·ro·ziez dis·ease
Du·temps sign
Dut·ton dis·ease
Du·val bac·il·lus
dwarf
dwarf·ism

dy·ad
   or di·ad
dy·ad·ic
   or di·ad·ic
dy·clo·nine
dy·dro·ges·ter·one
dy·man·thine
dy·nam·e·ter
dy·nam·ic
dy·nam·ics
dy·na·mo·gen·e·sis
   pl dy·na·mo·gen·e·ses
dy·na·mo·gen·ic
   or dy·na·mog·e·nous
dy·na·mog·e·nous
   or dy·na·mo·gen·ic
dy·na·mog·e·ny
   pl dy·na·mog·e·nies
dy·nam·o·graph
dy·na·mog·ra·phy
dy·na·mom·e·ter
dy·nam·o·met·ric
dy·na·mom·e·try
   pl dy·na·mom·e·tries
dy·na·o·neure
dy·na·moph·a·ny
dy·nam·o·scope
dy·na·mos·co·py
dy·na·therm
dyne
dy·phyl·line
dys·a·cou·si·a
   or dys·a·cou·sis
   or dys·a·cu·si·a
dys·a·cou·sis
   pl dys·a·cou·ses
   or dys·a·cou·si·a
dys·a·cous·ma
dys·a·cu·si·a
   or dys·a·cou·si·a
   or dys·a·cou·sis
dys·a·cu·sis
dys·ad·ap·ta·tion
dys·ad·re·nal·ism
dys·ad·re·ni·a
dys·ae·mi·a
   var of dys·e·mi·a
dys·aes·the·si·a
   var of dys·es·the·si·a

dys·an·ag·no·si·a
dys·an·ti·graph·i·a
dys·a·phe·a
dys·ap·ta·tion
dys·ar·te·ri·ot·o·my
   pl dys·ar·te·ri·ot·o·nies
dys·ar·thri·a
dys·ar·thric
dys·ar·thro·sis
   pl dys·ar·thro·ses
dys·au·di·a
dys·au·to·no·mi·a
dys·au·to·nom·ic
dys·bar·ism
dys·ba·si·a
dys·bou·li·a
   or dys·bu·li·a
dys·bu·li·a
   or dys·bou·li·a
dys·ce·pha·li·a
   man·dib·u·lo·oc·u·lo·fa·
   ci·a·lis
dys·ceph·a·ly
dys·chei·ri·a
   or dys·chi·ri·a
dys·che·si·a
   or dys·che·zi·a
dys·che·zi·a
   or dys·che·si·a
dys·che·zic
dys·chi·ri·a
   or dys·chei·ri·a
dys·cho·li·a
dys·chon·dro·pla·si·a
dys·chro·a
dys·chro·i·a
dys·chro·ma·to·der·mi·a
dys·chro·ma·tope
dys·chro·ma·top·si·a
dys·chro·ma·top·tic
dys·chro·mi·a
dys·chro·mo·der·mi·a
dys·chro·na·tion
dys·chro·nism
dys·chro·nous
dys·ci·ne·si·a
dys·co·ri·a
   or dis·co·ri·a
dys·cor·ti·cism

dys·cra·si·a
dys·cra·sic
dys·crat·ic
dys·cri·nism
dys·di·ad·o·cho·ki·ne·si·a
   or dys·di·ad·o·ko·ki·ne·
   si·a
dys·di·ad·o·ko·ki·ne·si·a
   or dys·dia·do·cho·ki·ne·
   si·a
dys·e·coi·a
dys·em·bry·o·ma
dys·em·bry·o·pla·si·a
dys·e·me·si·a
dys·em·e·sis
dys·e·mi·a
dys·en·ce·pha·li·a
   splanch·no·cys·ti·ca
dys·en·do·crine
dys·en·do·cri·ni·a·sis
dys·en·do·crin·ism
dys·en·do·cri·si·a·sis
dys·en·te·ri·a
dys·en·ter·ic
dys·en·ter·y
   pl dys·en·ter·ies
dys·er·e·the·si·a
dys·er·ga·si·a
dys·er·ga·sy
dys·er·gi·a
   or dys·er·gy
dys·er·gy
   pl dys·er·gies
   or dys·er·gi·a
dys·es·the·si·a
dys·es·thet·ic
dys·func·tion
dys·ga·lac·ti·a
dys·gam·ma·glob·u·lin·e·
   mi·a
dys·gen·e·sis
   pl dys·gen·e·ses
dys·gen·ic
dys·gen·ics
dys·ger·mi·no·ma
   pl dys·ger·mi·no·mas
   or dys·ger·mi·no·ma·ta
dys·geu·si·a
dys·glan·du·lar

dys·glob·u·li·nae·mi·a
   var of dys·glob·u·li·ne·
   mi·a
dys·glob·u·li·ne·mi·a
dys·gly·ce·mi·a
dys·gnath·ic
dys·gno·si·a
dys·gon·ic
dys·gram·ma·tism
dys·graph·i·a
dys·hae·mo·poi·e·sis
   var of dys·he·mo·poi·e·sis
dys·hae·mo·poi·et·ic
   var of dys·he·mo·poi·et·ic
dys·he·mo·poi·e·sis
dys·he·mo·poi·et·ic
dys·hid·ri·a
dys·hi·dro·sis
   pl dys·hi·dro·ses
   or dys·i·dro·sis
   pl dys·i·dro·ses
dys·ho·ri·a
dys·i·dro·sis
   pl dys·i·dro·ses
   or dys·hi·dro·sis
   pl dys·hi·dro·ses
dys·in·su·lin·ism
dys·junc·tion
dys·kar·y·o·sis
dys·kar·y·ot·ic
dys·ker·a·to·ma
dys·ker·a·to·sis
   pl dys·ker·a·to·ses
dys·ker·a·tot·ic
dys·ki·ne·si·a
dys·ki·net·ic
dys·la·li·a
dys·lec·tic
dys·lex·i·a
dys·lex·i·ac
dyx·lex·ic
dys·lo·chi·a
dys·lo·gi·a
dys·ma·se·sis
dys·ma·tu·ri·ty
dys·me·li·a
dys·men·or·rhe·a
dys·men·or·rhoe·a
   var of dys·men·or·rhe·a

dys·men·or·rhe·al
   or dys·men·or·rhe·ic
dys·men·or·rhe·ic
   or dys·men·or·rhe·al
dys·mer·o·gen·e·sis
dys·mer·o·ge·net·ic
dys·met·ri·a
dys·mim·i·a
dys·mne·si·a
dys·mor·phi·a
dys·mor·phic
dys·mor·pho·pho·bi·a
dys·my·e·lin·o·gen·ic
dys·my·o·to·ni·a
dys·no·mi·a
dys·o·don·ti·a·sis
dys·on·to·gen·e·sis
dys·on·to·ge·net·ic
dys·o·pi·a
dys·o·rex·i·a
dys·os·mi·a
dys·os·te·o·gen·e·sis
dys·os·to·sis
   pl dys·os·to·ses
dys·ox·i·diz·a·ble
dys·pan·cre·a·tism
dys·par·a·thy·roid·ism
dys·pa·reu·ni·a
dys·pep·si·a
dys·pep·tic
   or dys·pep·ti·cal
dys·pep·ti·cal
   or dys·pep·tic
dys·pep·ti·cal·ly
dys·per·i·stal·sis
dys·pha·gi·a
dys·phag·ic
dys·pha·si·a
dys·pha·sic
dys·phe·mi·a
dys·phoi·te·sis
dys·pho·ni·a
dys·phon·ic
dys·pho·ri·a
dys·pho·ric
dys·pho·ti·a
dys·phra·si·a
dys·pig·men·ta·tion
dys·pi·tu·i·ta·rism

dys·pla·si·a
dys·plas·tic
dys·pne·a
dysp·ne·al
dysp·ne·ic
dysp·noe·a
   var of dysp·ne·a
dys·po·ne·sis
dysp·noe·ic
   var of dysp·ne·ic
dys·po·net·ic
dys·prac·tic
dys·pra·gi·a
dys·prax·i·a
dys·pro·si·um
dys·pro·te·in·e·mi·a
dys·ra·ph·i·a
dys·ra·phism
dys·rhyth·mi·a
dys·rhyth·mic
dys·se·ba·ce·a
dys·se·ba·ci·a
dys·se·cre·to·sis

dys·so·cial
dys·som·ni·a
dys·sper·ma·tism
dys·sper·mi·a
dys·splen·ism
dys·sta·si·a
dys·stat·ic
dys·syn·chro·nous
dys·syn·er·gi·a
   or dys·syn·er·gy
dys·syn·er·gic
dys·syn·er·gy
   pl dys·syn·er·gies
   or dys·syn·er·gi·a
dys·tax·i·a
dys·tec·ti·a
dys·tec·tic
dys·tha·na·si·a
dys·the·si·a
dys·thet·ic
dys·thy·mi·a
dys·thy·mic
dys·thy·roi·dal

dys·thy·roi·dism
dys·tith·i·a
dys·to·ci·a
   or dys·to·ki·a
dys·to·cic
dys·to·cial
dys·to·ki·a
   or dys·to·ci·a
dys·to·ni·a
dys·ton·ic
dys·to·pi·a
dys·top·ic
dys·tro·phi·a
   or dys·tro·phy
dys·troph·ic
dys·troph·o·neu·ro·sis
dys·tro·phy
   pl dys·tro·phies
   or dys·tro·phi·a
dys·tryp·si·a
dys·u·ri·a
dys·u·ric

E

E point
E wave
Ea·gle test
Eales dis·ease
ear
ear·ache
ear·drum
Earle L fi·bro·sar·co·ma
ear·lobe
ear·pick
ear·piece
ear·plug
ear·wax
Ea·ton vi·rus
Ea·ton-Lam·bert
  syn·drome

Eb·ers pa·py·rus
E·ber·thel·la
Eb·ner glands
e·bran·le·ment
e·bri·e·ty
   pl e·bri·e·ties
e·bri·ose
e·bri·ous
Eb·stein a·nom·a·ly
eb·ul·lism
eb·ur·nat·ed
e·bur·na·tion
e·bur·ne·ous
e·cau·date
Ec·bal·li·um
ec·bol·ic

ec·bo·vi·rus
ec·cen·tric
   or ex·cen·tric
ec·cen·tri·cal·ly
ec·cen·tro·chon·dro·os·te·
  o·dys·tro·phy
ec·cen·tro·chon·dro·pla·
  si·a
ec·cen·tro·os·te·o·chon·
  dro·dys·pla·si·a
ec·ceph·a·lo·sis
   pl ec·ceph·a·lo·ses
ec·chon·dro·ma
   pl ec·chon·dro·mas
   or ec·chon·dro·ma·ta

c·chon·dro·sis
  pl ec·chon·dro·ses
c·chon·dro·tome
c·chy·mo·ma
c·chy·mosed
c·chy·mo·sis
  pl ec·chy·mo·ses
c·chy·mot·ic
c·co·pro·ti·co·phor·ic
c·crine
c·cri·nol·o·gy
  pl ec·cri·nol·o·gies
c·cri·sis
c·crit·ic
c·cy·e·sis
  pl ec·cy·e·ses
c·dem·ic
c·dem·o·ma·ni·a
c·der·on
c·der·on·ic
c·do·vi·rus
c·dys·i·al
c·dy·sis
  pl ec·dy·ses
c·dy·sone
c·go·nine
·chid·nase
·chid·nin
·chid·noph·a·ga
·chid·no·tox·in
·ch·i·na·ce·a
·ch·i·nate
  or ech·i·nat·ed
·ch·i·nat·ed
  or ech·i·nate
·chi·no·chrome
·chi·no·coc·co·sis
  pl e·chi·no·coc·co·ses
·chi·no·coc·cus
  pl e·chi·no·coc·ci
·chi·no·derm
·chi·no·der·ma·ta
·chi·noi·de·a
·ch·i·nop·sine
·chi·no·rhyn·chus
·ch·i·no·sis
  pl ech·i·no·ses
·chi·no·sto·ma

e·chi·no·sto·mi·a·sis
  pl e·chi·no·sto·mi·a·ses
e·chin·u·late
  or e·chin·u·lat·ed
e·chin·u·lat·ed
  or e·chin·u·late
Ech·is
ech·o
  pl ech·oes
ech·o·a·cou·si·a
ech·o·a·or·tòg·ra·phy
ech·o·car·di·o·gram
ech·o·car·di·og·ra·phy
ech·o·en·ceph·a·lo·gram
ech·o·en·ceph·a·lo·graph
ech·o·en·ceph·a·log·ra·phy
  pl ech·o·en·ceph·a·log·ra·
    phies
ech·o·gram
ech·o·graph·i·a
e·chog·ra·phy
ech·o·ki·ne·si·a
  pl ech·o·ki·ne·si·as
  or echo·ki·ne·sis
  pl ech·o·ki·ne·ses
ech·o·ki·ne·sis
  pl ech·o·ki·ne·ses
  or ech·o·ki·ne·si·a
  pl ech·o·ki·ne·si·as
ech·o·la·li·a
ech·o·lal·ic
ech·o·la·lus
ech·o·lo·ca·tion
e·cho·ma·tism
ech·o·mim·i·a
ech·o·mo·tism
ech·op·a·thy
ech·oph·o·ny
ech·o·phot·o·ny
ech·o·phra·si·a
ech·o·prax·i·a
ech·o·prax·y
ech·o·re·no·gram
ech·o·son·o·en·ceph·a·lo·
    gram
ech·o·son·o·gram
ech·o·thi·o·phate i·o·dide
ech·o·u·ter·o·gram

ech·o·vi·rus
Eck fis·tu·la
Eck·er di·lut·ing flu·id.
ec·la·bi·um
ec·lamp·si·a
ec·lamp·sism
ec·lamp·tic
ec·lamp·to·gen·ic
ec·lec·tic
ec·lec·ti·cism
e·clipse
ec·ly·sis
  pl ec·ly·ses
ec·mne·si·a
ec·mo·vi·rus
e·coid
e·col·o·gy
e·co·ma·ni·a
E·con·o·mo dis·ease
ec·o·phys·i·ol·o·gist
é·cor·ché
e·cos·tate
e·cos·ta·tion
e·cos·ta·tism
ec·o·sys·tem
ec·pho·ri·a
  pl ec·pho·ri·as
  or ec·pho·ri·ae
ec·pho·rize
ec·phy·lax·is
e·cra·seur
ec·so·vi·rus
ec·sta·cy
  pl ec·sta·cies
  or ec·sta·sy
  pl ec·sta·sies
ec·sta·sy
  pl ec·sta·sies
  or ec·sta·cy
  pl ec·sta·cies
ec·stat·ic
ec·tad
ec·tal
ec·ta·si·a
ec·ta·sis
  pl ec·ta·ses
ec·tat·ic

ec·ten·tal
ect·eth·moid
    or ect·eth·moi·dal
    or ec·to·eth·moid
ec·teth·moi·dal
    or ect·eth·moid
    or ec·to·eth·moid
ec·thy·ma
ec·thy·ma·tous
ec·to·an·ti·gen
ec·to·bat·ic
ec·to·blast
ec·to·car·di·a
ec·to·cer·vix
ec·to·cho·roi·de·a
ec·to·ci·ne·re·a
ec·to·cor·ne·a
ec·to·cra·ni·al
ec·to·crine
ec·to·cyst
ec·to·derm
ec·to·der·mal
    or ec·to·der·mic
ec·to·der·mic
    or ec·to·der·mal
ec·to·der·mo·sis
    pl ec·to·der·mo·ses
ec·to·en·tad
ec·to·en·zyme
ec·to·eth·moid
    or ect·eth·moid
    or ect·eth·moi·dal
ec·to·gen·e·sis
ec·to·ge·net·ic
ec·to·gen·ic
ec·tog·e·nous
ec·to·glob·u·lar
ec·tog·o·ny
ec·to·hor·mon·al
ec·to·hor·mone
ec·to·loph
ec·to·men·inx
    pl ec·to·me·nin·ges
ec·to·mere
ec·to·mes·o·derm
ec·to·morph
ec·to·mor·phic
ec·to·mor·phy
ec·to·pa·gi·a

ec·top·a·gus
ec·top·a·gy
ec·to·par·a·site
ec·to·par·a·sit·ic
ec·to·phyte
ec·to·phyt·ic
ec·to·pi·a
ec·top·ic
ec·to·pla·cen·ta
ec·to·pla·cen·tal
ec·to·plasm
ec·to·plas·mat·ic
ec·to·plas·mic
ec·to·plast
ec·to·plas·tic
ec·to·pot·o·my
ec·to·py
ec·to·sarc
ec·tos·te·al
ec·to·sto·sis
    pl ec·to·sto·ses
ec·to·thrix
ec·to·zo·on
    pl ec·to·zo·a
ec·tro·dac·tyl·i·a
ec·tro·dac·ty·lism
ec·tro·dac·ty·ly
    pl ec·tro·dac·ty·lies
ec·tro·gen·ic
ec·trog·e·ny
ec·tro·me·li·a
ec·tro·me·lic
ec·trom·e·lus
ec·trom·e·ly
ec·tro·pi·on
ec·tro·pi·on·i·za·tion
ec·tro·pi·on·ize
ec·tro·pi·um
ec·trop·o·dism
ec·tro·syn·dac·ty·ly
ec·trot·ic
ec·ty·lot·ic
ec·tyl·u·re·a
ec·ze·ma
ec·zem·a·tid
ec·zem·a·ti·za·tion
ec·zem·a·toid
ec·zem·a·to·sis
ec·zem·a·tous

Ed·dowes dis·ease
Ed·dy·ism
Ed·e·bohl op·er·a·tion
Ed·el·mann sign
e·de·ma
    pl e·de·mas
    or e·de·ma·ta
e·dem·a·tous
E·den·ta·ta
e·den·tate
e·den·ti·a
e·den·tu·late
e·den·tu·lous
e·de·ol·o·gy
e·des·tin
ed·e·tate
e·det·ic
ed·i·ble
Ed·in·ger-West·phal
    nu·cle·us
ed·i·pal
    var of oed·i·pal
ed·i·pism
    var of oed·i·pism
e·dis·yl·ate
e·do·ceph·a·lus
e·do·ceph·a·ly
ed·ro·phon·i·um
ed·u·ca·ble
e·duct
e·duc·tion
Ed·wards syn·drome
Ed·win Smith pa·py·rus
ef·face·ment
ef·fect
ef·fec·tor
ef·fem·i·na·tion
ef·fer·ent
ef·fer·vesce
ef·fer·ves·cence
ef·fer·ves·cent
ef·fleu·rage
ef·flo·resce
ef·flo·res·cence
ef·flo·res·cent
ef·flu·ent
ef·flu·vi·um
    pl ef·flu·vi·ums
    or ef·flu·via

ef·fort
ef·fuse
ef·fu·sion
e·ga·grop·i·lus
e·ger·sis
e·ger·tic
e·ges·ta
e·ges·tion
egg
e·glan·du·lar
e·glan·du·lose
e·go
e·go·bron·choph·o·ny
e·go·cen·tric
e·go·cen·tric·i·ty
  pl e·go·cen·tric·i·ties
e·go·cen·trism
e·go·dys·to·ni·a
e·go·dys·ton·ic
e·go·i·den·ti·ty
e·go·ism
e·go·ist
e·go·is·tic
  or e·go·is·ti·cal
e·go·is·ti·cal
  or e·go·is·tic
e·go·is·ti·cal·ly
e·go·ma·ni·a
e·go·ma·ni·ac
e·go·ma·ni·a·cal
e·go·ma·ni·a·cal·ly
e·goph·o·ny
  pl e·goph·o·nies
e·go·strength
e·go·syn·to·ni·a
e·go·syn·ton·ic
e·go·syn·to·ny
  pl e·go·syn·to·nies
e·go·tism
e·go·tist
e·go·tis·tic
  or e·go·tis·ti·cal
e·go·tis·ti·cal
  or e·go·tis·tic
e·go·tis·ti·cal·ly
e·go·trop·ic
Eh·lers-Dan·los
  syn·drome
Eh·ren·rit·ter gan·gli·on

Ehr·lich test
Ehr·lich-Heinz gran·ules
ei·co·nom·e·ter
  or ei·ko·nom·e·ter
ei·co·sane
ei·det·ic
ei·do·gen
ei·dop·tom·e·try
Eijk·man test
ei·ko·nom·e·ter
  or ei·co·nom·e·ter
Ei·me·ri·a
Ei·me·ri·id·ae
Ein·horn meth·od
ein·stein
ein·stein·i·um
Ein·tho·ven e·qua·tion
ei·san·the·ma
Ei·sen·men·ger syn·drome
ei·sen·zuck·er
e·jac·u·late
e·jac·u·la·ti·o
e·jac·u·la·tion
e·jac·u·la·to·ry
e·jac·u·la·tor u·ri·nae
e·ject
e·jec·ta
e·jec·tion
e·jec·tor
e·ka·i·o·dine
e·kis·tics
e·lab·o·ra·tion
el·a·cin
el·ae·o·my·en·chy·sis
  var of el·e·o·my·en·chy·sis
el·ae·op·tene
  var of el·e·op·tene
el·ae·o·stear·ic
  var of el·e·o·stear·ic
el·a·id·ic
e·la·i·din
el·a·pid
E·lap·i·dae
e·las·tance
e·las·tase
e·las·tic
e·las·ti·ca
e·las·tic·i·ty
  pl e·las·tic·i·ties

e·las·tin
e·las·to·fi·bro·ma
  pl e·las·to·fi·bro·mas
  or e·las·to·fi·bro·ma·ta
e·las·toi·do·sis, nod·u·lar
e·las·to·ma
  pl e·las·to·mas
  or e·las·to·ma·ta
e·las·to·mer
e·las·to·mer·ic
e·las·tom·e·ter
e·las·tom·e·try
e·las·to·mu·cin
e·las·tor·rhex·is
e·las·tose
e·las·to·sis
  pl e·las·to·ses
e·lat·er·in
e·la·te·ri·um
e·la·tion
el·bow
el·co·sis
el·der
el·drin
el·e·cam·pane
E·lec·tra com·plex
e·lec·tric
  or e·lec·tri·cal
e·lec·tri·cal
  or e·lec·tric
e·lec·tri·cal al·ter·nans
e·lec·tri·fy
e·lec·tri·za·tion
e·lec·tro·af·fin·i·ty
e·lec·tro·an·aes·the·si·a
  var of e·lec·tro·an·es·the·
  si·a
e·lec·tro·a·nal·y·sis
e·lec·tro·an·es·the·si·a
e·lec·tro·bi·ol·o·gy
  pl e·lec·tro·bi·ol·o·gies
e·lec·tro·bi·os·co·py
e·lec·tro·cap·il·lar·i·ty
e·lec·tro·car·di·o·gram
e·lec·tro·car·di·o·graph
e·lec·tro·car·di·o·graph·ic
e·lec·tro·car·di·og·ra·phy
  pl e·lec·tro·car·di·og·ra·
  phies

e·lec·tro·car·di·o·pho·nog·ra·phy
e·lec·tro·car·di·o·scope
e·lec·tro·ca·tal·y·sis
e·lec·tro·cau·ter·i·za·tion
e·lec·tro·cau·ter·y
  pl e·lec·tro·cau·ter·ies
e·lec·tro·chem·is·try
e·lec·tro·chro·ma·tog·ra·phy
e·lec·tro·co·ag·u·la·tion
e·lec·tro·co·ma
e·lec·tro·con·duc·tiv·i·ty
e·lec·tro·con·trac·til·i·ty
  pl e·lec·tro·con·trac·til·i·ties
e·lec·tro·con·vul·sive
e·lec·tro·cor·ti·cal
e·lec·tro·cor·ti·co·gram
e·lec·tro·cor·ti·co·graph·ic
e·lec·tro·cor·ti·co·graph·i·cal·ly
e·lec·tro·cor·ti·cog·ra·phy
e·lec·tro·cor·tin
e·lec·tro·cute
e·lec·tro·cu·tion
e·lec·tro·cys·to·scope
e·lec·tro·cys·tos·co·py
e·lec·trode
e·lec·tro·dep·o·si·tion
e·lec·tro·der·mal
e·lec·tro·der·ma·tome
e·lec·tro·des·ic·ca·tion
e·lec·tro·di·ag·no·sis
e·lec·tro·di·ag·nos·tics
e·lec·tro·di·al·y·sis
  pl e·lec·tro·di·al·y·ses
e·lec·tro·di·a·ly·zer
e·lec·tro·di·a·phane
e·lec·tro·di·aph·a·ny
e·lec·tro·dy·nam·ics
e·lec·tro·dy·na·mom·e·ter
e·lec·tro·en·ceph·a·lo·gram
e·lec·tro·en·ceph·a·lo·graph
e·lec·tro·en·ceph·a·lo·graph·ic

e·lec·tro·en·ceph·a·log·ra·phy
  pl e·lec·tro·en·ceph·a·log·ra·phies
e·lec·tro·end·os·mose
  or e·lec·tro·end·os·mo·sis
e·lec·tro·end·os·mo·sis
  pl elec·tro·end·os·mo·ses
  or elec·tro·end·os·mose
e·lec·tro·fit
e·lec·tro·form
e·lec·tro·gas·tro·gram
e·lec·tro·gas·tro·graph
e·lec·tro·gas·tro·gra·phy
  pl e·lec·tro·gas·trog·ra·phies
e·lec·tro·gen·e·sis
  pl e·lec·tro·gen·e·ses
e·lec·tro·gen·ic
e·lec·tro·gram
e·lec·trog·ra·phy
  pl e·lec·trog·ra·phies
e·lec·tro·hae·mos·ta·sis
  var of e·lec·tro·he·mos·ta·sis
e·lec·tro·he·mos·ta·sis
e·lec·tro·hys·ter·o·graph
e·lec·tro·hys·ter·og·ra·phy
e·lec·tro·im·mu·no·dif·fu·sion
e·lec·tro·ki·net·ic
e·lec·tro·ki·net·ics
e·lec·tro·ky·mo·gram
e·lec·tro·ky·mo·graph
e·lec·tro·ky·mog·ra·phy
  pl e·lec·tro·ky·mog·ra·phies
e·lec·tro·li·thot·ri·ty
e·lec·trol·o·gist
e·lec·trol·o·gy
e·lec·trol·y·sis
  pl e·lec·trol·y·ses
e·lec·tro·lyte
e·lec·tro·lyt·ic
e·lec·tro·lyze
e·lec·tro·mag·net
e·lec·tro·mag·net·ic
e·lec·tro·mag·net·ism
e·lec·tro·mas·sage

e·lec·trom·e·ter
e·lec·tro·met·ric
e·lec·tro·mo·tive
e·lec·tro·mus·cu·lar
e·lec·tro·my·o·gram
e·lec·tro·my·o·graph
e·lec·tro·my·o·graph·ic
e·lec·tro·my·og·ra·phy
  pl e·lec·tro·my·og·ra·phies
e·lec·tron
e·lec·tro·nar·co·sis
  pl e·lec·tro·nar·co·ses
e·lec·tron-dense
e·lec·tro·neg·a·tive
e·lec·tro·neg·a·tiv·i·ty
e·lec·tro·neu·ro·my·og·ra·phy
e·lec·tron·ic
e·lec·tro·nys·tag·mog·ra·phy
e·lec·tro·oc·u·lo·gram
e·lec·tro·oc·u·lo·gra·phy
  pl e·lec·tro·oc·u·log·ra·phies
e·lec·tro·os·mose
  or e·lec·tro·os·mo·sis
  or e·lec·tros·mo·sis
e·lec·tro·os·mo·sis
  pl e·lec·tro·os·mo·ses
  or e·lec·tro·os·mose
  or e·lec·tros·mo·sis
e·lec·tro·ox·i·da·tion
e·lec·tro·ox·i·diz·a·ble
e·lec·tro·pa·thol·o·gy
e·lec·tro·pher·o·gram
e·lec·tro·phil·ic
e·lec·tro·pho·bi·a
e·lec·tro·pho·rese
e·lec·tro·pho·re·sis
  pl e·lec·tro·pho·re·ses
e·lec·tro·pho·ret·ic
e·lec·tro·pho·ret·o·gram
e·lec·tro·phor·o·rus
  pl e·lec·troph·o·ri
e·lec·tro·pho·to·ther·a·py
e·lec·tro·phren·ic
e·lec·tro·phys·i·ol·o·gy
  pl e·lec·tro·phys·i·ol·o·gies

e·lec·tro·plex·y
  pl e·lec·tro·plex·ies
e·lec·tro·pos·i·tive
e·lec·tro·punc·ture
e·lec·tro·py·rex·i·a
e·lec·tro·re·duc·i·ble
e·lec·tro·re·duc·tion
e·lec·tro·re·sec·tion
e·lec·tro·ret·i·no·gram
e·lec·tro·ret·i·no·graph
e·lec·tro·ret·i·no·graph·ic
e·lec·tro·ret·i·nog·ra·phy
  pl e·lec·tro·ret·i·nog·ra·
    phies
e·lec·tro·scis·sion
e·lec·tro·scope
e·lec·tro·sec·tion
e·lec·tro·shock
e·lec·tro·sleep
e·lec·tros·mo·sis
  pl e·lec·tros·mo·ses
  or e·lec·tro·os·mo·sis
  or e·lec·tro·os·mose
e·lec·tro·sol
e·lec·tro·some
e·lec·tro·stat·ic
e·lec·tro·stat·ics
e·lec·tro·steth·o·phone
e·lec·tro·stim·u·la·tion
e·lec·tro·stri·a·to·gram
e·lec·tro·stric·tion
e·lec·tro·sur·ger·y
  pl e·lec·tro·sur·ger·ies
e·lec·tro·sur·gi·cal
e·lec·tro·syn·the·sis
e·lec·tro·tax·is
  pl e·lec·tro·tax·es
e·lec·tro·thal·a·mo·gram
e·lec·tro·tha·na·si·a
e·lec·tro·ther·a·peu·tics
e·lec·tro·ther·a·py
  pl e·lec·tro·ther·a·pies
e·lec·tro·therm
e·lec·tro·ther·mal
e·lec·tro·ther·mic
e·lec·tro·ther·my
e·lec·tro·tome
e·lec·tro·ton·ic
e·lec·trot·o·nus

e·lec·tro·tro·pism
e·lec·tro·tur·bi·nom·e·ter
e·lec·tro·va·go·gram
e·lec·tro·va·lence
e·lec·tro·ver·sion
e·lec·tro·vert
e·lec·tro·vi·bra·to·ry
e·lec·tro·win
e·lec·tu·ar·y
  pl e·lec·tu·ar·ies
el·e·doi·sin
el·e·i·din
el·e·ment
el·e·men·tal
el·e·men·ta·ry
el·e·mi
el·e·o·ma
  pl el·e·o·mas
  or el·e·o·ma·ta
el·e·om·e·ter
el·e·o·my·en·chy·sis
el·e·op·ten
el·e·op·tene
el·e·o·stear·ic
el·e·o·ther·a·py
el·e·phan·ti·ac
el·e·phan·ti·as·ic
el·e·phan·ti·a·sis
  pl el·e·phan·ti·a·ses
el·e·phan·toid
e·leu·ther·a bark
el·e·va·tor
El·ford mem·brane
Elft·man-Elft·man
  meth·od
e·lim·i·nant
e·lim·i·nate
e·lim·i·na·tion
e·lim·i·na·tive
e·lin·gua·tion
e·li·sion
e·lix·ir
El·kin op·er·a·tion
El·li·ot op·er·a·tion
El·li·ott treat·ment
el·lip·sin
el·lip·sis
  pl el·lip·ses
el·lip·soid

el·lip·soi·dal
el·lip·tic
  or el·lip·ti·cal
el·lip·ti·cal
  or el·lip·tic
el·lip·to·cyte
el·lip·to·cy·to·sis
  pl el·lip·to·cy·to·ses
El·lis curve
El·lis-van Crev·eld
  syn·drome
Ells·worth-How·ard test
e·lon·gate
e·lon·ga·tion
e·lope
e·lope·ment
El·schnig pearls
el·u·ant
  or el·u·ent
el·u·ate
el·u·ent
  or el·u·ant
e·lu·sive
e·lute
e·lu·tion
e·lu·tri·a·tion
El·veh·jem and Ken·ne·dy
  meth·od
E·ly sign
e·ma·ci·ate
e·ma·ci·a·tion
e·mac·u·la·tion
e·mail·lo·blast
em·a·nate
em·a·na·tion
em·a·na·to·ri·um
e·man·ci·pate
e·man·ci·pa·tion
em·a·no·ther·a·py
e·man·si·o men·si·um
e·mas·cu·late
e·mas·cu·la·tion
e·mas·cu·la·tor
Em·ba·do·mo·nas
em·balm
em·bar·rass
em·bar·rass·ment
Emb·den-Mey·er·hof
  scheme

117

em·bed
   or im·bed
Em·be·li·a
em·bel·ic
em·be·lin
em·bo·lae·mi·a
   var of em·bo·le·mi·a
em·bo·la·li·a
   or em·bo·lo·la·li·a
em·bo·le
   or em·bo·ly
em·bo·lec·to·my
   pl em·bo·lec·to·mies
em·bo·le·mi·a
em·bol·ic
em·bol·i·form
em·bo·lism
em·bo·li·za·tion
em·bo·loid
em·bo·lo·la·li·a
   or em·bo·la·li·a
em·bo·lo·phra·si·a
em·bo·lus
   pl em·bo·li
em·bo·ly
   pl em·bo·lies
   or em·bo·le
em·bouche·ment
em·bra·sure
em·bro·cate
em·bro·ca·tion
em·bry·ec·to·my
em·bry·o
em·bry·o·blast
em·bry·o·car·di·a
em·bry·o·chem·i·cal
em·bry·o·ci·dal
em·bry·oc·ton·ic
em·bry·oc·to·ny
em·bry·o·gen·e·sis
   pl em·bry·o·gen·e·ses
em·bry·o·ge·net·ic
em·bry·o·gen·ic
em·bry·og·e·ny
   pl em·bry·og·e·nies
em·bry·oid
em·bry·o·lem·ma
   pl em·bry·o·lem·mas
   or em·bry·o·lem·ma·ta

em·bry·o·log·ic
   or em·bry·o·log·i·cal
em·bry·o·log·i·cal
   or em·bry·o·log·ic
em·bry·ol·o·gist
em·bry·ol·o·gy
   pl em·bry·ol·o·gies
em·bry·o·ma
   pl em·bry·o·mas
   or em·bry·o·ma·ta
em·bry·o·mor·phous
em·bry·on
em·bry·o·nal
em·bry·o·nate
em·bry·on·ic
em·bry·on·i·form
em·bry·o·ni·za·tion
em·bry·o·noid
em·bry·o·ny
em·bry·op·a·thy
   pl em·bry·op·a·thies
em·bry·o·phore
em·bry·o·plas·tic
em·bry·o·to·ci·a
em·bry·o·tome
em·bry·ot·o·my
   pl em·bry·ot·o·mies
em·bry·o·tox·ic·i·ty
em·bry·o·tox·on
em·bry·o·troph
   or em·bry·o·trophe
em·bry·o·trophe
   or em·bry·o·troph
em·bry·o·troph·ic
em·bry·ot·ro·phy
   pl em·bry·ot·ro·phies
em·bry·ul·ci·a
em·bry·ul·cus
e·med·ul·late
e·mer·gen·cy
e·mer·gent
em·e·sis
   pl em·e·ses
em·e·ta·mine
e·met·a·tro·phi·a
e·met·ic
em·e·tine
em·e·to·ca·thar·sis
   pl em·e·to·ca·thar·ses

em·e·to·ca·thar·tic
em·e·to·ma·ni·a
em·e·to·mor·phine
em·e·to·pho·bi·a
e·mic·tion
e·mic·to·ry
em·i·grate
em·i·gra·tion
em·i·nence
em·i·nen·ti·a
em·i·o·cy·to·sis
em·is·sar·i·um
   pl em·is·sar·i·a
em·is·sar·y
e·mis·sion
em·men·a·gog·ic
em·men·a·gogue
em·men·i·a
em·men·i·op·a·thy
em·me·nol·o·gy
em·me·trope
em·me·tro·pi·a
em·me·trop·ic
Em·mon·si·a par·va
em·o·din
em·o·din-L-rham·no·side
e·mol·lient
e·mo·ti·o·mo·tor
e·mo·ti·o·mus·cu·lar
e·mo·tion
e·mo·tion·al
e·mo·ti·o·vas·cu·lar
em·pasm
em·pas·ma
em·path·ic
em·pa·thize
em·pa·thy
   pl em·pa·thies
em·per·i·po·le·sis
em·phly·sis
em·phrac·tic
em·phrax·is
   pl em·phrax·es
em·phy·se·ma
em·phy·sem·a·tous
em·pir·ic
   or em·pir·i·cal
em·pir·i·cal
   or em·pir·ic

em·pir·i·cism
em·plas·tic
em·plas·trum
pl em·plas·tra
em·pros·thot·o·nos
or em·pros·thot·o·nus
em·pros·thot·o·nus
or em·pros·thot·o·nos
em·pros·tho·zy·go·sis
em·py·e·ma
pl em·py·e·mas
or em·py·e·ma·ta
em·py·e·ma·tous
em·py·e·mic
em·py·e·sis
pl em·py·e·ses
em·py·reu·ma
pl em·py·reu·ma·ta
em·py·reu·mat·ic
or em·py·reu·mat·i·cal
em·py·reu·mat·i·cal
or em·py·reu·mat·ic
e·mul·gent
e·mul·si·ble
e·mul·si·fi·ca·tion
e·mul·si·fi·er
e·mul·si·fy
e·mul·sin
e·mul·sion
e·mul·sive
e·mul·soid
e·munc·to·ry
pl e·munc·to·ries
em·yl·cam·ate
e·nam·el
e·nam·e·lo·blas·to·ma
pl e·nam·e·lo·blas·to·mas
or e·nam·e·lo·blas·to·ma·ta
e·nam·e·lo·ma
pl e·nam·e·lo·mas
or e·nam·e·lo·ma·ta
e·nam·e·lo·plas·ty
e·nam·e·lum
e·nan·thal·de·hyde
e·nan·thate
en·an·them
or en·an·the·ma
en·an·the·ma
pl en·an·the·mas

or en·an·the·ma·ta
or en·an·them
en·an·them·a·tous
e·nan·thic
en·an·ti·o·bio·sis
en·an·ti·o·dro·mi·a
en·an·ti·o·la·li·a
en·an·ti·o·mer
en·an·ti·o·morph
en·an·ti·o·mor·phic
en·an·ti·o·mor·phous
en·ar·thro·di·al
en·ar·thro·sis
pl en·ar·thro·ses
en·can·this
pl en·can·thi·des
en·cap·su·lant
en·cap·su·late
en·cap·su·la·tion
en·cap·sule
en·car·di·tis
en·ceinte
en·ceph·a·lal·gi·a
en·ceph·a·lat·ro·phy
en·ce·phal·ic
en·ceph·a·lit·ic
en·ceph·a·li·tis
pl en·ceph·a·li·ti·des
en·ceph·a·li·to·gen·ic
or en·ceph·a·li·tog·e·nous
en·ceph·a·li·tog·e·nous
var of en·ceph·a·li·to·genic
en·ceph·a·li·to·zo·on
pl en·ceph·a·li·to·zo·a
en·ceph·a·lo·cele
en·ceph·a·lo·clas·tic
en·ceph·a·lo·coele
en·ceph·a·lo·cra·ni·o·cu·
ta·ne·ous
en·ceph·a·lo·cys·to·cele
en·ceph·a·lo·cys·to·me·nin·
go·cele
en·ceph·a·lo·dys·pla·si·a
en·ceph·a·lo·fa·cial
en·ceph·a·lo·gram
en·ceph·a·lo·graph
en·ceph·a·log·ra·phy
pl en·ceph·a·log·ra·phies
en·ceph·a·loid

en·ceph·a·lo·lith
en·ceph·a·lol·o·gy
en·ceph·a·lo·ma
pl en·ceph·a·lo·mas
or en·ceph·a·lo·ma·ta
en·ceph·a·lo·ma·la·ci·a
en·ceph·a·lo·men·in·gi·tis
pl en·ceph·a·lo·men·in·gi·
ti·des
en·ceph·a·lo·me·nin·go·
cele
en·ceph·a·lo·men·in·gop·
a·thy
en·ceph·a·lo·mere
en·ceph·a·lo·mer·ic
en·ceph·a·lom·e·ter
en·ceph·a·lo·my·e·li·tis
pl en·ceph·a·lo·my·e·li·
ti·des
en·ceph·a·lo·my·e·lo·neu·
rop·a·thy
en·ceph·a·lo·my·e·lon·ic
en·ceph·a·lo·my·e·lop·a·
thy
en·ceph·a·lo·my·e·lo·ra·
dic·u·li·tis
en·ceph·a·lo·my·e·lo·ra·
dic·u·lop·a·thy
en·ceph·a·lo·my·e·lo·sis
en·ceph·a·lo·my·o·car·di·
tis
en·ceph·a·lon
pl en·ceph·a·la
en·ceph·a·lo·nar·co·sis
en·ceph·a·lop·a·thy
pl en·ceph·a·lop·a·thies
en·ceph·a·lo·punc·ture
en·ceph·a·lo·py·o·sis
en·ceph·a·lo·ra·chid·i·an
en·ceph·a·lor·rha·gi·a
en·ceph·a·lo·scle·ro·sis
en·ceph·a·lo·scope
en·ceph·a·los·co·py
en·ceph·a·lo·sep·sis
en·ceph·a·lo·sis
pl en·ceph·a·lo·ses
en·ceph·a·lo·spi·nal
en·ceph·a·lo·tome
en·ceph·a·lot·o·my

en·ceph·a·lo·tri·gem·i·nal
en·chon·dral
en·chon·dro·ma
  pl en·chon·dro·mas
  or en·chon·dro·ma·ta
en·chon·dro·ma·to·sis
en·chon·drom·a·tous
en·chon·dro·sar·co·ma
  pl en·chon·dro·sar·co·mas
  or en·chon·dro·sar·co·ma·ta
en·chon·dro·sis
  pl en·chon·dro·ses
en·chy·le·ma
en·clave
en·clit·ic
en·cod·ing
en·col·pi·tis
en·cop·re·sis
  pl en·cop·re·ses
en·coun·ter group
en·cra·ni·us
en·crust
en·crus·ta·tion
  or in·crus·ta·tion
en·crust·ed
en·cy·e·sis
en·cy·prate
en·cyst
en·cys·ta·tion
en·cyst·ed
en·cyst·ment
end·a·del·phos
end·a·del·phus
End·a·me·ba
  var of End·a·moe·ba
end·am·e·bi·a·sis
  var of en·da·moe·bi·a·sis
End·a·moe·ba
end·am·oe·bi·a·sis
end·an·ge·i·tis
  or end·an·gi·i·tis
end·an·gi·i·tis
  or end·an·ge·i·tis
en·dan·gi·um
end·a·or·ti·tis
end·ar·ter·ec·to·my
  pl end·ar·ter·ec·to·mies
end·ar·te·ri·al
end·ar·te·ri·ec·to·my

end·ar·te·ri·tis
end·ar·te·ri·tis ob·lit·er·ans
end·ar·te·ri·um
  pl end·ar·te·ri·a
end·ar·ter·y
end·au·ral
end·ax·o·neu·ron
end·bod·y
end·brain
end·bulb
en·dem·ic
en·de·mi·ol·o·gy
en·de·mo·ep·i·dem·ic
end·ep·i·der·mis
end·er·gon·ic
en·der·mic
en·der·mo·sis
end·feet
en·do·ab·dom·i·nal
en·do·an·eu·rys·mor·rha·
  phy
en·do·an·gi·i·tis
en·do·a·or·ti·tis
en·do·ap·pen·di·ci·tis
en·do·ar·te·ri·tis
en·do·bi·ot·ic
en·do·blast
en·do·bron·chi·al
en·do·bron·chi·tis
en·do·car·di·ac
en·do·car·di·al
en·do·car·di·tis
en·do·car·di·um
  pl en·do·car·di·a
en·do·carp
en·do·ce·li·ac
en·do·cel·lu·lar
en·do·cer·vi·cal
en·do·cer·vi·ci·tis
en·do·cer·vix
  pl en·do·cer·vi·ces
en·do·cho·le·doch·al
en·do·chon·dral
en·do·chon·dro·ma
  pl en·do·chon·dro·mas
  or en·do·chon·dro·ma·ta
en·do·coe·li·ac
  var of en·do·ce·li·ac
en·do·col·i·tis

en·do·col·pi·tis
en·do·cra·ni·al
en·do·cra·ni·tis
en·do·cra·ni·um
  pl en·do·cra·ni·a
en·do·cri·nas·the·ni·a
en·do·crine
en·do·crin·ic
en·do·crin·ism
en·do·cri·no·log·ic
  or en·do·cri·no·log·i·cal
en·do·cri·no·log·i·cal
  or en·do·cri·no·log·ic
en·do·cri·nol·o·gist
en·do·cri·nol·o·gy
  pl en·do·cri·nol·o·gies
en·do·cri·no·path·ic
en·do·cri·nop·a·thy
  pl en·do·cri·nop·a·thies
en·do·crin·o·ther·a·py
en·do·ci·nous
en·do·cy·ma
en·do·cyst
en·do·cys·ti·tis
en·do·cyte
en·do·cy·to·sis
en·do·derm
en·do·der·ma·to·zo·o·no·sis
en·do·der·mo·phy·to·sis
en·do·don·ti·a
en·do·don·tic
en·do·don·ti·cal·ly
en·do·don·tics
en·do·don·tist
en·do·don·ti·tis
en·do·don·ti·um
en·do·don·tol·o·gy
en·do·en·ter·i·tis
en·do·en·zyme
en·do·er·gic
en·do·e·ryth·ro·cyt·ic
en·do·e·soph·a·gi·tis
en·dog·a·mous
en·dog·a·my
  pl en·dog·a·mies
en·do·gas·tric
en·do·ge·net·ic
en·do·gen·ic
en·dog·e·nous

120

en·dog·e·ny
en·do·gna·thi·on
en·do·go·ni·um
en·do·in·tox·i·ca·tion
en·do·la·ryn·ge·al
En·do·li·max
en·do·lymph
en·do·lym·pha
en·do·lym·phan·ge·al
 or en·do·lym·phan·gi·al
en·do·lym·phan·gi·al
 or en·do·lym·phan·ge·al
en·do·lym·phat·ic
en·do·lym·phic
en·do·ly·sin
en·do·men·inx
 pl en·do·me·nin·ges
en·do·mes·o·derm
en·do·mes·o·vas·cu·li·tis
en·do·me·trec·to·my
en·do·me·tri·al
en·do·me·tri·oid
en·do·me·tri·o·ma
 pl en·do·me·tri·o·mas
 or en·do·me·tri·o·ma·ta
en·do·me·tri·o·sis
 pl en·do·me·tri·o·ses
en·do·me·tri·ot·ic
en·do·me·tri·tis
en·do·me·tri·um
 pl en·do·me·tri·a
en·dom·e·try
en·do·mi·to·sis
 pl en·do·mi·to·ses
en·do·mix·is
en·do·morph
en·do·mor·phic
en·do·mor·phy
en·do·my·o·car·di·tis
en·do·mys·i·um
 pl en·do·mys·i·a
en·do·na·sal
en·do·neu·ral
en·do·neu·ri·al
en·do·neu·ri·tis
en·do·neu·ri·um
 pl en·do·neu·ri·a
en·do·nu·cle·ase
en·do·nu·cle·o·lus

en·do·par·a·site
en·do·par·a·sit·ic
en·do·par·a·sit·ism
en·do·pel·vic
en·do·pep·ti·dase
en·do·per·i·car·di·tis
en·do·per·i·my·o·car·di·tis
en·do·per·i·to·ni·tis
en·do·pha·ryn·ge·al
en·do·phle·bi·tis
 pl en·do·phle·bi·ti·des
en·doph·thal·mi·tis
en·do·phyte
en·do·phyt·ic
en·do·plasm
en·do·plas·mic
en·do·plas·mic re·tic·u·lum
en·do·plast
en·do·plas·tic
en·do·pol·y·ploid
en·do·pol·y·ploi·dy
 pl en·do·pol·y·ploi·dies
en·do·ra·di·o·sonde
en·do·re·du·pli·ca·tion
en·do·sal·pin·gi·o·ma
 pl en·do·sal·pin·gi·o·mas
 or en·do·sal·pin·gi·o·ma·ta
en·do·sal·pin·gi·o·sis
en·do·sal·pin·gi·tis
en·do·sal·pin·go·ma
en·do·sal·pin·go·sis
en·do·sarc
en·do·scope
en·do·scop·ic
en·do·scop·i·cal·ly
en·dos·co·py
 pl en·dos·co·pies
en·do·sep·sis
 pl en·do·sep·ses
en·do·skel·e·ton
en·dos·mom·e·ter
en·dos·mose
en·dos·mo·sic
en·dos·mo·sis
 pl en·dos·mo·ses
en·dos·mot·ic
en·do·some
en·do·sperm
en·do·spore

en·do·spor·u·late
end·os·te·al
end·os·te·i·tis
 or end·os·ti·tis
end·os·te·o·ma
 pl end·os·te·o·mas
 or end·os·te·o·ma·ta
end·os·te·um
 pl end·os·te·a
end·os·ti·tis
 or end·os·te·i·tis
end·os·to·ma
 pl end·os·to·mas
 or end·os·to·ma·ta
en·do·sto·mus
 pl en·do·sto·mi
end·os·to·sis
 pl end·os·to·ses
en·do·ten·din·e·um
en·do·ten·on
en·do·the·li·al
en·do·the·li·o·an·gi·i·tis
en·do·the·li·o·cho·ri·al
en·do·the·li·o·cyte
en·do·the·li·oid
en·do·the·li·o·ly·sin
en·do·the·li·o·ma
 pl en·do·the·li·o·mas
 or en·do·the·li·o·ma·ta
en·do·the·li·o·ma·to·sis
en·do·the·li·o·sis
en·do·the·li·o·tox·in
en·do·the·li·um
 pl en·do·the·li·a
en·do·ther·mal
en·do·ther·mic
en·do·ther·my
 pl en·do·ther·mies
en·do·thrix
 pl en·do·thri·ces
en·do·tox·e·mia
en·do·tox·i·co·sis
en·do·tox·in
en·do·tha·che·al
en·do·tra·che·li·tis
en·do·vas·cu·li·tis
en·do·ve·nous
en·do·ven·tric·u·lar
en·drin

en·dy·ma
en·e·ma
 pl en·e·mas
 or en·e·ma·ta
en·er·get·ic
en·er·get·i·cal·ly
en·er·get·ics
en·er·gid
en·er·giz·er
en·er·gom·e·ter
en·er·gy
 pl en·er·gies
en·er·vate
en·er·va·tion
en·flag·el·la·tion
en·gage·ment
en·gas·tri·us
En·gel·mann dis·ease
En·gel·Reck·ling·hau·sen
 dis·ease
en·globe
en·globe·ment
en·gorge
en·gorge·ment
en·graft
en·gram
en·gramme
 var of en·gram
en·gra·phi·a
Eng·ström tech·nique
en·haem·a·to·spore
 var of en·hem·a·to·spore
en·hem·a·to·spore
en·hex·y·mal
en·ka·tar·rha·phy
en·large
en·large·ment
e·nol
e·no·li·za·tion
e·no·lize
e·nol·o·gy
 pl e·nol·o·gies
e·no·ma·ni·a
en·oph·thal·mos
 or en·oph·thal·mus
en·oph·thal·mus
 or en·oph·thal·mos
en·or·gan·ic

en·o·si·ma·ni·a
en·os·to·sis
 pl en·os·to·ses
En·roth sign
en·sheathe
 or in·sheathe
en·si·form
en·som·phal·ic
en·som·pha·lus
en·stro·phe
en·tad
en·tal
Ent·a·me·ba
 var of Ent·a·moe·ba
ent·a·me·bi·a·sis
 pl ent·a·me·bi·a·ses
Ent·a·moe·ba
ent·a·moe·bi·a·sis
 var of ent·a·me·bi·a·sis
 pl ent·a·me·bi·a·ses
en·ta·si·a
en·ta·sis
en·tat·ic
en·tel·e·chy
en·ter·al
en·ter·al·gi·a
en·ter·al·gic
en·ter·ec·ta·sis
 pl en·ter·ec·ta·ses
en·ter·ec·to·my
 pl en·ter·ec·to·mies
en·ter·el·co·sis
en·ter·e·pip·lo·cele
en·ter·ic
en·ter·ic-coat·ed
en·ter·i·coid
en·ter·i·tis
 pl en·ter·i·tis·es
 or en·ter·i·ti·des
en·ter·o·a·nas·to·mo·sis
 pl en·ter·o·a·nas·to·mo·ses
en·ter·o·an·the·lone
En·ter·o·bac·te·ri·a·ce·ae
en·ter·o·bac·te·ri·al
en·ter·o·bac·te·ri·um
 pl en·ter·o·bac·te·ri·a
en·ter·o·bi·a·sis
 pl en·ter·o·bi·a·ses
En·ter·o·bi·us

en·ter·o·cele
en·ter·o·cen·te·sis
 pl en·ter·o·cen·te·ses
en·ter·o·cep·tive
en·ter·o·chro·maf·fin
en·ter·oc·ly·sis
 pl en·ter·oc·ly·ses
en·ter·o·coc·cus
 pl en·ter·o·coc·ci
en·ter·o·coel
 var of en·ter·o·coele
en·ter·o·coele
en·ter·o·coe·lic
en·ter·o·coe·lous
en·ter·o·co·lec·to·my
en·ter·o·co·lic
en·ter·o·co·li·tis
en·ter·o·co·los·to·my
en·ter·o·crin·in
en·ter·o·cu·ta·ne·ous
en·ter·o·cyst
en·ter·o·cys·to·cele
en·ter·o·cys·to·ma
 pl en·ter·o·cys·to·mas
 or en·ter·o·cys·to·ma·ta
en·ter·o·cys·to·plas·ty
en·ter·o·dyn·i·a
en·ter·o·en·ter·ic
en·ter·o·en·ter·os·to·my
 pl en·ter·o·en·ter·os·to·mies
en·ter·o·e·pip·lo·cele
en·ter·o·gas·tri·tis
en·ter·o·gas·tro·cele
en·ter·o·gas·trone
en·ter·og·e·nous
en·ter·o·gram
en·ter·o·graph
en·ter·o·gra·phy
en·ter·o·hep·a·ti·tis
 pl en·ter·o·hep·a·ti·ti·des
en·ter·o·hep·a·to·cele
en·ter·o·hy·dro·cele
en·ter·o·in·su·lar
en·ter·o·ki·nase
en·ter·o·ki·ne·si·a
en·ter·o·ki·net·ic
en·ter·o·ki·nin
en·ter·o·lith
en·ter·o·li·thi·a·sis

en·ter·ol·o·gist
en·ter·ol·o·gy
en·ter·ol·y·sis
  pl en·ter·ol·y·ses
en·ter·o·meg·a·ly
en·ter·o·me·ro·cele
En·ter·o·mo·nas
en·ter·o·my·co·sis
  pl en·ter·o·my·co·ses
en·ter·o·my·i·a·sis
  pl en·ter·o·my·i·a·ses
en·ter·on
en·ter·o·pa·ral·y·sis
  pl en·ter·o·pa·ral·y·ses
en·ter·o·pa·re·sis
en·ter·o·path·o·gen
en·ter·o·path·o·gen·e·sis
en·ter·o·path·o·gen·ic
en·ter·op·a·thy
  pl en·ter·op·a·thies
en·ter·o·pep·ti·dase
en·ter·o·pex·y
  pl en·ter·o·pex·ies
en·ter·o·plas·tic
en·ter·o·plas·ty
  pl en·ter·o·plas·ties
en·ter·o·ple·gi·a
en·ter·o·proc·ti·a
en·ter·op·to·sis
  pl en·ter·op·to·ses
en·ter·op·tot·ic
en·ter·or·rha·gi·a
en·ter·or·rha·phy
  pl en·ter·or·rha·phies
en·ter·or·rhe·a
en·ter·or·rhex·is
  pl en·ter·or·rhex·es
en·ter·or·rhoe·a
  var of en·ter·or·rhe·a
en·ter·o·scope
en·ter·o·sep·sis
  pl en·ter·o·sep·ses
en·ter·o·sid·er·in
en·ter·o·spasm
en·ter·o·sta·sis
  pl en·ter·o·sta·ses
en·ter·o·ste·no·sis
  pl en·ter·o·ste·no·ses

en·ter·os·to·my
  pl en·ter·os·to·mies
em·ter·o·tome
en·ter·ot·o·my
  pl en·ter·ot·o·mies
en·ter·o·tox·e·mi·a
en·ter·o·tox·i·gen·ic
en·ter·o·tox·in
en·ter·o·tox·ism
en·ter·o·trop·ic
en·ter·o·vag·i·nal
en·ter·o·ves·i·cal
en·ter·o·vi·ral
en·ter·o·vi·rus
en·ter·o·zo·an
en·ter·o·zo·on
  pl en·ter·o·zo·a
en·thal·py
en·the·o·ma·ni·a
en·the·sis
  pl en·the·ses
en·thet·ic
ent·i·ris
en·to·blast
en·to·cele
en·to·cho·roi·de·a
en·to·cone
en·to·co·nid
en·to·cor·ne·a
en·to·derm
en·to·der·mal
en·to·ec·tad
en·to·mere
en·to·mi·on
  pl en·to·mi·a
en·to·mog·e·nous
en·to·mol·o·gist
en·to·mol·o·gy
  pl en·to·mol·o·gies
en·to·moph·i·lous
en·to·mo·pho·bi·a
En·to·moph·tho·ra
en·to·pe·dun·cu·lar
en·to·phyte
en·top·ic
en·to·plasm
ent·op·tic
ent·op·to·scop·ic

ent·op·tos·co·py
  pl ent·op·tos·co·pies
en·to·ret·i·na
en·to·sarc
ent·os·te·o·sis
ent·os·to·sis
  pl ent·os·to·ses
ent·ot·ic
en·to·zo·al
en·to·zo·ic
en·to·zo·on
  pl en·to·zo·a
en·train·ment
en·trap·ment
en·tro·pi·on
en·tro·pi·on·ize
en·tro·py
en·ty·py
  pl en·ty·pies
e·nu·cle·ate
e·nu·cle·a·tion
e·nu·cle·a·tor
en·u·re·sis
  pl en·u·re·ses
en·u·ret·ic
en·ven·om
en·ven·om·a·tion
en·ven·om·i·za·tion
en·vi·ron·ment
en·vi·ron·men·tal
en·vi·ron·men·tal·ism
en·vi·ron·men·tal·ist
en·vi·ron·men·tal·ly
en·zo·ot·ic
en·zy·got·ic
en·zy·mat·ic
  or en·zy·mic
en·zy·mat·i·cal·ly
  or en·zy·mi·cal·ly
en·zyme
en·zy·mic
  or en·zy·matic
en·zy·mi·cal·ly
  or en·zy·mat·i·cal·ly
en·zy·mol·o·gist
en·zy·mol·o·gy
  pl en·zy·mol·o·gies
en·zy·mol·y·sis
en·zy·mo·lyt·ic

en·zy·mop·a·thy
en·zy·mo·pe·ni·a
en·zy·mo·sis
en·zy·mu·ri·a
e·on·ism
e·o·sin
  or e·o·sine
e·o·sine
  or e·o·sin
e·o·sin·o·cyte
e·o·sin·o·pe·ni·a
e·o·sin·o·pe·nic
e·o·sin·o·phil
  or e·o·sin·o·phile
e·o·sin·o·phile
  or e·o·sin·o·phil
e·o·sin·o·phil·i·a
e·o·sin·o·phil·ic
e·o·sin·o·phil·o·cyt·ic
e·o·sin·o·tac·tic
ep·ac·mas·tic
ep·ac·mic
e·pac·tal
ep·ar·te·ri·al
ep·ax·i·al
  or ep·ax·on·ic
ep·ax·on·ic
  or ep·ax·i·al
ep·en·ceph·a·lon
  pl ep·en·ceph·a·la
ep·en·dy·ma
ep·en·dy·mal
ep·en·dy·mi·tis
  pl ep·en·dy·mi·ti·des
ep·en·dy·mo·blast
ep·en·dy·mo·blas·to·ma
  pl ep·en·dy·mo·blas·to·mas
  or ep·en·dy·mo·blas·to·ma-
    ta
ep·en·dy·mo·cyte
ep·en·dy·mo·ma
  pl ep·en·dy·mo·mas
  or ep·en·dy·mo·ma·ta
ep·en·dy·mop·a·thy
ep·e·ryth·ro·zo·on
  pl ep·e·ryth·ro·zo·a
ep·e·ryth·ro·zo·on·o·sis
  pl ep·e·ryth·ro·zo·on·o·ses
eph·apse

e·phe·bi·at·rics
e·phe·bic
eph·e·bo·gen·e·sis
eph·e·bo·lo·gy
E·phed·ra
e·phed·rine
e·phe·lis
  pl e·phe·li·des
e·phem·er·a
e·phem·er·al
eph·i·dro·sis
ep·i·ag·na·thus
ep·i·an·dros·ter·one
ep·i·blast
ep·i·blas·tic
ep·i·blas·to·trop·ic
ep·i·bleph·a·ron
e·pib·o·le
  var of e·pib·o·ly
e·pib·o·lic
e·pib·o·ly
  pl e·pib·o·lies
  or e·pib·o·le
ep·i·bran·chi·al
ep·i·bul·bar
ep·i·can·thal
ep·i·can·thic
ep·i·can·thus
ep·i·car·di·al
ep·i·car·di·um
  pl ep·i·car·di·a
ep·i·carp
ep·i·chord·al
ep·i·cho·ri·on
ep·i·co·lic
ep·i·co·mus
ep·i·con·dyl·al·gi·a
ep·i·con·dy·lar
ep·i·con·dyle
ep·i·con·dyl·i·an
e·pi·con·dyl·ic
ep·i·con·dy·li·tis
ep·i·con·dy·lus
  pl ep·i·con·dy·li
ep·i·cor·a·coid
  or ep·i·cor·a·coi·dal
ep·i·cor·a·coi·dal
  or ep·i·cor·a·coid
ep·i·cra·ni·al

ep·i·cra·ni·o·tem·po·ra·lis
ep·i·cra·ni·um
  pl ep·i·cra·ni·ums
  or ep·i·cra·ni·a
ep·i·cra·ni·us
ep·i·cri·sis
  pl ep·i·cri·ses
ep·i·crit·ic
ep·i·cys·ti·tis
ep·i·cys·tot·o·my
ep·i·cyte
ep·i·dem·ic
ep·i·de·mic·i·ty
  pl ep·i·de·mic·i·ties
ep·i·de·mi·o·gen·e·sis
ep·i·de·mi·og·ra·phy
ep·i·de·mi·o·log·ic
  or ep·i·de·mi·o·log·i·cal
ep·i·de·mi·o·log·i·cal
  or ep·i·de·mi·o·log·ic
ep·i·de·mi·o·log·i·cal·ly
ep·i·de·mi·ol·o·gist
ep·i·de·mi·ol·o·gy
  pl ep·i·de·mi·ol·o·gies
ep·i·derm
ep·i·der·mal
  or ep·i·der·mic
ep·i·der·mat·ic
ep·i·der·ma·to·plas·ty
ep·i·der·ma·to·zo·o·no·sis
ep·i·der·mic
  or ep·i·der·mal
ep·i·der·mi·dal·i·za·tion
ep·i·der·mi·do·sis
ep·i·der·mis
ep·i·der·mi·tis
ep·i·der·mi·za·tion
ep·i·der·mo·dys·pla·si·a
ep·i·der·moid
  or ep·i·der·moid·al
ep·i·der·moid·al
  or ep·i·der·moid
ep·i·der·moid·o·ma
  pl ep·i·der·moid·o·mas
  or ep·i·der·moid·o·ma·ta
ep·i·der·mol·y·sis
  pl ep·i·der·mol·y·ses

ep·i·der·mo·ma
  pl ep·i·der·mo·mas
  or ep·i·der·mo·ma·ta
ep·i·mo·my·co·sis
  pl ep·i·der·mo·my·co·ses
ep·i·der·moph·y·tid
ep·i·der·mo·phy·tin
ep·i·der·moph·y·ton
ep·i·der·mo·phy·to·sis
  pl ep·i·der·mo·phy·to·ses
ep·i·der·mo·sis
ep·i·di·a·scope
ep·i·did·y·mal
ep·i·did·y·mec·to·my
ep·i·did·y·mis
  pl ep·i·did·y·mi·des
ep·i·did·y·mi·tis
ep·i·did·y·mo·or·chi·dec·to·
  my
ep·i·did·y·mo·or·chi·tis
ep·i·did·y·mot·o·my
ep·i·did·y·mo·vas·os·to·my
ep·i·du·ral
ep·i·du·rog·ra·phy
ep·i·es·tri·ol
ep·i·fas·ci·al
ep·i·fol·lic·u·li·tis
ep·i·gas·trae·um
  var of ep·i·gas·tri·um
  pl ep·i·gas·tra·ea
ep·i·gas·tral
  or ep·i·gas·tric
  or ep·i·gas·tri·cal
ep·i·gas·tral·gi·a
ep·i·gas·tric
  or ep·i·gas·tri·cal
  or ep·i·gas·tral
ep·i·gas·tri·cal
  or ep·i·gas·tral
  or ep·i·gas·tric
ep·i·gas·tri·o·cele
ep·i·gas·tri·um
  pl ep·i·gas·tri·a
ep·i·gas·tri·us
ep·i·gas·tro·cele
ep·i·gen·e·sis
  pl ep·i·gen·e·ses
ep·i·ge·net·ic
ep·i·gen·i·tal

ep·i·glot·tal
  or ep·i·glot·tic
ep·i·glot·tic
  or ep·i·glot·tal
ep·i·glot·tid·e·an
ep·i·glot·ti·dec·to·my
ep·i·glot·ti·di·tis
ep·i·glot·tis
ep·i·glot·ti·tis
e·pig·na·thus
e·pig·o·nal
ep·i·gua·nine
ep·i·hy·al
ep·i·hy·oid
ep·i·la·mel·lar
ep·i·la·tion
ep·i·lem·ma
ep·i·lem·mal
ep·i·lep·si·a
ep·i·lep·sy
  pl ep·i·lep·sies
ep·i·lep·tic
ep·i·lep·ti·form
ep·i·lep·to·genic
ep·i·lep·tog·e·nous
ep·i·lep·toid
ep·i·lep·tol·o·gist
ep·i·lep·tol·ogy
ep·i·loi·a
ep·i·man·di·bu·lar
ep·i·men·or·rha·gi·a
ep·i·men·or·rhe·a
ep·i·mer
e·pim·er·ase
ep·i·mere
ep·i·mer·ic
ep·i·mer·ite
e·pim·er·i·za·tion
ep·i·mor·pho·sis
  pl ep·i·mor·pho·ses
ep·i·my·o·car·di·um
ep·i·mys·i·al
ep·i·mys·i·um
  pl ep·i·mys·i·a
ep·i·neph·rin
  or ep·i·neph·rine
ep·i·neph·ri·nae·mi·a
  var of ep·i·neph·ri·ne·mi·a

ep·i·neph·rine
  or ep·i·neph·rin
ep·i·neph·ri·ne·mi·a
ep·i·ne·phri·tis
ep·i·neph·ros
ep·i·neu·ral
ep·i·neu·ri·al
ep·i·neu·ri·um
ep·i·no·sis
ep·i·nych·i·um
  or ep·i·o·nych·i·um
  or ep·o·nych·i·um
ep·i·o·nych·i·um
  or ep·i·nych·i·um
  or ep·o·nych·i·um
ep·i·ot·ic
ep·i·pal·a·tum
ep·i·pas·tic
ep·i·pa·tel·lar
ep·i·per·i·car·di·al
ep·i·pha·ryn·ge·al
ep·i·phar·ynx
  pl ep·i·pha·ryn·ges
ep·i·phe·nom·e·nal·ism
ep·i·phe·nom·enon
  pl ep·i·phe·nom·e·na
e·piph·o·ra
ep·i·phre·nal
ep·i·phren·ic
ep·i·phy·lax·is
  pl ep·i·phy·lax·es
e·piph·y·se·al
  or ep·i·phys·ial
ep·i·phys·e·ol·y·sis
  or ep·i·phys·i·ol·y·sis
ep·i·phys·e·o·ne·cro·sis
  or ep·i·phys·i·o·ne·cro·sis
ep·i·phys·e·op·a·thy
ep·i·phys·i·al
  or e·piph·y·se·al
ep·i·phys·i·o·de·sis
  pl ep·i·phys·i·o·de·ses
ep·i·phys·i·o·lis·the·sis
  pl ep·i·phys·i·o·lis·the·ses
ep·i·phys·i·ol·y·sis
  pl ep·i·phys·i·ol·y·ses
  or ep·i·phys·e·o·ly·sis

ep·i·phys·i·o·ne·cro·sis
  or ep·i·phys·e·o·ne·cro·sis
e·piph·y·sis
  pl e·piph·y·ses
e·piph·y·si·tis
ep·i·phyte
ep·i·phyt·ic
ep·i·pi·al
ep·i·pleu·ral
e·pip·lo·cele
ep·i·plo·ec·to·my
e·pip·lo·en·ter·o·cele
ep·i·plo·ic
e·pip·lo·me·ro·cele
e·pip·lom·phal·o·cele
e·pip·lo·on
  pl e·pip·lo·a
e·pip·lo·pex·y
ep·i·plor·rha·phy
e·pip·los·che·o·cele
ep·i·pro·pi·dine
ep·ip·ter·ic
ep·i·py·gus
ep·i·scle·ra
  pl ep·i·scle·ras
  or ep·i·scle·rae
ep·i·scle·ral
ep·i·scle·ri·tis
e·pis·i·o·cli·si·a
e·pis·i·o·el·y·tror·rha·phy
e·pis·i·o·per·i·ne·o·plas·ty
e·pis·i·o·per·i·ne·or·rha·phy
e·pis·i·o·plas·ty
e·pis·i·or·rha·gi·a
e·pis·i·or·rha·phy
e·pis·i·o·ste·no·sis
  pl e·pis·i·o·ste·no·ses
e·pis·i·ot·o·my
  pl e·pis·i·ot·o·mies
ep·i·sode
ep·i·som·al
ep·i·som·al·ly
ep·i·some
ep·i·spa·di·a
ep·i·spa·di·ac
ep·i·spa·di·al
ep·i·spa·di·as
ep·i·spas·tic
ep·i·sphe·noid

ep·i·spi·nal
ep·i·sple·ni·tis
e·pis·ta·sis
  pl e·pis·ta·ses
e·pis·ta·sy
ep·i·stat·ic
e·pi·stax·is
e·pis·te·mo·phil·i·a
e·pis·te·mo·phil·i·ac
ep·i·ster·nal
ep·i·ster·num
  pl ep·i·ster·na
ep·i·stro·phe·us
ep·i·stroph·ic
ep·i·sym·pus di·pus
ep·i·tar·sus
ep·i·tax·y
  pl ep·i·tax·ies
ep·i·ten·din·e·um
ep·i·ten·on
ep·i·thal·a·mus
  pl ep·i·thal·a·mi
ep·i·tha·lax·i·a
ep·i·the·li·al
ep·i·the·li·al·i·za·tion
  or ep·i·the·li·za·tion
ep·i·the·li·al·ize
  or ep·i·the·lize
ep·i·the·li·i·tis
ep·i·the·li·o·cho·ri·al
ep·i·the·li·o·fi·bril
ep·i·the·li·o·ge·net·ic
ep·i·the·li·oid
ep·i·the·li·o·ly·sin
ep·i·the·li·o·ly·sis
ep·i·the·li·o·ma
  pl ep·i·the·li·o·mas
  or ep·i·the·li·o·ma·ta
ep·i·the·li·o·ma·to·sis
ep·i·the·li·om·a·tous
ep·i·the·li·o·my·o·sis
  pl ep·i·the·li·o·my·o·ses
ep·i·the·li·tis
ep·i·the·li·um
  pl ep·i·the·li·ums
  or ep·i·the·li·a
ep·i·the·li·za·tion
  or ep·i·the·li·al·i·za·tion

ep·i·the·lize
  or ep·i·the·li·al·ize
ep·i·them
ep·i·thi·a·zide
ep·i·ton·ic
ep·i·to·nos
ep·i·to·nus
ep·i·tope
ep·i·trich·i·al
ep·i·trich·i·um
ep·i·troch·le·a
ep·i·troch·le·ar
ep·i·troch·le·ar·is
ep·i·troch·le·o-
  o·lec·ra·no·sis
e·pi·tu·ber·cu·lo·sis
  pl ep·i·tu·ber·cu·lo·ses
ep·i·tym·pan·ic
ep·i·tym·pa·num
  pl ep·i·tym·pa·nums
  or ep·i·tym·pa·ni
ep·i·typh·li·tis
ep·i·vag·i·ni·tis
ep·i·zo·ic
ep·i·zo·i·cide
ep·i·zo·ol·o·gy
  pl ep·i·zo·ol·o·gies
  or ep·i·zo·ot·i·ol·o·gy
  pl ep·i·zo·ot·i·ol·o·gies
  or ep·i·zo·ot·ol·o·gy
  pl ep·i·zo·ot·ol·o·gies
ep·i·zo·on
  pl ep·i·zo·a
ep·i·zo·on·o·sis
  pl ep·i·zo·on·o·ses
ep·i·zo·ot·ic
ep·i·zo·ot·i·ol·o·gy
  pl ep·i·zo·ot·i·ol·o·gies
  or ep·i·zo·ot·ol·o·gy
  pl ep·i·zo·ot·ol·o·gies
  or epi·zo·ol·o·gy
  pl ep·i·zo·ol·o·gies
ep·i·zo·ot·ol·o·gy
  pl ep·i·zo·ot·ol·o·gies
  or ep·i·zo·ol·o·gy
  pl ep·i·zo·ol·o·gies
  or ep·i·zo·ot·i·ol·o·gy
  pl ep·i·zo·ot·i·ol·o·gies

ep·o·nych·i·um
   or ep·i·nych·i·um
   or ep·i·o·nych·i·um
ep·o·nym
ep·o·nym·ic
e·pon·y·mous
ep·o·oph·o·ral
ep·o·oph·o·rec·to·my
ep·o·oph·o·ron
ep·or·nit·ic
Ep·som salt
Ep·stein syn·drome
Ep·stein-Barr vi·rus
e·pu·lis
   pl e·pu·li·des
ep·u·lo·fi·bro·ma
   pl ep·u·lo·fi·bro·mas
   or ep·u·lo·fi·bro·ma·ta
ep·u·loid
ep·u·lo·sis
e·qual
e·qua·tion
e·qua·tion·al
e·qua·tion·al·ly
e·qua·tor
e·qua·to·ri·al
e·qui·ax·i·al
Eq·ui·dae
e·qui·dom·i·nant
eq·ui·len·in
e·quil·i·brate
e·quil·i·bra·tion
e·quil·i·bra·to·ry
e·qui·lib·ri·um
   pl e·qui·lib·ri·ums
   or e·qui·lib·ri·a
e·qui·lin
e·qui·mo·lec·u·lar
e·quine
e·quin·i·a
eq·ui·no·ca·vus
eq·ui·no·val·gus
eq·ui·no·var·us
e·qui·nus
e·qui·po·tent
e·qui·po·ten·tial
eq·ui·se·to·sis
Eq·ui·se·tum
e·quiv·a·lence

e·quiv·a·len·cy
   pl e·quiv·a·len·cies
e·quiv·a·lent
e·quiv·a·lent·ly
e·ra·sion
Er·a·ty·rus cus·pi·da·tus
Erb pal·sy
Erb-Char·cot dis·ease
Erb-Du·chenne pa·ral·y·sis
Er·ben sign
Erb-Gold·flam symp·tom
   com·plex
er·bi·um
Erb-Zim·mer·lin type
Erd·mann re·a·gent
e·rect
e·rec·tile
e·rec·til·i·ty
   pl e·rec·til·i·ties
e·rec·tion
e·rec·tor
er·e·ma·cau·sis
e·re·mi·o·pho·bi·a
e·re·mo·pho·bi·a
e·rep·sin
er·e·thism
er·e·this·mic
er·e·this·o·phre·ni·a
er·e·this·tic
er·e·thit·ic
e·reu·tho·pho·bi·a
erg
er·ga·si·a
er·ga·si·a·try
er·ga·si·o·ma·ni·a
er·ga·si·o·pho·bi·a
er·gas·the·ni·a
er·gas·tic
er·gas·to·plasm
er·go·ba·sine
er·go·ba·si·nine
er·go·cal·cif·er·ol
er·go·cor·nine
er·go·cor·ni·nine
er·go·cris·tine
er·go·cris·ti·nine
er·go·cryp·tine
er·go·cryp·ti·nine
er·go·gen·ic

er·go·graph
er·go·graph·ic
er·gom·e·ter
er·go·met·ric
er·go·met·rine
er·go·met·ri·nine
er·go·nom·ic
er·go·nom·ics
er·gon·o·mist
er·go·no·vine
er·go·pho·bi·a
er·go·phore
er·go·plasm
er·go·sine
er·go·si·nine
er·go·some
er·gos·ta·nol
er·go·stat
er·gos·te·nol
er·gos·ter·in
er·gos·ter·ol
er·go·stet·rine
er·got
er·got·a·mine
er·go·tam·i·nine
er·go·ther·a·py
   pl er·go·ther·a·pies
er·go·thi·o·ne·ine
er·got·in
er·got·i·nine
er·got·ism
er·got·ized
er·go·to·cin
er·go·tox·ine
Er·ich·sen dis·ease
er·i·gens
E·rig·er·on
er·i·o·dic·tin
er·i·o·dic·ty·ol
Er·i·o·dic·ty·on
er·i·om·e·ter
e·ris·i·phake
   or e·rys·i·phake
E·ris·ta·lis
Er·len·mey·er flask
e·rode
E·ro·di·um

er·o·gen·ic
  or e·rog·e·nous
e·rog·e·nous
  or er·o·gen·ic
er·o·ma·ni·a
e·ros
e·rose
e·rose·ly
e·ro·si·o in·ter·dig·i·ta·lis
  blas·to·my·ce·ti·ca
e·ro·sion
e·ro·sive
e·ros·ive·ness
e·ro·siv·i·ty
  pl e·ro·siv·i·ties
e·rot·ic
  or e·rot·i·cal
e·rot·i·ca
e·rot·i·cal
  or e·rot·ic
e·rot·i·cal·ly
e·rot·i·cism
e·rot·i·cist
e·rot·i·ci·za·tion
e·rot·i·cize
e·rot·i·co·ma·ni·a
er·o·tism
er·o·ti·za·tion
er·o·tize
e·ro·to·gen·e·sis
  pl e·ro·to·gen·e·ses
e·ro·to·gen·ic
e·ro·to·ma·ni·a
e·ro·to·ma·ni·ac
e·ro·to·path
er·o·to·path·ic
er·o·top·a·thy
  pl er·o·top·a·thies
e·ro·to·pho·bi·a
er·rat·ic
er·rhine
er·u·bes·cent
e·ru·cic
e·ruct
e·ruc·tate
e·ruc·ta·tion
er·u·ga·tion
e·ru·ga·to·ry
e·rup·tion

e·rup·tive
E·ryn·gi·um
er·ys·i·mum
er·y·si·pel·as
er·y·si·pel·a·tous
er·y·sip·e·loid
Er·y·sip·e·lo·thrix
e·rys·i·phake
  or e·ris·i·phake
er·y·the·ma
er·y·the·mal
er·y·the·ma·toid
er·y·the·ma·tous
er·y·the·moid
er·y·ther·mal·gi·a
er·y·thor·bate
er·y·thor·bic
er·y·thrae·mi·a
  var of er·y·thre·mi·a
er·y·thral·gi·a
er·y·thras·ma
e·ryth·re·de·ma
e·ryth·re·de·ma
  pol·y·neu·ro·pa·thy
er·y·thre·mi·a
er·y·thre·mic
er·y·thrin
Er·y·thri·na
e·ryth·rism
er·y·thris·tic
er·y·thrite
e·ryth·ri·tol
e·ryth·ri·tyl
e·ryth·ro·blast
e·ryth·ro·blas·te·mi·a
e·ryth·ro·blas·tic
e·ryth·ro·blas·to·ma
  pl e·ryth·ro·blas·to·mas
  or e·ryth·ro·blas·to·ma·ta
e·ryth·ro·blas·to·pe·ni·a
e·ryth·ro·blas·to·sis
  pl e·ryth·ro·blas·to·ses
e·ryth·ro·blas·to·sis
  fe·ta·lis
e·ryth·ro·blas·tot·ic
E·ryth·ro·ce·bus
e·ryth·ro·chlo·ro·pi·a
e·ryth·ro·chlo·rop·si·a
e·ryth·ro·chlo·ro·py

e·ryth·ro·chro·mi·a
er·y·thro·cla·sis
e·ryth·ro·conte
e·ryth·ro·cru·o·rin
e·ryth·ro·cu·pre·in
e·ryth·ro·cy·a·no·sis
  pl e·ryth·ro·cy·a·no·ses
e·ryth·ro·cyte
e·ryth·ro·cy·the·mi·a
e·ryth·ro·cyt·ic
e·ryth·ro·cy·tin
e·ryth·ro·cy·to·blast
e·ryth·ro·cy·tol·y·sin
e·ryth·ro·cy·tol·y·sis
  pl e·ryth·ro·cy·tol·y·ses
e·ryth·ro·cy·tom·e·ter
e·ryth·ro·cy·tom·e·try
e·ryth·ro·cy·to·op·so·nin
e·ryth·ro·cy·to·poi·e·sis
  pl e·ryth·ro·cy·to·poi·e·ses
e·ryth·ro·cy·to·poi·et·ic
e·ryth·ro·cy·tor·rhex·is
e·ryth·ro·cy·tos·chi·sis
e·ryth·ro·cy·to·sis
  pl e·ryth·ro·cy·to·ses
e·ryth·ro·do·gen·er·a·tive
e·ryth·ro·der·ma
  pl e·ryth·ro·der·mas
  or e·ryth·ro·der·ma·ta
e·ryth·ro·der·mi·a
e·ryth·ro·dex·trin
  or e·ryth·ro·dex·trine
e·ryth·ro·dex·trine
  or e·ryth·ro·dex·trin
e·ryth·ro·don·ti·a
e·ryth·roe·de·ma
  var of e·ryth·re·de·ma
e·ryth·ro·gen·e·sis
  pl e·ryth·ro·gen·e·ses
e·ryth·ro·gen·ic
e·ryth·ro·gone
  or e·ryth·ro·go·ni·um
e·ryth·ro·go·ni·um
  or e·ryth·ro·gone
er·y·throid
er·y·thro·i·dine
e·ryth·ro·ker·a·to·der·mi·a
e·ryth·ro·ki·net·ics
er·y·throl

128

ryth·ro·labe
ryth·ro·leu·co·sis
  var of e·ryth·ro·leu·ko·sis
ryth·ro·leu·ke·mi·a
ryth·ro·leu·ko·blas·to·sis
ryth·ro·leu·ko·sis
  pl e·ryth·ro·leu·ko·ses
·y·throl·y·sin
·y·throl·y·sis
  pl er·y·throl·y·ses
ryth·ro·ma·ni·a
ryth·ro·me·lal·gi·a
ryth·ro·me·li·a
·y·throm·e·ter
ryth·ro·my·cin
ryth·ro·my·e·lo·sis
·y·thron
ryth·ro·ne·o·cy·to·sis
r·y·thro·ni·um
ryth·ro·no·cla·si·a
ryth·ro·pe·ni·a
ryth·ro·phage
ryth·ro·pha·gi·a
ryth·ro·phag·o·cy·to·sis
  pl e·ryth·ro·phag·o·cy·to·
    ses
ryth·ro·phe·re·sis
ryth·ro·phil
ryth·ro·phile
  or er·yth·roph·i·lous
r·yth·roph·i·lous
  or e·ryth·ro·phile
ryth·ro·phle·ine
ryth·ro·pho·bi·a
ryth·ro·phore
ryth·ro·phose
ryth·ro·phthi·sis
r·y·thro·pi·a
  or er·y·throp·si·a
ryth·ro·pla·si·a
ryth·ro·plas·tid
ryth·ro·poi·e·sis
  pl e·ryth·ro·poi·e·ses
ryth·ro·poi·et·ic
ryth·ro·poi·e·tin
ryth·ro·pros·o·pal·gi·a
r·y·throp·si·a
  or er·y·thro·pi·a
r·y·throp·sin

e·ryth·ror·rhex·is
er·y·throse
e·ryth·ro·sed·i·men·ta·tion
e·ryth·ro·sin
e·ryth·ro·sin·o·phil
er·y·thro·sis
  pl er·y·thro·ses
e·ryth·ro·sta·sis
er·y·throx·y·lon
e·ryth·ru·lose
er·y·thru·ri·a
Es·bach meth·od
es·cape
es·cap·ee
es·cap·ism
es·cap·ist
es·char
es·cha·ro·sis
es·cha·rot·ic
Esch·e·rich·i·a
es·chro·la·li·a
es·cor·cin
es·cu·le·tin
es·cu·lin
es·cutch·eon
es·er·a·mine
es·er·i·dine
es·er·ine
Es·march ban·dage
e·sod·ic
es·o·eth·moid·i·tis
es·o·gas·tri·tis
e·soph·a·gal
  var of e·soph·a·ge·al
e·soph·a·gal·gi·a
e·soph·a·ge·al
e·soph·a·gec·ta·si·a
e·soph·a·gec·ta·sis
e·soph·a·gec·to·my
e·soph·a·gec·to·py
e·soph·a·gism
e·soph·a·gis·mus
e·soph·a·gi·tis
e·soph·a·go·bron·chi·al
e·soph·a·go·cele
e·soph·a·go·du·o·de·nos·
    to·my
e·soph·a·go·dyn·i·a
e·soph·a·go·en·ter·os·to·my

e·soph·a·go·e·soph·a·gos·
    to·my
e·soph·a·go·gas·trec·to·my
e·soph·a·go·gas·tric
e·soph·a·go·gas·tro·a·nas·
    to·mo·sis
e·soph·a·go·gas·tro·plas·ty
e·soph·a·go·gas·tro·scope
e·soph·a·go·gas·tros·co·py
e·soph·a·go·gas·tros·to·my
  pl e·soph·a·go·gas·tros·
    to·mies
e·soph·a·go·gram
e·soph·a·go·gra·phy
e·soph·a·go·hi·a·tal
e·soph·a·go·je·ju·nos·to·my
e·soph·a·go·ma·la·ci·a
e·soph·a·gom·e·ter
e·soph·a·go·my·ot·o·my
e·soph·a·gop·a·thy
e·soph·a·go·pha·ryn·ge·al
e·soph·a·go·plas·ty
e·soph·a·go·pli·ca·tion
e·soph·a·gop·to·sis
e·soph·a·go·res·pi·ra·to·ry
e·soph·a·go·sal·i·var·y
e·soph·a·go·scope
e·soph·a·gos·co·py
e·soph·a·go·spasm
e·soph·a·go·ste·no·sis
e·soph·a·gos·to·ma
e·soph·a·gos·to·mi·a·sis
e·soph·a·gos·to·my
e·soph·a·go·tome
e·soph·a·got·o·my
eso·pha·go·trach·eal
e·soph·a·gus
  pl e·soph·a·gi
e·soph·o·gram
es·o·pho·ri·a
es·o·sphe·noid·i·tis
es·o·tro·pi·a
es·o·tro·pic
es·pun·di·a
es·sence
es·sen·tial
Es·ser in·lay graft
Es·sick cell band
es·ter

129

es·ter·ase
es·ter·i·fi·ca·tion
es·ter·i·fy
es·them·a·tol·o·gy
es·the·si·a
es·the·si·o·gen·ic
es·the·si·ol·o·gy
es·the·si·om·e·ter
es·the·si·om·e·try
  pl es·the·si·om·e·tries
es·the·si·o·neu·ro·blas·
  to·ma
  pl es·the·si·o·neu·ro·blas·to·
    mas
  or es·the·si·o·neu·ro·
    blas·to·ma·ta
es·the·si·o·neu·ro·ep·i·the·
  li·o·ma
  pl es·the·si·o·neu·ro·ep·
    i·the·li·o·mas
  or es·the·si·o·neu·ro·ep·
    i·the·li·o·ma·ta
es·the·si·o·neu·ro·ma
  pl es·the·si·o·neu·ro·mas
  or es·the·si·o·neu·ro·ma·ta
es·the·si·o·phys·i·ol·o·gy
  pl es·the·si·o·phys·i·ol·
    o·gies
es·the·sis
  pl es·the·ses
es·the·sod·ic
es·thet·ics
es·thi·om·e·ne
es·ti·val
es·ti·vate
es·ti·va·tion
es·ti·vo·au·tum·nal
Est·lan·der op·er·a·tion
es·to·late
es·tra·di·ol
es·tral
es·trane
es·tra·zi·nol
es·tri·a·sis
es·trin
es·trin·i·za·tion
es·tri·ol
es·tro·gen

es·tro·gen·ic
es·tro·ge·nic·i·ty
  pl es·tro·ge·nic·i·ties
es·tro·gen·i·za·tion
es·trone
es·trous
es·tru·al
es·tru·a·tion
es·trum
  or es·trus
es·trus
  or es·trum
es·tu·ar·i·um
es·y·late
et·a·fed·rine
é·tat
eth·a·cry·nic
e·tham·bu·tol
e·tham·i·van
e·tham·syl·ate
eth·a·nal
eth·ane
eth·a·no·ic
eth·a·nol
eth·a·nol·a·mine
eth·chlor·vy·nol
eth·ene
eth·e·noid
eth·e·none
e·ther
e·the·re·al
  or e·the·ri·al
e·the·ri·al
  or e·the·re·al
e·ther·ide
e·ther·i·fi·ca·tion
e·ther·i·fy
e·ther·i·za·tion
e·ther·ize
eth·i·cal
eth·i·cal·i·ty
  pl eth·i·cal·i·ties
eth·i·cal·ly
eth·i·cal·ness
eth·ics
eth·i·dene
eth·i·nam·ate
eth·ine

e·thi·nyl
  or e·thy·nyl
e·thi·nyl tri·chlo·ride
e·thi·on·a·mide
e·thi·o·nine
e·this·ter·one
eth·mo·car·di·tis
eth·mo·ceph·a·lus
eth·mo·fron·tal
eth·moid
eth·moi·dal
eth·moid·ec·to·my
eth·moid·i·tis
eth·moid·ot·o·my
eth·mo·lac·ri·mal
eth·mo·max·il·lar·y
eth·mo·na·sal
eth·mo·sphe·noid
eth·mo·tur·bi·nal
eth·nic
eth·no·graph·ic
  or eth·no·graph·i·cal
eth·no·graph·i·cal
  or eth·no·graph·ic
eth·nog·ra·phy
eth·no·log·ic
  or eth·no·log·i·cal
eth·no·log·i·cal
  or eth·no·log·ic
eth·nol·o·gy
eth·o·caine
eth·o·hep·ta·zine
eth·o·hex·a·di·ol
e·thol·o·gy
  pl e·thol·o·gies
eth·o·nam
eth·o·pro·pa·zine
eth·o·sux·i·mide
eth·o·to·in
eth·ox·a·zene
eth·ox·y
eth·ox·zol·a·mide
eth·y·benz·tro·pine
eth·yl
eth·yl·ate
eth·yl·a·tion
eth·yl·cel·lu·lose
eth·yl·ene
eth·yl·ene·di·a·mine

eth·yl·ene·di·a·mine·tet·
  ra·a·ce·tic
eth·yl·e·phed·rine
eth·yl·es·tren·ol
eth·yl·hy·dro·cu·pre·ine
eth·yl·i·dene
eth·yl·mor·phine
eth·yl·nor·ep·i·neph·rine
eth·yl·stib·a·mine
eth·yne
e·thy·ner·one
e·thy·no·di·ol
e·thy·nyl
  or e·thi·nyl
e·thy·nyl·es·tra·di·ol
é·tin·ce·lage
e·ti·o·cho·lan·o·lone
e·ti·o·late
e·ti·o·la·tion
e·ti·o·log·ic
  or e·ti·o·log·i·cal
e·ti·o·log·i·cal
  or e·ti·o·log·ic
e·ti·ol·o·gy
  pl e·ti·ol·o·gies
e·ti·o·path·o·gen·e·sis
  pl e·ti·o·path·o·gen·e·ses
e·ti·o·por·phy·rin
e·tryp·ta·mine
eu·aes·the·si·a
  var of eu·es·the·si·a
Eu·bac·ter·ri·a·les
Eu·bac·te·ri·um
eu·bi·ot·ics
eu·caine
eu·ca·lyp·tene
eu·ca·lyp·tol
  or eu·ca·lyp·tole
eu·ca·lyp·tole
  or eu·ca·lyp·tol
eu·ca·lyp·tus
  pl eu·ca·lyp·ti
euc·at·ro·pine
Eu·ces·to·da
eu·chlor·hy·dri·a
eu·chol·i·a
eu·chro·mat·ic
eu·chro·ma·tin
eu·chro·ma·top·si·a

eu·chro·ma·top·sy
eu·chro·mo·some
eu·co·dal
eu·cor·tism
eu·cra·si·a
eu·di·e·mor·rhy·sis
eu·di·om·e·ter
eu·di·om·e·try
eu·dip·si·a
eu·er·ga·si·a
eu·es·the·si·a
Eu·ge·ni·a
eu·gen·ic
  or eu·gen·i·cal
eu·gen·i·cal
  or eu·gen·ic
eu·gen·i·cist
eu·gen·ics
eu·gen·ism
eu·ge·nol
Eu·gle·na
eu·glob·u·lin
eu·gly·ce·mi·a
eu·gnath·ic
eu·gon·ic
eu·kar·y·on
eu·kar·y·o·sis
eu·kar·y·ote
eu·kar·y·ot·ic
eu·ker·a·tin
eu·ki·ne·si·a
eu·lam·i·nate
Eu·len·burg dis·ease
eu·me·tri·a
eu·mor·phic
eu·my·cete
Eu·my·ce·tes
eu·noi·a
eu·nuch
eu·nuch·ism
eu·nuch·oid
eu·nuch·oi·dal
eu·nuch·oid·ism
eu·on·y·mus
eu·pan·cre·a·tism
eu·pa·ral
eu·pa·to·rin
Eu·pa·to·ri·um
eu·pep·si·a

eu·pep·tic
eu·phen·ic
eu·phen·ics
cu·pho·ni·a
Eu·phor·bi·a
Eu·phor·bi·a·ce·ae
eu·phor·bi·um
eu·pho·ret·ic
eu·pho·ri·a
eu·pho·ri·ant
eu·pho·ric
eu·pho·ric·al·ly
eu·phys·i·o·log·ic
eu·plas·tic
eu·ploid
eu·ploid·y
  pl eu·ploid·ies
eup·ne·a
eup·noe·a
  var of eup·ne·a
eu·prax·i·a
eu·pro·cin
Eu·proc·tis chrys·or·rhe·a
eu·py·rene
eu·rhyth·mi·a
eu·ro·pis·o·ceph·a·lus
  pl eu·ro·pis·o·ceph·a·li
eu·ro·pi·um
eu·ro·pro·ceph·a·lus
  pl eu·ro·pro·ceph·a·li
Eu·ro·ti·a·les
eu·ry·ce·phal·ic
  or eu·ry·ceph·a·lous
eu·ry·ceph·a·lous
  or eu·ry·ce·phal·ic
eu·ry·chas·mus
eu·ryc·ne·mic
eu·ryg·nath·ic
eu·ryg·na·thism
eu·ryg·na·thous
eu·ry·mer·ic
eu·ry·on
eu·ry·so·mat·ic
  or eu·ry·some
  or eu·ry·so·mic
eu·ry·some
  or eu·ry·so·matic
  or eu·ry·so·mic

eu·ry·so·mic
  or eu·ry·some
  or eu·ry·so·mat·ic
eu·ry·ther·mal
eu·ry·ther·mic
Eu·scor·pi·us
eu·sta·chi·an
Eu·stron·gy·lus gi·gas
eu·sys·to·le
eu·tec·tic
eu·tha·na·si·a
eu·the·na·sic
eu·then·ics
Eu·the·ri·a
eu·the·ri·an
eu·ther·mic
eu·the·si·a
eu·thy·roid
eu·thy·roid·ism
eu·to·ci·a
eu·trep·is·ty
Eu·tri·at·o·ma
Eu·trom·bic·u·la
eu·tro·phi·a
eu·tro·phic
eu·tro·phy
  pl eu·tro·phies
e·vac·u·ant
e·vac·u·ate
e·vac·u·a·tion
e·vac·u·a·tor
e·vag·i·nate
e·vag·i·na·tion
ev·a·nes·cent
Ev·ans blue
e·ven·tra·tion
Ev·ers·busch op·er·a·tion
e·ver·sion
ev·i·rate
ev·i·ra·tion
e·vis·cer·ate
e·vis·cer·a·tion
ev·o·ca·tion
ev·o·ca·tor
e·voke
ev·o·lu·tion
e·vul·sion
E·wald node

Ew·art sign
ewe·neck
ewe·necked
Ew·ing sar·co·ma, tu·mor
ex·ac·er·bate
ex·ac·er·ba·tion
ex·al·ta·tion
ex·am·i·na·tion
ex·am·ine
ex·am·in·ee
ex·am·in·er
ex·an·them
  pl ex·an·thems
  or ex·an·the·ma
ex·an·the·ma
  pl ex·an·the·mas
  or ex·an·the·ma·ta
  or ex·an·them
ex·an·the·mat·ic
ex·an·them·a·tous
ex·ar·te·ri·tis
ex·ar·tic·u·la·tion
ex·cal·a·tion
ex·ca·vate
ex·ca·va·ti·o
  pl ex·ca·va·ti·o·nes
ex·ca·va·tion
ex·ca·va·tor
ex·ce·men·to·sis
ex·cen·tric
  or ec·cen·tric
ex·cer·e·bra·tion
ex·cer·nent
ex·cip·i·ent
ex·cise
ex·ci·sion
ex·cit·a·ble
ex·cit·a·bil·i·ty
  pl ex·cit·a·bil·i·ties
ex·cit·ant
ex·ci·ta·tion
ex·cit·a·to·ry
ex·cite
ex·cite·ment
ex·ci·to·mo·tor
ex·ci·tor
ex·ci·to·se·cre·to·ry
ex·ci·to·vas·cu·lar

ex·clave
ex·clu·sion
ex·coch·le·a·tion
ex·con·ju·gant
ex·co·ri·ate
ex·co·ri·a·tion
ex·cre·ment
ex·cre·men·tal
ex·cre·men·ti·tious
ex·cres·cence
ex·cres·cent
ex·cre·ta
ex·cre·tal
ex·crete
ex·cret·er
ex·cre·tion
ex·cre·to·ry
ex·cur·sive
ex·cur·va·tion
ex·cur·va·ture
ex·cy·clo·pho·ri·a
ex·cy·clo·tro·pi·a
ex·cys·ta·tion
ex·cyst·ment
ex·ec·u·tant
ex·e·dens
ex·e·mi·a
ex·en·ce·pha·li·a
ex·en·ce·phal·ic
ex·en·ceph·a·lus
ex·en·ceph·a·ly
ex·en·ter·ate
ex·en·ter·a·tion
ex·en·ter·a·tive
ex·er·cise
ex·er·e·sis
  pl ex·er·e·ses
ex·er·gon·ic
ex·fe·ta·tion
ex·flag·el·la·tion
ex·fo·li·ate
ex·fo·li·a·tion
ex·fo·li·a·tive
ex·ha·la·tion
ex·hale
ex·haust
ex·haus·tion
ex·haus·tive

132

ex·hib·it
ex·hi·bi·tion
ex·hi·bi·tion·ism
ex·hi·bi·tion·ist
ex·hil·a·rant
ex·hil·a·rate
ex·hil·a·ra·tion
ex·hu·ma·tion
ex·hume
ex·is·ten·tial
ex·is·ten·tial·ism
ex·i·tus
   pl ex·i·tus
ex·o·bi·ol·o·gy
ex·o·car·di·a
ex·o·car·di·ac
ex·o·car·di·al
ex·o·cat·a·pho·ri·a
ex·oc·cip·i·tal
ex·o·cer·vix
   pl ex·o·cer·vix·es
   or ex·o·cer·vi·ces
ex·o·cho·ri·on
   pl ex·o·cho·ri·a
ex·o·coe·lom
ex·o·coe·lom·ic
ex·o·co·li·tis
ex·o·crine
ex·o·cri·nol·o·gy
   pl ex·o·cri·nol·o·gies
ex·o·cy·to·sis
ex·o·de·vi·a·tion
ex·od·ic
ex·o·don·ti·a
ex·o·don·tics
ex·o·don·tist
ex·o·en·zyme
ex·o·er·gic
ex·o·e·ryth·ro·cyt·ic
ex·og·a·mous
ex·og·a·my
   pl ex·og·a·mies
ex·o·gas·tru·la
ex·o·gas·tru·la·tion
ex·o·ge·net·ic
ex·o·gen·ic
ex·og·e·nous
ex·o·hys·ter·o·pex·y

ex·o·me·tri·tis
ex·om·pha·los
ex·o·nu·cle·ase
ex·o·pep·ti·dase
ex·o·pho·ri·a
ex·oph·thal·mic
ex·oph·thal·mom·e·ter
ex·oph·thal·mom·e·try
ex·oph·thal·mos
   or ex·oph·thal·mus
ex·oph·thal·mus
   or ex·oph·thal·mos
ex·o·phyt·ic
ex·o·plasm
ex·o·se·ro·sis
ex·o·skel·e·ton
ex·os·mom·e·ter
ex·os·mose
ex·os·mo·sis
   pl ex·os·mo·ses
ex·os·mot·ic
ex·o·som·aes·the·si·a
   var of ex·o·som·es·the·si·a
ex·o·som·es·the·si·a
ex·o·spore
ex·o·spo·ri·um
   pl ex·o·spo·ri·a
ex·os·to·sec·to·my
ex·os·tosed
ex·os·to·sis
   pl ex·os·to·ses
ex·os·tot·ic
ex·o·ter·ic
ex·o·ter·i·cal·ly
ex·o·ther·mal
ex·o·ther·mic
ex·o·tox·ic
ex·o·tox·in
ex·o·tro·pi·a
ex·o·tro·pic
ex·pan·der
ex·pan·sile
ex·pan·sive
ex·pec·tant
ex·pec·to·rant
ex·pec·to·rate
ex·pec·to·ra·tion
ex·pel

ex·pe·ri·en·tial
ex·per·i·ment
ex·per·i·men·tal
ex·per·i·men·ta·tion
ex·pert
ex·pi·ra·tion
ex·pi·ra·to·ry
ex·pire
ex·plant
ex·plan·ta·tion
ex·plode
ex·plo·ra·tion
ex·plor·a·to·ry
ex·plore
ex·plor·er
ex·plo·sion
ex·plo·sive
ex·pose
ex·po·sure
ex·press
ex·pres·sion
ex·pres·siv·i·ty
ex·pul·sion
ex·pul·sive
ex·san·gui·nate
ex·san·gui·na·tion
ex·san·guine
ex·san·guin·i·ty
ex·sect
ex·sec·tion
ex·sic·cant
ex·sic·cate
ex·sic·ca·tion
ex·sic·ca·tive
ex·sic·ca·tor
ex·sic·co·sis
   pl ex·sic·co·ses
ex·sorp·tion
ex·stro·phy
   pl ex·stro·phies
ex·suf·fla·tion
ex·suf·fla·tor
ex·ten·der
ex·ten·sion
ex·ten·sor
ex·te·ri·or
ex·te·ri·or·i·za·tion
ex·te·ri·or·ize

ex·tern
or ex·terne
ex·ter·nad
ex·ter·nal
ex·ter·nal·ize
ex·terne
or ex·tern
ex·ter·nus
ex·ter·o·cap·tive
ex·ter·o·cep·tor
ex·ter·o·fec·tive
ex·ti·ma
pl ex·ti·mas
or ex·ti·mae
ex·tinc·tion
ex·tin·guish
ex·tir·pate
ex·tir·pa·tion
Ex·ton and Rose test
Ex·ton meth·od
ex·tor·sion
ex·tra-ar·tic·u·lar
ex·tra-buc·cal
ex·tra-bul·bar
ex·tra-cam·pine
ex·tra-cap·su·lar
ex·tra-car·di·ac
ex·tra-car·di·al
ex·tra-car·pal
ex·tra-cel·lu·lar
ex·tra-cer·e·bral
ex·tra-chro·mo·so·mal
ex·tra-cor·po·ral
ex·tra-cor·po·re·al
ex·tra-cor·pus·cu·lar
ex·tra-cor·ti·co·spi·nal
ex·tra-cra·ni·al
ex·tract
ex·tract·ant
ex·trac·tion
ex·trac·tive
ex·trac·tor
ex·tra-cys·tic
ex·tra-du·ral
ex·tra-em·bry·on·al
or ex·tra-em·bry·on·ic
ex·tra-em·bry·on·ic
or ex·tra-em·bry·on·al

ex·tra-ep·i·phys·e·al
ex·tra-e·ryth·ro·cyt·ic
ex·tra-e·soph·a·ge·al
ex·tra-fas·ci·al
ex·tra-gen·i·tal
ex·tra-gin·gi·val
ex·tra-he·pat·ic
ex·tra-lig·a·men·tous
ex·tra-mal·le·o·lus
ex·tra-mam·ma·ry
ex·tra-mar·gin·al
ex·tra-mas·toi·di·tis
ex·tra-med·ul·lar·y
ex·tra-mi·to·chon·dri·al
ex·tra-mu·ral
ex·tra-nu·cle·ar
ex·tra-oc·u·lar
ex·tra-o·ral
ex·tra-os·se·ous
ex·tra-pa·ren·chy·mal
ex·tra-pel·vic
ex·tra-per·i·ne·al
ex·tra-per·i·to·ne·al
ex·tra-pla·cen·tal
ex·tra-pleu·ral
ex·trap·o·late
ex·trap·o·la·tion
ex·tra-pros·tat·ic
ex·tra-psy·chic
ex·tra-pul·mo·nar·y
ex·tra-py·ram·i·dal
ex·tra-re·nal
ex·tra-sen·so·ry
ex·tra-sphinc·ter·ic
ex·tra-spi·nal
ex·tra-sys·to·le
ex·tra-thy·roi·dal
ex·tra-tu·bal
ex·tra-u·ter·ine
ex·tra-vag·i·nal
ex·trav·a·sate
ex·trav·a·sa·tion
ex·tra-vas·cu·lar
ex·tra-ven·tric·u·lar
ex·tra-ver·sion
or ex·tro·ver·sion
ex·tra·ver·sive

ex·tra·vert
or ex·tro·vert
ex·tra·vis·u·al
ex·tre·mis
ex·trem·i·tas
pl ex·trem·i·ta·tes
ex·trem·i·ty
pl ex·trem·i·ties
ex·trin·sic
ex·tro·gas·tru·la·tion
ex·tro·spec·tion
ex·tro·ver·sion
or ex·tra·ver·sion
ex·tro·vert
or ex·tra·vert
ex·trude
ex·tru·do·clu·sion
ex·tru·sion
ex·tu·bate
ex·tu·ba·tion
ex·u·ber·ance
ex·u·ber·ant
ex·u·date
ex·u·da·tion
ex·u·da·tive
ex·ude
ex·um·bil·i·ca·tion
ex·u·vi·ae
ex·u·vi·al
ex·u·vi·ate
ex·u·vi·a·tion
eye
eye·ball
eye·brow
eye·cup
eye·drop·per
eye·drop·per·ful
eye·glas·ses
eye·ground
eye·lash
eye·lid
eye·piece
eye·point
eye·sight
eye·spot
eye·strain
eye·tooth
eye·wash

F

Fab frag·ment
fa·bel·la
  pl fa·bel·lae
Fa·ber a·ne·mi·a
Fa·bi·an·a
fa·bism
fa·bis·mus
fab·ri·ca·tion
Fa·bri·cus-Mol·ler test
Fa·bry dis·ease
fab·u·la·tion
face
face gri·pée
face·bow
face-lift·ing
fac·et
  or fa·cette
fac·e·tec·to·my
fa·cette
  or fac·et
fa·ci·a
  var of fas·ci·a
fa·cial
fa·ci·a·lis
fa·ci·al·ly
fa·ci·es
  pl fa·ci·es
fa·cil·i·ta·tion
fa·cil·i·ty
fac·ing
fa·ci·o·bra·chi·al
fa·ci·o·cer·vi·cal
fa·ci·o·lin·gual
fa·ci·o·plas·ty
fa·ci·o·ple·gi·a
fa·ci·o·ple·gic
fa·ci·o·scap·u·lo·hu·mer·al
F-ac·tin

fac·ti·tious
fac·tor
fac·to·ri·al
fac·ul·ta·tive
fac·ul·ty
fae·cal
  var of fe·cal
fae·ca·lith
  var of fe·ca·lith
fae·ces
  var of fe·ces
faec·u·lent
  var of fec·u·lent
faex
fa·ga·rine
fag·o·py·rism
Fah·rae·us
  sed·i·men·ta·tion test
Fahr·en·heit
fail·ure
faint
Fair·ley pig·ment
fal·cate
fal·cial
fal·ci·form
fal·cip·a·rum ma·lar·i·a
fal·cu·la
fal·cu·lar
fal·lo·pi·an
Fal·lot te·tral·o·gy
fall·out
Falls test
false
fal·si·fi·ca·tion
fal·si·fy
falx
  pl fal·ces
fa·mes

fa·mil·i·al
fam·i·ly
  pl fam·i·lies
fam·ine
fa·nat·i·cism
Fan·co·ni syn·drome
fang
fan·go
fan·go·ther·a·py
Fan·ni·a
fan·ning
fan·ta·size
fan·tasm
  var of phan·tasm
fan·tast
  var of phan·tast
fan·ta·sy
  pl fan·ta·sies
  or phan·ta·sy
  pl phan·ta·sies
fan·tom
  var of phan·tom
fan·tri·done
Fa·ra·beuf tri·an·gle
far·ad
far·a·da·ic
  or fa·rad·ic
far·a·day
fa·rad·ic
  or far·a·da·ic
far·a·dim·e·ter
fa·rad·i·punc·ture
far·a·dism
far·a·di·za·tion
far·a·dize
far·a·do·con·trac·til·i·ty
far·a·do·mus·cu·lar
far·a·do·ther·a·py

135

Far·ber dis·ease
far·cy
    pl far·cies
far·del-bound
fa·ri·na
far·i·na·ceous
Far·ley, St. Clair, and Rei·sin·ger meth·od
Far·mer and Abt meth·od
far·ne·sol
far·ne·syl
Farre white line
far·sight·ed
far·sight·ed·ness
fas·ci·a
    pl fas·ci·as
    or fas·ci·ae
fas·ci·al
fas·ci·cle
fas·ci·cled
fas·cic·u·lar
fas·cic·u·late
    or fas·cic·u·lat·ed
fas·cic·u·lat·ed
    or fas·cic·u·late
fas·cic·u·la·tion
fas·cic·u·li·tis
fas·cic·u·lus
    pl fas·cic·u·li
fas·ci·ec·to·my
    pl fas·ci·ec·to·mies
fas·ci·i·tis
fas·ci·num
fas·ci·od·e·sis
    pl fas·ci·od·e·ses
fas·ci·o·la
    pl fas·ci·o·las
    or fas·ci·o·lae
fas·ci·o·li·a·sis
    pl fas·ci·o·li·a·ses
Fas·ci·o·loi·des
fas·ci·o·lop·si·a·sis
    pl fas·ci·o·lop·si·a·ses
Fas·ci·o·lop·sis
fas·ci·o·plas·ty
fas·ci·or·rha·phy
fas·ci·o·scap·u·lo·hu·mer·al
fas·ci·ot·o·my

fas·ci·tis
fast
fas·tid·i·ous
fas·tid·i·um
fas·tig·i·al
fas·tig·i·o·bul·bar
fas·tig·i·um
fast·ness
fat
fa·tal
fa·tal·i·ty
    pl fa·tal·i·ties
fat·i·ga·bil·i·ty
    pl fat·i·ga·bil·i·ties
fat·i·ga·ble
fa·tigue
fat·si·a
fat·sol·u·ble
fat·ty
fau·ces
fau·cial
fau·na
    pl fau·nas
    or fau·nae
Faust meth·od
fa·vag·i·nous
fa·ve·o·late
fa·ve·o·lus
    pl fa·ve·o·li
fa·vid
fa·vi·des
fa·vism
Fa·vre dis·ease
fa·vus
Fa·zi·o-Londe at·ro·phy
fear
fea·ture
feb·ri·cide
fe·bric·u·la
feb·ri·fa·cient
fe·brif·ic
fe·brif·u·gal
feb·ri·fuge
feb·ri·fu·gine
fe·brile
fe·bris
fe·cal
fe·ca·lith

fe·ca·loid
fe·ca·lo·ma
fe·ca·lu·ri·a
fe·ces
Fech·ner law
fec·u·la
    pl fec·u·lae
fec·u·lent
fe·cun·date
fe·cun·da·tion
fe·cun·di·ty
    pl fe·cun·di·ties
Fe·de-Ri·ga dis·ease
fee·ble·mind·ed
fee·ble·mind·ed·ness
feed·back
feed·ing
feel
Feer dis·ease
Feh·ling so·lu·tion
Feil-Klip·pel syn·drome
fel
feld·sher
Fe·li·dae
fe·line
fel·late
fel·la·ti·o
    or fel·la·tion
fel·la·tion
    or fel·la·ti·o
fel·la·tor
fel·la·trice
Fell-O'Dwy·er meth·od
fel·o·de·se
    pl fel·o-nes-de-se
    or fel·o-de-se
fel·on
fe·lo·ni·ous
fel·o·ny
felt·work
Fel·ty syn·drome
fel·y·pres·sin
fe·male
fem·i·nine
fem·i·nism
fem·i·ni·za·tion
fem·i·nize
fem·o·ral

fem·o·ro·cele
fem·o·ro·pop·lit·e·al
fem·o·ro·tib·i·al
fe·mur
   pl fe·murs
   or fem·o·ra
fen·al·a·mide
fen·a·mole
fen·chone
fen·clo·nine
fe·nes·tra
   pl fe·nes·trae
fe·nes·tral
fen·es·trate
   or fen·es·trat·ed
fen·es·trat·ed
   or fen·es·trate
fen·es·tra·tion
fen·eth·yl·line
fen·flu·ra·mine
fen·i·mide
fen·met·ra·mide
fen·nel
fen·ta·nyl
fen·u·greek
Fen·wick dis·ease
fen·yr·i·pol
fe·ral
fer·de·lance
Fé·ré·ol node
Fer·gu·son op·er·a·tion
fer·ment
fer·men·ta·tion
fer·men·ta·tive
fer·mi
fer·mi·on
fer·mi·um
fern·ing
fer·rat·ed
fer·re·dox·in
fer·ric
fer·ri·cy·a·nide
fer·ri·hae·mo·glo·bin
   var of fer·ri·he·mo·glo·bin
fer·ri·heme
fer·ri·he·mo·glo·bin
fer·ri·por·phy·rin
fer·ri·pro·to·por·phy·rin

fer·ri·tin
fer·ro·cho·li·nate
fer·ro·cy·a·nide
fer·ro·hae·mo·glo·bin
   var of fer·ro·he·mo·glo·bin
fer·ro·heme
fer·ro·he·mo·glo·bin
fer·ro·ki·net·ics
fer·ro·mag·net·ic
fer·ro·por·phy·rin
fer·ro·pro·tein
fer·ro·pro·to·por·phy·rin
fer·ro·ther·a·py
fer·rous
fer·ru·gi·na·tion
fer·ru·gin·e·ous
   or fer·ru·gi·nous
fer·ru·gi·nous
   or fer·ru·gin·e·ous
fer·rule
fer·rum
fer·tile
fer·til·i·ty
   pl fer·til·i·ties
fer·til·i·za·tion
fer·til·ize
fer·ti·li·zin
Fer·u·la
fe·ru·lic
fer·ves·cence
fes·cue foot
fes·ter
fes·ti·nant
fes·ti·nate
fes·ti·na·tion
fes·toon
fe·tal
fe·tal·i·za·tion
fe·ta·tion
fet·ich
   var of fet·ish
fet·ich·ism
   var of fet·ish·ism
fe·ti·cide
fet·id
fet·ish
fet·ish·ism
fet·ish·ist

fet·lock
fe·to·am·ni·ot·ic
fe·to·glob·u·lin
fe·tog·ra·phy
fe·tol·o·gist
fe·tol·o·gy
   pl fe·tol·o·gies
fe·tom·e·try
   pl fe·tom·e·tries
fe·to·pla·cen·tal
fe·to·pro·te·in
fe·tor
fe·tox·y·late
fe·tu·in
fe·tus
fe·ver
fe·ver·et
fe·ver·ish
fe·ver·ous
fex·ism
fi·at
fi·ber
fi·ber·co·lon·o·scope
fi·ber·gas·tro·scope
fi·ber·op·tic
fi·ber·op·tics
fi·ber·scope
fi·bra
   pl fi·brae
fi·bre
   var of fi·ber
fi·bri·form
fi·bril
fi·bril·la
   pl fi·bril·lae
fi·bril·lar
fi·bril·lar·y
fi·bril·late
fi·bril·la·tion
fi·bril·lo·gen·e·sis
fi·brin
fi·brin·ase
fi·bri·no·cel·lu·lar
fi·brin·o·gen
fi·brin·o·ge·ne·mi·a
fi·bri·no·gen·e·sis
fi·brin·o·gen·ic
fi·brin·o·ge·nol·y·sis

fi·brin·o·gen·ol·y·tic
fi·brin·o·gen·o·pe·ni·a
fi·bri·nog·e·nous
fi·bri·no·hem·or·rha·gic
fi·bri·noid
fi·bri·no·ki·nase
fi·bri·nol·y·sin
fi·bri·nol·y·sis
   pl fi·bri·nol·y·ses
fi·bri·no·lyt·ic
fi·bri·no·pe·ni·a
fi·bri·no·pep·tide
fi·bri·no·plas·tin
fi·bri·no·pu·ru·lent
fi·bri·nos·co·py
fi·brin·ous
fi·bri·nu·ri·a
fi·bro·ad·e·no·ma
   pl fi·bro·ad·e·no·mas
   or fi·bro·ad·e·no·ma·ta
fi·bro·ad·i·pose
fi·bro·am·e·lo·blas·to·ma
   pl fi·bro·am·e·lo·blas·to·
    mas
   or fi·bro·am·e·lo·blas·to·
    ma·ta
fi·bro·an·gi·o·li·po·ma
   pl fi·bro·an·gi·o·li·po·mas
   or fi·bro·an·gi·o·li·po·ma·ta
fi·bro·an·gi·o·ma
   pl fi·bro·an·gi·o·mas
   or fi·bro·an·gi·o·ma·ta
fi·bro·a·re·o·lar
fi·bro·blast
fi·bro·blas·tic
fi·bro·blas·to·ma
   pl fi·bro·blas·to·mas
   or fi·bro·blas·to·ma·ta
fi·bro·bron·chi·tis
fi·bro·cal·car·e·ous
fi·bro·cal·cif·ic
fi·bro·car·ci·no·ma
   pl fi·bro·car·ci·no·mas
   or fi·bro·car·ci·no·ma·ta
fi·bro·car·ti·lage
fi·bro·car·ti·lag·i·nes
   in·ter·ver·te·bra·les
fi·bro·car·ti·lag·i·nous

fi·bro·car·ti·la·go
   pl fi·bro·car·ti·lag·i·nes
fi·bro·ca·se·ous
fi·bro·cav·i·tar·y
fi·bro·cel·lu·lar
fi·bro·ce·men·to·ma
   pl fi·bro·ce·men·to·mas
   or fi·bro·ce·men·to·ma·ta
fi·bro·chon·dri·tis
fi·bro·chon·dro·ma
   pl fi·bro·chon·dro·mas
   or fi·bro·chon·dro·ma·ta
fi·bro·chon·dro·os·te·o·ma
   pl fi·bro·chon·dro·os·te·o·
    mas
   or fi·bro·chon·dro·os·te·o·
    ma·ta
fi·bro·col·lag·e·nous
fi·bro·cyst
fi·bro·cys·tic
fi·bro·cys·to·ma
   pl fi·bro·cys·to·mas
   or fi·bro·cys·to·ma·ta
fi·bro·cyte
fi·bro·dys·pla·si·a
fi·bro·e·las·tic
fi·bro·e·las·to·sis
fi·bro·en·chon·dro·ma
   pl fi·bro·en·chon·dro·mas
   or fi·bro·en·chon·dro·ma·ta
fi·bro·ep·i·the·li·o·ma
   pl fi·bro·ep·i·the·li·o·mas
   or fi·bro·ep·i·the·li·o·ma·ta
fi·bro·fat·ty
fi·brog·li·a
fi·bro·gli·o·ma
   pl fi·bro·gli·o·mas
   or fi·bro·gli·o·ma·ta
fi·bro·hae·mo·tho·rax
   var of fi·bro·he·mo·tho·rax
fi·bro·he·mo·tho·rax
fi·broid
fi·broid·ec·to·my
fi·bro·in
fi·bro·lam·i·nar
fi·bro·lei·o·my·o·ma
   pl fi·bro·lei·o·my·o·mas
   or fi·bro·lei·o·my·o·ma·ta

fi·bro·li·po·ma
   pl fi·bro·li·po·mas
   or fi·bro·li·po·ma·ta
fi·bro·li·pom·a·tous
fi·bro·lip·o·sar·co·ma
   pl fi·bro·lip·o·sar·co·mas
   or fi·bro·lip·o·sar·co·ma·ta
fi·brol·y·sis
fi·bro·ma
   pl fi·bro·mas
   or fi·bro·ma·ta
fi·bro·ma·to·gen·ic
fi·bro·ma·toid
fi·bro·ma·to·sis
   pl fi·bro·ma·to·ses
fi·brom·a·tous
fi·brome en pas·tille
fi·bro·mus·cu·lar
fi·bro·my·i·tis
fi·bro·my·o·ma
   pl fi·bro·my·o·mas
   or fi·bro·my·o·ma·ta
fi·bro·my·o·mec·to·my
fi·bro·my·o·si·tis
fi·bro·myx·o·li·po·ma
   pl fi·bro·myx·o·li·po·mas
   or fi·bro·myx·o·li·po·ma·ta
fi·bro·myx·o·ma
   pl fi·bro·myx·o·mas
   or fi·bro·myx·o·ma·ta
fi·bro·myx·o·sar·co·ma
   pl fi·bro·myx·o·sar·co·mas
   or fi·bro·myx·o·sar·co·ma·
    ta
fi·bro·neu·ro·ma
   pl fi·bro·neu·ro·mas
   or fi·bro·neu·ro·ma·ta
fi·bro·os·te·o·chon·dro·ma
   pl fi·bro·os·te·o·chon·
    dro·mas
   or fi·bro·os·te·o·chon·
    dro·ma·ta
fi·bro·os·te·o·ma
   pl fi·bro·os·te·o·mas
   or fi·bro·os·te·o·ma·ta
fi·bro·os·te·o·sar·co·ma
   pl fi·bro·os·te·o·sar·co·mas
   or fi·bro·os·te·o·sar·co·ma·
    ta

fi·bro·pap·il·lo·ma
  pl fi·bro·pap·il·lo·mas
  or fi·bro·pap·il·lo·ma·ta
fi·bro·pla·si·a
fi·bro·plas·tic
fi·bro·plate
fi·bro·psam·mo·ma
  pl fi·bro·psam·mo·mas
  or fi·bro·psam·mo·ma·ta
fi·bro·pu·ru·lent
fi·bro·sar·co·ma
  pl fi·bro·sar·co·mas
  or fi·bro·sar·co·ma·ta
fi·bro·sar·com·a·tous
fi·brose
fi·bro·se·rous
fi·bro·sis
  pl fi·bro·ses
fi·bro·sit·ic
fi·bro·si·tis
fi·bro·tho·rax
fi·brot·ic
fi·brous
fi·bro·vas·cu·lar
fi·bro·xan·tho·ma
  pl fi·bro·xan·tho·mas
  or fi·bro·xan·tho·ma·ta
fi·bro·xan·thom·a·tous
fib·u·la
  pl fib·u·las
  or fib·u·lae
fib·u·lar
fib·u·lo·cal·ca·ne·al
fib·u·lo·cal·ca·ne·us
fib·u·lo·tib·i·a·lis
fi·cin
Fick prin·ci·ple
fi·co·sis
Fied·ler dis·ease
field of vi·sion
fi·èv·re bou·ton·neuse
fig
fig·ure
fig·ure-ground
fig·wort
fi·la·ceous
fil·a·ment
fil·a·men·ta·ry
fil·a·men·ta·tion

fil·a·men·tous
fil·a·men·tum
fi·lar
fi·lar·i·a
  pl fi·lar·i·ae
fi·lar·i·al
fil·a·ri·a·sis
  pl fil·a·ri·a·ses
  or fil·ar·i·o·sis
  pl fil·ar·i·o·ses
fi·lar·i·ci·dal
fi·lar·i·cide
fi·lar·i·form
fi·lar·i·id
fil·a·rin
Fi·lar·i·oi·de·a
fil·ar·i·o·sis
  pl fil·ar·i·o·ses
  or fil·a·ri·a·ses
  pl fil·a·ri·a·ses
Fil·a·tov dis·ease
Fil·a·tov-Dukes dis·ease
fil·i·al
fi·lic·ic
fil·i·cin
fil·i·cin·ic
fil·i·form
fil·i·pin
Fi·lip·o·wicz sign
fil·i·punc·ture
fil·let
fill·ing
film
fil·o·pod
  pl fil·o·pods
  or fil·o·po·di·um
  pl fil·o·po·dia
fi·lo·po·di·um
  pl fil·o·po·dia
  or fi·lo·pod
  pl fi·lo·pods
fi·lo·pres·sure
fil·ter
fil·ter·a·bil·i·ty
  pl fil·ter·a·bil·i·ties
fil·ter·a·ble
  or fil·tra·ble
fil·tra·ble
  or fil·ter·a·ble

fil·trate
fil·tra·tion
fil·trum
  pl fil·tra
fi·lum
  pl fi·la
fim·bri·a
  pl fim·bri·ae
fim·bri·ae tu·bae u·ter·i·nae
fim·bri·al
fim·bri·ate
  or fim·bri·at·ed
fim·bri·at·ed
  or fim·bri·ate
fim·bri·a·tion
fim·bri·ec·to·my
fim·bri·o·cele
fim·bri·o·den·tate
Find·lay op·er·a·tion
fin·ger
fin·gered
fin·ger·nail
fin·ger·print
fin·ger·print·ing
fin·ger·tip
Fin·kel·dey cells
Fin·ney op·er·a·tion
Fin·ney-von Ha·ber·er op·
  er·a·tion
Fi·no·chet·ti stir·rup
fire·bug
fire·damp
first aid
first-de·gree
first set
Fish·berg test
fish·ber·ry
fis·sile
fis·sion
fis·sion·a·ble
fis·sip·a·rous
fis·su·la
  pl fis·su·lae
fis·su·ra
  pl fis·su·rae
fis·su·rae cer·e·bel·li
fis·su·ral
fis·su·ra·tion
fis·sure

fis·tu·la
pl fis·tu·las
or fis·tu·lae
fis·tu·lar
fis·tu·late
fis·tu·la·tion
fis·tu·la·tome
fis·tu·lec·to·my
fis·tu·li·za·tion
fis·tu·lize
fis·tu·lo·en·ter·os·to·my
fis·tu·lo·gram
fis·tu·lot·o·my
pl fis·tu·lot·o·mies
fis·tu·lous
fit
Fitz·ger·ald-Gard·ner
syn·drome
Fitz-Hugh–Cur·tis
syn·drome
fix·ate
fix·a·tion
fix·a·tive
fix·ing
fla·bel·lum
pl fla·bel·la
flac·cid
flac·cid·i·ty
pl flac·cid·i·ties
Flack node
flag·el·lant
flag·el·lant·ism
fla·gel·lar
Flag·el·la·ta
Flag·el·la·tae
flag·el·late
flag·el·la·tion
fla·gel·li·form
flag·el·lo·ma·ni·a
flag·el·lo·sis
pl flag·el·lo·ses
fla·gel·lo·spore
fla·gel·lum
pl fla·gel·lums
or fla·gel·la
Flagg re·sus·ci·ta·tion
flail
Fla·ja·ni dis·ease
flam·ma·ble

flange
flank
flap
flare
flash·eye
flask
flat
Fla·tau law
Fla·tau-Schil·der dis·ease
flat·foot
flat·foot·ed
flat·ness
flat·sedge
flat·u·lence
pl flat·u·len·ces
or flat·u·len·cies
or flat·u·len·cy
flat·u·len·cy
or flat·u·lence
flat·u·lent
fla·tus
flat·worm
fla·va·none
fla·ve·do
fla·vi·an·ic
fla·vin
fla·vine
fla·vi·vi·rus
Fla·vo·bac·te·ri·um
fla·vo·ki·nase
fla·vone
fla·vo·noid
fla·vo·nol
fla·vo·none
fla·vo·pro·tein
fla·vor
fla·vo·xan·thin
fla·vox·ate
flax·seed
flea
flea·bane
flea·bite
flea-bit·ten
Flech·sig tract
flec·tion
or flex·ion
fleck·fie·ber
fleck·milz of Fei·tis
Flei·scher-Kay·ser ring

flesh
fletch·er·ism
fletch·er·ize
flex
flex·i·bil·i·tas ce·re·a
flex·i·bil·i·ty
flex·i·ble
flex·ile
flex·im·e·ter
flex·ion
or flec·tion
Flex·ner re·port
Flex·ner-Job·ling
car·ci·no·sar·co·ma
flex·or
flex·u·ous
flex·u·ra
pl flex·u·rae
flex·ur·al
flex·ure
flick·er
Flindt spots
Flink mur·mur
floa·ta·tion
var of flo·ta·tion
float·ers
float·ing
floc
floc·cil·la·tion
floc·cose
floc·cu·lar
floc·cu·late
floc·cu·la·tion
floc·cule
floc·cu·lence
floc·cu·lent
floc·cu·lo·nod·u·lar
floc·cu·lus
pl floc·cu·li
flo·ra
pl flo·ras
or flo·rae
flor·an·ty·rone
Flor·ence flask
flo·ren·ti·um
flo·res
Flo·rey u·nit
flo·rid
flo·ri·form

loss
lo·ta·tion
low
low·er bas·ket of Boch·
   da·lek
low·er in·dex
low·me·ter
lox·u·ri·dine
lu
lu·ban·i·late
luc·tu·ance
luc·tu·ant
luc·tu·ate
luc·tu·a·tion
lu·do·rex
lu·dro·cor·ti·sone
lu·fen·am·ic
luh·mann test
lu·id
lu·id·ex·tract
lu·id·gly·cer·ate
lu·id·i·ty
   pl flu·id·i·ties
lu·id·ounce
lu·i·drachm
   var of flu·i·dram
lu·i·dram
luke
lu·men
   pl flu·mi·na
lu·meth·a·sone
lu·me·thi·a·zide
lu·met·ra·mide
lu·mi·na
lu·min·o·rex
lu·nid·a·zole
lu·o·cin·o·lone
   a·cet·o·nide
lu·o·cor·to·lone
lu·or
lu·or·ap·a·tite
lu·or·chrome
lu·o·rene
lu·o·res·ce·in
lu·o·res·cence
lu·o·res·cent
lu·o·res·cin
luor·i·date
luor·i·da·tion

flu·o·ride
fluor·i·di·za·tion
fluor·i·dize
flu·o·rim·e·ter
   or flu·o·rom·e·ter
flu·o·rim·e·try
   pl flu·o·rim·e·tries
   or flu·o·rom·e·try
   pl flu·o·rom·e·tries
fluor·i·nate
fluor·i·na·tion
flu·o·rine
flu·o·rite
flu·o·ro·a·ce·tic
flu·o·ro·car·bon
flu·o·ro·car·di·o·gram
flu·o·ro·car·di·o·graph
flu·o·ro·car·di·og·ra·phy
fluor·o·chrome
fluor·o·gen
flu·o·ro·graph·ic
flu·o·rog·ra·phy
flu·o·rom·e·ter
   or flu·o·rim·e·ter
flu·o·ro·meth·o·lone
flu·o·ro·met·ric
flu·o·rom·e·try
   pl flu·o·rom·e·tries
   or flu·o·rim·e·try
   pl flu·o·rim·e·tries
flu·o·ro·phos·phate
flu·o·ro·pho·to·met·ric
flu·o·ro·pho·tom·e·try
flu·o·ro·roent·ge·nog·ra·
   phy
flu·o·ro·sal·an
fluor·o·scope
fluor·o·scop·ic
fluor·o·scop·i·cal·ly
fluor·os·co·pist
fluor·os·co·py
   pl fluor·os·co·pies
flu·o·ro·sis
   pl flu·o·ro·ses
flu·o·ro·u·ra·cil
flu·ox·y·mes·ter·one
flu·per·o·lone
flu·phen·a·zine
flu·pred·nis·o·lone

flu·ran·dren·o·lide
flu·raz·e·pam
flu·ro·ges·tone
flu·ro·thyl
flu·rox·ene
Flu·ry strain
flush
flut·ter
flut·ter-fi·bril·la·tion
flux
fly
fly·belt
Fo·à-Kur·loff cell
foam
fo·cal
fo·cal·i·za·tion
fo·cal·ize
fo·cim·e·ter
   or fo·com·e·ter
fo·com·e·ter
   or fo·cim·e·ter
fo·cus
   pl fo·cus·es
   or fo·ci
foen·u·greek
   var of fen·u·greek
Foer·ster sign
Foer·ster-Pen·field
   op·er·a·tion
foe·tal
   var of fe·tal
foe·ti·cide
   var of fe·ti·cide
foet·id
   var of fet·id
foe·to·glob·u·lin
   var of fe·to·glob·u·lin
foe·tor
   var of fe·tor
foe·tus
   pl foe·tus·es
   or foe·ti
   var of fe·tus
fog·ging
fo·go sel·va·gem
foil
Foix syn·drome
Foix-A·la·jou·a·nine
   syn·drome

fo·la·cin
fo·late
fold
Fo·ley Y-plas·ty
fo·li·a cer·e·bel·li
fo·li·a·ceous
fo·li·ate
fo·lic
fo·lie
fo·lie à deux
    pl fo·lies à deux
Fo·lin and Den·is meth·od
Fo·lin and Far·mer meth·od
Fo·lin and Schaf·fer meth·od
Fo·lin and Young·burg meth·od
Fo·lin meth·od
Fo·lin, Can·non and Den·is meth·od
Fo·lin-Cio·cal·teu re·a·gent
fo·lin·ic
Fo·lin-Mc·Ell·roy test
Fo·lin-Wu test
fo·li·ose
    or fo·li·ous
fo·li·ous
    or fo·li·ose
fo·li·um
    pl fo·li·a
fol·li·cle
fol·li·clis
fol·lic·u·lar
fol·lic·u·late
    or fol·lic·u·lat·ed
fol·lic·u·lat·ed
    or fol·lic·u·late
fol·lic·u·li
fol·lic·u·lin
fol·lic·u·li·tis
fol·lic·u·loid
fol·lic·u·lo·ma
    pl fol·lic·u·lo·mas
    or fol·lic·u·lo·ma·ta
fol·lic·u·lo·sis
fol·lic·u·lus
    pl fol·lic·u·li
fol·low-up

fo·ment
fo·men·ta·tion
fo·mes
    pl fom·i·tes
Fong le·sion
Fon·se·ca dis·ease
Fon·se·cae·a
Fon·ta·na spa·ces
fon·ta·nel
    or fon·ta·nelle
fon·ta·nelle
    or fon·ta·nel
fon·tic·u·li cra·ni·i
fon·tic·u·lus
    pl fon·tic·u·li
foot-and-mouth dis·ease
foot·bath
foot-can·dle
foot·ling
foot-pound
foot·print
foots
foot·sore
foot·sore·ness
fo·ra·men
    pl fo·ra·mens
    or fo·ram·i·na
fo·ra·men mag·num
fo·ra·men o·va·le
fo·ram·i·nal
fo·ra·mi·nif·er·ous
fo·ram·i·not·o·my
fo·ra·min·u·late
fo·ra·min·u·lum
    pl fo·ra·min·u·la
Forbes dis·ease
Forbes-Al·bright syn·drome
force
for·ceps
    pl for·ceps
    or for·ceps·es
    or for·cip·es
Forch·hei·mer sign
for·ci·pate
    or for·ci·pat·ed
for·ci·pat·ed
    or for·ci·pate
for·cip·i·tal

for·ci·pres·sure
For·dyce dis·ease
fore·arm
fore·brain
fore·con·scious
fore·fin·ger
fore·foot
    pl fore·feet
fore·gut
fore·head
for·eign
fore·kid·ney
Fo·rel bun·dle
fore·leg
fore·limb
fore·milk
fo·ren·sic
fo·ren·si·cal·ly
fore·paw
fore·play
fore·pleas·ure
fore·skin
fore·stom·ach
fore·top
fore·wa·ters
form
for·mal·de·hyde
form·am·ide
for·ma·lin
for·ma·lin·ize
for·mate
for·ma·ti·o
    pl for·ma·ti·o·nes
for·ma·tion
for·ma·tive
for·ma·zan
forme fruste
    pl formes frustes
for·mic
for·mi·cant
for·mi·ca·tion
for·mi·ci·a·sis
for·mim·i·no·glu·tam·ic
for·mim·i·no·glu·tam·ic·ac·i·du·ri·a
for·mim·i·no·trans·fer·ase
for·mo·cre·sol
for·mol
for·mol-gel

for·mol·ize
for·mo·ni·trile
for·mox·yl
for·mu·la
  pl for·mu·las
  or for·mu·lae
for·mu·lar·y
  pl for·mu·lar·ies
for·mu·la·tion
for·myl
for·myl·am·ide
for·myl·ase
for·myl·a·tion
for·myl·fo·lic
for·myl·for·mic
for·myl·gly·cine
for·myl·pte·ro·ic
for·ni·cal
for·ni·cate
for·ni·ca·tion
for·ni·ca·tor
for·ni·ca·trix
  pl for·ni·ca·tri·ces
for·nix
  pl for·ni·ces
For·o·blique
Fors·gren meth·od
Forss·man an·ti·gens
Fort Bragg fe·ver
Fosh·ay test
fos·pi·rate
fos·sa
  pl fos·sae
fos·sette
fos·su·la
  pl fos·su·lae
fos·su·late
Fos·ter rule
Fos·ter-Ken·ne·dy
  syn·drome
Fother·gill dis·ease
Fou·chet re·a·gent
fou·droy·ant
foul
foul brood
fou·lage
foun·der
four·chet
  var of four·chette

four·chette
fo·ve·a
  pl fo·ve·ae
fo·vea cen·tra·lis
fo·ve·al
fo·ve·ate
  or fo·ve·at·ed
fo·ve·at·ed
  or fo·ve·ate
fo·ve·a·tion
fo·ve·i·form
fo·ve·o·la
  pl fo·ve·o·las
  or fo·ve·o·lae
fo·ve·o·lae
fo·ve·o·lar
fo·ve·o·late
Fo·ville pa·ral·y·sis
Fow·ler po·si·tion
fox·glove
frac·tion·al
frac·tion·ate
frac·tion·a·tion
frac·ture
frad·i·cin
Fraenk·el glands
Fraentz·el mur·mur
fraen·u·lum
  pl fraen·u·la
  var of fren·u·lum
frae·num
  pl frae·nums
  or frae·na
  var of fre·num
frag·ile
fra·gil·i·tas
fra·gil·i·tas os·si·um
fra·gil·i·ty
  pl fra·gil·i·ties
fra·gil·o·cyte
fra·gil·o·cy·to·sis
  pl fra·gil·o·cy·to·ses
frag·men·ta·tion
fraise
fram·be·si·a
fram·be·si·o·ma
fram·boe·si·a
  var of fram·be·si·a

Frame, Rus·sell, and Wil·
  hel·mi meth·od
frame·shift
frame·work
Fran·ce·schet·ti syn·drome
Fran·ci·sel·la tu·la·ren·sis
Fran·cis test
fran·ci·um
Fran·çois syn·drome
fran·gu·la
fran·gu·lin
fran·gu·lo·side
frank
Frank op·er·a·tion
Franke meth·od
Frank·en·häu·ser
  gan·gli·on
Frank·fort ho·ri·zon·tal
  plane
frank·in·cense
frank·lin·ic
fra·ter·nal
frat·ri·cide
Fraun·ho·fer lines
frax·in
freckle
Fre·det-Ram·stedt
  op·er·a·tion
free-as·so·ci·ate
free-float·ing
free-liv·ing
Free·man rule
free-mar·tin
freeze
  froze
freeze-dry
  freeze-dried
freeze-etch·ing
Frei test
Frei·berg dis·ease
frem·i·tus
fre·nal
fre·nec·to·my
fre·net·ic
  var of phre·net·ic
fre·no·plas·ty
fre·not·o·my
fren·u·lum
  pl fren·u·la

143

fre·num
  pl fre·nums
  or fre·na
fren·zied
fren·zy
  pl fren·zies
fre·quen·cy
Frer·ich the·o·ry
fre·tum
  pl fre·ta
Freud·i·an
Freud·i·an·ism
Freund ad·ju·vant
Freund·lich ad·sorp·tion
  e·qua·tion
Frey syn·drome
fri·a·bil·i·ty
  pl fri·a·bil·i·ties
fri·a·ble
fri·a·ble·ness
fric·tion
fric·tion·al
Frid·er·ich·sen syn·drome
Fried rule
Frie·de·mann-Grae·ser
  meth·od
Frie·den·wald no·mo·gram
Fried·länd·er ba·cil·lus
Fried·man test
Fried·mann va·so·mo·tor
  symp·tom com·plex
Fried·reich a·tax·i·a
Fried·rich-Bau·er
  op·er·a·tion
frig·id
fri·gid·i·ty
  pl fri·gid·i·ties
frig·o·la·bile
frig·o·rif·ic
frig·o·sta·ble
frig·o·ther·a·py
fringe
Frisch ba·cil·lus
frit
Froh·de re·a·gent
Fröh·lich syn·drome
Froin syn·drome
frole·ment
Fro·ment sign

From·mel dis·ease
frons
  pl fron·tes
fron·tad
fron·tal
fron·ta·lis
fron·tal·ly
front·let
fron·to·eth·moid
fron·to·lac·ri·mal
fron·to·ma·lar
fron·to·max·il·lar·y
fron·to·men·tal
fron·to·na·sal
fron·to·oc·cip·i·tal
fron·to·pa·ri·e·tal
fron·to·pon·tine
fron·to·pon·to·cer·e·bel·lar
fron·to·sphe·noid
fron·to·tem·po·ral
fron·to·tem·po·ra·le
  pl fron·to·tem·po·ra·li·a
fron·to·zy·go·mat·ic
Fro·riep gan·gli·on
frost·bite
  frost·bit
frot·tage
frot·teur
fruc·tiv·o·rous
fruc·to·fu·ran·o·san
fruc·to·fu·ra·nose
fruc·to·fu·ran·o·side
fruc·to·ki·nase
fruc·to·py·ra·nose
fruc·to·san
fruc·tose
fruc·tose 1,6-di·phos·
  phate
fruc·tose 1-phos·phate
fruc·tose 6-phos·phate
fruc·to·se·mi·a
fruc·to·side
fruc·to·su·ri·a
fru·giv·o·rous
fru·men·ta·ceous
fru·men·tum
frus·trate
frus·tra·tion
Fuchs dys·tro·phy

fuch·sin
  or fuch·sine
fuch·sine
  or fuch·sin
fuch·sin·o·phil
fuch·sin·o·phil·i·a
fuch·sin·o·phil·ic
fu·co·san
fu·cose
fu·co·si·dase
fu·co·si·do·sis
fu·cus
Fuer·bring·er sign
fu·ga·cious
fu·gac·i·ty
  pl fu·gac·i·ties
fu·gal
fu·gi·tive
Fu·gu
fugue
ful·crum
  pl ful·crums
  or ful·cra
ful·gu·rant
ful·gu·rate
ful·gu·ra·tion
fu·lig·i·nous
full-blood·ed
full-mouth·ed
full-thick·ness graft
ful·mi·nant
ful·mi·nate
fu·ma·gil·lin
fu·ma·rase
fu·ma·rate
Fu·mar·i·a·ce·ae
fu·mar·ic
fu·mig·a·cin
fu·mi·gant
fu·mi·gate
fu·mi·ga·tion
fum·ing
func·ti·o
func·ti·o lae·sa
func·tion
func·tion·al
func·tion·al·ly
fun·dal
fun·da·ment

n·da·men·tal
n·dec·to·my
  pl fun·dec·to·mies
n·dic
n·di·form
n·do·plas·ty
n·do·pli·ca·tion
n·do·scop·ic
  var of fun·du·scop·ic
n·dos·co·py
  var of fun·dus·co·py
n·du·lus
  pl fun·du·lus
n·dus
  pl fun·di
n·du·scope
n·du·scop·ic
n·dus·co·py
  pl fun·dus·co·pies
n·du·sec·to·my
n·gae·mi·a
  var of fun·ge·mi·a
n·gal
n·gate
n·ge·mi·a
un·gi Im·per·fec·ti
n·gi·ci·dal
n·gi·cid·al·ly
n·gi·cide
n·gi·ci·din
n·gi·form
n·gi·sta·sis
n·gi·stat
n·gi·stat·ic
n·gi·tox·ic
n·gi·tox·ic·i·ty
  pl fun·gi·tox·ic·i·ties
n·goid

fun·gos·i·ty
  pl fun·gos·i·ties
fun·gous
fun·gus
  pl fun·gus·es
  or fun·gi
fu·nic
fu·ni·cle
fu·nic·u·lar
fu·nic·u·li·tis
fu·nic·u·lus
  pl fu·nic·u·li
fu·nis
fun·nel
fu·ral
fu·ran
fu·ra·nose
fu·ra·zol·i·done
fu·ra·zo·li·um
fur·az·o·sin
fur·ca
  pl fur·cae
fur·cal
fur·ca·lis
fur·cate
fur·ca·tion
fur·co·cer·cous
fur·cu·la
  pl fur·cu·lae
fur·fur
  pl fur·fu·res
fur·fu·ra·ceous
fur·fu·ral
fur·fur·al·de·hyde
fur·fu·ryl
fu·ri·bund
fu·ro·ic
fu·ror

fu·ro·sem·ide
  or fur·se·mide
fu·ro·yl
fur·sa·lan
fur·se·mide
  or fu·ro·sem·ide
fu·run·cle
fu·run·cu·lar
fu·run·cu·loid
fu·run·cu·lo·sis
  pl fu·run·cu·lo·ses
fu·run·cu·lous
fu·run·cu·lus
  pl fu·run·cu·li
fu·ryl
Fu·sar·i·um
  pl Fu·sar·i·a
fus·cin
fus·co·cae·ru·li·us
  oph·thal·mo·max·il·lar·
  is of O·ta
fuse
fu·seau
  pl fu·seaux
fu·sel
fu·si·ble
fu·sid·ic
fu·si·form
Fu·si·for·mis
fu·si·mo·tor
fu·sion
fu·sion·al
fu·so·bac·te·ri·um
  pl fu·so·bac·te·ri·a
fu·so·cel·lu·lar
fu·so·spi·ril·lo·sis
fu·so·spi·ro·che·tal
fu·so·spi·ro·che·to·sis
fus·ti·ga·tion
fuzz

G

G ac·id
G-ac·tin
gad·fly
   pl·gad·flies
Gad·i·dae
gad·o·le·ic
gad·o·lin·i·um
Ga·dus
Gaert·ner to·no·me·ter
Gaff·ky·a
gag
gage
   var of gauge
gain
Gais·böck syn·drome
gait
ga·lac·ta·cra·si·a
gal·ac·tae·mi·a
   var of gal·ac·te·mi·a
ga·lac·ta·gogue
   or ga·lac·to·gogue
ga·lac·tan
ga·lac·tase
gal·ac·te·mi·a
ga·lact·hi·dro·sis
ga·lac·tic
ga·lac·tin
gal·ac·tis·chi·a
ga·lac·to·blast
ga·lac·to·bol·ic
ga·lac·to·cele
ga·lac·to·fla·vin
ga·lac·to·gen
ga·lac·to·gogue
   or ga·lac·ta·gogue
ga·lac·toid
ga·lac·to·ki·nase
ga·lac·to·lip·id
   or ga·lac·to·lip·ide
   or ga·lac·to·lip·in
ga·lac·to·lip·ide
   or ga·lac·to·lip·in
   or ga·lac·to·lip·id
ga·lac·to·lip·in
   or ga·lac·to·lip·id
   or ga·lac·to·lip·ide
gal·ac·to·ma
   pl gal·ac·to·mas

or gal·ac·to·ma·ta
gal·ac·tom·e·ter
ga·lac·to·meth·yl·ose
gal·ac·ton·ic
gal·ac·toph·a·gous
gal·ac·toph·ly·sis
ga·lac·to·phore
gal·ac·toph·o·ri·tis
gal·ac·toph·o·rous
gal·ac·toph·thi·sis
gal·ac·toph·y·gous
ga·lac·to·pla·ni·a
ga·lac·to·poi·e·sis
   pl ga·lac·to·poi·e·ses
ga·lac·to·poi·et·ic
ga·lac·to·py·ra
gal·ac·to·py·ra·nose
ga·lac·to·py·re·tic
ga·lac·tor·rhea
ga·lac·tor·rhoe·a
   var of ga·lac·tor·rhe·a
ga·lac·to·sac·char·ic
ga·lac·tos·ae·mi·a
   var of ga·lac·to·se·mi·a
ga·lac·to·sa·mine
ga·lac·to·san
gal·ac·tos·che·sis
ga·lac·to·scope
ga·lac·tose
ga·lac·to·se·mi·a
ga·lac·to·se·mic
ga·lac·to·sid·ase
ga·lac·to·side
gal·ac·to·sis
   pl gal·ac·to·ses
ga·lac·to·sphin·go·side
ga·lac·to·sta·si·a
gal·ac·tos·ta·sis
ga·lac·tos·u·ri·a
ga·lac·to·ther·a·py
   pl ga·lac·to·ther·a·pies
ga·lac·to·tox·i·con
ga·lac·to·tox·in
ga·lac·to·tox·ism
   or ga·lac·tox·ism
gal·ac·tot·ro·phy
ga·lac·tox·ism
   or ga·lac·to·tox·ism
ga·lac·to·zy·mase

gal·ac·tu·ri·a
ga·lac·tu·ron·ic
Ga·la·go
Gal·ant re·flex
gal·ba·num
ga·le·a
   pl ga·le·as
   or ga·le·ae
ga·le·a ap·o·neu·rot·i·ca
gal·e·an·thro·py
Ga·le·ga
ga·le·na
ga·len·ic
   or ga·len·i·cal
ga·len·i·cal
   or ga·len·ic
ga·len·ics
ga·len·ism
gal·e·o·phil·i·a
gal·e·o·pho·bi·a
gal·e·ro·pi·a
gall
gal·la
gal·la·mine tri·eth·i·o·dide
gal·late
gall·blad·der
gal·le·in
gal·ler·y
gal·lic
Gal·lie-Le Me·su·ri·er
   op·er·a·tion
Gal·li·for·mes
gal·li·na·ceous
gal·li·um
gal·lo·cy·a·nin
gal·lon
gal·lop
gal·lo·tan·nic
gall·stone
gal·siek·te
Gal·ton law
gal·van·ic
gal·va·nism
gal·va·ni·za·tion
gal·va·nize
gal·va·no·cau·ter·y
   pl gal·va·no·cau·ter·ies
gal·va·no·con·trac·til·i·ty
gal·va·nom·e·ter

gal·va·no·mus·cu·lar
gal·va·no·ner·vous
gal·va·no·pal·pa·tion
gal·va·no·punc·ture
gal·va·no·scope
gal·va·nos·co·py
gal·va·no·sur·ger·y
   pl gal·va·no·sur·ger·ies
gal·va·no·tax·is
   pl gal·va·no·tax·es
gal·va·no·ther·a·py
gal·va·no·ther·my
gal·va·no·ton·ic
gal·va·not·o·nus
gal·va·no·trop·ic
gal·va·not·ro·pism
gal·vo
gam·a·soi·do·sis
   pl gam·a·soi·do·ses
Gam·bi·an
   try·pan·o·so·mi·a·sis
gam·bir
gam·boge
Gam·bu·si·a
gam·e·tan·gi·um
   pl gam·e·tan·gi·a
gam·ete
ga·met·ic
ga·met·i·cal·ly
ga·me·to·cide
ga·me·to·cyte
ga·me·to·gen·e·sis
   pl ga·me·to·gen·e·ses
ga·me·to·gen·ic
   or gam·e·tog·e·nous
gam·e·tog·e·nous
   or ga·me·to·gen·ic
gam·e·tog·e·ny
   pl gam·e·tog·e·nies
   or ga·me·tog·o·ny
   pl ga·me·tog·o·nies
ga·me·to·go·ni·um
   pl ga·me·to·go·ni·a
gam·e·tog·o·ny
   pl gam·e·tog·o·nies
   or gam·e·tog·e·ny
   pl gam·e·tog·e·nies
gam·e·toid
ga·me·to·ki·net·ic

ga·me·to·phyte
ga·me·to·phyt·ic
gam·fex·ine
gam·ic
gam·ma ben·zene
   hex·a·chlo·ride
gam·ma glob·u·lin
gam·ma·cism
   or gam·ma·cis·mus
gam·ma·cis·mus
   or gam·ma·cism
gam·ma·glob·u·lin·op·
   a·thy
Gam·mel syn·drome
gam·mop·a·thy
Gam·na dis·ease
Gam·na-Fa·vre bod·ies
Gam·na-Gan·dy bod·ies
gam·o·gen·e·sis
   pl gam·o·gen·e·ses
gam·o·ge·net·ic
gam·o·ge·net·i·cal·ly
gam·o·ma·ni·a
gam·one
gam·ont
gam·o·pet·al·ous
gam·o·pho·bi·a
gam·o·sep·al·ous
Gam·per bow·ing re·flex
Gam·strop dis·ease
Gan·dy-Gam·na nod·ules
gan·glia
gan·gli·al
gan·gli·ar
gan·gli·ate
   or gan·gli·at·ed
gan·gli·at·ed
   or gan·gli·ate
gan·gli·ec·to·my
gan·gli·form
   or gan·gli·o·form
gan·gli·i·tis
gan·gli·o·blast
gan·gli·o·cyte
gan·gli·o·cy·to·ma
   pl gan·gli·o·cy·to·mas
   or gan·gli·o·cy·to·ma·ta

gan·gli·o·cy·to·neu·ro·ma
   pl gan·gli·o·cy·to·neu·
     ro·mas
   or gan·gli·o·cy·to·neu·
     ro·ma·ta
gan·gli·o·form
   or gan·gli·form
gan·gli·oid
gan·gli·o·ma
   pl gan·gli·o·mas
   or gan·gli·o·ma·ta
gan·gli·on
   pl gan·gli·ons
   or gan·gli·a
gan·gli·o·nate
   or gan·gli·o·nat·ed
gan·gli·o·nat·ed
   or gan·gli·o·nate
gan·gli·o·nec·to·my
   pl gan·gli·o·nec·to·mies
Gan·gli·o·ne·ma
gan·gli·o·neu·ro·blas·to·ma
   pl gan·gli·o·neu·ro·blas·
     to·mas
   or gan·gli·o·neu·ro·blas·
     to·ma·ta
gan·gli·o·neu·ro·cy·to·ma
   pl gan·gli·o·neu·ro·cy·
     to·mas
   or gan·gli·o·neu·ro·cy·
     to·ma·ta
gan·gli·o·neu·ro·ma
   pl gan·gli·o·neu·ro·mas
   or gan·gli·o·neu·ro·ma·ta
gan·gli·on·ic
gan·gli·on·i·tis
gan·gli·o·nos·to·my
gan·gli·o·ple·gic
gan·gli·o·side
gan·gli·o·si·do·sis
   pl gan·gli·o·si·do·ses
gan·gli·o·sym·path·
   i·co·blas·to·ma
   pl gan·gli·o·sym·path·i·
     co·blas·to·mas
   or gan·gli·o·sym·path·
     i·co·blas·to·ma·ta
gan·go·sa
gan·grae·na o·ris

gan·grene
gan·gre·no·sis
gan·gre·nous
gangue
gan·o·blast
Gan·ser syn·drome
Gant op·er·a·tion
Gant·zer mus·cle
gap
gape·worm
Gar·cin·i·a
Gard·ner syn·drome
gar·get
gar·gle
gar·goyl·ism
Gar·land tri·an·gle
Gar·ré dis·ease
Gar·rod test
gar·ru·li·ty
    pl gar·ru·li·ties
Gart·ner duct
gas
gas·e·ous
gas·kin
gas·om·e·ter
gas·o·met·ric
gasp
gas·se·ri·an
gas·ter
Gas·ter·oph·i·lus
gas·tra·den·i·tis
gas·tral
gas·tral·gi·a
gas·tral·gic
gas·tral·go·ke·no·sis
gas·tras·the·ni·a
gas·tra·tro·phi·a
gas·trec·ta·si·a
gas·trec·ta·sis
    pl gas·trec·ta·ses
gas·trec·to·my
    pl gas·trec·to·mies
gas·tric
gas·tric·sin
gas·trin
gas·trin·o·ma
gas·trit·ic
gas·tri·tis
    pl gas·trit·i·des

gas·tro·a·ceph·a·lus
    pl gas·tro·a·ceph·a·li
gas·tro·a·mor·phus
    pl gas·tro·a·mor·phi
gas·tro·a·nas·to·mo·sis
    pl gas·tro·a·nas·to·mo·ses
gas·tro·cam·er·a
gas·tro·car·di·ac
gas·tro·cele
gas·tro·cne·mi·al
gas·tro·cne·mi·us
    pl gas·tro·cne·mi·i
gas·tro·coel
    or gas·tro·coele
gas·tro·coele
    or gas·tro·coel
gas·tro·col·ic
gas·tro·co·li·tis
gas·tro·co·lot·o·my
    pl gas·tro·co·lot·o·mies
gas·tro·col·pot·o·my
gas·tro·cu·ta·ne·ous
gas·tro·di·a·phane
gas·tro·di·aph·a·nos·co·py
    pl gas·tro·di·aph·a·nos·
        co·pies
gas·tro·di·a·pha·ny
gas·tro·did·y·mus
gas·tro·dis·ci·a·sis
Gas·tro·dis·coi·des
Gas·tro·dis·cus hom·i·nis
gas·tro·disk
gas·tro·du·o·de·nal
gas·tro·du·o·de·ni·tis
gas·tro·du·o·de·nos·co·py
gas·tro·du·o·de·nos·to·my
    pl gas·tro·du·o·de·nos·
        to·mies
gas·tro·dy·ni·a
gas·tro·en·ter·al·gi·a
gas·tro·en·ter·ic
gas·tro·en·ter·it·ic
gas·tro·en·ter·i·tis
    pl gas·tro·en·ter·i·tis·es
    or gas·tro·en·ter·i·ti·des
gas·tro·en·ter·o·a·
    nas·to·mo·sis
gas·tro·en·ter·o·co·li·tis
gas·tro·en·ter·ol·o·gist

gas·tro·en·ter·ol·o·gy
    pl gas·tro·en·ter·ol·o·gies
gas·tro·en·ter·op·a·thy
    pl gas·tro·en·ter·op·a·thies
gas·tro·en·ter·op·to·sis
gas·tro·en·ter·os·to·my
    pl gas·tro·en·ter·os·to·mies
gas·tro·en·ter·ot·o·my
gas·tro·ep·i·plo·ic
gas·tro·e·soph·a·ge·al
gas·tro·e·soph·a·gi·tis
gas·tro·e·soph·a·gos·to·my
gas·tro·e·soph·a·go·plas·ty
gas·tro·fi·ber·scope
gas·tro·gas·tros·to·my
gas·tro·ga·vage
gas·tro·gen·ic
gas·tro·graph
gas·tro·he·pat·ic
gas·tro·hep·a·ti·tis
gas·tro·hy·per·ton·ic
gas·tro·il·e·ac
gas·tro·il·e·i·tis
gas·tro·il·e·os·to·my
gas·tro·in·tes·ti·nal
gas·tro·je·ju·nal
gas·tro·je·ju·ni·tis
gas·tro·je·ju·no·col·ic
gas·tro·je·ju·nos·to·my
    pl gas·tro·je·ju·nos·to·mies
gas·tro·lav·age
gas·tro·li·e·nal
gas·tro·lith
gas·tro·li·thi·a·sis
gas·trol·o·gist
gas·trol·o·gy
    pl gas·trol·o·gies
gas·trol·y·sis
    pl gas·trol·y·ses
gas·tro·ma·la·ci·a
gas·tro·meg·a·ly
gas·trom·e·lus
gas·tro·mes·en·ter·ic
gas·tro·my·co·sis
    pl gas·tro·my·co·ses
gas·tro·my·ot·o·my
gas·tro·myx·or·rhe·a
gas·trone

gas·tro·oe·soph·a·ge·al
  var of gas·tro·e·soph·a·ge·al
gas·tro·oe·soph·a·go·
  plas·ty
  var of gas·tro·e·soph·a·go·
  plas·ty
gas·tro·pan·cre·at·ic
gas·tro·pa·ral·y·sis
gas·tro·par·a·si·tus
gas·tro·par·e·sis
gas·tro·pa·thy
gas·tro·pex·y
  pl gas·tro·pex·ies
Gas·troph·i·lus
gas·tro·pho·tor
gas·tro·phren·ic
gas·tro·plas·ty
gas·tro·ple·gi·a
gas·tro·pli·ca·tion
Gas·trop·o·da
gas·trop·o·dous
gas·tro·pore
gas·trop·to·sis
  pl gas·trop·to·ses
gas·tro·pul·mo·nar·y
gas·tro·py·lo·rec·to·my
gas·tro·py·lor·ic
gas·tror·rha·gi·a
gas·tror·rha·phy
  pl gas·tror·rha·phies
gas·tror·rhe·a
gas·tror·rhoe·a
  var of gas·tror·rhe·a
gas·tro·sal·i·var·y
gas·tros·chi·sis
  pl gas·tros·chi·ses
gas·tro·scope
gas·tro·scop·ic
gas·tros·co·py
  pl gas·tros·co·pies
gas·tro·spasm
gas·tro·splen·ic
gas·tro·stax·is
gas·tro·ste·no·sis
gas·tros·to·ga·vage
gas·tros·to·la·vage
gas·tros·to·my
  pl gas·tros·to·mies
gas·tro·suc·cor·rhe·a

gas·tro·suc·cor·rhoe·a
  var of gas·tro·suc·cor·rhe·a
gas·tro·tho·ra·cop·a·gus
gas·trot·o·my
  pl gas·trot·o·mies
gas·tro·to·nom·e·ter
gas·tro·tox·ic
gas·tro·tox·in
gas·tro·trop·ic
gas·tro·tym·pa·ni·tes
gas·trox·yn·sis
gas·tru·la
  pl gas·tru·las
  or gas·tru·lae
gas·tru·la·tion
gas·tru·late
Gatch bed
gat·o·phil·i·a
gat·o·pho·bi·a
Gaucher dis·ease
gauge
Gault re·flex
gaul·the·ri·a
gaul·the·rin
gaul·the·ro·lin
gaunt·let
gauss
Gaus·sel sign
Gauss·i·an points
gauze
ga·vage
gaze
g-com·po·nent
Gee-Her·ter dis·ease
geel·dik·kop
Gee-Thay·sen dis·ease
Ge·gen·baur mus·cle
ge·gen·hal·ten
Gei·gel re·flex
Gei·ger count·er
  or Gei·ger-Mül·ler
  count·er
Geiger-Mül·ler counter
  or Gei·ger count·er
gei·so·ma
gel
gel·as·ma
ge·las·mus
ge·las·tic

gel·ate
ge·lat·i·fi·ca·tion
gel·a·tin
  or gel·a·tine
ge·lat·i·nase
gel·a·tine
  or gel·a·tin
ge·la·ti·nif·er·ous
ge·la·ti·ni·za·tion
ge·lat·i·nize
ge·lat·i·noid
ge·lat·i·no·lyt·ic
ge·lat·i·no·sa
ge·lat·i·nous
ge·la·tion
gel·a·tose
geld
Ge·li·neau syn·drome
Ge·li·neau Red·lich
  syn·drome
Ge·le test
gel·o·ple·gi·a
gel·ose
gel·o·sin
ge·lo·sis
gel·o·to·lep·sy
gel·se·mine
gel·se·mi·um
gem·el·lol·o·gy
ge·mel·lus
  pl ge·mel·lus·es
  or ge·mel·li
gem·i·nate
gem·i·nate·ly
gem·i·na·tion
gem·i·nous
ge·mis·to·cyte
ge·mis·to·cyt·ic
gem·ma
  pl gem·mae
gem·mate
gem·ma·tion
gem·mu·la·tion
gem·mule
ge·na
  pl ge·nae
ge·nal
gen·der
Gen·dre fix·ing flu·id

gene
ge·ne·al·o·gy
  pl ge·ne·al·o·gies
gen·er·al
gen·er·al·i·za·tion
gen·er·al·ize
gen·er·a·tion
gen·er·a·tive
gen·er·a·tive·ly
gen·er·a·tor
ge·ner·ic
gen·es·er·ine
ge·ne·si·al
ge·nes·ic
ge·ne·si·ol·o·gy
gen·e·sis
  pl gen·e·ses
ge·net·ic
ge·net·i·cist
ge·net·ics
gen·et·o·troph·ic
gen·e·tous
ge·ni·al
gen·ic
gen·i·cal·ly
ge·nic·u·lar
ge·nic·u·late
  or ge·nic·u·lat·ed
ge·nic·u·lat·ed
  or ge·nic·u·late
ge·nic·u·late·ly
ge·nic·u·lo·cal·ca·rine
ge·nic·u·lo·tem·po·ral
ge·nic·u·lum
  pl ge·nic·u·la
ge·ni·o·glos·sus
  pl ge·ni·o·glos·si
ge·ni·o·hy·o·glos·sus
  pl ge·ni·o·hy·o·glos·sus
ge·ni·o·hy·oid
ge·ni·on
ge·ni·o·plas·ty
  pl ge·ni·o·plas·ties
ge·ni·pha·ryn·ge·us
gen·i·tal
gen·i·ta·li·a
gen·i·tal·i·ty
  pl gen·i·tal·i·ties
gen·i·tal·oid

gen·i·tals
gen·i·to·cru·ral
gen·i·to·fem·o·ral
gen·i·to·plas·ty
gen·i·to·u·ri·nar·y
gen·i·to·ves·i·cal
gen·ius
gen·o·blast
gen·o·cide
gen·o·cop·y
gen·o·der·ma·to·sis
  pl gen·o·der·ma·to·ses
ge·nom
  or genome
ge·nome
  or ge·nom
ge·nom·ic
gen·o·pho·bia
gen·o·type
gen·o·typ·ic
  or gen·o·typ·i·cal
gen·o·typ·i·cal
  or ge·no·typ·ic
gen·ta·mi·cin
gen·tian
gen·tian·o·phil·ic
gen·tian·o·pho·bic
gen·ti·o·bi·ose
gen·ti·o·pic·rin
gen·tis·ic
gen·ti·sin
ge·nu
  pl gen·u·a
ge·nu val·gum
ge·nu var·um
gen·u·al
gen·u·cu·bi·tal
gen·u·fa·cial
gen·u·pec·to·ral
ge·nus
  pl gen·er·a
gen·y·chei·lo·plas·ty
gen·y·plas·ty
  pl gen·y·plas·ties
ge·ode
ge·o·med·i·cine
ge·o·met·ric
  or ge·o·met·ri·cal

ge·o·met·ri·cal
  or ge·o·met·ric
ge·o·met·ric-op·tic
ge·o·pa·thol·o·gy
  pl ge·o·pa·thol·o·gies
ge·o·pha·gia
  or ge·oph·a·gy
ge·oph·a·gism
ge·oph·a·gist
ge·oph·a·gous
ge·oph·a·gy
  pl geo·pha·gies
  or geo·pha·gi·a
Ge·oph·i·lus
Geor·gi-Sachs test
ge·o·tax·is
ge·ot·ri·cho·sis
  pl ge·ot·ri·cho·ses
Ge·ot·ri·chum
ge·o·trop·ic
ge·o·trop·i·cal·ly
ge·ot·ro·pism
ge·phy·ro·pho·bi·a
Ger·agh·ty op·er·a·tion
ge·ra·ni·al
ge·ra·ni·ol
ge·rat·ic
ger·a·tol·o·gy
  pl ger·a·tol·o·gies
ger·bil
  pl ger·bil·le
ger·bil·le
  or ger·bil
ger·e·ol·o·gy
Ger·hardt dis·ease
ger·i·at·ric
ger·i·a·tri·cian
ger·i·at·rics
ger·i·a·trist
ger·i·o·don·tics
ger·i·o·psy·cho·sis
  pl ger·i·o·psy·cho·ses
Ger·lach val·ue
Ger·li·er dis·ease
germ
germ plasm
Ger·man mea·sles
ger·ma·nin
ger·ma·ni·um

germ·cell
germ·free
ger·mi·cid·al
ger·mi·cide
ger·mi·nal
ger·mi·nate
ger·mi·na·tion
ger·mi·na·tive
ger·mine
ger·mi·no·ma
  pl ger·mi·no·mas
  or ger·mi·no·ma·ta
germ·layer
germ·proof
germ·y
ger·o·co·mi·a
ger·o·com·i·cal
ge·roc·o·my
ger·o·der·ma
  or ger·o·der·mi·a
ger·o·der·mi·a
  ger·o·der·ma
ger·o·don·ti·a
ger·o·don·tics
ger·o·don·tol·o·gy
ger·o·ma·ras·mus
ger·o·mor·phism
ge·ron·tal
ge·ron·tic
ger·on·tol·o·gy
  pl ger·on·tol·o·gies
ge·ron·to·phil·i·a
ge·ron·to·pho·bi·a
ge·ron·to·pi·a
ge·ron·to·ther·a·peu·tics
ge·ron·to·ther·a·py
  pl ge·ron·to·ther·a·pies
ger·on·tox·on
Ge·ro·ta fas·ci·a
Gersh-Ma·cal·lum
  meth·od
Gerst·mann syn·drome
Ge·sell de·vel·op·men·tal
  sched·ule
ges·ta·gen
ge·stalt
  pl ge·stalts
  or ge·stalt·en
ge·stalt·ism

ge·stalt·ist
ges·tate
ges·ta·tion
ges·ta·tion·al
ges·to·sis
  pl ges·to·ses
Get·so·wa ad·e·no·ma
geu·ma·pho·bi·a
ghat·ti
Ghon com·plex
Gia·co·mi·ni band
Gian·nuz·zi cells
gi·ant
gi·ant·ism
Gi·ar·di·a
gi·ar·di·a·sis
  pl gi·ar·di·a·ses
  or gi·ar·di·o·sis
  pl gi·ar·di·o·ses
gi·ar·di·o·sis
  pl gi·ar·di·o·ses
  or gi·ar·di·a·sis
  pl gi·ar·di·a·ses
gib·ber·el·lic
gib·ber·el·lin
gib·bon
Gib·bon-Lan·dis test
gib·bos·i·ty
  pl gib·bos·i·ties
gib·bous
Gibbs ad·sorp·tion law
Gibbs-Don·nan
  e·qui·lib·ri·um
Gibbs-Helm·holtz
  e·qua·tion
gib·bus
Gi·bral·tar fe·ver
Gib·son ban·dage
gid
gid·di·ness
gid·dy
Giem·sa stain
Gier·ke cor·pus·cles
Gif·ford op·er·a·tion
gi·gan·tism
gi·gan·to·blast
gi·gan·to·chro·mo·blast
gi·gan·to·cyte
gi·gan·to·mas·ti·a

Gi·gli op·er·a·tion
Gil·bert syn·drome
Gil·christ dis·ease
gild·ing
Gil·e·ad balm
Gil·ford-Hutch·in·son
  dis·ease
gill arch
gill cleft
gill slit
Gil·le·ni·a
Gilles de la Tou·rette syn·
  drome
Gil·lies op·er·a·tion
Gill·more nee·dles
gilt
Gim·ber·nat lig·a·ment
gin·ger
gin·gi·va
  pl gin·gi·vae
gin·gi·val
gin·gi·val·gi·a
gin·gi·val·ly
gin·gi·vec·to·my
  pl gin·gi·vec·to·mies
gin·gi·vi·tis
gin·gi·vo·buc·cal
gin·gi·vo·glos·sal
gin·gi·vo·glos·si·tis
gin·gi·vo·la·bi·al
gin·gi·vo·plas·ty
  pl gin·gi·vo·plas·ties
gin·gi·vo·sis
gin·gi·vo·sto·ma·ti·tis
  pl gin·gi·vo·sto·ma·ti·ti·des
  or gin·gi·vo·sto·ma·ti·tis·es
gin·gly·form
gin·gly·mo·ar·thro·dia
gin·gly·mo·ar·thro·di·al
gin·gly·moid
gin·gly·mus
  pl gin·gly·mi
Gi·ral·dès or·gan
Gi·rard re·a·gent
gir·dle
Gir·dle·stone op·er·a·tion
git·al·in
gith·a·gism
Gith·lin syn·drome

151

git·o·gen·in
git·o·nin
gi·tox·i·gen·in
gi·tox·in
git·ter
git·ter·fa·sern
giz·zard
gla·bel·la
    pl gla·bel·lae
gla·bel·lar
gla·brate
gla·brous
gla·cial
glad·i·ate
glad·i·ol·ic
glad·i·o·lus
    pl glad·i·o·li
giair·in
glair·y
gland
gland of Bar·tho·lin
glan·der·ous
glan·ders
glan·di·lem·ma
glands
glan·du·la
    pl glan·du·lae
glan·du·lar
glan·du·lous
glans
    pl glan·des
glans cli·to·ri·dis
glans pe·nis
Glas·ser dis·ease
Gla·se·ri·an fis·sure
glass·es
Glau·ber salt
glau·ca·ru·bin
glau·co·ma
glau·co·ma·to·cy·clit·ic
glau·co·ma·tous
gleet
gleet·y
glen·o·hu·mer·al
gle·noid
gli·a
gli·a·cyte
gli·a·din
gli·al

gli·o·bac·te·ri·a
gli·o·blas·to·ma
    pl gli·o·blas·to·mas
    or gli·o·blas·to·ma·ta
gli·o·coc·cus
    pl gli·o·coc·ci
gli·o·cyte
gli·o·cy·to·ma
gli·og·e·nous
gli·o·ma
    pl gli·o·mas
    or gli·o·ma·ta
gli·o·ma·to·sis
    pl gli·o·ma·tos·es
gli·om·a·tous
gli·o·neu·ro·ma
    pl gli·o·neu·ro·mas
    or gli·o·neu·ro·ma·ta
gli·o·sar·co·ma
    pl gli·o·sar·co·mas
    or gli·o·sar·co·ma·ta
gli·o·sis
    pl gli·o·ses
gli·o·some
gli·o·tox·in
Glis·son cap·sule
glis·son·i·tis
Glo·bid·i·um
glo·bin
glo·bi·nom·e·ter
glo·bose
glo·bose·ly
glo·bo·side
glo·bos·i·ty
    pl glo·bos·i·ties
glob·u·lar
glob·ule
glob·u·lin
glob·u·lin·u·ri·a
glo·bus
glo·bus hys·ter·i·cus
glo·bus pal·li·dus
glo·mal
glo·man·gi·o·ma
    pl glo·man·gi·o·mas
    or glo·man·gi·o·ma·ta
glome
glo·mec·to·my
    pl glo·mec·to·mies

glom·er·ate
glo·mer·u·lar
glo·mer·u·li
glo·mer·u·li·tis
glo·mer·u·lo·ne·phri·tis
    pl glo·mer·u·lo·ne·phri·
    ti·des
glo·mer·u·lop·a·thy
glo·mer·u·lo·scle·ro·sis
    pl glo·mer·u·lo·scle·ro·ses
glo·mer·u·lose
glo·mer·u·lus
    pl glo·mer·u·li
glo·mus
    pl glom·er·a
    or glo·mi
glo·mus ca·rot·i·cum
glos·sa
    pl glos·sas
    or glos·sae
glos·sal
gloss·al·gi·a
glos·san·thrax
glos·sec·to·my
Glos·si·na
glos·si·tis
glos·so·cele
glos·so·dy·na·mom·e·ter
gloss·o·dyn·i·a
glos·so·ep·i·glot·tid·e·an
glos·so·graph
glos·so·hy·al
glos·so·kin·es·thet·ic
glos·so·la·li·a
glos·sol·o·gy
    pl glos·sol·o·gies
glos·so·pal·a·ti·nus
    pl glos·so·pal·a·ti·ni
glos·sop·a·thy
    pl glos·sop·a·thies
glos·so·pha·ryn·ge·al
glos·so·plas·ty
glos·sor·rha·phy
glos·so·spasm
glos·sot·o·my
glos·so·trich·i·a
glot·tal
glot·tic

glot·tis
pl glot·tis·es
or glot·ti·des
glot·tol·o·gy
pl glot·tol·o·gies
glu·ca·gon
glu·ca·gon·o·ma
glu·car·ic
glu·cide
glu·cin·i·um
glu·co·a·scor·bic
glu·co·cer·e·bro·side
glu·co·cor·ti·coid
glu·co·fu·ra·nose
glu·co·gen·ic
glu·co·ki·nase
glu·co·kin·in
glu·co·lip·id
or glu·co·lip·ide
glu·co·lip·ide
or glu·co·lip·id
glu·col·y·sis
pl glu·col·y·ses
glu·co·ne·o·gen·e·sis
pl glu·co·ne·o·gen·e·ses
glu·con·ic
glu·co·phore
glu·co·pro·te·in
glu·co·py·ra·nose
glu·co·sa·mine
glu·co·san
glu·cose
glu·cose-1-phos·phate
glu·cose-6-phos·phate
glu·co·si·dase
glu·co·side
glu·co·sid·ic
glu·co·sid·i·cal·ly
glu·co·sin
glu·co·sone
glu·co·sul·fone
glu·cos·u·ri·a
glu·cu·ron·ic
glu·cu·ron·i·dase
glu·cu·ro·nide
glu·ta·mate
glu·tam·ic
glu·tam·i·nase
glu·ta·mine

glu·ta·min·ic
glu·tam·yl
glu·ta·ral·de·hyde
glu·tar·ic
glu·ta·thi·one
glu·te·al
glu·te·lin
glu·ten
glu·te·nin
glu·te·o·fem·o·ral
glu·te·o·tro·chan·ter·ic
glu·teth·i·mide
glu·te·us
pl glu·te·i
glu·tin
glu·ti·nous
glu·ti·tis
glu·tose
glut·ton·y
gly·bu·ride
gly·cae·mi·a
var of gly·cem·i·a
gly·can
gly·case
gly·ce·mi·a
gly·ce·mic
glyc·er·al·de·hyde
gly·cer·ic
glyc·er·i·dase
glyc·er·ide
glyc·er·id·ic
glyc·er·in
or glyc·er·ine
glyc·er·in·at·ed
glyc·er·ine
or glyc·er·in
glyc·er·ite
glyc·er·o·gel·a·tin
glyc·er·ol
glyc·er·o·phos·pha·tase
glyc·er·o·phos·phate
glyc·er·o·phos·pho·ric
glyc·er·ose
glyc·er·yl
gly·ci·nate
gly·cine
gly·ci·nin
gly·ci·nu·ri·a
Gly·ciph·a·gus

gly·co·bi·ar·sol
gly·co·ca·lyx
gly·co·chol·ate
gly·co·chol·ic
gly·co·coll
gly·co·cy·a·mine
gly·co·gen
gly·co·ge·nase
gly·co·gen·e·sis
pl gly·co·gen·e·ses
gly·co·ge·net·ic
gly·co·gen·ic
gly·co·ge·nol·y·sis
pl gly·co·ge·nol·y·ses
gly·co·gen·o·lyt·ic
gly·co·gen·o·sis
gly·cog·e·nous
gly·cog·e·ny
gly·co·geu·si·a
gly·co·hae·mi·a
var of gly·co·he·mi·a
gly·co·he·mi·a
gly·co·his·tech·i·a
gly·col
gly·col·al·de·hyde
gly·co·late
gly·col·ic
or gly·col·lic
gly·co·lip·id
or gly·co·lip·ide
gly·co·lip·ide
or gly·co·lip·id
gly·co·lip·in
gly·col·lic
or gly·col·ic
gly·co·lyl
gly·col·y·sis
pl gly·col·y·ses
gly·co·lyt·ic
gly·co·met·a·bol·ic
gly·co·me·tab·o·lism
gly·co·ne·o·gen·e·sis
pl gly·co·ne·o·gen·e·ses
gly·co·nin
gly·co·nu·cle·o·pro·te·in
gly·co·pe·ni·a
gly·co·pep·tide
gly·co·pex·is
gly·co·phil·i·a

153

gly·co·pro·te·in
gly·co·pty·a·lism
gly·co·pyr·ro·late
gly·cor·rha·chi·a
gly·cor·rhe·a
gly·cor·rhoe·a
  var of gly·cor·rhe·a
gly·co·sae·mi·a
  var of gly·co·se·mi·a
gly·co·sa·mine
gly·co·se·cre·to·ry
gly·co·se·mi·a
gly·co·si·al·i·a
gly·co·si·a·lor·rhe·a
gly·co·si·dal
gly·co·si·dase
gly·co·side
gly·co·sid·ic
gly·co·som·e·ter
gly·co·sphin·go·lip·id
gly·co·sphin·go·side
gly·co·stat·ic
gly·cos·u·ri·a
gly·cos·u·ric
gly·co·troph·ic
  or gly·co·trop·ic
gly·co·trop·ic
  or gly·co·troph·ic
glyc·u·re·sis
  pl glyc·u·re·ses
gly·cu·ron·ic
gly·cu·ron·idase
gly·cu·ro·nide
gly·cu·ro·nu·ri·a
gly·cyl
glyc·yr·rhe·tic
glyc·yr·rhe·tin·ic
glyc·yr·rhi·za
glyc·yr·rhi·zic
glyc·yr·rhi·zin
gly·hex·a·mide
gly·o·ca·lyx
gly·oc·ta·mide
gly·ox·al
gly·ox·a·lase
gly·ox·a·late
gly·ox·a·line
gly·ox·yl·ic
gly·par·a·mide

Gmel·in test
gnat
gnath·al
  or gnath·ic
gna·thal·gi·a
gnath·ic
  or gna·thal
gna·thi·on
gna·thi·tis
gnath·o·ceph·a·lus
gnath·o·dy·na·mom·e·ter
gnath·o·dyn·i·a
gnath·ol·o·gy
gna·thop·a·gus
  par·a·sit·i·cus
gnath·o·pal·a·tos·chi·ses
gna·tho·plas·ty
gna·thos·chi·sis
Gna·thos·to·ma
gna·thos·to·mi·a·sis
  pl gna·thos·to·mi·a·ses
gno·si·a
gno·sis
  pl gno·ses
gnos·tic
gno·to·bi·ol·o·gy
  pl gno·to·bi·ol·o·gies
gno·to·bi·o·ta
gno·to·bi·ote
gno·to·bi·ot·ic
gno·to·bi·ot·i·cal·ly
gno·to·bi·ot·ics
Go·a pow·der
gob·let cell
go·det
Godt·fred·sen syn·drome
Goetsch test
Gof·man test
go·go
goi·ter
goi·ter·o·gen·ic
  or goi·tro·gen·ic
goi·tre
  var of goi·ter
goi·trin
goi·tro·gen
goi·tro·gen·ic
  or goi·ter·o·gen·ic

goi·tro·ge·nic·i·ty
  pl goi·tro·ge·nic·i·ties
goi·trous
Gold·ber·ger limb lead
Gold·blatt kid·ney
Gol·den·har syn·drome
gold·en·rod
gold·en·seal
Gold·flam dis·ease
Gold·schei·der dis·ease
Gold·stein ca·tas·tro·phic
  re·ac·tion
Gold·stein-Schee·rer tests
Gold·thwait op·er·a·tion
Gol·gi ap·pa·ra·tus, bod·y,
  com·plex
Gol·gi-Maz·zo·ni
  cor·pus·cle
gol·gi·o·ki·ne·sis
Gol·gi-Rez·zon·i·co
  spi·rals
Goll tract
Goltz syn·drome
Gom·bault neu·ri·tis
Gom·bault-Phi·lippe
  tri·an·gle
go·mit·o·li
gom·pho·sis
  pl gom·pho·ses
gon·a·cra·ti·a
go·nad
go·nad·al
go·nad·ec·to·my
  pl go·nad·ec·to·mies
go·nad·ec·to·mize
go·nad·o·blas·to·ma
  pl go·nad·o·blas·to·mas
  or go·nad·o·blas·to·ma·ta
go·nad·o·cen·tric
go·nad·o·ther·a·py
go·nad·o·tro·phic
  or go·nad·o·tro·pic
go·nad·o·tro·phin
  or go·nad·o·tro·pin
go·nad·o·trop·ic
  or go·nad·o·tro·phic
go·nad·o·tro·pin
  or go·nad·o·tro·phin

gon·a·duct
  or gon·o·duct
go·nag·ra
go·nal·gi·a
gon·an·gi·ec·to·my
gon·ar·thri·tis
gon·ar·throc·ace
gon·ar·throt·o·my
  pl gon·ar·throt·o·mies
go·nat·o·cele
Gon·da re·flex
gon·e·cyst
gon·e·cys·tic
gon·e·cys·ti·tis
gon·e·cys·to·lith
gon·e·cys·to·py·o·sis
gon·e·poi·e·sis
  pl gon·e·poi·e·ses
Gon·gy·lo·ne·ma
gon·gy·lo·ne·mi·a·sis
go·ni·al
gon·ic
go·nid·i·al
go·nid·i·um
  pl go·nid·i·a
go·ni·o·chei·los·chi·sis
go·ni·o·cra·ni·om·e·try
  pl go·ni·o·cra·ni·om·e·tries
go·ni·om·e·ter
go·ni·on
  pl go·ni·a
go·ni·o·punc·ture
go·ni·o·scope
go·ni·o·scop·ic
go·ni·os·co·py
  pl go·ni·os·co·pies
go·ni·ot·o·my
go·ni·tis
go·ni·um
gon·o·blast
gon·o·coc·cae·mi·a
  var of gon·o·coc·ce·mi·a
gon·o·coc·cal
  or gon·o·coc·cic
gon·o·coc·ce·mi·a
gon·o·coc·cic
  or gon·o·coc·cal
gon·o·coc·cide

gon·o·coc·cus
  pl gon·o·coc·ci
gon·o·cyte
gon·o·cy·to·ma
  pl gon·o·cy·to·mas
  or gon·o·cy·to·ma·ta
gon·o·duct
  or gon·a·duct
gon·o·gen·e·sis
  pl gon·o·gen·e·ses
go·nom·er·y
  pl go·nom·er·ies
gon·o·phore
gon·or·rhe·a
gon·or·rhe·al
gon·or·rhoe·a
  var of gon·or·rhe·a
gon·or·rhoe·al
  var of gon·or·rhe·al
gon·y·al·gi·a par·es·
  thet·i·ca
Gon·y·au·lax
gon·y·camp·sis
gon·y·o·cele
gon·y·on·cus
Gon·za·les blood group
Gooch cru·ci·ble, fil·ter
Good syn·drome
Goo·dell sign
Good·e·nough test
Good·pas·ture syn·drome
Good·sall rule
goose bumps
goose pim·ples
goose-flesh
Gop·a·lan syn·drome
Gor·di·a·ce·a
Gor·don re·flex
gorge
gor·get
go·ril·la
Gor·lin syn·drome
go·ron·dou
Gos·syp·i·um
gos·sy·pol
Gott·leib cut·i·cle
gouge
Gou·ger·ot-Blum dis·ease

Gou·ger·ot-Hou·wer-
  Sjö·gren syn·drome
Gou·lard extract
goun·dou
gout
gout·i·ness
gou·ty
Gow·er tract
Gow·er-Hen·ry re·flex
Gow·ers-col·umn
graaf·ian fol·li·cle
grac·ile
grac·i·lis
gra·da·tim
Gra·de·ni·go syn·drome
gra·di·ent
grad·u·ate
grad·u·at·ed
Grae·fe sign
Grae·ser meth·od
Graff meth·od
graft
Gra·ham law
Gra·ham-Cole test
Gra·ham Steell mur·mur
grain
grainage
gram
Gram meth·od, so·lu·tion,
  stain
Gram-Clau·di·us stain
gram·i·ci·din
gram·i·niv·o·rous
gram·me
  var of gram
gram·me·ter
gram·mol·e·cule
gram·neg·a·tive
gram·pos·i·tive
gram·var·i·a·ble
gra·na·tum
Gran·cher pneu·mon·i·a
grand mal
Gran·dry-Mer·kel
  cor·pus·cle
Gran·ger line
gran·u·la
gran·u·lar
gran·u·late

gra·nu·la·ti·o
   pl gra·nu·la·ti·o·nes
gran·u·la·tion
gran·u·la·ti·o·nes
   a·rach·noi·de·a·les
gran·ule
gran·u·li·form
gran·u·lo·ad·i·pose
gran·u·lo·blast
gran·u·lo·blas·tic
gran·u·lo·blas·to·sis
   pl gran·u·lo·blas·to·ses
gran·u·lo·cyte
gran·u·lo·cyt·ic
gran·u·lo·cy·to·pe·ni·a
gran·u·lo·cy·to·poi·e·sis
   pl gran·u·lo·cy·to·poi·e·ses
gran·u·lo·cy·to·poi·et·ic
gran·u·lo·cy·to·sis
   pl gran·u·lo·cy·to·ses
gran·u·lo·fil
gran·u·lo·ma
   pl gran·u·lo·mas
   or gran·u·lo·ma·ta
gran·u·lo·ma in·gui·na·le
gran·u·lo·ma
   py·o·gen·i·cum
gran·u·lo·ma·to·sis
   pl gran·u·lo·ma·to·ses
gran·u·lom·a·tous
gran·u·lo·mere
gran·u·lo·pec·tic
gran·u·lo·pe·ni·a
gran·u·lo·pex·is
gran·u·lo·pex·y
gran·u·lo·phil
gran·u·lo·plasm
gran·u·lo·plas·tic
gran·u·lo·poi·e·sis
   pl gran·u·lo·poi·e·ses
gran·u·lo·sa
gran·u·lose
gran·u·lo·sis
   pl gran·u·lo·ses
gra·num
   pl gra·na
graph
graph·aes·the·si·a
   var of graph·es·the·si·a

graph·an·aes·the·si·a
   var of graph·an·es·the·sia
graph·an·es·the·si·a
graph·es·the·si·a
graph·ic
graph·ite
gra·phit·ic
graph·o·log·i·cal
gra·phol·o·gy
   pl gra·phol·o·gies
graph·o·ma·ni·a
graph·o·ma·ni·ac
graph·o·mo·tor
graph·o·pho·bi·a
graph·or·rhe·a
graph·or·rhoe·a
   var of graph·or·rhe·a
graph·o·spasm
Gra·ser di·ver·tic·u·lum
Gras·set law
Gras·set-Gaus·sel
   phe·nom·e·non
gra·ti·o·la
Gra·tio·let op·tic
   ra·di·a·tion
grat·tage
grave
gra·ve·do
grav·el
grav·el-blind
Graves dis·ease
grav·id
grav·i·da
   pl grav·i·das
   or grav·i·dae
gra·vid·ic
gra·vid·i·ty
   pl gra·vid·i·ties
grav·id·ness
grav·i·do·car·di·ac
gra·vim·e·ter
grav·i·met·ric
   or grav·i·met·ri·cal
grav·i·met·ri·cal
   or grav·i·met·ric
grav·i·met·ri·cal·ly
gra·vim·e·try
   pl gra·vim·e·tries

gra·vis ne·o·na·to·rum
   jaun·dice
grav·i·stat·ic
grav·i·tate
grav·i·ta·tion
grav·i·ta·tion·al
grav·i·ty
   pl grav·i·ties
Gra·witz tu·mor
Gray stain
gray·out
grease
Green·berg meth·od
Green·field dis·ease
green·sick·ness
green·stick frac·ture
gref·fo·tome
greg·a·loid
Greg·a·ri·na
greg·a·rine
greg·a·rin·i·an
Greg·a·rin·i·da
greg·a·ri·no·sis
   pl greg·a·ri·no·ses
gre·gar·i·ous·ness
Greg·er·sen test
Greg·o·ry pow·der
Greig hy·per·tel·or·ism
grenz
Grey Tur·ner sign
grid
Grie·sing·er dis·ease
Grif·fith meth·od
grin·de·li·a
grind·ing
grip
   or grippe
gripe
grip·pal
grippe
   or grip
gris·e·o·ful·vin
Gri·solle sign
gris·tle
Gri·ti-Stokes am·pu·ta·tion
gro·cer's itch
Groc·co sign
Groen·blad-Strand·berg
   syn·drome

Groe·nouw cor·ne·al dys·tro·phy
groin
group prac·tice
group ther·a·py
grow
growth
Gru·ber li·ga·ment
Grüb·ler stain
grume
gru·mose
gru·mous
Grün·wald stain
Gryn·feltt tri·an·gle
gry·o·chrome
gry·po·sis
pl gry·po·ses
G-stro·phan·thin
gua·co
guai·ac
or guai·a·cum
guai·a·col
guai·a·cum
or guai·ac
gua·na·cline
gua·na·drel
gua·nase
gua·na·zo·lo
guan·cy·dine
guan·eth·i·dine
gua·ni·dine
gua·ni·di·no·a·ce·tic
gua·nine
guan·i·so·quin
gua·no·clor
guan·oc·tine
gua·no·phore
gua·no·sine
guan·ox·an
guan·ox·y·fen
gua·nyl·ic
gua·ra·na
gua·ra·nine
Guar·nie·ri bod·ies
gua·za
gu·ber·nac·u·lar
gu·ber·nac·u·lum
pl gu·ber·nac·u·la
Gud·den com·mis·sure

Gu·der·natsch test
Gue·neau de Mus·sy point
gue·non
Gue·rin fold
Guil·lain-Bar·ré syn·drome
Guil·lain sign
guil·lo·tine
guin·ea pig
guin·ea worm
gu·lar
Guld·berg-Waa·ge law
Gull and Sut·ton dis·ease
Gull dis·ease
gul·let
gu·lose
gum ar·a·bic
gum·boil
gum·ma
pl gum·mas
or gum·ma·ta
gum·ma·tous
gum·my
Gum·precht sha·dows
gun·cot·ton
gun·jah
Gün·ther dis·ease
gur·ney
Gur·vich ra·di·a·tion
gus·ta·tion
gus·ta·tive
gus·ta·to·ri·al
gus·ta·to·ri·al·ly
gus·ta·to·ri·ly
gus·ta·to·ry
gus·to·lac·ri·mal
gut
Guth·rie test
Gut·stein stain
gut·ta
pl gut·tae
gut·ta-per·cha
gut·tate
gut·ta·tion
gut·ter
gut·tie
gut·ti·form
Gutt·mann sign
gut·tur·al

gut·tur·oph·o·ny
gut·tur·o·tet·a·ny
Gut·zeit test
Gwath·mey meth·od
gym·no·cyte
gym·no·pho·bi·a
gym·no·spore
gy·nan·der
gy·nan·dri·a
gy·nan·drism
gy·nan·dro·blas·to·ma
pl gy·nan·dro·blas·to·mas
or gy·nan·dro·blas·to·ma·ta
gy·nan·droid
gy·nan·dro·morph
gy·nan·dro·mor·phic
gy·nan·dro·mor·phism
gy·nan·dro·mor·phous
gy·nan·dro·mor·phy
gy·nan·drous
gy·nan·dry
gy·nan·thro·pus
gyn·a·tre·si·a
gy·ne·cic
gy·ne·co·gen·ic
gy·ne·cog·ra·phy
pl gy·ne·cog·ra·phies
gy·ne·coid
gy·ne·co·log·ic
or gy·ne·co·log·i·cal
gy·ne·co·log·i·cal
or gy·ne·co·log·ic
gy·ne·col·o·gist
gy·ne·col·o·gy
pl gy·ne·col·o·gies
gy·ne·co·ma·ni·a
gy·ne·co·mas·ti·a
gy·ne·co·ma·zi·a
gy·ne·cop·a·thy
gy·ne·co·pho·bi·a
gy·ne·pho·gi·a
gy·ne·pho·ric
gy·ni·at·rics
gy·nism
gy·no·gam·one
gy·no·gen·e·sis
pl gy·no·gen·e·ses
gy·nog·ra·phy

gyn·o·mer·o·gon
gyn·o·me·rog·o·ny
gyn·o·path·ic
gy·no·plas·tic
gy·no·plas·ty
gyp·sum
gy·ral
gy·rate
gy·ra·tion
Gy·rau·lus sai·go·nen·sis

gyre
gy·rec·to·my
    pl gy·rec·to·mies
gyr·en·ceph·a·late
    or gyr·en·ce·phal·ic
    or gyr·en·ceph·a·lous
gyr·en·ce·phal·ic
    or gyr·en·ceph·a·late
    or gyr·en·ceph·a·lous

gy·ren·ceph·a·lous
    or gyr·en·ce·phal·ic
    or gyr·en·ceph·a·late
gy·ri
gy·rose
gy·ro·spasm
gy·rous
gy·rus
    pl gy·ri

H

H an·ti·gen
Haab re·flex
Haa·se rule
ha·be·na
ha·be·nar
ha·ben·u·la
    pl ha·ben·u·lae
ha·ben·u·lar
ha·ben·u·lo·pe·dun·cu·lar
ha·bil·i·ta·tion
hab·it
hab·i·tat
hab·it-form·ing
ha·bit·u·al
ha·bit·u·ate
hab·it·u·a·tion
hab·i·tus
    pl hab·i·tus
Hab·ro·ne·ma
hab·ro·ne·mi·a
    or hab·ro·ne·mo·sis
hab·ro·ne·mi·a·sis
    pl hab·ro·ne·mi·a·ses
hab·ro·ne·mic
hab·ro·ne·mo·sis
    or hab·ro·ne·mi·a
hache·ment

hack·ing
Ha·den-Haus·ser meth·od
ha·de·pho·bi·a
haem
    var of heme
Hae·ma·cha·tes
Hae·ma·dip·sa
Hae·ma·gog·us
Hae·ma·moe·ba
Hae·ma·phy·sa·lis
Hae·ma·to·bi·a ir·ri·tans
Hae·ma·to·pi·nus
Hae·ma·to·si·phon
Hae·ma·to·ther·ma
hae·ma·tox·y·lon
hae·min
    var of he·min
hae·mo·bar·ton·el·la
    pl hae·mo·bar·ton·el·lae
hae·mo·glo·bin
    var of he·mo·glo·bin
Hae·mo·greg·a·ri·na
hae·mo·greg·a·rine
    var of he·mo·greg·a·rine
Hae·mon·chus
Hae·mo·pro·te·us
haem·or·rha·gi·a

Hae·mo·spo·rid·i·a
hae·mo·spo·rid·i·an
Hae·nel sign
Hae·ser co·ef·fi·cient
Haff dis·ease
Haff·kine vac·cine
haf·ni·um
Hag·e·dorn and Jen·sen
    meth·od
Hag·e·dorn nee·dle
Ha·ge·man fac·tor
Hag·ner bag
Hahn·e·mann·ism
Hai·din·ger brushes
Hai·ley-Hai·ley dis·ease
Haines test
Haj·ek op·er·a·tion
ha·la·tion
hal·a·zone
Hal·ber·staedt·er bod·ies
Hal·dane cham·ber
half-blood·ed
half-bred
half-breed
half-caste
half-life
half-sib·ling

half·val·ue
hal·i·but-liver oil
hal·ide
hal·i·ste·re·sis
   pl hal·i·ste·re·ses
hal·i·ste·ret·ic
hal·ite
hal·i·to·sis
   pl hal·i·to·ses
hal·i·tus
Hall mus·cle
hal·la·chrome
Hal·le point
Hal·ler ha·ben·u·la
Hal·ler·mann-Streiff-Fran·çois syn·drome
Hal·ler·vor·den-Spatz dis·ease
Hal·lion law
Hal·lo·peau dis·ease
hal·lu·cal
hal·lu·ci·nate
hal·lu·ci·na·tion
hal·lu·ci·na·tive
hal·lu·ci·na·to·ry
hal·lu·ci·no·gen
hal·lu·ci·no·gen·ic
hal·lu·ci·no·sis
   pl hal·lu·ci·no·ses
hal·lux
   pl hal·lu·ces
hal·ma·to·gen·e·sis
   pl hal·ma·to·gen·e·ses
ha·lo
hal·o·chro·mism
hal·o·gen
hal·o·gen·ate
hal·o·ge·ton
hal·oid
ha·lom·e·ter
ha·lo·per·i·dol
hal·o·phil
hal·o·phile
hal·o·phil·ic
   or hal·o·phil·ous
hal·o·phil·ous
   or hal·o·phil·ic
hal·o·pro·ges·ter·one
hal·o·pro·gin

hal·o·thane
hal·qui·nols
Hal·stead tests
Hal·sted
hal·zoun
Ham·a·me·lis
ha·mar·ti·a
ha·mar·to·blas·to·ma
   pl ha·mar·to·blas·to·mas
   or ha·mar·to·blas·to·ma·ta
ham·ar·to·ma
   pl ham·ar·to·mas
   or ham·ar·to·ma·ta
ham·ar·tom·a·tous
ha·mar·to·pho·bi·a
ha·mate
ha·ma·tum
   pl ha·ma·tums
   or ha·ma·ta
Ham·burg·er rule
Ham·il·ton sign
Ham·man dis·ease
Ham·man-Rich syn·drome
Ham·mar·sten test
ham·mer
Ham·mer·schlag meth·od
ham·mer·toe
Ham·mond dis·ease
Hamp·ton ma·neu·ver
ham·ster
ham·string
ham·u·lar
ham·u·late
ham·u·lus
   pl ham·u·li
ha·my·cin
hand
hand·ed·ness
hand·i·cap
Hand·ley meth·od
hand·piece
hand·print
Hand-Schül·ler-Chris·tian dis·ease
Han·ger test
hang·nail
hang·o·ver
hang-up
Han·ot cir·rho·sis

Han·sen dis·ease
han·se·nid
han·se·no·sis
han·se·not·ic
hap·a·lo·nych·i·a
haph·al·ge·si·a
haph·e·pho·bi·a
hap·lo·dont
hap·lo·don·ty
   pl hap·lo·don·ties
hap·loid
hap·loi·dy
   pl hap·loi·des
hap·lol·o·gy
   pl hap·lol·o·gies
hap·lo·my·co·sis
hap·lont
hap·lon·tic
hap·lo·pi·a
hap·lo·scope
hap·lo·scop·ic
hap·lo·type
hap·lo·typ·ic
hap·ten
   or hap·tene
hap·tene
   or hap·ten
hap·ten·ic
hap·te·pho·bi·a
hap·tic
   or hap·ti·cal
hap·ti·cal
   or hap·tic
hap·tics
hap·to·dys·pho·ri·a
hap·to·glo·bin
hap·to·phore
Ha·ra·da syn·drome
Har·den-Young es·ter
hard·en·ing
Har·de·ri·an gland
Har·ding-Pas·sey mel·a·no·ma
hard·ness
hard-of-hear·ing
Har·dy-Wein·berg prin·ci·ple, law
Hare syn·drome
hare·lip

hare·lip·ped
Har·kins meth·od
har·le·quin
Har·ley dis·ease
har·ma·line
har·ma·lol
har·mine
har·mo·ni·a
har·mon·ic
har·mo·ny
   pl har·mo·nies
har·pax·o·pho·bi·a
har·poon
Har·ring·ton op·er·a·tion
Har·ris and Ben·e·dict
   stan·dards
Har·ris he·ma·tox·y·lin
Har·ri·son groove
Har·row·er-Er·ick·son test
Hart·ley-Krause
   op·er·a·tion
Hart·mann fos·sa
Hart·man·nel·la
Hart·nup dis·ease
harts·horn
hash·eesh
   var of hash·ish
Hash·i·mo·to dis·ease
hash·ish
Has·kins test
Has·ner valve
Has·sall bod·y
Has·sall-Hen·le warts
Hau·dek niche
haunch
Haus·ser meth·od
haus·to·ri·um
   pl haus·to·ri·a
haus·tra co·li
haus·tral
haus·trat·ed
haus·tra·tion
haus·trum
   pl haus·tra
haus·tus
   pl haus·tus
haut mal
Ha·ver·hill fe·ver
Ha·vers glands

ha·ver·sian
Haxt·hau·sen dis·ease
Hay·em cor·pus·cle
Hay·em-Wi·dal syn·drome
Hay·garth nodes
Haynes op·er·a·tion
head
head·ache
head·ach·y
head·lock
head·shrink·er
heal
health
health·ful
health·y
hear
heart
heart·beat
heart·block
heart·burn
heart·lung
heart·wa·ter
heart·worm
heat·stroke
heaves
hea·vy chain
he·be·phre·ni·a
he·be·phren·ic
Heb·er·den node
Heb·er·den-
   Ro·sen·bach node
he·bet·ic
heb·e·tude
heb·e·tu·di·nous
he·bi·at·rics
he·bos·te·ot·o·my
he·bot·o·my
Heb·ra pit·y·ri·a·sis
hec·a·ter·om·er·al
hec·a·ter·o·mer·ic
   or hec·a·to·mer·ic
hec·a·to·mer·ic
   or hec·a·ter·o·mer·ic
Hecht-Schla·er
   ad·ap·tom·e·ter
hec·tic
hec·ti·cal·ly
hec·to·gram
hec·to·li·ter

hec·tom·e·ter
Hed·blom syn·drome
he·de·o·ma
he·do·ni·a
he·don·ic
he·don·i·cal·ly
he·don·ism
he·don·ist
he·don·is·tic
he·do·no·pho·bi·a
heel
Heer·fordt dis·ease
Hef·ke-Tur·ner sign
he·gem·o·ny
Hegg·lin a·nom·a·ly
Hei·den·hain cells
Heim-Krey·sig sign
Hei·ne·ke-Mik·u·licz
   op·er·a·tion
Hei·ne-Med·in dis·ease
Hei·ner syn·drome
Heinz bod·ies
Heinz-Ehr·lich bod·ies
Heis·ter valve
Hek·toen phe·nom·e·non
hel·coid
hel·co·ma
   pl hel·co·mas
   or hel·co·ma·ta
hel·cot·ic
Held spa·ces
he·li·an·thin
   or he·li·an·thine
he·li·an·thine
   or he·li·an·thin
hel·i·cal
hel·ic·i·form
hel·i·cine
hel·i·cis
hel·i·coid
   or hel·i·coi·dal
hel·i·coi·dal
   or hel·i·coid
hel·i·co·pod
hel·i·co·po·di·a
hel·i·co·ru·bin
hel·i·co·tre·ma
he·li·en·ceph·a·li·tis
he·li·o·phage

e·li·o·phobe
e·li·o·pho·bi·a
e·li·o·sis
pl he·li·o·ses
e·li·o·stat
e·li·o·tax·is
pl he·li·o·tax·es
e·li·o·ther·a·py
pl he·li·o·ther·a·pies
e·li·o·trop·ic
e·li·o·trop·i·cal·ly
e·li·o·tro·pin
e·li·ot·ro·pism
le·li·o·zo·a
e·li·o·zo·an
e·li·o·zo·ic
e·li·um
e·lix
pl he·lix·es
or he·li·ces
e·lix·in
lel·ke·si·mas·tix
el·le·bore
el·le·bor·ine
el·le·bor·ism
lel·ler test
lel·li·ge meth·od
lel·lin law
lel·ly fix·ing flu·id
lelm·holtz the·o·ry of
ac·com·mo·da·tion
el·minth
el·min·tha·gogue
el·min·them·e·sis
lel·min·thi·a·sis
pl hel·min·thi·a·ses
el·min·thic
lel·minth·ism
el·min·thoid
lel·min·tho·log·ic
lel·min·thol·o·gist
lel·min·thol·o·gy
pl hel·min·thol·o·gies
el·min·tho·ma
pl hel·min·tho·mas
or hel·min·tho·ma·ta
el·min·tho·pho·bi·a
el·min·thous
le·lo·der·ma

he·lo·ma
pl he·lo·mas
or he·lo·ma·ta
he·lo·ni·as
he·lot·o·my
pl he·lot·o·mies
hel·vol·ic
Hel·weg bun·dle
hem·a·ba·rom·e·ter
he·ma·chro·ma·to·sis
he·ma·chrome
hem·a·chro·sis'
he·ma·cy·tom·e·ter
or he·mo·cy·tom·e·ter
he·ma·cy·to·zo·on
he·mad
he·ma·drom·o·graph
he·ma·dro·mom·e·ter
hem·ad·sorp·tion
he·ma·dy·na·mom·e·ter
he·mag·glu·ti·nate
he·mag·glu·ti·na·tion
he·mag·glu·ti·nin
or he·mo·ag·glu·ti·nin
he·mal
he·mal·um
hem·a·nal·y·sis
pl hem·a·nal·y·ses
he·man·gi·ec·ta·si·a
he·man·gi·ec·ta·sis
pl he·man·gi·ec·ta·ses
he·man·gi·ec·tat·ic
he·man·gi·o·am·e·
lo·blas·to·ma
pl he·man·gi·o·am·e·
lo·blas·to·mas
or he·man·gi·o·am·e·lo·
blas·to·ma·ta
he·man·gi·o·blas·to·ma
pl he·man·gi·o·blas·to·mas
or he·man·gi·o·blas·to·ma·ta
he·man·gi·o·e·las·to·
myx·o·ma
pl he·man·gi·o·e·las·to·
myx·o·mas
or he·man·gi·o·e·las·to·
myx·o·ma·ta
he·man·gi·o·en·do·the·
li·o·blas·to·ma

pl he·man·gi·o·en·do·
the·li·o·blas·to·mas
or he·man·gi·o·en·do·
the·li·o·blas·to·ma·ta
he·man·gi·o·en·do·the·li·
o·ma
pl he·man·gi·o·en·do·the·li·
o·mas
or he·man·gi·o·en·do·the·li·
o·ma·ta
he·man·gi·o·en·do·the·li·o·
sar·co·ma
pl he·man·gi·o·en·do·the·li·
o·sar·co·mas
or he·man·gi·o·en·do·the·li·
o·sar·co·ma·ta
he·man·gi·o·fi·bro·ma
pl he·man·gi·o·fi·bro·mas
or he·man·gi·o·fi·bro·ma·ta
he·man·gi·o·li·po·ma
pl he·man·gi·o·li·po·mas
or he·man·gi·o·li·po·ma·ta
he·man·gi·o·ma
pl he·man·gi·o·mas
or he·man·gi·o·ma·ta
he·man·gi·o·ma·to·sis
pl he·man·gi·o·ma·to·ses
he·man·gi·om·a·tous
he·man·gi·o·my·o·li·po·ma
pl he·man·gi·o·my·o·li·po·
mas
or he·man·gi·o·my·o·li·po·
ma·ta
he·man·gi·o·per·i·cy·to·ma
pl he·man·gi·o·per·i·cy·to·
mas
or he·man·gi·o·per·i·cy·to·
ma·ta
he·man·gi·o·sar·co·ma
pl he·man·gi·o·sar·co·mas
or he·man·gi·o·sar·co·ma·ta
hem·a·phe·in
he·ma·poi·e·sis
pl he·ma·poi·e·sis
or he·mo·poi·e·sis
pl he·mo·poi·e·ses
hem·a·poph·y·sis
pl hem·a·poph·y·ses

hem·ar·thro·sis
pl hem·ar·thro·ses
he·ma·te·in
he·ma·tem·e·sis
hem·at·en·ceph·a·lon
he·ma·therm
he·ma·ther·mal
or he·ma·ther·mous
he·ma·ther·mous
or he·ma·ther·mal
he·mat·hi·dro·sis
he·mat·ic
he·ma·tid
hem·at·i·dro·sis
he·ma·tim·e·ter
he·ma·tim·e·try
hem·a·tin
hem·a·ti·ne·mi·a
hem·a·tin·ic
hem·a·ti·nom·e·ter
hem·a·ti·no·met·ric
hem·a·ti·nu·ri·a
hem·a·tite
hem·a·to·aer·om·e·ter
hem·a·to·bil·i·a
hem·a·to·blast
hem·a·to·blas·tic
hem·a·to·cele
hem·a·to·che·zi·a
hem·a·to·chro·ma·to·sis
hem·a·to·chy·lo·cele
he·ma·to·chy·lu·ri·a
he·ma·to·coe·li·a
hem·a·to·col·po·me·tra
hem·a·to·col·pos
or hem·a·to·col·pus
hem·a·to·col·pus
or hem·a·to·col·pos
hem·a·to·crit
hem·a·to·cry·al
hem·a·to·crys·tal·lin
hem·a·to·cy·a·nin
hem·a·to·cyst
hem·a·to·cyte
hem·a·to·cy·tol·y·sis
pl hem·a·to·cy·tol·y·ses
hem·a·to·cy·tom·e·ter
hem·a·to·cy·to·zo·on

hem·a·to·cy·tu·ri·a
hem·a·to·dy·nam·ics
hem·a·to·dy·na·mom·e·ter
hem·a·to·dys·cra·si·a
hem·a·to·en·ce·phal·ic
hem·a·to·gen·e·sis
hem·a·to·gen·ic
hem·a·tog·e·nous
hem·a·to·glo·bin
hem·a·to·gone
or hem·a·to·go·ni·a
hem·a·to·go·ni·a
or hem·a·to·gone
hem·a·to·hi·dro·sis
hem·a·to·his·tone
he·ma·toid
he·ma·toi·din
he·ma·to·lith
he·ma·to·log·ic
or he·ma·to·log·i·cal
he·ma·to·log·i·cal
or he·ma·to·log·ic
he·ma·tol·o·gist
he·ma·tol·o·gy
pl he·ma·tol·o·gies
hem·a·to·lymph·an·gi·o·ma
pl hem·a·to·lymph·an·gi·o·
mas
or hem·a·to·lymph·an·gi·o·
ma·ta
hem·a·to·lymph·u·ri·a
he·ma·tol·y·sis
pl he·ma·tol·y·ses
hem·a·to·lyt·ic
hem·a·to·lyt·o·poi·e·tic
he·ma·to·ma
pl he·ma·to·mas
or he·ma·to·ma·ta
hem·a·to·me·di·as·ti·num
he·ma·tom·e·ter
he·ma·to·me·tra
he·ma·tom·e·try
he·ma·to·mole
hem·at·om·phal·o·cele
hem·a·to·my·e·li·a
hem·a·to·my·e·li·tis
pl hem·a·to·my·e·li·tis·es
or hem·a·to·my·e·li·ti·des

hem·a·to·my·el·o·pore
he·ma·ton·ic
he·ma·ton·o·sis
hem·a·to·pa·thol·o·gy
he·ma·to·pa·thy
hem·a·to·per·i·car·di·um
hem·a·to·per·i·to·ne·um
hem·a·to·phage
hem·a·to·pha·gi·a
hem·a·toph·a·gous
hem·a·toph·a·gus
hem·a·to·phil·i·a
hem·a·to·pho·bi·a
hem·a·to·phyte
hem·a·to·plas·tic
hem·a·to·poi·e·sis
pl hem·a·to·poi·e·ses
hem·a·to·poi·et·ic
hem·a·to·poi·et·i·cal·ly
hem·a·to·por·phyr·i·a
hem·a·to·por·phy·rin
hem·a·to·por·phy·ri·ne·
mi·a
hem·a·to·por·phy·ri·nu·ri·a
hem·a·to·pre·cip·i·tin
hem·a·tor·rha·chis
hem·a·tor·rhe·a
hem·a·to·sal·pinx
pl hem·a·to·sal·pin·ges
hem·a·tos·che·o·cele
hem·a·to·scope
hem·a·tos·co·py
hem·a·tose
hem·a·to·si·pho·ni·a·sis
he·ma·to·sis
hem·a·to·spec·tro·scope
hem·a·to·spec·tros·co·py
hem·a·to·sper·ma·to·cele
hem·a·to·sper·mi·a
hem·a·to·stat·ic
hem·a·tos·te·on
hem·a·to·ther·a·py
hem·a·to·ther·mal
hem·a·to·ther·mous
hem·a·to·tho·rax
hem·a·to·tox·ic
hem·a·to·tox·ic·i·ty
hem·a·to·tox·i·co·sis
hem·a·to·tra·che·los

hem·a·to·trop·ic
hem·a·to·tym·pa·num
he·ma·tox·y·lin
he·ma·tox·y·lin·o·phil·ic
hem·a·to·zo·al
hem·a·to·zo·an
hem·a·to·zo·ic
hem·a·to·zo·on
   pl hem·a·to·zo·a
hem·a·tu·ri·a
hem·au·to·graph
hem·au·to·graph·ic
hem·au·tog·ra·phy
heme
hem·er·a·lo·pi·a
hem·er·a·lop·ic
hem·er·a·pho·ni·a
hem·i·a·blep·si·a
hem·i·a·car·di·us
hem·i·a·ceph·a·lus
hem·i·ac·e·tal
hem·i·a·chro·ma·top·si·a
hem·i·a·gen·e·sis
hem·i·a·geu·si·a
hem·i·al·bu·mose
hem·i·al·bu·mo·su·ri·a
hem·i·am·bly·o·pi·a
hem·i·a·my·os·the·ni·a
hem·i·an·a·cu·si·a
hem·i·an·aes·the·si·a
   var of hem·i·an·es·the·si·a
hem·i·an·al·ge·si·a
hem·i·an·en·ceph·a·ly
hem·i·an·es·the·si·a
hem·i·an·o·pi·a
   or hem·i·an·op·si·a
hem·i·an·op·si·a
   or hem·i·an·o·pia
hem·i·an·op·tic
hem·i·an·os·mi·a
hem·i·a·prax·i·a
hem·i·a·tax·i·a
hem·i·ath·e·to·sis
   pl hem·i·ath·e·to·ses
hem·i·at·ro·phy
   pl hem·i·at·ro·phies
hem·i·az·y·gos
hem·i·bal·lism
   or hem·i·bal·lis·mus

hem·i·bal·lis·mus
   or hem·i·bal·lism
he·mic
hem·i·car·di·a
hem·i·cel·lu·lose
hem·i·cel·lu·los·ic
hem·i·cen·trum
   pl hem·i·cen·trums
   or hem·i·cen·tra
hem·i·ceph·a·lia
hem·i·ceph·a·lus
hem·i·ceph·a·ly
hem·i·ce·re·brum
   pl hem·i·ce·re·brums
   or hem·i·ce·re·bra
hem·i·cho·re·a
hem·i·chro·ma·top·si·a
hem·i·co·lec·to·my
   pl hem·i·co·lec·to·mies
hem·i·col·lin
hem·i·con·vul·sion
hem·i·cra·ni·a
hem·i·cra·ni·o·sis
hem·i·cys·tec·to·my
hem·i·de·cor·ti·ca·tion
hem·i·des·mus
hem·i·di·a·pho·re·sis
hem·i·di·a·phragm
hem·i·dro·sis
hem·i·dys·es·the·si·a
hem·i·dys·tro·phy
   pl hem·i·dys·tro·phies
hem·i·ec·tro·me·li·a
hem·i·e·las·tin
hem·i·el·lip·tic
hem·i·ep·i·lep·sy
hem·i·fa·cial
hem·i·gas·trec·to·my
hem·i·geu·si·a
hem·i·glo·bin
hem·i·glos·sec·to·my
   pl hem·i·glos·sec·to·mies
hem·i·glos·si·tis
hem·i·glos·so·ple·gi·a
hem·i·gna·thi·a
hem·i·gnath·us
hem·i·hi·dro·sis
hem·i·hyp·aes·the·si·a
   var of hem·i·hyp·es·the·si·a

hem·i·hyp·al·ge·si·a
hem·i·hy·per·aes·the·si·a
   var of hem·i·hy·per·
     es·the·si·a
hem·i·hy·per·es·the·si·a
hem·i·hy·per·hi·dro·sis
hem·i·hy·per·to·ni·a
hem·i·hy·per·tro·phy
   pl hem·i·hy·per·tro·phies
hem·i·hyp·es·the·si·a
hem·i·hy·po·to·ni·a
hem·i·kar·y·on
hem·i·kar·y·ot·ic
hem·i·lab·y·rin·thec·to·my
hem·i·lam·i·nec·to·my
   pl hem·i·lam·i·nec·to·mies
hem·i·lar·yn·gec·to·my
   pl hem·i·lar·yn·gec·to·mies
hem·i·lar·ynx
hem·i·lat·er·al
hem·i·le·sion
hem·i·mac·ro·ceph·a·ly
hem·i·man·dib·u·lec·to·my
   pl hem·i·man·dib·u·lec·to·
     mies
hem·i·man·dib·u·lo·glos·
   sec·to·my
hem·i·max·il·lec·to·my
hem·i·me·li·a
hem·i·me·lus
   pl hem·i·me·li
hem·i·me·tab·o·lous
he·min
hem·i·ne·phrec·to·my
   pl hem·i·ne·phrec·to·mies
hem·i·o·pi·a
   or hem·i·op·si·a
hem·i·op·ic
hem·i·op·si·a
   or hem·i·o·pi·a
he·mip·a·gus
hem·i·pal·a·tec·to·my
hem·i·pal·a·to·la·ryn·go·
   ple·gi·a
hem·i·pa·ral·y·sis
hem·i·par·an·es·the·si·a
hem·i·par·a·ple·gi·a
hem·i·pa·re·sis
   pl hem·i·par·e·ses

hem·i·pa·ret·ic
hem·i·par·kin·son·ism
hem·i·pel·vec·to·my
   pl hem·i·pel·vec·to·mies
hem·i·pel·vis
hem·i·pin·to
hem·i·pla·cen·ta
hem·i·ple·gi·a
hem·i·ple·gic
He·mip·ter·a
he·mip·ter·an
  or he·mip·ter·on
he·mip·ter·on
  or he·mip·ter·an
he·mip·ter·ous
hem·i·ra·chis·chi·sis
hem·i·sco·to·sis
hem·i·sect
hemi·sec·tion
hem·i·so·mus
hem·i·spasm
hem·i·sphae·ri·a
  bul·bi·u·re·thrae
hem·i·sphae·ri·um
hem·i·sphere
hem·i·spher·ec·to·my
  pl hem·i·spher·ec·to·mies
hem·i·spher·ic
  or hem·i·spher·i·cal
hem·i·spher·i·cal
  or hem·i·spher·ic
hem·i·sphe·ri·um
hem·i·spo·ro·sis
hem·i·sy·ner·gi·a
hem·i·sys·to·le
hem·i·ter·a·ta
hem·i·te·rat·ic
hem·i·ter·pene
hem·i·tho·rax
  pl hem·i·tho·rax·es
  or hem·i·tho·ra·ces
hem·i·thy·roi·dec·to·my
hem·i·ver·te·bra
hem·i·zy·gos·i·ty
hem·i·zy·gote
hem·i·zy·gous
hem·lock
Hem·me·ler
  throm·bop·a·thy

he·mo·ag·glu·ti·nin
  or he·mag·glu·tin·in
he·mo·al·ka·lim·e·ter
he·mo·bil·i·a
he·mo·bil·i·ru·bin
he·mo·blast
he·mo·blas·tic
he·mo·blas·to·sis
he·mo·ca·ther·e·sis
he·mo·che·zi·a
he·mo·cho·ri·al
he·mo·chro·ma·to·sis
  pl he·mo·chro·ma·to·ses
he·mo·chro·ma·tot·ic
he·mo·chrome
he·mo·chro·mo·gen
he·mo·chro·mom·e·ter
he·mo·cla·si·a
he·moc·la·sis
he·mo·clas·tic
he·mo·co·ag·u·la·tion
he·mo·co·ag·u·lin
he·mo·coe·lom
he·mo·con·cen·tra·tion
he·mo·co·ni·a
  or he·mo·ko·ni·a
he·mo·co·ni·o·sis
  pl he·mo·co·ni·o·ses
he·mo·cry·os·co·py
he·mo·cry·stal·lin
he·mo·cu·pre·in
he·mo·cy·a·nin
he·mo·cyte
he·mo·cy·to·blast
he·mo·cy·to·blas·tic
he·mo·cy·to·blas·to·ma
  pl he·mo·cy·to·blas·to·mas
  or he·mo·cy·to·blas·
    to·ma·ta
he·mo·cy·to·ca·ther·e·sis
he·mo·cy·to·gen·e·sis
he·mo·cy·tol·o·gy
he·mo·cy·tol·y·sis
  pl he·mo·cy·tol·y·ses
he·mo·cy·tom·e·ter
  or he·ma·cy·tom·e·ter
he·mo·cy·tom·e·try
he·mo·cy·to·poi·e·sis
he·mo·cy·to·trip·sis

he·mo·cy·to·zo·on
  pl he·mo·cy·to·zo·a
he·mo·di·ag·no·sis
  pl he·mo·di·ag·no·ses
he·mo·di·al·y·sis
  pl he·mo·di·al·y·ses
he·mo·di·a·lyz·er
he·mo·di·a·stase
he·mo·di·lu·tion
he·mo·drom·o·graph
he·mo·dro·mom·e·ter
he·mo·dro·mom·e·try
he·mo·dy·nam·ic
he·mo·dy·nam·i·cal·ly
he·mo·dy·nam·ics
he·mo·dy·na·mom·e·ter
he·mo·dy·na·mom·e·try
he·mo·en·do·the·li·al
he·mo·e·rthy·rin
he·mo·fer·rum
he·mo·fil·tra·tion
he·mo·flag·el·late
he·mo·fus·cin
he·mo·gen·e·sis
he·mo·gen·ic
he·mog·e·nous
he·mo·glo·bin
he·mo·glo·bi·ne·mi·a
he·mo·glo·bin·ic
he·mo·glo·bi·nif·er·ous
he·mo·glo·bi·nol·y·sis
he·mo·glo·bi·nom·e·ter
he·mo·glo·bi·nom·e·try
  pl he·mo·glo·bi·nom·e·tries
he·mo·glo·bin·op·a·thy
  pl he·mo·glo·bin·op·a·thies
he·mo·glo·bi·no·phil·i·a
he·mo·glo·bi·no·phil·ic
he·mo·glo·bi·nous
he·mo·glo·bi·nu·ri·a
he·mo·glo·bi·nu·ric
he·mo·gram
he·mo·greg·a·rine
he·mo·his·ti·o·blast
he·mo·hy·dro·sal·pinx
he·moid
he·mo·ki·ne·sis
he·mo·ko·ni·a
  or he·mo·con·i·a

he·mo·ko·ni·o·sis
he·mo·lith
he·mo·lymph
he·mo·lym·phan·gi·o·ma
he·mol·y·sate
he·mol·y·sin
he·mol·y·sis
   pl he·mol·y·ses
he·mol·y·soid
he·mo·lyt·ic
he·mo·lyt·o·poi·et·ic
he·mo·ly·za·tion
he·mo·lyze
he·mo·ma·nom·e·ter
he·mo·me·di·as·ti·num
he·mo·met·a·ki·ne·si·a
he·mo·met·a·ki·ne·sis
he·mom·e·ter
he·mo·me·tra
he·mo·met·ric
he·mom·e·try
   pl he·mom·e·tries
he·mo·my·e·lo·gram
he·mo·ne·phro·sis
he·mo·pa·thol·o·gy
he·mop·a·thy
   pl he·mop·a·thies
he·mo·per·i·car·di·um
   pl he·mo·per·i·car·di·a
he·mo·per·i·to·ne·um
   pl he·mo·per·i·to·ne·ums
   or he·mo·per·i·to·ne·a
he·mo·pex·in
he·mo·pex·is
he·mo·phage
he·mo·pha·gi·a
he·mo·phag·ic
he·mo·phag·o·cyte
he·mo·phag·o·cyt·ic
he·moph·a·gous
he·mo·phil
he·mo·phile
he·mo·phil·i·a
he·mo·phil·i·ac
he·mo·phil·ic
he·mo·phil·i·oid
He·moph·i·lus
he·mo·pho·bi·a
he·mo·phor·ic

he·moph·thal·mi·a
he·moph·thal·mos
he·moph·thi·sis
he·mo·plas·tic
he·mo·pleu·ra
he·mo·pneu·mo·per·i·car·
   di·um
he·mo·pneu·mo·tho·rax
   pl he·mo·pneu·mo·tho·rax·
   es
   or he·mo·pneu·mo·tho·ra·
   ces
he·mo·poi·e·sis
   pl he·mo·poi·e·ses
   or he·ma·poi·e·sis
   pl he·mo·poi·e·ses
he·mo·poi·et·ic
he·mo·poi·e·tin
he·mo·por·phy·rin
he·mo·po·si·a
he·mo·pre·cip·i·tin
he·mo·pro·te·in
He·mo·pro·te·us
he·mo·pro·to·zo·a
he·mop·so·nin
he·mop·ty·sis
   pl he·mop·ty·ses
he·mo·pyr·role
hem·or·rhage
hem·or·rha·gen·ic
hem·or·rhag·ic
hem·or·rhag·in
hem·or·rhe·a
he·mor·rhe·ol·o·gy
hem·or·rhoid
hem·or·rhoi·dal
hem·or·rhoi·dec·to·my
   pl hem·or·rhoi·dec·to·mies
hem·or·rhoids
he·mo·sal·pinx
   pl he·mo·sal·pin·ges
he·mo·sid·er·in
he·mo·sid·er·i·nu·ri·a
he·mo·sid·er·o·sis
   pl he·mo·sid·er·o·ses
he·mo·sid·e·rot·ic
he·mo·sper·mi·a
He·mo·spo·rid·i·a
he·mo·sta·si·a

he·mo·sta·sis
   pl he·mo·sta·ses
he·mo·stat
he·mo·stat·ic
he·mo·styp·tic
he·mo·ta·chom·e·ter
he·mo·ta·chom·e·try
he·mo·ther·a·py
he·mo·tho·rax
   pl he·mo·tho·rax·es
   or he·mo·tho·ra·ces
he·mo·tox·ic
he·mo·tox·ic·i·ty
he·mo·tox·in
he·mo·troph
he·mot·ro·phe
he·mo·troph·ic
he·mo·tym·pa·num
he·mo·zo·in
he·mo·zo·on
   pl he·mo·zo·a
hen·bane
Hench and Al·drich test
hen·dec·yl
Hen·der·son-Has·sel·balch
   e·qua·tion
Hen·der·son op·er·a·tion
Hen·le loop, sheath
Hen·ne·berg dis·ease
Hen·och-Schön·lein
   pur·pu·ra
hen·pu·e
Hen·ri·ques-Sor·en·sen
   meth·od
hen·ry
   pl hen·rys
   or hen·ries
Hen·ry law
Hen·sen ca·nal
he·par
hep·a·rin
hep·a·ri·nae·mi·a
   var of hep·a·ri·ne·mi·a
hep·a·ri·ne·mi·a
hep·a·rin·i·za·tion
hep·a·rin·ize
hep·a·rin·o·cyte
hep·a·rin·oid
hep·a·ri·tin

hep·a·ri·ti·nu·ri·a
hep·a·tal·gi·a
hep·a·ta·tro·phi·a
hep·a·tec·to·phi·a
hep·a·tec·to·my
    pl hep·a·tec·to·mies
he·pat·ic
He·pat·i·ca
he·pat·i·co·du·o·de·nos·to·my
    pl he·pat·i·co·du·o·de·nos·to·mies
he·pat·i·co·en·ter·os·to·my
he·pat·i·co·gas·tros·to·my
he·pat·i·co·je·ju·nos·to·my
he·pat·i·co·li·thot·o·my
    pl he·pat·i·co·li·thot·o·mies
he·pat·i·co·lith·o·trip·sy
he·pat·i·co·pan·cre·at·ic
he·pat·i·co·re·nal
he·pat·i·cos·to·my
he·pat·i·cot·o·my
hep·a·ti·tis
    pl hep·a·ti·tis·es
    or hep·a·tit·i·des
hep·a·ti·za·tion
hep·a·tize
hep·a·to·blas·to·ma
hep·a·to·can·a·lic·u·lar
hep·at·o·cele
hep·a·to·cel·lu·lar
hep·a·to·chol·an·gi·o·du·o·de·nos·to·my
hep·a·to·chol·an·gi·o·en·ter·os·to·my
hep·a·chol·an·gi·o·gas·tros·to·my
hep·a·to·chol·an·gi·o·je·ju·nos·to·my
hep·a·to·cho·lan·gi·tis
hep·a·to·cir·rho·sis
hep·a·to·col·ic
he·pa·to·cu·pre·in
hep·a·to·cys·tic
hep·a·to·cyte
hep·a·to·du·o·de·nal
hep·a·to·du·o·de·nos·to·my
hep·a·to·dyn·i·a
hep·a·to·fla·vin

hep·a·to·gas·tric
hep·a·to·gen·ic
    or hep·a·tog·e·nous
hep·a·tog·e·nous
    or hep·a·to·gen·ic
hep·a·to·gram
hep·a·tog·ra·phy
hep·a·toid
hep·a·to·je·ju·nal
hep·a·to·jug·u·lar
hep·a·to·len·tic·u·lar
hep·a·to·li·e·nal
hep·a·to·li·e·nog·ra·phy
hep·a·to·lith
hep·a·to·li·thec·to·my
hep·a·to·li·thi·a·sis
hep·a·tol·o·gy
hep·a·tol·y·sin
hep·a·tol·y·sis
hep·a·to·ma
    pl hep·a·to·mas
    or hep·a·to·ma·ta
hep·a·to·ma·la·ci·a
hep·a·to·me·ga·li·a
hep·a·to·me·gal·ic
hep·a·to·meg·a·ly
    pl hep·a·to·meg·a·lies
hep·a·to·mel·a·no·sis
hep·a·tom·phal·o·cele
hep·a·to·neph·ric
hep·a·to·pan·cre·at·ic
hep·a·top·a·thy
    pl hep·a·top·a·thies
hep·a·to·pex·y
    pl hep·a·to·pex·ies
hep·a·to·pleu·ral
hep·a·to·pneu·mon·ic
hep·a·to·por·tal
hep·a·top·to·sis
he·pa·to·pul·mo·nar·y
hep·a·to·re·nal
hep·a·tor·rha·phy
hep·a·tor·rhex·is
    pl hep·a·tor·rhex·es
hep·a·to·scan
hep·a·tos·co·py
    pl hep·a·tos·co·pies
hep·a·to·sis
    pl hep·a·to·ses

hep·a·to·sple·ni·tis
hep·a·to·sple·nog·ra·phy
hep·a·to·sple·no·meg·a·ly
    pl hep·a·to·sple·no·meg·a·lies
hep·a·to·sple·nop·a·thy
hep·a·to·ther·a·py
hep·a·to·tot·o·my
hep·a·to·tox·e·mi·a
hep·a·to·tox·ic
hep·a·to·tox·ic·i·ty
    pl hep·a·to·tox·ic·i·ties
hep·a·to·tox·in
hep·a·to·u·ro·log·ic
hep·ta·bar·bi·tal
hep·ta·chro·mic
hep·tad
hept·al·de·hyde
hep·tane
hep·tose
hep·tu·lose
hep·tyl
her·a·pa·thite
her·ba·ceous
her·bal
her·bal·ist
her·bi·cid·al
her·bi·cid·al·ly
her·bi·cide
her·bi·vore
her·biv·o·rous
Herbst bod·ies
he·red·i·tar·i·an
he·red·i·tar·i·an·ism
he·red·i·tar·i·ly
he·red·i·ta·ry
he·red·i·ty
    pl he·red·i·ties
her·e·do·de·gen·er·a·tion
her·e·do·de·gen·er·a·tive
her·e·do·fa·mil·i·al
her·e·do·mac·u·lar
her·e·do·path·i·a a·tac·ti·ca
    pol·y·neu·ri·ti·for·mis
Her·ing ca·nal
Her·ing-Breu·er re·flex
her·i·ta·bil·i·ty
    pl her·i·ta·bil·i·ties
her·i·ta·ble

her·i·tage
Her·man·sky-Pud·lak
 syn·drome
her·maph·ro·dism
her·maph·ro·dite
her·maph·ro·dit·ic
her·maph·ro·dit·ism
Her·me·ti·a
her·met·ic
 or her·met·i·cal
her·met·i·cal
 or her·met·ic
her·met·i·cal·ly
her·nia
 pl her·ni·as
 or her·ni·ae
her·ni·al
her·ni·ate
her·ni·at·ed
her·ni·a·tion
her·ni·oid
her·ni·ol·o·gy
her·ni·o·plas·ty
her·ni·or·rha·phy
 pl her·ni·or·rha·phies
her·ni·o·tome
her·ni·ot·o·my
 pl her·ni·ot·o·mies
her·o·in
her·o·in·ism
her·pan·gi·na
her·pes
her·pes sim·plex
her·pes·vi·rus
her·pet·ic
her·pet·i·form
her·pe·tol·o·gy
Her·pe·tom·o·nas
Her·rick a·ne·mi·a
Her·ring bod·ies
Hers dis·ease
her·sage
Her·ter in·fan·til·ism
Her·ter-Fos·ter meth·od
Hert·wig epi·the·li·al root
 sheath
hertz
Hertz·i·an waves

Herx·hei·mer-Mans·feld
 phe·nom·e·non
Her·yng sign
herz·stoss
Hesch·l gy·ri
hes·per·e·tin
 or hes·per·i·tin
hes·per·i·din
hes·per·i·tin
 or hes·per·e·tin
Hes·sel·bach lig·a·ment
het·a·cil·lin
het·er·a·del·phi·a
het·er·a·del·phus
het·er·a·de·ni·a
het·er·a·den·ic
het·er·aes·the·si·a
 var of het·er·es·the·si·a
Het·er·a·kis gal·li·nae
het·er·a·li·us
het·er·aux·e·sis
het·er·ax·i·al
het·er·e·cious
het·er·er·gic
het·er·es·the·si·a
het·er·o·ag·glu·ti·na·tion
het·er·o·ag·glu·ti·nin
het·er·o·al·bu·mose
het·er·o·al·bu·mo·su·ri·a
het·er·o·al·lele
het·er·o·an·ti·bod·y
het·er·o·an·ti·gen
het·er·o·at·om
het·er·o·au·to·tro·phic
het·er·o·aux·in
het·er·o·aux·one
het·er·o·blas·tic
het·er·o·blas·ty
 pl het·er·o·blas·ties
het·er·o·car·y·on
 or het·er·o·kar·y·on
het·er·o·car·y·o·sis
 or het·er·o·kar·y·o·sis
het·er·o·car·y·ot·ic
 or het·er·o·kar·y·ot·ic
het·er·o·cel·lu·lar
het·er·o·ceph·a·lus
het·er·o·chro·mat·ic
het·er·o·chro·ma·tin

het·er·o·chro·mi·a
het·er·o·chro·mic
 or het·er·o·chro·mous
het·er·o·chro·mo·some
het·er·o·chro·mous
 or het·er·o·chro·mic
het·er·o·chro·ni·a
het·er·o·chron·ic
het·er·och·ro·nism
 or het·er·och·ro·ny
het·er·och·ro·nous
het·er·och·ro·ny
 pl het·er·och·ro·nies
 or het·er·och·ro·nism
het·er·och·tho·nous
het·er·o·crine
het·er·o·cy·cle
het·er·o·cy·clic
het·er·o·cyst
het·er·o·cy·to·trop·ic
Het·er·od·er·a
het·er·o·der·mic
het·er·o·dont
het·er·od·ro·mous
het·er·od·y·mus
het·er·oe·cious
 var of het·er·e·cious
het·er·o·e·rot·ic
het·er·o·er·o·tism
het·er·o·fer·men·ta·tive
het·er·o·gam·ete
het·er·o·ga·met·ic
het·er·o·gam·e·try
het·er·og·a·mous
het·er·og·a·my
 pl het·er·og·a·mies
het·er·o·ge·ne·i·ty
 pl het·er·o·ge·ne·i·ties
het·er·o·ge·ne·ous
het·er·o·ge·ne·ous·ness
het·er·o·gen·e·sis
 pl het·er·o·gen·e·ses
het·er·o·ge·net·ic
het·er·o·gen·ic
het·er·og·e·nous
het·er·o·geu·si·a
het·er·o·gon·ic
het·er·og·o·ny
 pl het·er·og·o·nies

167

het·er·o·graft
het·er·og·ra·phy
het·er·o·haem·ag·glu·ti·nin
    var of het·er·o·hem·ag·
    glu·ti·nin
het·er·o·hae·mol·y·sin
    var of het·er·o·he·mol·y·sin
het·er·o·hem·ag·glu·ti·na·
    tion
het·er·o·hem·ag·glu·ti·nin
het·er·o·he·mol·y·sin
het·er·o·hyp·no·sis
het·er·oid
het·er·o·im·mu·ni·ty
het·er·o·in·tox·i·ca·tion
het·er·o·i·on
het·er·o·kar·y·on
    or het·er·o·car·y·on
het·er·o·kar·y·o·sis
    or het·er·o·car·y·o·sis
het·er·o·kar·y·ot·ic
    or het·er·o·car·y·ot·ic
het·er·o·ker·a·to·plas·ty
het·er·o·ki·ne·si·a
het·er·o·ki·ne·sis
het·er·o·lac·tic
het·er·o·la·li·a
het·er·o·lat·er·al
het·er·ol·o·gous
het·er·ol·o·gy
    pl het·er·ol·o·gies
het·er·o·ly·sin
het·er·o·ly·sis
    pl het·er·o·ly·ses
het·er·o·lyt·ic
het·er·o·mas·ti·gate
    or het·er·o·mas·ti·gate
het·er·o·mas·ti·gote
    or het·er·o·mas·ti·gate
het·er·o·mer·ic
het·er·om·er·ous
het·er·o·met·a·pla·si·a
het·er·o·met·ric
het·er·o·me·tro·pi·a
het·er·o·mor·phic
    or het·er·o·mor·phous
het·er·o·mor·phism
het·er·o·mor·pho·sis
    pl het·er·o·mor·pho·ses

het·er·o·mor·phous
    or het·er·o·mor·phic
het·er·on·o·mous
het·er·on·y·mous
het·er·o·os·te·o·plas·ty
het·er·op·a·gus
het·er·o·path·ic
het·er·op·a·thy
het·er·o·pha·si·a
het·er·o·phe·mi·a
het·er·o·phe·my
    pl het·er·o·phe·mies
het·er·o·phil
    or het·er·o·phile
het·er·o·phile
    or het·er·o·phil
het·er·o·phil·ic
het·er·o·pho·ni·a
het·er·o·pho·ral·gi·a
het·er·o·pho·ri·a
het·er·o·phor·ic
het·er·oph·thal·mi·a
Het·er·oph·y·es
het·er·o·phy·i·a·sis
het·er·o·phy·id
het·er·o·phy·id·i·a·sis
het·er·o·pla·si·a
het·er·o·plasm
het·er·o·plas·tic
het·er·o·plas·ti·cal·ly
het·er·o·plas·ty
    pl het·er·o·plas·ties
het·er·o·ploid
het·er·o·ploi·dy
    pl het·er·o·ploi·dies
het·er·o·pol·y·ac·id
het·er·o·pol·y·sac·cha·ride
het·er·o·pro·so·pus
het·er·o·pro·te·ose
het·er·op·si·a
Het·er·op·ter·a
het·er·op·tics
het·er·o·pyc·no·sis
    or het·er·o·pyk·no·sis
het·er·o·pyc·not·ic
    or het·er·o·pyk·not·ic
het·er·o·pyk·no·sis
    or het·er·o·pyc·no·sis

het·er·o·pyk·not·ic
    or het·er·o·pyc·not·ic
het·er·o·sac·cha·ride
het·er·o·scope
het·er·os·co·py
    pl het·er·os·co·pies
het·er·o·sex·u·al
het·er·o·sex·u·al·i·ty
    pl het·er·o·sex·u·al·i·ties
het·er·o·sex·u·al·ly
het·er·o·side
het·er·o·sis
    pl het·er·o·ses
het·er·os·mi·a
het·er·o·some
het·er·os·po·rous
het·er·o·stim·u·la·tion
het·er·o·sug·ges·ti·bil·i·ty
het·er·o·sug·ges·tion
het·er·o·tax·i·a
    or het·er·o·tax·is
het·er·o·tax·ic
het·er·o·tax·is
    pl het·er·o·tax·es
    or het·er·o·tax·i·a
het·er·o·therm
het·er·o·ther·my
het·er·o·to·ni·a
het·er·o·to·pi·a
    or het·er·ot·o·py
het·er·o·top·ic
het·er·ot·o·pous
het·er·ot·o·py
    pl het·er·ot·o·pies
    or het·er·o·to·pi·a
het·er·o·tox·in
het·er·o·trans·plant
het·er·o·trans·plan·ta·tion
het·er·o·tri·cho·sis
    pl het·er·o·tri·cho·ses
het·er·o·troph
het·er·o·tro·phic
het·er·o·tro·phi·cal·ly
het·er·ot·ro·phims
het·er·ot·ro·phy
    pl het·er·ot·ro·phies
het·er·o·tro·pi·a
het·er·o·typ·ic
    or het·er·o·typ·i·cal

het·er·o·typ·i·cal
or het·er·o·typ·ic

het·er·o·ty·pus

het·er·o·xan·thine
or het·er·o·xan·thin

het·er·o·xan·thin
or het·er·o·xan·thine

het·er·ox·e·nous

het·er·ox·e·ny

het·er·o·zy·go·sis
pl het·er·o·zy·go·ses

het·er·o·zy·gos·i·ty
pl het·er·o·zy·gos·i·ties

het·er·o·zy·gote

het·er·o·zy·got·ic

het·er·o·zy·gous

Heth·er·ing·ton stain

Heub·ner dis·ease

Heub·ner-Herter dis·ease

Heu·ser mem·brane

hex·a·bi·ose
or hex·o·bi·ose

hex·a·canth
or hex·a·can·thous

hex·a·can·thous
or hex·a·canth

hex·a·clor·eth·ane
or hex·a·chlo·ro·eth·ane

hex·a·chlo·ro·cy·clo·
hex·ane

hex·a·chlo·ro·eth·ane
or hex·a·chlor·eth·ane

hex·a·chlo·ro·phene

hex·a·chro·mic

hex·ad

hex·a·dac·ty·lism

hex·a·dac·ty·ly

hex·a·dec·a·no·ic

hex·a·dec·yl

hex·a·di·meth·rine

hex·a·eth·yl·tet·ra·
phos·phate

hex·a·flu·o·re·ni·um

hex·a·flu·o·ro·di·eth·yl

hex·a·gen·ic

hex·a·hy·dric

hex·a·hy·dro·hem·a·to·
por·phy·rin

hex·a·hy·dro·phe·nol

hex·a·hy·drox·y·cy·clo·
hex·ane

hex·al·de·hyde

hex·a·me·tho·ni·um

hex·a·meth·yl·en·a·mine

hex·a·meth·yl·ene·tet·
ra·mine

hex·a·mine

Hex·am·i·ta

hex·am·i·ti·a·sis

hex·a·nal

hex·ane

hex·ane·di·o·ic

hex·a·no·ic

hex·a·ploid

hex·a·ploi·dy

hex·a·va·lent

hex·a·vi·ta·min

hex·ax·i·al

hex·es·trol

hex·e·thal

hex·et·i·dine

hex·o·bar·bi·tal

hex·o·bar·bi·tone

hex·o·bi·ose
or hex·a·bi·ose

hex·o·cy·cli·um

hex·oes·trol
var of hex·es·tral

hex·o·ki·nase

hex·one

hex·os·a·mine

hex·o·san

hex·ose

hex·u·lose

hex·u·ron·ic

hex·yl

hex·yl·caine

hex·yl·re·sor·ci·nol

Hey am·pu·ta·tion

hi·a·tal

hi·a·tus
pl hi·a·tus·es

Hibbs op·er·a·tion

hi·ber·nate

hi·ber·na·tion

hi·ber·no·ma
pl hi·ber·no·mas
or hi·ber·no·ma·ta

hic·cough
or hip·cup

hip·cup
or hic·cough

Hicks sign

hi·drad·e·ni·tis
or hy·drad·e·ni·tis

hi·drad·e·no·car·ci·no·ma
pl hi·drad·e·no·car·ci·
no·mas
or hi·drad·e·no·car·ci·
no·ma·ta

hi·drad·e·no·cyte

hi·drad·e·no·cyt·ic

hi·drad·e·noid

hi·drad·e·no·ma
pl hi·drad·e·no·mas
or hi·drad·e·no·ma·ta
or hy·drad·e·no·ma

hi·dro·a

Hid·ro·cyst·ad·e·no·ma
pl hid·ro·cyst·ad·e·no·mas
or hid·ro·cyst·ad·e·
no·ma·ta

hid·ro·cys·to·ma
pl hid·ro·cys·to·mas
or hid·ro·cys·to·ma·ta

hid·ro·poi·e·sis

hid·ro·poi·et·ic

hid·ror·rhe·a

hid·ror·rhoe·a
var of hid·ror·rhe·a

hi·dros·ad·e·ni·tis
or hy·dros·ad·e·ni·tis

hi·dros·che·sis

hi·drose

hi·dro·sis
pl hi·dro·ses

hy·drot·ic
or hy·drot·ic

hi·er·al·gi·a

hi·er·ic

hi·er·o·lis·the·sis

hi·er·on·o·sus

hi·er·o·pho·bi·a

high-en·er·gy

high-strung

hi·lar

hi·li·tis

Hill re·ac·tion
Hill sign
Hill-Flack sign
Hil·liard lu·pus
hill·ock
Hil·ton law
hi·lum
   pl hi·la
hi·lus
   pl hi·li
hind·brain
hind·foot
hind·gut
Hines and Brown test
Hin·kle pill
Hin·ton test
hip
hip·bone
hip·pan·thro·py
Hip·pe·la·tes
Hip·pel-Lin·dau dis·ease
Hip·po·bos·ca
hip·po·bos·cid
Hip·po·bos·ci·dae
hip·po·cam·pal
hip·po·cam·pus
   pl hip·po·cam·pi
Hip·poc·ra·tes
hip·po·crat·ic
hip·poc·ra·tism
hip·po·lith
hip·pol·o·gy
   pl hip·pol·o·gies
hip·po·myx·o·ma
hip·pu·rase
hip·pu·rate
hip·pu·ri·a
hip·pu·ric
hip·pu·ri·case
hip·pus
hir·cis·mus
hir·cus
   pl hir·ci
Hirsch·berg re·flex
Hirsch·feld nerve
Hirsch·sprung dis·ease
hir·sute
hir·sute·ness
hir·su·tic

hir·su·ti·es
   pl hir·su·ti·es
hir·sut·ism
hir·tel·lous
Hirtz rale
hi·ru·di·cide
hi·ru·din
Hir·u·din·e·a
hir·u·din·e·an
hir·u·di·ni·a·sis
   pl hir·u·di·ni·a·ses
Hir·u·din·i·dae
Hi·ru·do
His spa·ces
His-Held spa·ces
Hiss ser·um wa·ter
His·ta·dyl
his·ta·mi·nase
his·ta·mine
his·tam·i·ne·mi·a
his·tam·i·ner·gic
his·ta·min·ic
his·ta·min·o·lyt·ic
his·ta·nox·i·a
His-Ta·wa·ra node
his·ti·dase
his·ti·di·nae·mi·a
   var of his·ti·di·ne·mi·a
his·ti·dine
his·ti·di·ne·mi·a
his·ti·di·nu·ri·a
his·ti·dyl
his·ti·o·cyte
his·ti·o·cyt·ic
his·ti·o·cy·toid
his·ti·o·cy·to·ma
   pl his·ti·o·cy·to·mas
   or his·ti·o·cy·to·ma·ta
his·ti·o·cy·to·sar·co·ma
   pl his·ti·o·cy·to·sar·co·mas
   or his·ti·o·cy·to·sar·co·ma·ta
his·ti·o·cy·to·sis
   pl his·ti·o·cy·to·ses
his·ti·o·gen·ic
his·ti·oid
his·ti·o·ma
   pl his·ti·o·mas
   or his·ti·o·ma·ta

his·ti·o·troph·ic
his·to·blast
his·to·chem·i·cal
his·to·chem·i·cal·ly
his·to·chem·is·try
   pl his·to·chem·is·tries
his·to·chem·o·graph
his·to·che·mog·ra·phy
   pl his·to·che·mog·ra·phies
his·to·com·pat·i·bil·i·ty
   pl his·to·com·pat·i·bil·i·ties
his·to·com·pat·i·ble
his·to·cyte
his·to·di·al·y·sis
his·to·dif·fer·en·ti·a·tion
his·to·flu·o·res·cence
his·to·gen·e·sis
   pl his·to·gen·e·ses
his·to·ge·net·ic
his·to·ge·net·i·cal·ly
his·to·gen·ic
his·tog·e·nous
his·tog·e·ny
   pl his·tog·e·nies
his·to·gram
his·tog·ra·phy
his·to·haem·a·tin
   var of his·to·he·ma·tin
his·to·hem·a·tin
his·toid
his·to·in·com·pat·i·bil·i·ty
his·to·in·com·pat·i·ble
his·to·ki·ne·sis
his·to·log·ic
   or his·to·log·i·cal
his·to·log·i·cal
   or his·to·log·ic
his·to·log·i·cal·ly
his·tol·o·gist
his·tol·o·gy
   pl his·tol·o·gies
his·tol·y·sis
   pl his·tol·y·ses
his·to·lyt·ic
his·to·ma
   pl his·to·mas
   or his·to·ma·ta
his·to·met·a·plas·tic
His·to·mo·nas

170

his·to·mo·ni·a·sis
his·to·mor·phol·o·gy
his·to·my·co·sis
his·tone
his·to·neu·rol·o·gy
his·ton·o·my
his·to·nu·ri·a
his·to·path·o·log·ic
 or his·to·path·o·lo·gi·cal
his·to·path·o·log·i·cal
 or his·to·path·o·log·ic
his·to·path·o·log·i·cal·ly
his·to·pa·thol·o·gist
his·to·pa·thol·o·gy
 pl his·to·pa·thol·o·gies
his·to·phys·i·o·log·ic
 or his·to·phys·i·o·log·i·cal
his·to·phys·i·o·log·i·cal
 or his·to·phys·i·o·lo·gic
his·to·phys·i·ol·o·gy
 pl his·to·phys·i·ol·o·gies
His·to·plas·ma
his·to·plas·min
his·to·plas·mo·ma
 pl his·to·plas·mo·mas
 or his·to·plas·mo·ma·ta
his·to·plas·mo·sis
 pl his·to·plas·mo·ses
his·to·ra·di·og·ra·phy
his·tor·rhex·is
his·to·ry
 pl his·to·ries
his·to·spec·tros·co·py
his·to·ther·a·py
his·to·throm·bin
his·to·tome
his·tot·o·my
his·to·tox·ic
his·to·tox·in
his·to·trip·sy
his·to·troph
 or his·to·trophe
his·to·trophe
 or his·to·troph
his·to·troph·ic
his·to·trop·ic
his·tot·ro·pism
his·to·zo·ic
his·to·zyme

his·tri·on·ic
his·tri·o·nism
His-Wer·ner dis·ease
Hitch·cock re·a·gent
Hit·zig cen·ter
hives
Hjär·re dis·ease
hoarse
hoarse·ness
hoar·y
hob·ble
Hoch·sin·ger sign
hock
Hodg·kin dis·ease
Hodg·son di·sease
ho·do·neu·ro·mere
ho·do·pho·bi·a
hoe
Hoeh·ne sign
hof
Hof·bau·er cell
Hof·fa dis·ease
Hoff·mann duct
Hoff·mann-Werd·nig
 syn·drome
Hof·meis·ter se·ries
Hö·gyes treat·ment
Hoke op·er·a·tion
hol·an·dric
hol·an·dry
 pl hol·an·dries
hol·ar·thri·tis
hol·er·ga·si·a
Hol·ger Niel·sen meth·od
ho·lid·ic
ho·lism
ho·lis·tic
ho·lis·ti·cal·ly
Hol·la dis·ease
Hol·lan·der test
Hol·len·horst bod·ies
Holmes sign
Holm·gren test
Holm·gren-Gol·gi ca·nals
hol·mi·um
hol·o·a·car·di·us
hol·o·a·cra·ni·a
hol·o·blas·tic
hol·o·blas·ti·cal·ly

hol·o·ce·phal·ic
hol·o·crine
ho·loc·ri·nous
hol·o·di·as·tol·ic
hol·o·en·dem·ic
hol·o·en·zyme
ho·log·a·mous
ho·log·a·my
 pl ho·log·a·mies
hol·o·gas·tros·chi·sis
hol·o·gram
hol·o·graph
ho·lo·graph·ic
ho·lo·graph·i·cal·ly
ho·log·ra·phy
 pl ho·log·ra·phies
hol·o·gyn·ic
ho·log·y·ny
 pl ho·log·y·nies
ho·lo·mas·ti·gote
hol·o·met·a·bol·ic
hol·o·me·tab·o·lous
hol·o·mi·crog·ra·phy
ho·lo·mor·pho·sis
 pl ho·lo·mor·pho·ses
ho·lo·phyt·ic
ho·lo·pros·en·ceph·a·ly
hol·o·ra·chis·chi·sis
hol·o·sac·cha·ride
hol·o·side
hol·o·so·mat·ic
hol·o·sys·tol·ic
hol·o·zo·ic
Holt-O·ram syn·drome
Holt·er-Doyle meth·od
hom·a·lo·ceph·a·lus
 pl hom·a·lo·ceph·a·li
hom·a·lo·cor·y·phus
hom·a·lo·me·to·pus
hom·a·lo·pis·tho·cra·ni·us
hom·a·lu·ra·nus
hom·a·lu·ri·a
Ho·mans sign
ho·ma·rine
ho·mat·ro·pine
hom·ax·i·al
hom·ax·o·ni·al
Home gland
ho·me·o·chrome

171

ho·me·o·ki·ne·sis
pl ho·me·o·ki·ne·sis
ho·me·o·met·ric
ho·me·o·mor·phous
ho·me·o·path
ho·me·o·path·ic
ho·me·o·path·i·cal·ly
ho·me·op·a·thist
ho·me·op·a·thy
pl ho·me·op·a·thies
ho·me·o·pla·si·a
ho·me·o·plas·tic
ho·me·o·sis
ho·me·o·sta·sis
pl ho·me·o·sta·ses
ho·me·o·stat·ic
ho·me·o·ther·a·py
ho·me·o·ther·mal
ho·me·o·ther·mic
or ho·moi·o·ther·mic
or ho·moi·o·ther·mal
ho·me·o·typ·ic
ho·me·o·typ·i·cal
hom·er·gic
home·sick
home·sick·ness
ho·mich·lo·pho·bi·a
hom·i·ci·dal
hom·i·cid·al·ly
hom·i·cide
hom·in·i·an
or hom·i·nid
hom·i·nid
or ho·min·i·an
Ho·min·i·dae
hom·i·nized
hom·i·noid
Hom·i·noi·de·a
ho·mo
ho·mo·al·lele
ho·mo·bi·o·tin
ho·mo·blas·tic
ho·mo·cen·tric
or ho·mo·cen·tri·cal
ho·mo·cen·tri·cal
or ho·mo·cen·tric
ho·mo·chrome
ho·mo·chro·mo·i·som-
  er·ism

ho·moch·ro·nous
ho·mo·clad·ic
ho·mo·cy·clic
ho·mo·cys·te·ine
ho·mo·cys·tine
ho·mo·cys·ti·nu·ri·a
ho·mo·cy·to·trop·ic
ho·mo·dont
ho·mod·ro·mous
ho·mo·dy·nam·ic
ho·mo·dy·na·my
ho·moe·o·mor·phous
  var of ho·me·o·mor·phous
ho·moe·o·path
  var of ho·me·o·path
ho·moe·o·path·ic
  var of ho·me·o·path·ic
ho·moe·op·a·thist
  var of ho·me·op·a·thist
ho·moe·op·a·thy
  var of ho·me·op·a·thy
ho·moe·o·pla·si·a
  var of ho·me·o·pla·si·a
ho·moe·o·plas·tic
  var of ho·me·o·plas·tic
ho·moe·o·sis
  var of ho·me·o·sis
ho·mo·e·rot·ic
ho·mo·e·rot·i·cism
  or ho·mo·er·o·tism
ho·mo·er·o·tism
  or ho·mo·er·ot·i·cism
ho·mo·fer·men·ta·tive
ho·mo·ga·met·ic
ho·mo·gam·ic
  or ho·mog·a·mous
ho·mog·a·mous
  or ho·mo·gam·ic
ho·mog·a·my
  pl ho·mog·a·mies
ho·mog·a·nate
ho·mo·ge·ne·i·ty
ho·mo·ge·neous
ho·mo·ge·ne·ous·ly
ho·mo·ge·ne·ous·ness
ho·mo·gen·e·sis
  pl ho·mo·gen·e·ses
ho·mo·ge·net·ic
  or ho·mo·ge·net·i·cal

ho·mo·ge·net·i·cal
  or ho·mo·ge·net·ic
ho·mo·gen·ic
ho·mo·gen·i·tal·i·ty
ho·mog·e·ni·za·tion
ho·mog·e·nize
ho·mog·e·nous
ho·mo·gen·tis·ic
ho·mog·e·ny
  pl ho·mog·e·nies
ho·mo·glan·du·lar
ho·mo·graft
ho·moi·o·therm
ho·moi·o·ther·mal
  or ho·moi·o·ther·mic
  or ho·me·o·ther·mic
ho·moi·o·ther·mic
  or ho·me·o·ther·mic
  or ho·moio·ther·mal
ho·moi·o·ther·my
ho·moi·o·top·ic
ho·mo·lac·tic
ho·mo·la·li·a
ho·mo·lat·er·al
ho·mo·lec·i·thal
ho·mo·log
ho·mo·log·ic
ho·mol·o·gize
ho·mol·o·giz·er
ho·mol·o·gous
ho·mo·logue
  var of ho·mo·log
ho·mol·o·gy
  pl ho·mol·o·gies
ho·mol·y·sin
ho·mol·y·sis
  pl ho·mol·y·ses
ho·mo·lyt·ic
ho·mo·mor·phic
ho·mon·o·mous
ho·mon·y·mous
ho·mon·y·my
ho·mo·phile
ho·mo·phil·ic
ho·mo·pho·bi·a
ho·mo·pho·bic
ho·mo·plast
ho·mo·plas·tic
ho·mo·plas·ti·cal·ly

ho·mo·plas·ty
ho·mo·po·lar
ho·mo·pol·y·mer
ho·mo·pol·y·sac·cha·ride
Ho·mop·ter·a
ho·mo·qui·nine
hom·or·gan·ic
ho·mo·ser·ine
ho·mo·sex·u·al
ho·mo·sex·u·al·i·ty
  pl ho·mo·sex·u·al·i·ties
ho·mo·sex·u·al·ly
ho·mo·spo·rous
ho·mo·spo·ry
  pl ho·mo·spo·ries
ho·mo·therm
ho·mo·ther·mal
  or ho·mo·ther·mous
  or ho·mo·ther·mic
ho·mo·ther·mic
  or ho·mo·ther·mal
  or ho·mo·ther·mous
ho·mo·ther·mous
  or ho·mo·ther·mal
  or ho·mo·ther·mic
hom·o·tope
ho·mo·top·ic
ho·mo·trans·plant
ho·mo·trans·plan·ta·tion
ho·mo·typ·al
ho·mo·type
ho·mo·typ·ic
ho·mo·vi·tal
ho·mo·zy·go·sis
  pl ho·mo·zy·go·ses
ho·mo·zy·gos·i·ty
ho·mo·zy·gote
ho·mo·zy·got·ic
ho·mo·zy·gous
ho·mo·zy·gous·ly
ho·mun·cu·lus
  pl ho·mun·cu·li
hoof-and-mouth dis·ease
hoof·bound
Hooke law
Hook·er meth·od
hook·let
hook·worm
hoove

hoo·ven
Hoo·ver sign
hop
Hope mur·mur
Hopf dis·ease
Hop·kins-Cole re·ac·tion
Hop·mann pol·yp
Hop·pe-Gold·flam
  dis·ease
ho·qui·zil
ho·ra
hor·de·in
hor·de·nine
hor·de·o·lum
  pl hor·de·o·la
Hor·de·um
ho·ris·ma·scope
ho·ri·zon
hor·i·zon·tal
hor·me·pho·bi·a
hor·me·sis
hor·mi·on
Hor·mo·den·dron
Hor·mo·den·drum
hor·mon·a·gogue
hor·mo·nal
hor·mon·al·ly
hor·mone
hor·mon·ic
hor·mo·no·poi·e·sis
hor·mo·no·poi·et·ic
Hor·ner syn·drome
horn·i·fi·ca·tion
ho·rop·ter
hor·op·ter·ic
hor·rip·i·la·tion
horse·fly
horse·foot
horse·pox
horse·rad·ish
horse·shoe
Hors·ley op·er·a·tion
Hor·te·ga cell
Hor·ton syn·drome
hos·pi·tal
hos·pi·tal·ism
hos·pi·tal·i·za·tion
hos·pi·tal·ize
hos·tile

hos·til·i·ty
Hotch·kiss meth·od
Hot·ten·tot ap·ron
hot·ten·tot·ism
house·fly
house·maids knee
Hous·say phe·nom·e·non
Hous·ton fold
hove
ho·ven
How·ard meth·od
How·ard-Dol·man depth
  per·cep·tion test
How·ell-Jol·ly bod·ies
How·ship la·cu·nas
How·ship-Rom·berg
  syn·drome
Hr fac·tor
H-sub·stance
Hu·chard dis·ease
Hud·dle·son test
Hud·son line
hue
Hug·gins test
Hug·gins-Mil·ler-Jen·sen
  test
Hughes re·flex
Hu·guier ca·nal
Huh·ner test
hu·man
hu·man·o·scope
hu·mate
hu·mec·tant
hu·mec·ta·tion
hu·mer·al
hu·mer·o·ra·di·al
hu·mer·o·scap·u·lar
hu·mer·o·ul·nar
hu·mer·us
  pl hu·me·ri
hu·mic
hu·mic·o·lin
hu·mid
hu·mid·i·fi·ca·tion
hu·mid·i·fi·er
hu·mid·i·fy
hu·mid·i·ty
  pl hu·mid·i·ties
hu·mid·ly

hu·min
hu·mor
hu·mor·al
hu·mour
 var of hu·mor
hump·back
hump·backed
Hum·phry op·er·a·tion
hu·mu·lene
hu·mu·lus
hu·mus
hunch·back
hunch·backed
hun·ger
Hun·ner ul·cer
Hunt at·ro·phy
Hun·ter ca·nal
Hun·ter·i·an chan·cre
Hun·ter-Schre·ger bands
Hun·ting·ton cho·re·a
Hup·pert test
Hur·ler syn·drome
Hürth·le cells
Husch·ke car·ti·lage
Hutch·in·son teeth
Hutch·in·son tri·ad
Hutch·in·son-Boeck
 dis·ease
Hutch·in·son-Gil·ford
 syn·drome
hutch·in·so·ni·an teeth
Hutch·i·son type
huy·gen·i·an eye·piece
hy·al
hy·a·lin
 or hy·a·line
hy·a·line
 or hy·a·lin
hy·a·lin·i·za·tion
hy·a·lin·ize
hy·a·li·no·sis
 pl hy·a·li·no·ses
hy·a·li·nu·ri·a
hy·a·li·tis
hy·a·lo·cap·su·li·tis
hy·al·o·gen
hy·a·loid
hy·a·loi·de·o·cap·su·lar
hy·a·lo·mere

Hy·a·lom·ma
hy·a·lo·mu·coid
hy·a·lo·nyx·is
hy·a·lo·pha·gi·a
hy·a·lo·plasm
hy·a·lo·se·ro·si·tis
hy·al·o·some
hy·a·lu·ro·nate
hy·a·lu·ron·ic
hy·a·lu·ron·i·dase
hy·ben·zate
hy·brid
hy·brid·ism
hy·brid·i·ty
hy·brid·i·za·tion
hy·brid·ize
hy·can·thone
hy·clate
hy·dan·to·ic
hy·dan·to·in
hy·dan·to·in·ate
hy·dat·ic
hy·dat·id
hy·dat·id of Mor·ga·gni
hy·da·tid·i·form
 or hy·dat·i·form
hy·da·tid·o·cele
hy·da·ti·do·sis
 pl hy·da·ti·do·ses
hy·da·ti·dos·to·my
hy·dat·i·form
 or hy·da·tid·i·form
Hyde dis·ease
hyd·no·car·pic
hyd·no·car·pus
hy·dra·bam·ine
hy·dra·ce·tin
hy·drac·id
hy·drad·e·ni·tis
 or hi·drad·e·ni·tis
hy·drad·e·no·ma
 pl hy·drad·e·no·mas
 or hy·drad·e·no·ma·ta
 or hi·drad·e·no·ma
hy·drae·mi·a
 var of hy·dre·mia
hy·drae·mic
 var of hy·dre·mic
hy·dra·er·o·per·i·to·ne·um

hy·dra·gog
hy·dra·gogue
 var of hy·dra·gog
hy·dra·la·zine
hy·dram·ni·on
hy·dram·ni·os
hy·dran·en·ceph·a·ly
hy·dran·ge·a
hy·drar·gyr·i·a
 or hy·drar·gyr·i·a·sis
hy·drar·gyr·i·a·sis
 or hy·drar·gyr·i·a
hy·drar·gyr·ism
hy·drar·gy·ro·pho·bi·a
hy·drar·gyr·oph·thal·mi·a
hy·drar·gy·rum
hy·drar·thro·sis
 pl hy·drar·thro·ses
hy·drase
hy·dras·tine
hy·dras·ti·nine
hy·dras·tis
hy·dra·tase
hy·drate
hy·dra·tion
hy·dra·tor
hy·drau·lic
hy·drau·lics
hy·dra·zide
hy·dra·zine
hy·dra·zone
hy·dre·lat·ic
hy·dre·mi·a
hy·dre·mic
hy·dren·ceph·a·lo·cele
hy·dren·ceph·a·lo·me·nin·
 go·cele
hy·dren·ceph·a·lus
 pl hy·dren·ceph·a·li
 or hy·dren·ceph·a·ly
 pl hy·dren·ceph·a·lies
hy·dren·ceph·a·ly
 pl hy·dren·ceph·a·lies
 or hy·dren·ceph·a·lus
 pl hy·dren·ceph·a·li
hy·dri·a·try
hy·dric
hy·dride
hy·dri·od·ic

hy·dri·o·dide
hy·dri·on
hy·dro·a
hy·dro·ab·do·men
hy·dro·al·co·hol·ic
hy·dro·bil·i·ru·bin
hy·dro·bro·mate
hy·dro·bro·mic
hy·dro·bro·mide
hy·dro·ca·lix
   or hy·dro·ca·lyx
hy·dro·cal·y·co·sis
hy·dro·ca·lyx
   or hy·dro·ca·lix
hy·dro·car·bon
hy·dro·cele
hy·dro·ce·lec·to·my
hy·dro·ce·phal·ic
hy·dro·ceph·a·lo·cele
hy·dro·ceph·a·loid
hy·dro·ceph·a·lus
  pl hy·dro·ceph·a·li
   or hy·dro·ceph·a·ly
  pl hy·dro·ceph·a·lies
hy·dro·ceph·a·ly
  pl hy·dro·ceph·a·lies
   or hy·dro·ceph·a·lus
  pl hy·dro·ceph·a·li
hy·dro·chlo·ric
hy·dro·chlo·ride
hy·dro·chlo·ro·thi·a·zide
hy·dro·cho·le·cys·tis
hy·dro·chol·er·e·sis
  pl hy·dro·chol·e·re·ses
hy·dro·cho·le·ret·ic
hy·dro·cin·chon·i·dine
hy·dro·cin·cho·nine
hy·dro·cir·so·cele
hy·dro·co·done
hy·dro·col·li·dine
hy·dro·col·loid
hy·dro·col·loi·dal
hy·dro·col·pos
hy·dro·co·ni·on
hy·dro·con·qui·nine
hy·dro·cor·ta·mate
hy·dro·cor·ti·sone
hy·dro·co·tar·nine
Hy·dro·cot·y·le

hy·dro·cy·an·ic
hy·dro·cyst
hy·dro·dip·so·ma·ni·a
hy·dro·dy·nam·ic
hy·dro·dy·nam·ics
hy·dro·en·ceph·a·lo·cele
hy·dro·er·got·i·nine
hy·dro·flu·me·thi·a·zide
hy·dro·flu·or·ic
hy·dro·gel
hy·dro·gen
hy·dro·gen·ase
hy·dro·gen·ate
hy·dro·gen·a·tion
hy·dro·gen·ly·ase
hy·dro·glos·sa
hy·dro·gym·nas·tics
hy·dro·haem·a·to·ne·phro·
  sis
  var of hy·dro·hem·a·to·ne·
   phro·sis
hy·dro·haem·a·to·sal·pinx
  var of hy·dro·hem·a·to·sal·
   pinx
hy·dro·hem·a·to·ne·phro·
  sis
hy·dro·hem·a·to·sal·pinx
hy·dro·hep·a·to·sis
hy·dro·ki·net·ic
hy·dro·ki·net·ics
hy·drol
hy·dro·lac·tom·e·ter
hy·dro·lase
hy·dro·ly·ase
hy·drol·o·gy
hy·dro·lymph
hy·drol·y·sate
  or hy·drol·y·zate
hy·dro·lyse
  or hy·dro·lyze
hy·drol·y·sis
  pl hy·drol·y·ses
hy·dro·lyte
hy·dro·lyt·ic
hy·dro·lyz·able
hy·drol·y·zate
  or hy·drol·y·sate
hy·dro·lyze
  or hy·dro·lyse

hy·dro·ma
hy·dro·ma·ni·a
hy·dro·mas·sage
hy·dro·mel
hy·dro·men·in·gi·tis
  pl hy·dro·men·in·git·i·des
hy·dro·me·nin·go·cele
hy·drom·e·ter
hy·dro·me·tra
hy·dro·met·ric
hy·dro·me·tro·col·pos
hy·drom·e·try
hy·dro·mi·cro·ceph·a·ly
hy·dro·mor·phone
hy·drom·pha·lus
hy·dro·my·e·li·a
hy·dro·my·e·lo·cele
hy·dro·my·e·lo·me·ning·o·
  cele
hy·dro·my·o·ma
hy·dro·my·rinx
hy·dro·ne·phro·sis
  pl hy·dro·ne·phro·ses
hy·dro·ne·phrot·ic
hy·dro·ni·um
hy·dro·nol
hy·dro·path·ic
hy·dro·path·i·cal·ly
hy·drop·a·thy
  pl hy·drop·a·thies
hy·dro·pel·vis
hy·dro·per·i·car·di·tis
hy·dro·per·i·car·di·um
  pl hy·dro·per·i·car·di·a
hy·dro·per·i·on
hy·dro·per·i·to·ne·um
  pl hy·dro·per·i·to·ne·ums
   or hy·dro·per·i·to·ne·a
Hy·droph·i·dae
hy·dro·phil
hy·dro·phile
  or hy·dro·phil·ic
hy·dro·phil·i·a
hy·dro·phil·ic
  or hy·dro·phile
hy·droph·i·lism
hy·droph·i·lous
hy·dro·phobe
hy·dro·pho·bi·a

hy·dro·pho·bic
hy·dro·pho·bic·i·ty
pl hy·dro·pho·bic·i·ties
hy·dro·phone
hy·droph·thal·mos
hy·dro·phy·so·me·tra
hy·drop·ic
hy·dro·pleu·ra
hy·dro·pneu·ma·to·sis
hy·dro·pneu·mo·go·ny
hy·dro·pneu·mo·per·i·car·di·um
hy·dro·pneu·mo·per·i·to·ne·um
hy·dro·pneu·mo·tho·rax
pl hy·dro·pneu·mo·tho·rax·es
or hy·dro·pneu·mo·tho·ra·ces
hy·drops
or hy·drop·sy
pl hy·drop·ses
pl hy·drop·sies
hy·drops fe·tal·is
hy·drop·sy
pl hy·drop·sies
or hy·drops
pl hy·drop·ses
hy·dro·py·o·ne·phro·sis
hy·dro·quin·i·dine
hy·dro·quin·ine
hy·dro·quin·ol
hy·dro·qui·none
hy·dror·rhe·a
hy·dror·rhoe·a
var of hy·dror·rhe·a
hy·dros·ad·e·ni·tis
or hi·dros·ad·e·ni·tis
hy·dro·sal·pinx
pl hy·dro·sal·pin·ges
hy·dro·sar·co·cele
hy·dros·che·o·cele
hy·dro·sol
hy·dro·sol·ic
hy·dro·sol·u·ble
hy·dro·sper·ma·to·cele
hy·dro·sper·ma·to·cyst
hy·dro·spi·rom·e·ter
hy·dro·stat

hy·dro·stat·ic
hy·dro·stat·ics
hy·dro·sul·fu·ric
hy·dro·sy·rin·go·my·e·li·a
hy·dro·tac·tic
hy·dro·tax·is
pl hy·dro·tax·es
hy·dro·ther·a·peu·tic
or hy·dro·ther·a·peu·ti·cal
hy·dro·ther·a·peu·ti·cal
or hy·dro·ther·a·peu·tic
hy·dro·ther·a·peu·tics
hy·dro·ther·a·pist
hy·dro·ther·a·py
pl hy·dro·ther·a·pies
hy·dro·ther·mal
hy·dro·ther·mal·ly
hy·dro·thi·o·ne·mi·a
hy·dro·thi·o·nu·ri·a
hy·dro·tho·rac·ic
hy·dro·tho·rax
pl hy·dro·tho·rax·es
or hy·dro·tho·ra·ces
hy·drot·ic
or hi·drot·ic
hy·dro·tis
hy·dro·trop·ic
hy·dro·trop·i·cal·ly
hy·drot·ro·pism
hy·drot·ro·py
hy·dro·tym·pa·num
hy·dro·u·re·ter
hy·dro·u·re·ter·o·ne·phro·sis
hy·dro·u·re·ter·o·sis
hy·drous
hy·dro·va·ri·um
hy·drox·ide
hy·drox·o·co·bal·a·min
hy·drox·y
hy·drox·y·a·ce·tic
hy·drox·y·am·phet·a·mine
hy·drox·y·ap·a·tite
hy·drox·y·ben·zene
hy·drox·y·ben·zo·ic
hy·drox·y·bu·tyr·ic
hy·drox·y·chlo·ro·quine
hy·drox·y·cor·ti·cos·ter·one

hy·drox·y·di·one
hy·drox·y·eth·ane
hy·drox·y·in·dole·a·ce·tic
hy·drox·yl
hy·drox·yl·a·mine
hy·drox·yl·ase
hy·drox·yl·at·ed
hy·drox·yl·a·tion
hy·drox·y·ly·sine
hy·drox·y·phen·a·mate
hy·drox·y·pro·ges·ter·one
hy·drox·y·pro·li·nae·mi·a
var of hy·drox·y·pro·li·ne·mi·a
hy·drox·y·pro·line
hy·drox·y·pro·li·ne·mi·a
hy·drox·y·quin·o·line
hy·drox·y·ste·a·rin
hy·drox·y·stil·bam·i·dine
hy·drox·y·tryp·ta·mine
hy·drox·y·u·re·a
hy·drox·y·zine
Hy·dro·zo·a
hy·dro·zo·an
hy·dro·zo·on
pl hy·dro·zo·ons
or hy·dro·zo·an
hy·dru·ri·a
hy·dru·ric
hy·e·tom·e·try
hy·ge·ian
hy·giene
hy·gi·en·ic
or hy·gi·en·i·cal
hy·gi·en·i·cal
or hy·gi·en·ic
hy·gi·en·i·cal·ly
hy·gi·en·ics
hy·gien·ist
hy·gien·i·za·tion
hy·gre·che·ma
hy·gric
hy·grine
hy·gro·ble·phar·ic
hy·gro·ma
pl hy·gro·mas
or hy·gro·ma·ta
hy·grom·a·tous
hy·grom·e·ter

176

y·gro·met·ric
  or hy·gro·met·ri·cal
y·gro·met·ri·cal
  or hy·gro·met·ric
y·grom·e·try
  pl hy·grom·e·tries
y·gro·my·cin
y·gro·pho·bi·a
y·gro·scope
y·gro·scop·ic
y·gro·scop·i·cal·ly
y·gro·sco·pic·i·ty
  pl hy·gro·sco·pic·i·ties
y·gros·co·py
y·gro·sto·mi·a
y·lic
y·lo·pho·bi·a
y·lo·trop·ic
y·lo·zo·ism
y·men
y·men·al
y·men·ec·to·my
y·men·i·tis
y·men·oid
y·me·no·le·pi·a·sis
  pl hy·me·no·le·pi·a·ses
y·me·no·le·pid·i·dae
y·me·nol·e·pis
y·me·nol·o·gy
y·me·nop·ter·a
y·me·nop·ter·an
y·me·nop·ter·on
  pl hy·me·nop·ter·ons
  or hy·me·nop·tera
y·me·nop·ter·ous
y·men·or·rha·phy
y·men·o·tome
y·men·ot·o·my
  pl hy·men·ot·o·mies
y·o·de·ox·y·cho·lic
  or hy·o·des·ox·y·cho·lic
y·o·des·ox·y·cho·lic
  or hy·o·de·ox·y·cho·lic
y·o·ep·i·glot·tic
  or hy·o·ep·i·glot·tid·e·an
y·o·ep·i·glot·tid·e·an
  or hy·o·ep·i·glot·tic
y·o·glos·sal

hy·o·glos·sus
  pl hy·o·glos·si
hy·oid
  or hy·oi·dal
  or hy·oi·de·an
hy·oi·dal
  or hy·oid
  or hy·oi·de·an
hy·oi·de·an
  or hy·oi·dal
  or hy·oid
hy·o·man·dib·u·lar
hy·o·scine
hy·o·scy·a·mine
hy·o·scy·a·mus
hy·o·sta·pe·di·al
Hy·o·stron·gy·lus
hy·o·thy·roid
hyp·ac·ou·sic
  or hy·a·cu·sic
hyp·a·cu·si·a
hyp·a·cu·sic
  or hyp·ac·ou·sic
hyp·a·cu·sis
hyp·aes·the·si·a
  var of hyp·es·the·si·a
hyp·aes·the·sic
  var of hy·pes·the·sic
hyp·aes·thet·ic
  var of hyp·es·thet·ic
hyp·al·bu·mi·nae·mi·a
  var of hyp·al·bu·mi·ne·mi·a
hyp·al·bu·mi·ne·mi·a
hyp·al·bu·mi·no·sis
hyp·al·ge·si·a
  or hyp·al·gi·a
hyp·al·ge·sic
hyp·al·gi·a
  or hyp·al·ge·si·a
hyp·am·ni·on
hy·pam·ni·os
hy·pan·a·ki·ne·sis
hyp·an·i·sog·na·thism
hyp·an·i·sog·na·thous
hy·paph·o·rine
hyp·ar·ter·i·al
hyp·as·the·ni·a
hyp·ax·i·al
  or hyp·ax·on·ic

hyp·ax·on·ic
  or hyp·ax·i·al
hyp·az·o·tu·ri·a
hy·pen·gy·o·pho·bi·a
hyp·e·o·sin·o·phil
  or hyp·e·o·sin·o·phile
hyp·e·o·sin·o·phile
  or hyp·e·o·sin·o·phil
hy·per·ab·duc·tion
hy·per·ac·id
hy·per·ac·id·am·i·nu·ri·a
hy·per·a·cid·i·ty
  pl hy·per·a·cid·i·ties
hy·per·ac·tive
hy·per·ac·tiv·i·ty
  pl hy·per·ac·tiv·i·ties
hy·per·a·cu·i·ty
hy·per·a·cu·si·a
hy·per·a·cu·sis
hy·per·ad·e·no·sis
hy·per·a·di·po·sis
hy·per·a·dre·nal·cor·ti·cal·
  ism
hy·per·a·dre·nal·ism
hy·per·a·dre·ni·a
hy·per·a·dre·no·cor·ti·cism
hy·per·ae·mi·a
  var of hy·per·e·mi·a
hy·per·ae·mic
  var of hy·per·e·mic
hy·per·aer·a·tion
hy·per·aes·the·si·a
  var of hy·per·es·the·si·a
hy·per·aes·thet·ic
  var of hy·per·es·thet·ic
hy·per·af·fec·tiv·i·ty
hy·per·al·do·ster·o·nism
hy·per·al·ge·si·a
hy·per·al·ge·sic
hy·per·al·i·men·ta·tion
hy·per·al·i·men·to·sis
hy·per·am·i·no·ac·id·u·ri·a
hy·per·am·mo·nae·mi·a
  var of hy·per·am·mo·
  ne·mi·a
hy·per·am·mo·ne·mi·a
hy·per·am·ne·si·a

177

hy·per·am·y·la·sae·mi·a
var of hy·per·am·y·la·se·mi·a
hy·per·am·y·la·se·mi·a
hy·per·an·a·ki·ne·si·a
hy·per·a·phi·a
hy·per·aph·ic
hy·per·az·o·tae·mi·a
var of hy·per·az·o·te·mi·a
hy·per·az·o·te·mi·a
hy·per·az·o·tu·ri·a
hy·per·bar·ic
hy·per·bar·i·cal·ly
hy·per·bar·ism
hy·per·be·ta·al·a·ni·nae·mi·a
var of hy·per·be·ta·al·a·ni·ne·mi·a
hy·per·be·ta·al·a·ni·ne·mi·a
hy·per·bet·a·lip·o·pro·te·in·e·mi·a
hy·per·bil·i·ru·bi·nae·mi·a
var of hy·per·bil·i·ru·bi·ne·mi·a
hy·per·bil·i·ru·bi·ne·mi·a
hy·per·brach·y·ceph·al
hy·per·brach·y·ce·phal·ic
hy·per·brach·y·ceph·a·ly
pl hy·per·brach·y·ceph·a·lies
hy·per·brach·y·cra·ni·al
hy·per·bu·li·a
hy·per·cal·cae·mi·a
var of hy·per·cal·ce·mi·a
hy·per·cal·ce·mi·a
hy·per·cal·ce·mic
hy·per·cal·ci·nu·ri·a
hy·per·cap·ni·a
hy·per·cap·nic
hy·per·car·bi·a
hy·per·car·o·te·nae·mi·a
var of hy·per·car·o·te·ne·mi·a
hy·per·car·o·te·ne·mi·a
hy·per·ca·thar·sis
hy·per·ca·thar·tic
hy·per·ca·thex·is
pl hy·per·ca·thex·es
hy·per·cel·lu·lar·i·ty

hy·per·ce·men·to·sis
pl hy·per·ce·men·to·ses
hy·per·ce·nes·the·si·a
hy·per·cham·aer·rhine
hy·per·chlo·rae·mi·a
var of hy·per·chlo·re·mi·a
hy·per·chlo·rae·mic
var of hy·per·chlo·re·mic
hy·per·chlo·re·mi·a
hy·per·chlo·re·mic
hy·per·chlor·hy·dri·a
hy·per·cho·les·ter·ae·mi·a
var of hy·per·cho·les·ter·e·mi·a
hy·per·cho·les·ter·e·mi·a
hy·per·cho·les·ter·e·mic
hy·per·cho·les·ter·ol·ae·mi·a
var of hy·per·cho·les·ter·ol·e·mi·a
hy·per·cho·les·ter·ol·e·mi·a
or hy·per·cho·les·ter·e·mi·a
hy·per·cho·les·ter·ol·e·mic
hy·per·cho·li·a
hy·per·chro·ma·si·a
hy·per·chro·mat·ic
hy·per·chro·ma·tism
hy·per·chro·ma·to·sis
pl hy·per·chro·ma·to·ses
hy·per·chro·me·mi·a
hy·per·chro·mi·a
hy·per·chro·mic
hy·per·chy·li·a
hy·per·chy·lo·mi·cro·nae·mi·a
var of hy·per·chy·lo·mi·cro·ne·mi·a
hy·per·chy·lo·mi·cro·ne·mi·a
hy·per·co·ag·u·la·bil·i·ty
hy·per·coe·naes·the·si·a
var of hy·per·ce·nes·the·si·a
hy·per·cor·ti·cism
hy·per·cry·aes·the·si·a
var of hy·per·cry·es·the·si·a
hy·per·cry·al·ge·si·a
hy·per·cry·es·the·si·a
hy·per·cu·pre·mi·a

hy·per·cu·pri·u·ri·a
hy·per·cy·a·not·ic
hy·per·cy·the·mi·a
hy·per·cy·to·sis
hy·per·dac·tyl·i·a
hy·per·dac·ty·ly
hy·per·di·crot·ic
hy·per·di·cro·tism
hy·per·dip·loid
hy·per·dip·loi·dy
pl hy·per·dip·loi·dies
hy·per·dis·ten·tion
hy·per·di·u·re·sis
hy·per·dol·i·cho·cra·ni·al
hy·per·dy·na·mi·a
hy·per·dy·nam·ic
hy·per·e·che·ma
hy·per·e·las·tic
hy·per·e·las·tic·i·ty
hy·per·em·e·sis
pl hy·per·em·e·ses
hy·per·em·e·sis grav·i·dar·um
hy·per·e·met·ic
hy·per·e·mi·a
hy·per·e·mic
hy·per·en·ceph·a·lus
hy·per·en·dem·ic
hy·per·en·dem·ic·i·ty
pl hy·per·en·dem·ic·i·ties
hy·per·e·o·sin·o·phil·i·a
hy·per·ep·i·thy·mi·a
hy·per·e·qui·lib·ri·um
hy·per·er·ga·si·a
hy·per·er·gi·a
hy·per·er·gic
hy·per·er·gy
pl hy·per·er·gies
hy·per·e·ryth·ro·cy·the·mi·a
hy·per·es·o·pho·ri·a
hy·per·es·the·si·a
hy·per·es·thet·ic
hy·per·es·tri·ne·mi·a
hy·per·es·trin·ism
hy·per·es·tro·ge·ne·mi·a
hy·per·es·tro·gen·ism
hy·per·ex·cit·a·bil·i·ty
pl hy·per·ex·cit·a·bil·i·ties

hy·per·ex·o·pho·ri·a
hy·per·ex·ten·si·ble
hy·per·ex·ten·sion
hy·per·fer·rae·mi·a
var of hy·per·fer·re·mi·a
hy·per·fer·re·mi·a
hy·per·fi·brin·o·ge·ne·mi·a
hy·per·fi·bri·nol·y·sis
hy·per·flex·ion
hy·per·fo·cal
hy·per·fo·lic·ac·id·ae·mi·a
var of hy·per·fo·lic·ac·
id·e·mi·a
hy·per·fo·lic·ac·id·e·mi·a
hy·per·func·tion
hy·per·ga·lac·ti·a
hy·per·ga·lac·to·sis
hy·per·gam·ma·glob·u·li·
nae·mi·a
var of hy·per·gam·ma·
glob·u·li·ne·mi·a
hy·per·gam·ma·glob·u·li·
ne·mi·a
hy·per·gen·e·sis
hy·per·ge·net·ic
hy·per·gen·i·tal·ism
hy·per·geu·ses·the·si·a
hy·per·geu·si·a
hy·per·gi·a
hy·per·glan·du·lar
hy·per·glo·bu·li·a
hy·per·glob·u·li·nae·mi·a
var of hy·per·glob·u·li·
ne·mi·a
hy·per·glob·u·lin·e·mi·a
hy·per·gly·cae·mi·a
var of hy·per·gly·ce·mi·a
hy·per·gly·cae·mic
var of hy·per·gly·ce·mic
hy·per·gly·ce·mi·a
hy·per·gly·ce·mic
hy·per·glyc·er·i·de·mi·a
hy·per·gly·ci·nae·mi·a
var of hy·per·gly·ci·ne·mi·a
hy·per·gly·ci·ne·mi·a
hy·per·gly·co·ge·nol·y·sis
hy·per·gly·cor·rha·chi·a
hy·per·gly·co·su·ri·a
hy·per·gly·ox·a·la·tu·ri·a

hy·per·go·nad·ism
hy·per·go·ni·a
hy·per·hae·mo·lyt·ic
var of hy·per·he·mo·lyt·ic
hy·per·he·do·ni·a
hy·per·he·don·ism
hy·per·he·mo·glo·bi·ne·
mi·a
hy·per·he·mo·lyt·ic
hy·per·hep·a·ri·nae·mi·a
var of hy·per·hep·a·ri·
ne·mi·a
hy·per·hep·a·ri·ne·mi·a
hy·per·hep·a·ri·ne·mic
hy·per·hi·dro·sis
pl hy·per·hi·dro·ses
or hy·per·i·dro·sis
pl hy·per·i·dro·ses
hy·per·his·ta·mi·nae·mi·a
var of hy·per·his·ta·mi·ne·
mi·a
hy·per·his·ta·mi·ne·mi·a
hy·per·hor·mo·nal
hy·per·hy·dra·tion
hy·per·i·cin
Hy·per·i·cum
hy·per·i·dro·sis
pl hy·per·i·dro·ses
or hy·per·hi·dro·sis
pl hy·per·hi·dro·ses
hy·per·im·mune
hy·per·im·mu·no·glob·
u·li·nae·mi·a
var of hy·per·im·mu·no·
glob·u·li·ne·mi·a
hy·per·im·mu·no·glob·u·li·
ne·mi·a
hy·per·in·fla·tion
hy·per·in·o·sae·mi·a
var of hy·per·in·o·se·mi·a
hy·per·in·o·se·mi·a
hy·per·in·su·lin·ism
hy·per·in·vo·lu·tion
hy·per·ir·ri·ta·bil·i·ty
hy·per·ir·ri·ta·ble
hy·per·i·so·ton·ic
hy·per·ka·lae·mi·a
var of hy·per·ka·le·mi·a

hy·per·ka·lae·mic
var of hy·per·ka·le·mic
hy·per·ka·le·mi·a
hy·per·ka·le·mic
hy·per·ker·a·tin·i·za·tion
hy·per·ker·a·to·sis
pl hy·per·ker·a·to·ses
hy·per·ker·a·tot·ic
hy·per·ke·to·nae·mi·a
var of hy·per·ke·to·ne·mi·a
hy·per·ke·to·ne·mi·a
hy·per·ke·to·nu·ri·a
hy·per·ki·nae·mi·a
var of hy·per·ki·ne·mi·a
hy·per·ki·ne·mi·a
hy·per·ki·ne·si·a
hy·per·ki·ne·sis
hy·per·ki·net·ic
hy·per·lac·ta·tion
hy·per·lep·tor·rhine
hy·per·leu·ko·cy·to·sis
hy·per·li·pae·mi·a
var of hy·per·li·pe·mi·a
hy·per·li·pae·mic
var of hy·per·li·pe·mic
hy·per·li·pe·mi·a
hy·per·li·pe·mic
hy·per·lip·i·dae·mi·a
var of hy·per·lip·i·de·mi·a
hy·per·lip·i·de·mi·a
hy·per·lip·i·de·mic
hy·per·lip·o·pro·te·
in·ae·mi·a
var of hy·per·lip·o·
pro·te·in·e·mi·a
hy·per·lip·o·pro·te·in·e·
mi·a
hy·per·li·po·sis
hy·per·li·thu·ri·a
hy·per·lo·gi·a
hy·per·lu·cen·cy
hy·per·ly·si·nae·mi·a
var of hy·per·ly·si·ne·mi·a
hy·per·ly·si·ne·mi·a
hy·per·mag·ne·sae·mi·a
var of hy·per·mag·ne·
se·mi·a
hy·per·mag·ne·se·mi·a
hy·per·ma·ni·a

hy·per·man·ic
hy·per·mas·ti·a
hy·per·ma·ture
hy·per·meg·a·so·ma
hy·per·mel·a·no·sis
hy·per·mel·a·not·ic
hy·per·men·or·rhe·a
hy·per·men·or·rhoe·a
   var of hy·per·men·or·rhe·a
hy·per·met·a·bol·ic
hy·per·me·tab·o·lism
hy·per·met·a·mor·pho·sis
   pl hy·per·met·a·mor·pho·
   ses
hy·per·me·tri·a
hy·per·met·rope
hy·per·me·tro·pi·a
hy·per·me·tro·pic
hy·perm·ne·si·a
hy·perm·ne·sic
hy·perm·ne·sis
hy·per·morph
hy·per·mo·til·i·ty
hy·per·my·o·to·ni·a
hy·per·my·o·tro·phy
hy·per·na·trae·mi·a
   var of hy·per·na·tre·mi·a
hy·per·na·tre·mi·a
hy·per·ne·a
hy·per·ne·o·cy·to·sis
hy·per·neph·roid
hy·per·ne·phro·ma
   pl hy·per·ne·phro·mas
   or hy·per·ne·phro·ma·ta
hy·per·noe·a
   var of hy·per·ne·a
hy·per·noi·a
hy·per·nu·tri·tion
hy·per·oes·tri·nae·mi·a
   var of hy·per·es·tri·ne·mi·a
hy·per·oes·trin·ism
   var of hy·per·es·trin·ism
hy·per·oes·tro·ge·nae·mi·a
   var of hy·per·es·tro·ge·
   ne·mi·a
hy·per·oes·tro·gen·ism
   var of hy·per·es·tro·
   gen·ism
hy·per·on

hy·per·on·to·morph
hy·per·o·nych·i·a
hy·per·ope
hy·per·oph·thal·mo·path·ic
hy·per·o·pi·a
hy·per·op·ic
hy·per·or·chi·dism
hy·per·o·rex·i·a
hy·per·or·tho·cy·to·sis
hy·per·or·thog·na·thous
hy·per·or·thog·na·thy
hy·per·os·mi·a
hy·per·os·mic
hy·per·os·mo·lar·i·ty
hy·per·os·te·og·e·ny
hy·per·os·to·sis
   pl hy·per·os·to·ses
hy·per·os·tot·ic
hy·per·ox·ae·mi·a
   var of hy·per·ox·e·mi·a
hy·per·ox·a·lu·ri·a
hy·per·ox·e·mi·a
hy·per·ox·i·a
hy·per·ox·y·gen·a·tion
hy·per·par·a·site
hy·per·par·a·sit·ic
hy·per·par·a·sit·ism
hy·per·par·a·thy·roid·ism
hy·per·path·i·a
hy·per·path·ic
hy·per·pep·sin·i·a
hy·per·per·i·stal·sis
   pl hy·per·per·i·stal·ses
hy·per·pex·i·a
hy·per·pha·gi·a
hy·per·pha·gic
hy·per·pha·lan·gi·a
hy·per·pha·lan·gism
hy·per·pha·lan·gy
hy·per·pha·si·a
hy·per·phen·yl·al·a·ni·
   nae·mi·a
   var of hy·per·phen·yl·
   al·a·ni·ne·mi·a
hy·per·phen·yl·al·a·ni·ne·
   mi·a
hy·per·pho·ne·sis
hy·per·pho·ni·a
hy·per·pho·ri·a

hy·per·phos·pha·tae·mi·a
   var of hy·per·phos·pha·
   te·mi·a
hy·per·phos·pha·te·mi·a
hy·per·phos·pha·tu·ri·a
hy·per·phre·ni·a
hy·per·pi·e·si·a
   or hy·per·pi·e·sis
hy·per·pi·e·sis
   or hy·per·pi·e·si·a
hy·per·pi·et·ic
hy·per·pig·men·ta·tion
hy·per·pi·tu·i·ta·rism
hy·per·pi·tu·i·tary
hy·per·pla·si·a
hy·per·plas·mi·a
hy·per·plas·tic
hy·per·plat·y·mer·ic
hy·per·ploid
hy·per·ploi·dy
   pl hy·per·ploi·dies
hy·per·pne·a
hy·per·pne·ic
hy·per·pnoe·a
   var of hy·per·pne·a
hy·per·po·lar·i·za·tion
hy·per·po·lar·ize
hy·per·po·ne·sis
hy·per·po·ro·sis
hy·per·po·si·a
hy·per·po·tas·sae·mi·a
   var of hy·per·po·tas·se·mi·a
hy·per·po·tas·se·mi·a
hy·per·pra·gi·a
hy·per·prag·ic
hy·per·prax·i·a
hy·per·pre·be·ta·lip·o·pro·
   te·in·e·mi·a
hy·per·pres·by·o·pi·a
hy·per·pro·cho·re·sis
hy·per·pro·li·nae·mi·a
   var of hy·per·pro·li·ne·mi·a
hy·per·pro·li·ne·mi·a
hy·per·pro·sex·i·a
hy·per·pro·te·in·ae·mi·a
   var of hy·per·pro·te·
   in·e·mi·a
hy·per·pro·te·in·e·mi·a
hy·per·pro·te·o·sis

hy·per·psy·cho·sis
hy·per·py·ret·ic
hy·per·py·rex·i·a
hy·per·re·ac·tive
hy·per·re·flex·i·a
hy·per·re·flex·ic
hy·per·res·o·nance
hy·per·res·o·nant
hy·per·ru·gos·i·ty
hy·per·sal·e·mi·a
hy·per·sal·i·va·tion
hy·per·se·cre·tion
hy·per·se·cre·to·ry
hy·per·seg·men·ta·tion
hy·per·sen·si·tive
hy·per·sen·si·tive·ness
hy·per·sen·si·tiv·i·ty
  pl hy·per·sen·si·tiv·i·ties
hy·per·sen·si·ti·za·tion
hy·per·sen·si·tize
hy·per·ser·o·to·ni·nae·mi·a
  var of hy·per·ser·o·to·ni·
  ne·mi·a
hy·per·ser·o·to·ni·ne·mi·a
hy·per·sex·u·al
hy·per·sex·u·al·i·ty
  pl hy·per·sex·u·al·i·ties
hy·per·si·a·lo·sis
hy·per·som·ni·a
hy·per·son·ic
hy·per·sple·nic
hy·per·sple·nism
hy·per·sthe·ni·a
hy·per·sthe·nic
hy·per·sus·cep·ti·bil·i·ty
  pl hy·per·sus·cep·ti·
  bil·i·ties
hy·per·syn·chro·ny
hy·per·tel·o·rism
Hy·per·ten·sin
hy·per·ten·sin·ase
hy·per·ten·sin·o·gen
hy·per·ten·sion
hy·per·ten·sive
hy·per·ten·sor
hy·per·the·co·sis
hy·per·the·li·a
hy·per·therm·al·ge·si·a
hy·per·ther·mes·the·si·a

hy·per·ther·mi·a
hy·per·ther·mic
hy·per·ther·mo·aes·the·si·a
  var of hy·per·ther·mo·es·
  the·si·a
hy·per·ther·mo·es·the·si·a
hy·per·ther·my
hy·per·throm·bi·ne·mi·a
hy·per·thy·mi·a
hy·per·thy·mism
hy·per·thy·mi·za·tion
hy·per·thy·re·o·sis
  pl hy·per·thy·re·o·ses
  or hy·per·thy·ro·sis
  pl hy·per·thy·ro·ses
hy·per·thy·roid
hy·per·thy·roid·ism
hy·per·thy·ro·sis
  pl hy·per·thy·ro·ses
  or hy·per·thy·re·o·sis
  pl hy·per·thy·re·o·ses
hy·per·thy·ro·tro·pin·ism
hy·per·thy·rox·i·ne·mi·a
hy·per·to·ni·a
  or hy·per·to·ny
hy·per·ton·ic
hy·per·to·nic·i·ty
  pl hy·per·to·nic·i·ties
hy·per·to·nus
hy·per·to·ny
  pl hy·per·to·nies
  or hy·per·to·ni·a
hy·per·tri·cho·sis
  pl hy·per·tri·cho·ses
hy·per·tri·glyc·er·i·dae·
  mi·a
  var of hy·per·tri·glyc·er·
  i·de·mi·a
hy·per·tri·glyc·er·i·de·mi·a
hy·per·tro·phic
hy·per·trophy
  pl hy·per·tro·phies
hy·per·tro·pi·a
hy·per·ty·ro·si·nae·mi·a
  var of hy·per·ty·ro·si·
  ne·mi·a
hy·per·ty·ro·si·ne·mi·a
hy·per·u·re·sis

hy·per·u·ri·cae·mi·a
  var of hy·per·u·ri·ce·mi·a
hy·per·u·ri·ce·mi·a
hy·per·val·i·nae·mi·a
  var of hy·per·val·i·ne·mi·a
hy·per·val·i·ne·mi·a
hy·per·vas·cu·lar
hy·per·veg·e·ta·tive
hy·per·ven·ti·la·tion
hy·per·vis·cos·i·ty
hy·per·vis·cous
hy·per·vi·ta·min·o·sis
  pl hy·per·vi·ta·min·o·ses
hy·per·vo·lae·mi·a
  var of hy·per·vo·le·mi·a
hy·per·vo·lae·mic
  var of hy·per·vo·le·mic
hy·per·vo·le·mi·a
hy·per·vo·le·mic
hy·per·vo·lu·mic
hyp·es·the·si·a
hyp·es·the·sic
hyp·es·thet·ic
hy·pha
  pl hy·phae
hy·phae·ma
  var of hy·phe·ma
hy·phae·mi·a
  var of hy·phe·mi·a
hy·phal
hyp·he·do·ni·a
hy·phe·ma
hy·phe·mi·a
hyp·hi·dro·sis
  pl hyp·hi·dro·ses
hy·pho·gen·ic
Hy·pho·my·ce·tes
hy·pho·my·co·sis
hyp·na·gog·ic
  or hyp·no·gog·ic
hyp·na·gogue
hyp·nal·gi·a
hyp·nic
hyp·no·a·nal·y·sis
  pl hyp·no·a·nal·y·ses
hyp·no·don·tics
hyp·no·gen·e·sis
  pl hyp·no·gen·e·ses
hyp·no·ge·net·ic

hyp·no·ge·net·i·cal·ly
hyp·no·gen·ic
hyp·nog·e·nous
hyp·no·gog·ic
  or hyp·na·gog·ic
hyp·noid
  or hyp·noi·dal
hyp·noi·dal
  or hyp·noid
hyp·no·lep·sy
hyp·nol·o·gy
  pl hyp·nol·o·gies
hyp·no·nar·co·sis
hyp·no·pho·bi·a
  or hyp·no·pho·by
hyp·no·pho·bic
hyp·no·pho·by
  pl hyp·no·pho·bies
  or hyp·no·pho·bi·a
hyp·no·phre·no·sis
  pl hyp·no·phre·no·ses
hyp·no·pom·pic
hyp·no·si·gen·e·sis
hyp·no·sis
  pl hyp·no·ses
hyp·no·ther·a·py
  pl hyp·no·ther·a·pies
hyp·not·ic
hyp·no·tise
  var of hyp·no·tize
hyp·no·tism
hyp·no·tist
hyp·no·tize
hyp·no·toid
hyp·no·tox·in
hy·po
hy·po·a·cid·i·ty
  pl hy·po·a·cid·i·ties
hy·po·ac·tiv·i·ty
hy·po·a·cu·si·a
hy·po·a·cu·sis
hy·po·a·dren·a·li·ne·mi·a
hy·po·a·dre·nal·ism
hy·po·a·dre·ni·a
hy·po·a·dre·no·cor·ti·cism
hy·po·aes·the·si·a
  var of hy·po·es·the·si·a
hy·po·af·fec·ti·vi·ty
hy·po·ag·na·thus

hy·po·al·bu·mi·nae·mi·a
  var of hy·po·al·bu·mi·
  ne·mi·a
hy·po·al·bu·mi·ne·mi·a
hy·po·al·bu·mi·no·sis
hy·po·al·do·ster·o·nism
hy·po·al·i·men·ta·tion
hy·po·al·ler·gen·ic
hy·po·az·o·tu·ri·a
hy·po·bar·ic
hy·po·bar·ism
hy·po·ba·rop·a·thy
hy·po·bil·i·ru·bi·nae·mi·a
  var of hy·po·bil·i·ru·bi·
  ne·mi·a
hy·po·bil·i·ru·bi·ne·mi·a
hy·po·blast
hy·po·blas·tic
hy·po·bran·chi·al
hy·po·bro·mite
hy·po·bro·mous
hy·po·bu·li·a
hy·po·bu·lic
hy·po·cal·cae·mi·a
  var of hy·po·cal·ce·mi·a
hy·po·cal·cae·mic
  var of hy·po·cal·ce·mic
hy·po·cal·ce·mi·a
hy·po·cal·ce·mic
hy·po·cal·cif·ic
hy·po·cal·ci·fi·ca·tion
hy·po·cal·ci·fy
hy·po·cal·ci·u·ri·a
hy·po·cap·ni·a
hy·po·car·bi·a
hy·po·ca·thex·is
hy·po·ce·lom
hy·po·ce·ru·lo·plas·mi·nae·
  mi·a
  var of hy·po·ce·ru·lo·
  plas·mi·ne·mi·a
hy·po·ce·ru·lo·plas·mi·ne·
  mi·a
hy·po·chlo·rae·mi·a
  var of hy·po·chlo·re·mi·a
hy·po·chlo·re·mi·a
hy·po·chlo·re·mic
hy·po·chlor·hy·dri·a
hy·po·chlor·hy·dric

hy·po·chlo·rite
hy·po·chlo·ri·za·tion
hy·po·chlo·rous
hy·po·chlor·u·ri·a
hy·po·cho·les·ter·o·lae·
  mi·a
  var of hy·po·cho·les·ter·o·
  le·mi·a
hy·po·cho·les·ter·o·le·mi·a
hy·po·chon·dri·a
hy·po·chon·dri·ac
hy·po·chon·dri·a·cal
hy·po·chon·dri·a·cal·ly
hy·po·chon·dri·al
hy·po·chon·dri·a·sis
  pl hy·po·chon·dri·a·ses
hy·po·chon·dri·um
  pl hy·po·chon·dri·a
hy·po·chord·al
hy·po·chro·ma·si·a
hy·po·chro·mat·ic
hy·po·chro·ma·tism
hy·po·chro·ma·to·sis
hy·po·chro·me·mi·a
hy·po·chro·mi·a
hy·po·chro·mic
hy·po·chy·li·a
hy·po·ci·ne·si·a
hy·po·coe·lom
  var of hy·po·ce·lom
hy·po·com·ple·men·te·mi·a
hy·po·cone
hy·po·con·id
hy·po·con·ule
hy·po·con·u·lid
hy·po·cri·nism
hy·po·cu·prae·mi·a
  var of hy·po·cu·pre·mi·a
hy·po·cu·pre·mi·a
hy·po·cu·prae·mic
  var of hy·po·cu·pre·mic
hy·po·cu·pre·mic
hy·po·cy·clo·sis
  pl hy·po·cy·clo·ses
hy·po·cy·thae·mi·a
  var of hy·po·cy·the·mi·a
hy·po·cy·the·mi·a
hy·po·dac·ty·ly
hy·po·derm

Hy·po·der·ma
hy·po·der·mal
hy·po·der·mat·ic
hy·po·der·mat·i·cal·ly
hy·po·der·ma·toc·ly·sis
hy·po·der·mi·a·sis
hy·po·der·mic
hy·po·der·mi·cal·ly
hy·po·der·mis
hy·po·der·moc·ly·sis
  pl hy·po·der·moc·ly·ses
hy·po·der·mo·li·thi·a·sis
hy·po·dip·loid
hy·po·dip·loi·dy
  pl hy·po·dip·loi·dies
hy·po·dip·si·a
hy·po·don·ti·a
hy·po·dy·na·mi·a
hy·po·dy·nam·ic
hy·po·ec·cri·si·a
hy·po·en·doc·ri·nism
hy·po·er·gi·a
hy·po·er·gic
hy·po·er·gy
  pl hy·po·er·gies
hy·po·es·o·pho·ri·a
hy·po·es·the·si·a
hy·po·es·trin·ism
hy·po·ex·o·pho·ri·a
hy·po·fer·rae·mi·a
  var of hy·po·fer·re·mi·a
hy·po·fer·re·mi·a
hy·po·fi·bri·no·ge·nae·mi·a
  var of hy·po·fi·bri·no·ge·
  ne·mi·a
hy·po·fi·bri·no·ge·ne·mi·a
hy·po·func·tion
hy·po·func·tion·al
hy·po·ga·lac·ti·a
hy·po·gam·ma·glob·u·li·
  nae·mi·a
  var of hy·po·gam·ma·
  glob·u·li·ne·mi·a
hy·po·gam·ma·glob·u·li·ne·
  mi·a
hy·po·gas·tric
hy·po·gas·tri·um
  pl hy·po·gas·tri·a
hy·po·gas·tro·did·y·mus

hy·po·gas·trop·a·gus
hy·po·gas·tros·chi·sis
hy·po·gen·e·sis
  pl hy·po·gen·e·ses
hy·po·ge·net·ic
hy·po·gen·i·tal·ism
hy·po·geu·si·a
hy·po·glos·sal
hy·po·glos·sis
hy·po·glos·si·tis
hy·po·glos·sus
  pl hy·po·glos·si
hy·po·glot·tis
  pl hy·po·glot·tis·es
  or hy·po·glot·ti·des
hy·po·gly·cae·mi·a
  var of hy·po·gly·ce·mi·a
hy·po·gly·cae·mic
  var of hy·po·gly·ce·mic
hy·po·gly·ce·mi·a
hy·po·gly·ce·mic
hy·po·gly·ce·mo·sis
hy·po·gly·cin
hy·po·gly·co·ge·nol·y·sis
hy·po·gly·cor·rha·chi·a
hy·pog·na·thous
hy·pog·na·thus
hy·po·go·nad·ism
hy·po·gon·a·do·trop·ic
hy·po·gran·u·lo·cy·to·sis
hy·po·hi·dro·sis
  pl hy·po·hi·dro·ses
hy·po·in·su·lin·ism
hy·po·ka·le·mi·a
hy·po·ka·le·mic
hy·po·ker·a·to·sis
hy·po·ki·ne·si·a
hy·po·ki·ne·sis
  pl hy·po·ki·ne·ses
hy·po·ki·net·ic
hy·po·lem·mal
hy·po·lep·si·o·ma·ni·a
hy·po·leu·ko·cyt·ic
hy·po·ley·dig·ism
hy·po·li·pae·mi·a
  var of hy·po·li·pe·mi·a
hy·po·li·pae·mic
  var of hy·po·li·pe·mic
hy·po·li·pe·mi·a

hy·po·li·pe·mic
hy·po·lo·gi·a
hy·po·mag·ne·sae·mi·a
  var of hy·po·mag·ne·se·
  mi·a
hy·po·mag·ne·se·mi·a
hy·po·mag·ne·se·mic
hy·po·ma·ni·a
hy·po·man·ic
hy·po·mas·ti·a
hy·po·ma·ture
hy·po·ma·zi·a
hy·po·mel·a·no·sis
hy·po·mel·a·not·ic
hy·po·men·or·rhe·a
hy·po·men·or·rhoe·a
  var of hy·po·men·or·rhe·a
hy·po·mere
hy·po·me·tab·o·lism
hy·po·me·tri·a
hy·po·me·tro·pi·a
hy·po·mi·cro·gnath·us
hy·po·mi·cron
hy·po·mi·cro·so·ma
hy·pom·ne·si·a
hy·po·morph
hy·po·morph·ic
hy·po·mo·til·i·ty
  pl hy·po·mo·til·i·ties
hy·po·my·o·to·ni·a
hy·po·myx·i·a
hy·po·na·trae·mi·a
  var of hy·po·na·tre·mi·a
hy·po·na·tre·mi·a
hy·po·ne·o·cy·to·sis
hy·po·ni·trous
hy·po·noi·a
hy·po·nych·i·al
hy·po·nych·i·um
hy·po·oes·trin·ism
  var of hy·po·es·trin·ism
hy·po·or·tho·cy·to·sis
hy·po·os·to·sis
  pl hy·po·os·to·ses
hy·po·os·tot·ic
hy·po·o·var·i·an·ism
hy·po·pan·cre·a·tism
hy·po·par·a·thy·roid
hy·po·par·a·thy·roid·ism

hy·po·per·fu·sion
hy·po·per·me·a·bil·i·ty
hy·po·pha·lan·gism
hy·po·phar·yn·gi·tis
hy·po·phar·yn·gos·co·py
hy·po·phar·ynx
   pl hy·po·phar·ynx·es
   or hy·po·pha·ryn·ges
hy·po·pho·ne·sis
hy·po·pho·ni·a
hy·po·pho·ri·a
hy·po·phos·pha·tae·mi·a
   var of hy·po·phos·pha·te·
   mi·a
hy·po·phos·pha·ta·si·a
hy·po·phos·pha·te·mi·a
hy·po·phos·pha·tu·ri·a
hy·po·phos·phite
hy·po·phos·pho·rous
hy·po·phre·ni·a
hy·po·phren·ic
hy·po·phre·no·sis
   pl hy·po·phre·no·ses
hy·poph·y·se·al
   or hy·poph·y·si·al
hy·poph·y·sec·to·mize
hy·poph·y·sec·to·my
   pl hy·poph·y·sec·to·mies
hy·poph·y·se·o·por·tal
hy·po·phys·e·o·priv·ic
   or hy·po·phys·i·o·priv·ic
hy·poph·y·si·al
   or hy·poph·y·se·al
hy·po·phys·i·o·priv·ic
   or hy·po·phys·e·o·priv·ic
hy·poph·y·sis
   pl hy·poph·y·ses
hy·poph·y·sis cer·e·bri
hy·po·pi·e·si·a
hy·po·pi·e·sis
hy·po·pig·men·ta·tion
hy·po·pin·e·al·ism
hy·po·pi·tu·i·ta·rism
hy·po·pi·tu·i·tar·y
hy·po·pla·si·a
hy·po·plas·tic
hy·po·plas·ty
hy·po·ploid

hy·po·ploi·dy
   pl hy·po·ploi·dies
hy·po·pne·a
hy·po·po·ro·sis
hy·po·po·si·a
hy·po·po·tas·sae·mi·a
   var of hy·po·po·tas·se·mi·a
hy·po·po·tas·se·mi·a
hy·po·po·tas·se·mic
hy·po·prax·i·a
hy·po·pro·sex·i·a
hy·po·pros·o·dy
hy·po·pro·te·in·ae·mi·a
   var of hy·po·pro·te·in·e·
   mi·a
hy·po·pro·te·in·e·mi·a
hy·po·pro·te·in·e·mic
hy·po·pro·throm·bi·nae·
   mi·a
   var of hy·po·pro·throm·bi·
   ne·mi·a
hy·po·pro·throm·bi·ne·mi·a
hy·po·pro·throm·bi·ne·mic
hy·po·psel·a·phe·si·a
hy·po·psy·cho·sis
hy·pop·ty·a·lism
hy·po·py·on
hy·po·re·ac·tive
hy·po·re·flex·i·a
hy·po·re·flex·ic
hy·po·ri·bo·fla·vin·o·sis
   pl hy·po·ri·bo·fla·vin·o·ses
hy·po·sa·le·mi·a
hy·po·sal·i·va·tion
hy·po·scle·ral
hy·po·se·cre·tion
hy·po·sen·si·tive
hy·po·sen·si·tiv·i·ty
   pl hy·po·sen·si·tiv·i·ties
hy·po·sen·si·ti·za·tion
hy·po·sen·si·tize
hy·pos·mi·a
hy·pos·mo·lar·i·ty
hy·po·som·ni·a
hy·po·spa·di·a
   or hy·po·spa·di·as
hy·po·spa·di·ac
hy·po·spa·di·as
   or hy·po·spa·di·a

hy·po·sper·ma·to·gen·e·sis
hy·po·sphre·si·a
hy·pos·ta·sis
   pl hy·pos·ta·ses
hy·po·stat·ic
hy·po·sthe·ni·a
hy·po·sthe·ni·ant
hy·po·sthen·ic
hy·pos·the·nu·ri·a
hy·pos·the·nu·ric
hy·po·sto·mi·a
hy·po·styp·sis
hy·po·styp·tic
hy·po·sul·fite
   or hy·po·sul·phite
hy·po·sul·phite
   or hy·po·sul·fite
hy·po·syn·er·gi·a
hy·po·tax·i·a
hy·po·tax·is
hy·po·tel·o·rism
hy·po·ten·sion
hy·po·ten·sive
hy·po·ten·sor
hy·po·tha·lam·ic
hy·po·thal·a·mo·hy·poph·y·
   se·al
hy·po·thal·a·mus
   pl hy·po·thal·a·mi
hy·po·the·nar
hy·po·therm·aes·the·si·a
   var of hy·po·therm·es·
   the·si·a
hy·po·ther·mal
hy·po·therm·es·the·si·a
hy·po·ther·mi·a
hy·po·ther·mic
hy·po·ther·my
hy·poth·e·sis
   pl hy·poth·e·ses
hy·po·throm·bi·ne·mi·a
hy·po·thy·mi·a
hy·po·thy·mism
hy·po·thy·roid
hy·po·thy·roid·ism
hy·po·thy·ro·sis
hy·po·to·ni·a
   or hy·pot·o·ny
hy·po·ton·ic

hy·po·ton·i·cal·ly
hy·po·to·nic·i·ty
  pl hy·po·to·nic·i·ties
hy·po·to·nus
hy·po·to·ny
  pl hy·po·to·nies
  or hy·po·to·ni·a
hy·po·tox·ic·i·ty
hy·po·trans·fer·ri·ne·mi·a
hy·po·tri·cho·sis
  pl hy·po·tri·cho·sis·es
  or hy·po·tri·cho·ses
hy·po·tri·chot·ic
hy·pot·ro·phy
  pl hy·pot·ro·phies
hy·po·tro·pi·a
hy·po·tym·pan·ic
hy·po·tym·pan·ot·o·my
hy·po·tym·pa·num
  pl hy·po·tym·pa·nums
  or hy·po·tym·pa·na
hy·po·va·so·pres·si·nae·
  mi·a
  var of hy·po·va·so·pres·si·
  ne·mi·a
hy·po·va·so·pres·si·ne·mi·a
hy·po·veg·e·ta·tive
hy·po·ven·ti·la·tion
hy·po·vi·ta·min·o·sis
  pl hy·po·vi·ta·min·o·sis·es
  or hy·po·vi·ta·min·o·ses
hy·po·vi·ta·min·ot·ic
hy·po·vo·lae·mi·a
  var of hy·po·vo·le·mi·a
hy·po·vo·lae·mic
  var of hy·po·vo·le·mic
hy·po·vo·le·mi·a
hy·po·vo·le·mic
hy·po·vo·li·a
hy·po·vo·lu·mic
hy·pox·ae·mi·a
  var of hy·pox·e·mi·a
hy·pox·ae·mic
  var of hy·pox·e·mic
hy·po·xan·thine
hy·po·xan·thyl·ic
hy·pox·e·mi·a
hy·pox·e·mic
hy·pox·i·a

hy·pox·ic
hyp·sa·rhyth·mi·a
  var of hyp·sar·rhyth·mi·a
hyp·sa·rhyth·moid
  var of hyp·sar·rhyth·moid
hyp·sar·rhyth·mi·a
hyp·sar·rhyth·moid
hyp·si·brach·y·ce·phal·ic
hyp·si·brach·y·ceph·al·ism
hyp·si·ce·phal·ic
  or hyp·si·ceph·a·lous
hyp·si·ceph·a·lous
  or hyp·si·ce·phal·ic
hyp·si·ceph·a·ly
hyp·si·conch
hyp·si·loid
hyp·si·sta·phyl·i·a
hyp·si·sta·phyl·ic
hyp·si·staph·y·line
hyp·so·chrome
hyp·so·chro·mic
hyp·so·dont
hyp·so·don·tism
hyp·so·ki·ne·sis
hyp·so·pho·bi·a
Hyrtl loop
hys·sop
hys·ter·al·gi·a
hys·ter·al·gic
hys·ter·a·tre·si·a
hys·ter·ec·to·mize
hys·ter·ec·to·my
  pl hys·ter·ec·to·mies
hys·ter·e·sis
  pl hys·ter·e·ses
hys·ter·eu·ryn·ter
hys·ter·eu·ry·sis
hys·te·ri·a
hys·ter·i·ac
hys·ter·ic
  or hys·ter·i·cal
hys·ter·i·cal
  or hys·ter·ic
hys·ter·i·cal·ly
hys·ter·i·cism
hys·ter·ics
hys·ter·i·form
hys·ter·i·tis
hys·ter·o·bu·bon·o·cele

hys·ter·o·cat·a·lep·sy
hys·ter·o·cele
hys·ter·o·clei·sis
hys·ter·o·cys·tic
hys·ter·o·cys·to·pex·y
hys·ter·o·de·mo·nop·a·thy
hys·ter·o·dyn·i·a
hys·ter·o·ep·i·lep·sy
  pl hys·ter·o·ep·i·lep·sies
hys·ter·o·ep·i·lep·tic
hys·ter·o·fren·a·to·ry
hys·ter·o·fren·ic
hys·ter·o·gen·ic
hys·ter·og·e·nous
hys·ter·og·e·ny
hys·ter·o·gram
hys·ter·o·graph
hys·ter·og·ra·phy
  pl hys·ter·og·ra·phies
hys·ter·oid
  or hys·ter·oi·dal
hys·ter·oi·dal
  or hys·ter·oid
hys·ter·o·lap·a·rot·o·my
hys·ter·o·lith
hys·ter·o·li·thi·a·sis
  pl hys·ter·o·li·thi·a·ses
hys·ter·ol·o·gy
  pl hys·ter·ol·o·gies
hys·ter·ol·y·sis
  pl hys·ter·ol·y·ses
hys·ter·o·ma·ni·a
hys·ter·om·e·ter
hys·ter·om·e·try
hys·ter·o·my·o·ma
  pl hys·ter·o·my·o·mas
  or hys·ter·o·my·o·ma·ta
hys·ter·o·my·o·mec·to·my
hys·ter·o·my·ot·o·my
hys·ter·o·
  o·o·pho·rec·to·my
  pl hys·ter·o·
  o·o·pho·rec·to·mies
hys·ter·o·path·ic
hys·ter·op·a·thy
hys·ter·o·pex·y
  pl hys·ter·o·pex·ies
hys·ter·o·phil·i·a
hys·ter·o·pi·a

hys·ter·o·plas·ty
hys·ter·op·to·sis
hys·ter·or·rha·phy
  pl hys·ter·or·rha·phies
hys·ter·or·rhex·is
  pl hys·ter·or·rhex·es
hys·ter·o·sal·pin·gec·to·my
  pl hys·ter·o·sal·pin·gec·
  to·mies
hys·ter·o·sal·pin·gog·ra·
  phy
  pl hys·ter·o·sal·pin·gog·ra·
  phies
hys·ter·o·sal·pin·go-
  o·o·pho·rec·tomy

pl hys·ter·o·sal·pin·go-
  o·o·pho·rec·to·mies
hys·ter·o·sal·pin·gos·to·my
hys·ter·o·scope
hys·ter·o·scop·ic
hys·ter·os·co·py
  pl hys·ter·os·co·pies
hys·ter·o·spasm
hys·ter·o·sto·mat·o·my
  pl hys·ter·o·sto·mat·o·mies
hys·ter·o·tel·y
  pl hys·ter·o·tel·ies
hys·ter·o·tome
hys·ter·ot·o·my
  pl hys·ter·ot·o·mies

hys·ter·o·tra·che·lec·to·my
  pl hys·ter·o·tra·che·lec·
  to·mies
hys·ter·o·tra·che·lo·plas·ty
hys·ter·o·tra·che·lor·rha·
  phy
  pl hys·ter·o·tra·che·lor·
  rha·phies
hys·ter·o·tra·che·lot·o·my
  pl hys·ter·o·tra·che·lot·
  o·mies
hys·ter·o·trau·mat·ic
hys·ter·o·trau·ma·tism
hys·tero·tu·bog·ra·phy
hys·trix
hy·ther

I

I band
I e·lec·tro·ret·i·no·gram
i·am·a·tol·o·gy
i·at·ric
  or i·at·ri·cal
i·at·ri·cal
  or i·at·ric
i·at·ro·chem·i·cal
i·at·ro·chem·is·try
  pl i·at·ro·chem·is·tries
i·at·ro·gen·e·sis
i·at·ro·gen·ic
i·at·ro·gen·i·cal·ly
i·at·ro·ge·nic·i·ty
  pl i·at·ro·ge·nic·i·ties
i·at·ro·math·e·mat·ics
i·at·ro·phys·i·cist
iat·ro·phys·ics
i·at·ro·tech·ni·cal
i·at·ro·tech·nics
i·bo·ga·ine

i·bu·fe·nac
i·bu·pro·fen
Ice·land dis·ease
ich·no·gram
i·chor
i·chor·oid
i·chor·ous
i·chor·rhae·mi·a
  var of i·chor·rhe·mi·a
i·chor·rhe·a
i·chor·rhe·mi·a
i·chor·rhoe·a
  var of i·chor·rhe·a
ich·tham·mol
ich·thy·ism
  or ich·thy·is·mus
ich·thy·is·mus
  or ich·thy·ism
ich·thy·o·col
  or ich·thy·o·coll
  or ich·thy·o·col·la

ich·thy·o·coll
  or ich·thy·o·col
  or ich·thy·o·col·la
ich·thy·o·col·la
  or ich·thy·o·col
  or ich·thy·o·coll
ich·thy·oid
ich·thy·oi·dal
ich·thy·ol·o·gy
ich·thy·oph·a·gous
ich·thy·o·pho·bi·a
ich·thy·o·sar·co·tox·in
ich·thy·o·sar·co·tox·ism
ich·thy·o·si·form
ich·thy·o·sis
  pl ich·thy·o·ses
ich·thy·ot·ic
ich·thy·o·tox·in
ich·thy·o·tox·ism
ich·thy·o·tox·is·mus
i·con

i·con·ic
i·co·nog·ra·phy
i·con·o·lag·ny
i·con·o·ma·ni·a
ic·tal
ic·ter·ic
ic·ter·i·tious
   or ic·ter·i·tous
ic·ter·i·tous
   or ic·ter·i·tious
ic·ter·o·a·ne·mi·a
ic·ter·o·gen·ic
   or ic·ter·og·e·nous
ic·ter·og·e·nous
   or ic·ter·o·gen·ic
ic·ter·o·he·mo·lyt·ic
ic·ter·o·hem·or·rhag·ic
ic·ter·o·hep·a·ti·tis
ic·ter·oid
ic·ter·us
ic·ter·us grav·is
ic·ter·us in·dex
ic·tus
id
i·de·al·i·za·tion
i·de·a·tion
i·de·a·tion·al
i·dée fixe
   pl i·dées fixes
i·den·ti·cal
i·den·ti·fi·ca·tion
i·den·ti·fy
i·den·ti·ty
   pl i·den·ti·ties
i·de·o·ge·net·ic
id·e·og·e·nous
id·e·o·glan·du·lar
id·e·o·ki·net·ic
id·e·ol·o·gy
id·e·o·met·a·bol·ic
id·e·o·me·tab·o·lism
i·de·o·mo·tion
id·e·o·mo·tor
id·e·o·mus·cu·lar
id·e·o·pho·bi·a
id·e·o·plas·tic
id·e·o·plas·ty
id·e·o·syn·chy·si·a
id·e·o·syn·chy·sis

id·e·o·vas·cu·lar
id·i·o·blast
id·i·o·chro·mo·some
id·i·o·cra·si·a
id·i·oc·ra·sy
   pl id·i·oc·ra·sies
id·i·o·crat·ic
   or id·i·o·crat·i·cal
id·i·o·crat·i·cal
   or id·i·o·crat·ic
id·i·oc·to·ni·a
id·i·o·cy
   pl id·i·o·cies
id·i·og·a·mist
id·i·o·gen·e·sis
   pl id·i·o·gen·e·ses
id·i·o·ge·net·ic
id·i·o·glos·si·a
id·i·o·glot·tic
id·i·o·gram
id·i·o·hyp·no·tism
id·i·o·la·li·a
id·i·ol·o·gism
id·i·o·me·tri·tis
id·i·o·mus·cu·lar
id·i·o·neu·ro·sis
id·i·o·pa·thet·ic
id·i·o·path·ic
id·i·o·path·i·cal·ly
id·i·op·a·thy
   pl id·i·op·a·thies
id·i·o·plasm
id·i·o·plas·mat·ic
id·i·o·psy·chol·o·gy
id·i·o·re·flex
id·i·o·ret·i·nal
id·i·o·some
id·i·o·spasm
id·i·o·spas·tic
id·i·o·syn·cra·cy
   pl id·i·o·syn·cra·cies
   or id·i·o·syn·cra·sy
   pl id·i·o·syn·cra·sies
id·i·o·syn·cra·sy
   or id·i·o·syn·cra·cy
   pl id·i·o·syn·cra·sies
   pl id·i·o·syn·cra·cies
id·i·o·syn·crat·ic
id·io·syn·cra·ti·cal·ly

id·i·ot
id·i·ot·ic
   or id·i·ot·i·cal
id·i·ot·i·cal
   id·i·ot·ic
id·i·ot·i·cal·ly
id·i·o·troph·ic
id·i·ot sa·vant
   pl id·i·ots sa·vants
   or id·i·ot sa·vants
id·i·o·ven·tric·u·lar
id·i·tol
i·do·lo·ma·ni·a
id·ose
i·dox·u·ri·dine
ig·na·ti·a
ig·ni·punc·ture
ig·ni·tion
il·e·ac
   or il·e·al
il·e·al
   or il·e·ac
il·e·ec·to·my
   pl il·e·ec·to·mies
il·e·it·ic
il·e·i·tis
   pl il·e·it·i·des
il·e·o·ap·pen·dic·u·lar
il·e·o·cae·cal
   var of il·e·o·ce·cal
il·e·o·cae·cos·to·my
   var of il·e·o·ce·cos·to·my
il·e·o·cae·cum
   var of il·e·o·ce·cum
il·e·o·ce·cal
il·e·o·ce·cos·to·my
   pl il·e·o·ce·cos·to·mies
il·e·o·ce·cum
   pl il·e·o·ce·ca
il·e·o·co·lic
il·e·o·co·li·tis
il·e·o·co·lon·ic
il·e·o·co·los·to·my
   pl il·e·o·co·los·to·mies
il·e·o·co·lot·o·my
il·e·o·cu·ta·ne·ous
il·e·o·cys·to·plas·ty
il·e·o·cys·tos·to·my
il·e·o·il·e·al

il·e·o·il·e·os·to·my
il·e·op·a·gus
   or il·i·op·a·gus
il·e·o·proc·tos·to·my
il·e·o·rec·tal
il·e·or·rha·phy
il·e·o·sig·moid·os·to·my
il·e·os·to·my
   pl il·e·os·to·mies
il·e·ot·o·my
il·e·o·trans·verse
il·e·o·trans·ver·sos·to·my
il·e·o·typh·li·tis
il·e·o·ves·i·cal
il·e·um
   pl il·e·a
il·e·us
il·i·ac
il·i·a·cus
   pl il·i·a·ci
il·i·a·del·phus
il·i·o·cap·su·lar·is
il·i·o·cap·su·lo·tro·chan·ter·i·cus
il·i·o·coc·cyg·e·al
il·i·o·coc·cyg·e·us
il·i·o·cos·ta·lis
il·i·o·cos·to·cer·vi·ca·lis
il·i·o·fem·o·ral
il·i·o·hy·po·gas·tric
il·i·o·in·gui·nal
il·i·o·lum·bar
il·i·op·a·gus
   or il·e·op·a·gus
il·i·o·par·a·si·tus
il·i·o·pec·tin·e·al
il·i·o·pso·as
il·i·o·pso·at·ic
il·i·o·pu·bic
il·i·o·sa·cra·lis
il·i·o·tho·ra·cop·a·gus
il·i·o·tib·i·al
il·i·o·tro·chan·ter·ic
il·i·o·xi·phop·a·gus
il·i·um
   pl il·i·a
ill
il·laq·ue·ate

il·laq·ue·a·tion
ill-bred
il·le·git·i·ma·cy
   pl il·le·git·i·ma·cies
il·le·git·a·mate
Il·lic·i·um
il·li·ni·tion
il·lin·i·um
ill·ness
il·lu·mi·nance
il·lu·mi·nate
il·lu·mi·na·tion
il·lu·mi·nism
il·lu·sion
il·lu·sion·al
il·lu·sion·ar·y
il·lu·so·ry
i·ma
im·age
im·ag·ery
   pl im·ag·er·ies
i·mag·i·nal
i·mag·i·nar·y
i·mag·i·na·tion
i·mag·i·na·tive
i·mag·ine
i·ma·go
   pl i·ma·goes
   or i·mag·i·nes
im·a·pun·ga
im·a·zine
im·bal·ance
im·be·cile
im·be·cil·ic
im·be·cil·i·ty
   pl im·be·cil·i·ties
im·bed
   or em·bed
im·bibe
im·bi·bi·tion
im·bri·cate
im·bri·ca·tion
im·i·daz·o·le
im·i·daz·o·line
im·i·daz·o·lyl
im·ide
i·mi·do
i·mid·o·line

im·i·naz·ole
im·ine
im·i·no
im·i·no·u·re·a
i·mip·ra·mine
im·i·tate
im·i·ta·tion
im·i·ta·tive
im·ma·ture
im·ma·tu·ri·ty
   pl im·ma·tu·ri·ties
im·me·di·ate
im·med·i·ca·ble
im·merse
im·mer·sion
im·mis·ci·ble
im·mis·ci·bly
im·mo·bil·i·ty
   pl im·mo·bil·i·ties
im·mo·bi·li·za·tion
im·mo·bi·lize
im·mor·tal
im·mor·tal·i·ty
   pl im·mor·tal·i·ties
im·mune
im·mu·ni·ty
   pl im·mu·ni·ties
im·mu·ni·fa·cient
im·mu·ni·ty
im·mu·ni·za·tion
im·mu·nize
im·mu·no·as·say
im·mu·no·as·say·a·ble
im·mu·no·bi·ol·o·gy
im·mu·no·blast
im·mu·no·chem·is·try
   pl im·mu·no·chem·is·tries
im·mu·no·com·pe·tence
im·mu·no·com·pe·tent
im·mu·no·con·glu·ti·nin
im·mu·no·cyte
im·mu·no·cy·to·chem·i·cal
im·mu·no·cy·to·chem·i·cal·ly
im·mu·no·cy·to·chem·is·try
   pl im·mu·no·cy·to·chem·is·tries

im·mu·no·de·fi·cien·cy
pl im·mu·no·de·fi·cien·cies
im·mu·no·dif·fu·sion
im·mu·no·e·lec·tro·pho·re·sis
pl im·mu·no·e·lec·tro·pho·re·ses
im·mu·no·e·lec·tro·pho·ret·ic
im·mu·no·e·lec·tro·pho·ret·i·cal·ly
im·mu·no·fer·ri·tin
im·mu·no·fil·tra·tion
im·mu·no·flu·o·res·cence
im·mu·no·flu·o·res·cent
im·mu·no·gen
im·mu·no·gen·e·sis
pl im·mu·no·gen·e·ses
im·mu·no·ge·net·ic
im·mu·no·ge·net·i·cal·ly
im·mu·no·ge·net·ics
im·mu·no·gen·ic
im·mu·no·gen·ic·i·ty
im·mu·no·glob·u·lin
im·mu·no·gran·u·lom·a·tous
im·mu·no·hae·ma·tol·o·gy
var of im·mu·no·he·ma·tol·o·gy
im·mu·no·he·ma·to·log·ic
or im·mu·no·he·ma·to·log·i·cal
im·mu·no·he·ma·to·log·i·cal
or im·mu·no·he·ma·to·log·ic
im·mu·no·he·ma·tol·o·gist
im·mu·no·he·ma·tol·o·gy
pl im·mu·no·he·ma·tol·o·gies
im·mu·no·he·mo·lyt·ic
im·mu·no·his·to·chem·i·cal
im·mu·no·his·to·chem·i·cal·ly
im·mu·no·his·to·chem·is·try
pl im·mu·no·his·to·chem·is·tries

im·mu·no·his·to·log·ic
im·mu·no·his·to·log·i·cal
im·mu·no·his·to·log·i·cal·ly
im·mu·no·his·tol·o·gy
pl im·mu·no·his·tol·o·gies
im·mu·no·log·ic
or im·mu·no·log·i·cal
im·mu·no·log·i·cal
or im·mu·no·log·ic
im·mu·no·log·i·cal·ly
im·mu·nol·o·gist
im·mu·nol·o·gy
pl im·mu·nol·o·gies
im·mu·no·path·o·log·ic
or im·mu·no·path·o·log·i·cal
im·mu·no·path·o·log·i·cal
or im·mu·no·path·o·log·ic
im·mu·no·pa·thol·o·gist
im·mu·no·pa·thol·o·gy
pl im·mu·no·pa·thol·o·gies
im·mu·no·pho·re·sis
im·mu·no·pre·cip·i·ta·tion
im·mun·o·pro·lif·er·a·tive
im·mu·no·re·ac·tive
im·mu·no·re·ac·tiv·i·ty
pl im·mu·no·re·ac·tiv·i·ties
im·mu·no·sor·bent
im·mu·no·sup·pres·sant
im·mu·no·sup·pres·sion
im·mu·no·sup·pres·sive
im·mu·no·sur·veil·lance
im·mu·no·ther·a·peu·tic
im·mu·no·ther·a·py
pl im·mu·no·ther·a·pies
im·mu·no·tox·in
im·mu·no·trans·fu·sion
im·pact·ed
im·pac·tion
im·pair·ment
im·pal·pa·ble
im·par
im·par·i·dig·i·tate
im·passe
im·pa·tent
im·ped·ance
im·ped·i·ment
im·per·ative

im·per·cep·ti·ble
im·per·cep·tion
im·per·fo·rate
im·per·fo·ra·tion
im·per·me·a·ble
im·per·me·a·bil·i·ty
pl im·per·me·a·bil·i·ties
im·per·me·a·bly
im·per·vi·ous
im·pe·tig·i·ni·za·tion
im·pe·tig·i·nized
im·pe·tig·i·noid
im·pe·tig·i·nous
im·pe·ti·go
im·pe·tus
im·ping·er
Im·plac·en·ta·li·a
im·plant
im·plan·ta·tion
im·po·tence
or im·po·ten·cy
im·po·ten·cy
pl im·po·ten·cies
or im·po·tence
im·po·tent
im·po·tent·ly
im·preg·nate
im·preg·na·tion
im·pres·si·o
pl im·pres·si·o·nes
im·pres·sion
im·pres·si·o·nes dig·i·ta·tae
im·print
im·print·ing
im·pro·cre·ance
im·pro·cre·ant
im·pu·ber·al
im·pu·bic
im·pulse
im·pul·sion
im·pul·sive
im·pu·ta·bil·i·ty
im·vic
in di·es
in ex·tre·mis
in si·tu
in u·te·ro
in vac·u·o

in vi·tro
in vi·vo
in·a·cid·i·ty
in·ac·tion
in·ac·ti·vate
in·ac·ti·va·tion
in·ac·tive
in·ac·tiv·i·ty
   pl in·ac·tiv·i·ties
in·ad·e·qua·cy
   pl in·ad·e·qua·cies
in·ad·e·quate
in·ad·e·quate·ly
in·al·i·men·tal
in·an·i·mate
in·a·ni·tion
in·ap·par·ent
in·ap·pe·tence
in·ar·tic·u·late
in·ar·tic·u·late·ly
in·ar·ti·cu·lo mor·tis
in·as·sim·i·la·ble
in·born
in·breathe
in·bred
in·breed
in·breed·er
In·ca bone
in·ca·nous
in·ca·pac·i·tant
in·ca·pac·i·tate
in·ca·pac·i·ta·tion
in·ca·pac·i·ta·tor
in·cap·a·ri·na
in·car·cer·ate
in·car·cer·a·tion
in·car·i·al
in·car·nant
in·car·na·tive
in·cen·di·ar·ism
in·cen·di·ar·y
   pl in·cen·di·ar·ies
in·cep·tion
in·cep·tus
in·cest
in·ces·tu·ous
in·ces·tu·ous·ly
in·ci·den·ce
in·ci·dent

in·ci·den·tal
in·cin·er·ate
in·cin·er·a·tion
in·cin·er·a·tor
in·cip·i·ence
in·cip·i·en·cy
in·cip·i·ent
in·ci·sal
in·cise
in·ci·sion
in·ci·sive
in·ci·si·vus
in·ci·so·la·bi·al
in·ci·so·lin·gual
in·ci·so·prox·i·mal
in·ci·sor
in·ci·su·ra
   pl in·ci·sur·rae
   or in·ci·sure
in·ci·su·rae
in·ci·su·ral
in·ci·sure
   or in·ci·su·ra
in·cli·na·ti·o
   pl in·cli·na·ti·o·nes
in·cli·na·tion
in·cline
in·cli·nom·e·ter
in·clu·sion
in·co·ag·u·la·bil·i·ty
in·co·ag·u·la·ble
in·co·her·ence
in·co·her·ent
in·com·pat·i·bil·i·ty
   pl in·com·pat·i·bil·i·ties
in·com·pat·i·ble
in·com·pat·i·bly
in·com·pen·sa·tion
in·com·pe·tence
in·com·pe·ten·cy
   pl in·com·pe·ten·cies
in·com·pe·tent
in·com·plete
in·con·gru·ence
in·con·gru·ent
in·con·gru·i·ty
in·con·stant
in·con·ti·nence
in·con·ti·nent

in·con·ti·nen·ti·a pig·men·ti
in·co·or·di·nate
in·co·or·di·na·tion
in·cor·po·rate
in·cor·po·ra·tion
in·co·sta·pe·di·al
in·cre·ment
in·cre·men·tal
in·cre·tion
in·cre·to·ry
in·cross
in·cross·bred
in·crust
   or en·crust
in·crus·ta·tion
   or en·crus·ta·tion
in·cu·bate
in·cu·ba·tion
in·cu·ba·tor
in·cu·bus
   pl in·cu·bus·es
   or in·cu·bi
in·cu·dal
in·cu·dec·to·my
in·cu·di·form
in·cu·do·mal·le·al
in·cu·do·sta·pe·di·al
in·cur·a·ble
in·cur·a·bly
in·cur·vate
in·cur·va·tion
in·cus
   pl in·cu·des
in·cy·clo·pho·ri·a
in·cy·clo·tro·pi·a
in·da·ga·tion
in·da·mine
in·de·cent
In·de·cid·u·a
in·de·ci·sion
in·dent
in·den·ta·tion
in·dex
   pl in·dex·es
   or in·di·ces
In·dex Med·i·cus
In·di·a ink meth·od
in·di·can

in·di·cant
in·di·ca·nu·ri·a
in·di·cate
in·di·ca·tion
in·di·ca·tor
in·do·co·phose
In·di·el·la
in·dif·fer·ent
in·dif·fer·ent·ism
in·dig·e·nous
in·di·ges·ti·bil·i·ty
   pl in·di·gest·i·bil·i·ties
in·di·gest·i·ble
in·di·ges·tion
in·dig·i·ta·tion
in·di·go
in·dig·o·tin
in·di·go·u·ri·a
in·di·rect
in·di·ru·bin
in·dis·crim·i·nate
in·dis·crim·i·nate·ly
in·dis·posed
in·dis·po·si·tion
in·di·um
in·di·vid·u·al·i·za·tion
in·di·vid·u·al·ize
in·di·vid·u·a·tion
in·do·cy·a·nine green
in·dol·ac·e·tu·ri·a
in·dole
in·dole·a·ce·tic
in·dole·bu·tyr·ic
in·do·lence
in·do·lent
in·dole·pro·pi·on·ic
in·dole·py·ru·vic
in·do·log·e·nous
in·do·lu·ri·a
in·do·lyl·a·cryl·o·yl·gly·
   cine
in·do·lyl·a·cryl·o·yl·gly·ci·
   nu·ri·a
in·do·meth·a·cin
in·do·phe·nol
in·dox·ole
in·dox·yl
in·dox·y·log·e·nous
in·dox·yl·sul·fate

in·dox·yl·sul·fu·ric
in·dox·yl·u·ri·a
in·dri·line
in·duce
in·duc·er
in·duc·i·ble
in·duc·tance
in·duc·tion
in·duc·tive
in·duc·to·py·rex·i·a
in·duc·tor
in·duc·to·ri·um
in·duc·to·ther·my
   pl in·duc·to·ther·mies
in·du·lin
   or in·du·line
in·du·line
   or in·du·lin
in·du·rate
in·du·ra·tion
in·du·ra·tive
in·du·si·um
   pl in·du·si·a
in·du·si·um gris·e·um
in·dwell·ing
in·e·bri·ant
in·e·bri·ate
in·e·bri·a·tion
in·e·bri·e·ty
   pl in·e·bri·e·ties
in·ef·fi·ca·cious
in·ef·fi·ca·cy
in·e·las·tic
in·ert
in·er·tia
   pl in·er·tias
   or in·er·ti·ae
in·fan·cy
   pl in·fan·cies
in·fant
in·fan·ti·cide
in·fan·tile
in·fan·til·ism
in·farct
in·farc·tec·to·my
in·farct·ed
in·farc·tion
in·fect
in·fec·tion

in·fec·tious
in·fec·tious·ly
in·fec·tive
in·fec·tiv·i·ty
   pl in·fec·tiv·i·ties
in·fe·cun·di·ty
   pl in·fe·cun·di·ties
in·fe·ri·or
in·fe·ri·or·i·ty
   pl in·fe·ri·or·i·ties
in·fe·ro·lat·er·al
in·fe·ro·me·di·al
in·fe·ro·pa·ri·e·tal
in·fe·ro·pos·te·ri·or
in·fer·tile
in·fer·til·i·ty
   pl in·fer·til·i·ties
in·fest
in·fes·ta·tion
in·fes·tive
in·fib·u·la·tion
in·fil·trate
in·fil·tra·tion
in·fin·i·ty
in·firm
in·fir·ma·ry
   pl in·fir·ma·ries
in·fir·mi·ty
   pl in·fir·mi·ties
in·flame
in·flam·ma·ble
in·flam·ma·tion
in·flam·ma·to·ry
in·flate
in·fla·ter
   or in·fla·tor
in·fla·tion
in·fla·tor
   or in·fla·ter
in·flec·tion
in·flex·ion
   var of in·flec·tion
in·flo·res·cence
in·flu·en·za
in·flu·en·zal
in·fold
in·foot·ed
in·fra·al·ve·o·lar
in·fra·au·ric·u·lar

in·fra·ax·il·lar·y
in·fra·bo·ny
in·fra·bulge
in·fra·car·di·ac
in·fra·cla·vic·u·lar
in·fra·cla·vic·u·lar·is
in·fra·cli·noid
in·fra·clu·sion
in·fra·con·dy·lism
in·fra·cos·tal
in·frac·tion
in·fra·den·ta·le
in·fra·di·a·phrag·mat·ic
in·fra·gle·noid
in·fra·glot·tic
in·fra·gran·u·lar
in·fra·hy·oid
in·fra·mam·ma·ry
in·fra·mar·gin·al
in·fra·max·il·lar·y
in·fra·na·sal
in·fra·na·tant
in·fra·nu·cle·ar
in·fra·oc·clu·sion
in·fra·or·bit·al
in·fra·pa·tel·lar
in·fra·phys·i·o·log·ic
in·fra·place·ment
in·fra·red
in·fra·roent·gen
in·fra·scap·u·lar
in·fra·son·ic
in·fra·spi·na·tus
    pl in·fra·spi·na·ti
in·fra·spi·nous
in·fra·ster·nal
in·fra·tem·po·ral
in·fra·tem·po·ra·le
in·fra·ten·to·ri·al
in·fra·troch·le·ar
in·fra·um·bil·i·cal
in·fra·vag·i·nal
in·fra·ver·sion
in·fra·ves·i·cal
in·fra·zy·go·mat·ic
in·fric·tion
in·fun·dib·u·lar
in·fun·dib·u·li·form

in·fun·dib·u·lo·ma
    pl in·fun·dib·u·lo·mas
    or in·fun·dib·u·lo·ma·ta
in·fun·dib·u·lo·pel·vic
in·fun·dib·u·lo·ven·tric·u·lar
in·fun·dib·u·lum
    pl in·fun·dib·u·la
in·fuse
in·fus·i·ble
in·fu·sion
In·fu·so·ri·a
in·fu·so·ri·al
in·fu·so·ri·an
in·gest
in·ges·ta
in·ges·tant
in·gest·i·ble
in·ges·tion
in·ges·tive
in·glu·vi·es
    pl in·glu·vi·es
In·gras·si·a wings
in·gra·ves·cent
in·gre·di·ent
in·grow·ing
in·grown
in·growth
in·guen
    pl in·gui·na
in·gui·nal
in·gui·no·cru·ral
in·gui·no·dyn·i·a
in·gui·no·la·bi·al
in·gui·no·scro·tal
in·hal·ant
in·ha·la·tion
in·ha·la·tor
in·hale
in·hal·er
in·her·ent
in·her·ent·ly
in·her·it
in·her·it·a·bil·i·ty
    pl in·her·it·a·bil·i·ties
in·her·it·a·ble
in·her·i·tance
in·hib·in
in·hib·it

in·hib·i·ter
    or in·hib·i·tor
in·hi·bi·tion
in·hib·i·tive
in·hib·i·tor
    or in·hib·i·ter
in·hib·i·to·ry
in·ho·mo·ge·ne·i·ty
    pl in·ho·mo·ge·ne·i·ties
in·ho·mo·ge·ne·ous
in·i·ac
    or in·i·al
in·i·al
    or in·i·ac
in·i·en·ceph·a·lus
in·i·en·ceph·a·ly
in·i·od·y·mus
in·i·on
in·i·op·a·gus
in·i·ops
i·ni·tial
i·ni·ti·a·tor
i·ni·tis
in·ject
in·ject·a·ble
in·jec·tant
in·jec·ted
in·jec·tion
in·jec·tor
in·jure
in·ju·ri·ous
in·ju·ry
    pl in·ju·ries
ink·blot
in·lay
in·let
in·ly·ing
in·nate
in·ner ear
in·ner-di·rect·ed
in·ner·vate
in·ner·va·tion
in·ner·va·tion·al
in·nid·i·a·tion
in·no·cent
in·noc·u·ous
in·nom·i·nate
in·nox·ious
in·nu·tri·tion

192

o·blast
oc·ci·pit·i·a
o·chon·dri·tis
oc·u·la·bil·i·ty
oc·u·la·ble
oc·u·lant
oc·u·late
oc·u·la·tion
oc·u·la·tive
oc·u·la·tor
oc·u·lum
pl in·oc·u·la
o·cyte
o·gen
o·gen·e·sis
og·e·nous
og·li·a
o·kom·ma
op·er·a·ble
or·gan·ic
or·gan·i·cal·ly
o·sae·mi·a
var of in·o·se·mi·a
os·co·py
os·cu·late
os·cu·la·tion
ose
o·se·mi·a
o·sine
o·sin·ic
no·si·tol
no·si·tol·hex·a·phos·phor·
ic
o·si·tu·ri·a
o·su·ri·a
o·trop·ic
pa·tient
put
quest
qui·line
sal·i·vate
sal·i·va·tion
sa·lu·bri·ous
sa·lu·bri·ty
pl in·sa·lu·bri·ties
sane
sane·ly
sane·ness
san·i·tar·y

in·san·i·ta·tion
in·san·i·ty
pl in·san·i·ties
in·scrip·ti·o
pl in·scrip·ti·o·nes
in·scrip·tion
in·sect
In·sec·ta
in·sec·ti·ci·dal
in·sec·ti·cid·al·ly
in·sec·ti·cide
in·sec·ti·fuge
in·se·cure
in·se·cure·ly
in·se·cu·ri·ty
pl in·se·cu·ri·ties
in·sem·in·ate
in·sem·i·na·tion
in·sen·si·bil·i·ty
in·sen·si·ble
in·sen·si·bly
in·ser·tion
in·sheathe
or en·sheathe
in·sid·i·ous
in·sight
in·sip·id
in·so·bri·e·ty
pl in·so·bri·e·ties
in·so·la·tion
in·sol·u·bil·i·ty
pl in·sol·u·bil·i·ties
in·sol·u·ble
in·som·ni·a
in·som·ni·ac
in·sorp·tion
in·spec·tion
in·sper·sion
in·spi·ra·tion
in·spi·ra·tor
in·spi·ra·to·ry
in·spire
in·spi·rom·e·ter
in·spis·sate
in·spis·sa·tion
in·spis·sa·tor
in·sta·bil·i·ty
pl in·sta·bil·i·ties
in·stance

in·star
in·step
in·stil
or in·still
in·still
or in·stil
in·stil·la·tion
in·stil·la·tor
in·stinct
in·stinc·tive
in·stinc·tive·ly
in·stinc·tu·al
in·sti·tutes
in·stru·ment
in·stru·men·tal
in·stru·men·tar·i·um
pl in·stru·men·tar·i·a
in·stru·men·ta·tion
in·su·date
in·su·da·tion
in·suf·fi·cien·cy
pl in·suf·fi·cien·cies
in·suf·fi·cient
in·suf·fi·cient·ly
in·suf·flate
in·suf·fla·tion
in·suf·fla·tor
in·su·la
pl in·su·lae
in·su·lar
in·su·late
in·su·la·tion
in·su·la·tor
in·su·lin
in·su·li·nae·mi·a
var of in·su·li·ne·mi·a
in·su·li·nase
in·su·li·ne·mi·a
in·su·li·no·gen·e·sis
in·su·li·no·ma
pl in·su·li·no·mas
or in·su·li·no·ma·ta
in·su·li·tis
in·su·lo·ma
pl in·su·lo·mas
or in·su·lo·ma·ta
in·sult
in·sus·cep·ti·bil·i·ty
pl in·sus·cep·ti·bil·i·ties

in·sus·cep·ti·ble
in·tact
in·te·grate
in·te·gra·tion
in·teg·ri·ty
   pl in·teg·ri·ties
in·teg·u·ment
in·teg·u·men·tal
   or in·teg·u·men·ta·ry
in·teg·u·men·ta·ry
   or in·teg·u·men·tal
in·teg·u·men·tum
in·tel·lect
in·tel·lec·tu·al
in·tel·lec·tu·al·i·za·tion
in·tel·lec·tu·al·ize
in·tel·li·gence
in·tel·li·gence quo·tient
in·tel·li·gent
in·tem·per·ance
in·tem·per·ate
in·tem·per·ate·ly
in·tem·per·ate·ness
in·tense
in·ten·si·fi·ca·tion
in·ten·si·fy
in·ten·sim·e·ter
in·ten·sive
in·ten·tion
in·ten·tion·al
in·ter·ac·ces·so·ry
in·ter·ac·i·nar
   or in·ter·ac·i·nous
in·ter·ac·i·nous
   or in·ter·ac·i·nar
in·ter·al·ve·o·lar
in·ter·an·nu·lar
in·ter·ar·tic·u·lar
in·ter·ar·y·te·noid
in·ter·ar·y·te·noi·de·us
in·ter·a·tri·al
in·ter·ax·o·nal
in·ter·blink
in·ter·bod·y
in·ter·brain
in·ter·breed
in·ter·ca·la·ry

in·ter·ca·late
in·ter·can·a·lic·u·lar
in·ter·cap·il·lar·y
in·ter·ca·rot·id
in·ter·car·pal
in·ter·car·ti·lag·i·nous
in·ter·cav·er·nous
in·ter·cel·lu·lar
in·ter·cen·tral
in·ter·ce·re·bral
in·ter·chon·dral
in·ter·cil·i·um
in·ter·cla·vi·cle
in·ter·cla·vic·u·lar
in·ter·cli·noid
in·ter·coc·cyg·e·al
in·ter·co·lum·nal
   or in·ter·co·lum·nar
in·ter·co·lum·nar
   or in·ter·co·lum·nal
in·ter·con·dy·lar
in·ter·con·dy·loid
in·ter·cor·o·nar·y
in·ter·cos·tal
in·ter·cos·tal·ly
in·ter·cos·to·bra·chi·al
in·ter·cou·pler
in·ter·course
in·ter·cri·co·thy·rot·o·my
in·ter·cris·tal
in·ter·cross
in·ter·cru·ral
in·ter·cur·rent
in·ter·cus·pa·tion
in·ter·cusp·ing
in·ter·den·tal
in·ter·den·ti·um
in·ter·dic·tion
in·ter·dig·i·tal
in·ter·dig·i·tate
in·ter·dig·i·ta·tion
in·ter·dis·ci·pli·nar·y
in·ter·duc·tal
in·ter·face
in·ter·fa·cial
in·ter·fas·cic·u·lar
in·ter·fem·o·ral
in·ter·fere

in·ter·fer·ence
in·ter·fer·o·gen·e·sis
in·ter·fe·rom·e·ter
in·ter·fer·o·met·ric
in·ter·fer·o·met·ri·cal·ly
in·ter·fe·rom·e·try
   pl in·ter·fe·rom·e·tries
in·ter·fer·on
in·ter·fer·on·o·gen
in·ter·fer·tile
in·ter·fer·til·i·ty
   pl in·ter·fer·til·i·ties
in·ter·fi·bril·lar
in·ter·fi·lar
in·ter·fol·lic·u·lar
in·ter·fo·ve·o·lar
in·ter·fron·tal
in·ter·fur·ca
   pl in·ter·fur·cae
in·ter·gem·mal
in·ter·glob·u·lar
in·ter·glu·te·al
in·ter·go·ni·al
in·ter·grade
in·ter·he·mal
in·ter·hem·i·sphe·ric
in·ter·ic·tal
in·te·ri·or
in·ter·ja·cent
in·ter·ki·ne·sis
   pl in·ter·ki·ne·ses
in·ter·la·bi·al
in·ter·la·mel·lar
in·ter·lam·i·nar
in·ter·lig·a·men·ta·ry
in·ter·lig·a·men·tous
In·ter·lin·gua
in·ter·lo·bar
in·ter·lo·bi·tis
in·ter·lob·u·lar
in·ter·mam·ma·ry
in·ter·mar·riage
in·ter·max·il·la
   pl in·ter·max·il·las
   or in·ter·max·il·lae
in·ter·max·il·lar·y
in·ter·med·i·ar·y
in·ter·me·di·ate

in·ter·me·din
in·ter·me·di·o·lat·er·al
in·ter·me·di·o·me·di·al
in·ter·me·di·us
in·ter·mem·bra·nous
in·ter·men·in·ge·al
in·ter·men·stru·al
in·ter·ment
in·ter·mes·o·blas·tic
in·ter·met·a·car·pal
in·ter·met·a·mer·ic
in·ter·met·a·tar·sal
in·ter·mi·cel·lar
in·ter·mis·sion
in·ter·mi·tot·ic
in·ter·mit·tence
in·ter·mit·ten·cy
   pl in·ter·mit·ten·cies
in·ter·mit·tent
in·ter·mu·ral
in·ter·mus·cu·lar
in·tern
in·ter·nal
in·ter·nal·i·za·tion
in·ter·nal·ize
in·ter·nar·i·al
in·ter·na·sal
in·ter·na·tal
in·ter·na·tion·al u·nit
in·terne
   var of in·tern
in·ter·neu·ral
in·ter·neu·ron
   or in·ter·neu·rone
in·ter·neu·ro·nal
in·ter·neu·rone
   or in·ter·neu·ron
in·ter·nist
in·ter·no·dal
in·ter·node
in·tern·ship
in·ter·nu·cle·ar
in·ter·nun·ci·al
in·ter·nus
in·ter·oc·clu·sal
in·ter·o·cep·tive
in·ter·o·cep·tor
in·ter·o·fec·tion

in·ter·o·fec·tive
in·ter·o·ges·tate
in·ter·ol·i·var·y
in·ter·or·bi·tal
in·ter·os·se·us
   pl in·ter·os·se·i
in·ter·pal·a·tine
in·ter·pal·pe·bral
in·ter·pap·il·lar·y
in·ter·pa·ri·e·tal
in·ter·par·ox·ys·mal
in·ter·pe·dun·cu·lar
in·ter·pel·vi·o·ab·dom·i·nal
in·ter·per·son·al
in·ter·pha·lan·ge·al
in·ter·phase
in·ter·pha·sic
in·ter·plant
in·ter·plas·mic
in·ter·pleu·ral
in·ter·po·late
in·ter·po·la·tion
in·ter·pose
in·ter·po·si·tion
in·ter·pre·ta·tion
in·ter·pris·mat·ic
in·ter·prox·i·mal
   or in·ter·prox·i·mate
in·ter·prox·i·mate
   or in·ter·prox·i·mal
in·ter·pu·bic
in·ter·pu·pil·lar·y
in·ter·py·ram·i·dal
in·ter·ra·di·al
in·ter·ra·dic·u·lar
in·ter·re·nal
in·ter·re·tic·u·lar
in·ter·scap·u·lar
in·ter·scap·u·lo·tho·rac·ic
in·ter·sect
in·ter·sec·ti·o
   pl in·ter·sec·ti·o·nes
in·ter·sec·ti·o·nes ten·din·
   e·ae
in·ter·sec·tion
in·ter·seg·men·tal
in·ter·sen·so·ry
in·ter·sep·tal

in·ter·sep·to·val·vu·lar
in·ter·sex
in·ter·sex·u·al
in·ter·sex·u·al·ism
in·ter·sex·u·al·i·ty
   pl in·ter·sex·u·al·i·ties
in·ter·sex·u·al·ly
in·ter·sig·moid
in·ter·space
in·ter·sphe·noid
in·ter·spi·nal
   or in·ter·spi·nous
in·ter·spi·na·lis
   pl in·ter·spi·na·les
in·ter·spi·nous
   or in·ter·spi·nal
in·ter·stage
in·ter·ster·ile
in·ter·ste·ril·i·ty
   pl in·ter·ste·ril·i·ties
in·ter·sti·cial
   or in·ter·sti·tial
in·ter·stice
   pl in·ter·stic·es
in·ter·sti·tial
   or in·ter·sti·cial
in·ter·sti·ti·o·ma
   pl in·ter·sti·ti·o·mas
   or in·ter·sti·ti·o·ma·ta
in·ter·sti·ti·o·spi·nal
in·ter·sti·ti·um
   pl in·ter·sti·tia
in·ter·sub·car·di·nal
in·ter·sys·tol·ic
in·ter·tar·sal
in·ter·ter·ri·to·ri·al
in·ter·tho·rac·i·co·scap·u·
   lar
in·ter·tra·gic
in·ter·trans·ver·sa·les
in·ter·trans·ver·sar·i·i
in·ter·trans·ver·sa·lis
in·ter·trans·verse
in·ter·tri·gem·i·nal
in·ter·trig·i·nous
in·ter·tri·go
in·ter·tro·chan·ter·ic
in·ter·tu·ber·al

in·ter·tu·ber·cu·lar
in·ter·tu·bu·lar
in·ter·u·re·ter·al
in·ter·u·re·ter·ic
in·ter·vag·i·nal
in·ter·val
in·ter·val·vu·lar
in·ter·vas·cu·lar
in·ter·ve·nous
in·ter·ven·tion
in·ter·ven·tric·u·lar
in·ter·ver·te·bral
in·ter·vil·lous
in·ter·zo·nal
in·tes·ti·nal
in·tes·ti·nal·ly
in·tes·tine
in·tes·ti·num
   pl in·tes·ti·na
in·ti·ma
   pl in·ti·mas
   or in·ti·mae
in·ti·mal
in·ti·mec·to·my
in·ti·mi·tis
in·tine
in·toed
in·toe·ing
in·tol·er·ance
in·tor·sion
   or in·tor·tion
in·tort
in·tort·er
in·tor·tion
   or in·tor·sion
in·tox·i·cant
in·tox·i·cate
in·tox·i·ca·tion
in·tra vi·tam
in·tra·ab·dom·i·nal
in·tra·ac·i·nar
in·tra·al·ve·o·lar
in·tra·ar·te·ri·al
in·tra·ar·te·ri·al·ly
in·tra·ar·tic·u·lar
in·tra·a·tri·al
in·tra·bron·chi·al
in·tra·bron·chi·o·lar
in·tra·cal·y·ce·al

in·tra·can·a·lic·u·lar
in·tra·cap·su·lar
in·tra·car·di·ac
in·tra·car·di·al·ly
in·tra·car·ti·lag·i·nous
in·tra·cav·er·nous
in·tra·cav·i·tar·y
in·tra·cel·lu·lar
in·tra·cer·e·bel·lar
in·tra·cer·e·bral
in·tra·cer·vi·cal
in·tra·cho·ri·on·ic
in·tra·cho·roi·dal
in·tra·cis·ter·nal
in·tra·cis·ter·nal·ly
in·tra·cor·ne·al
in·tra·cor·pus·cu·lar
in·tra·cra·ni·al
in·tra·cra·ni·al·ly
in·trac·ta·ble
in·tra·cu·ta·ne·ous
in·tra·cu·tic·u·lar
in·tra·cys·tic
in·tra·cy·to·plas·mic
in·tra·der·mal
   or in·tra·der·mic
in·tra·der·mic
   or in·tra·der·mal
in·tra·duc·tal
in·tra·du·ral
in·tra·em·bry·on·ic
in·tra·ep·i·der·mal
in·tra·ep·i·the·li·al
in·tra·e·ryth·ro·cyt·ic
in·tra·e·soph·a·ge·al
in·tra·fa·cial
in·tra·fas·cic·u·lar
in·tra·fu·sal
in·tra·gem·mal
in·tra·ge·ner·ic
in·tra·gen·ic
in·tra·glu·te·al
in·tra·group
   or in·tra·group·al
in·tra·group·al
   or in·tra·group
in·tra·he·pat·ic
in·tra·jug·u·lar
in·tra·lam·i·nar

in·tra·le·sion·al
in·tra·lig·a·men·ta·ry
in·tra·lig·a·men·tous
in·tra·lo·bar
in·tra·lob·u·lar
in·tra·lu·mi·nal
in·tra·mam·ma·ry
in·tra·med·ul·lar·y
in·tra·mem·bra·nous
in·tra·men·stru·al
in·tra·mo·lec·u·lar
in·tra·mu·co·sal
in·tra·mu·ral
in·tra·mus·cu·lar
in·tra·my·o·car·di·al
in·tra·my·o·me·tri·al
in·tra·na·sal
in·tra·na·tal
in·tra·neu·ral
in·tra·nu·cle·ar
in·tra·oc·u·lar
in·tra·op·er·a·tive
in·tra·op·er·a·tive·ly
in·tra·op·tic
in·tra·o·ral
in·tra·or·bit·al
in·tra·pan·cre·at·ic
in·tra·pa·ren·chy·mal
in·tra·pa·ri·e·tal
in·tra·par·tum
in·tra·pel·vic
in·tra·per·i·car·di·ac
in·tra·per·i·car·di·al
in·tra·per·i·to·ne·al
in·tra·pha·lan·ge·al
in·tra·pi·al
in·tra·pleu·ral
in·tra·psy·chic
   or in·tra·psy·chi·cal
in·tra·psy·chi·cal
   or in·tra·psy·chic
in·tra·pul·mo·nar·y
in·tra·pul·mon·ic
in·tra·re·nal
in·tra·scap·u·lar
in·tra·scle·ral
in·tra·scro·tal
in·tra·seg·men·tal
in·tra·sel·lar

in·tra·spi·nal
in·tra·spi·nous
in·tra·sple·nic
in·tra·ster·nal
in·tra·stro·mal
in·tra·syn·o·vi·al
in·tra·the·cal
in·tra·tho·rac·ic
in·tra·ton·sil·lar
in·tra·tra·che·al
in·tra·tro·chan·ter·ic
in·tra·tu·bal
in·tra·tu·bu·lar
in·tra·tym·pan·ic
in·tra·um·bil·i·cal
in·tra·u·re·ter·al
in·tra·u·re·thral
in·tra·u·ter·ine
in·tra·vag·i·nal
in·trav·a·sate
in·trav·a·sa·tion
in·tra·vas·cu·lar
in·tra·vas·cu·lar·ly
in·tra·ve·nous
in·tra·ve·nous·ly
in·tra·ven·tric·u·lar
in·tra·ver·te·bral
in·tra·ves·i·cal
in·tra·vi·tal
in·tra·vi·tel·line
in·tra·vit·re·ous
in·trin·sic
in·trin·si·cal·ly
in·trin·si·coid
in·tro·ces·sion
in·tro·fi·er
in·tro·flex·ion
in·troi·tal
in·troi·tus
   pl in·troi·tus
in·tro·ject
in·tro·jec·tion
in·tro·mis·sion
in·tro·mit·tent
in·tro·spect
in·tro·spec·tion
in·tro·spec·tive
in·tro·sus·cep·tion
in·tro·ver·sion

in·tro·ver·sive
in·tro·vert
in·trude
in·tu·bate
in·tu·ba·tion
in·tu·ba·tor
in·tu·i·tion
in·tu·i·tive
in·tu·mesce
in·tu·mes·cence
in·tu·mes·cent
in·tu·mes·cen·ti·a
   pl in·tu·mes·cen·ti·ae
in·tus·sus·cept
in·tus·sus·cep·tion
in·tus·sus·cep·tum
   pl in·tus·sus·cep·ta
in·tus·sus·cip·i·ens
   pl in·tus·sus·cip·i·en·tes
in·u·la
in·u·lase
   or in·u·lin·ase
in·u·lin
in·u·lin·ase
   or in·u·lase
in·unc·tion
in·vade
in·vad·er
in·vag·i·nate
in·vag·i·na·tion
in·va·lid
in·va·lid·ism
in·va·sin
in·va·sion
in·va·sive
in·va·sive·ness
in·ven·to·ry
in·verse
in·ver·sion
in·ver·sive
in·vert
in·ver·tase
in·ver·te·bral
In·ver·te·bra·ta
in·ver·te·brate
in·vert·ed
in·ver·tin
in·ver·tor
in·ver·tose

in·vest
in·vest·ment
in·vet·er·ate
in·vi·a·bil·i·ty
   pl in·vi·a·bil·i·ties
in·vi·a·ble
in·vi·ril·i·ty
in·vis·ca·tion
in·vo·lu·cre
in·vo·lu·crum
   pl in·vo·lu·cra
in·vol·un·tar·y
in·vo·lute
in·vo·lu·tion
in·vo·lu·tion·al
i·o·ben·zam·ic
i·o·ce·tam·ic
i·o·da·mide
I·o·da·moe·ba
i·o·date
i·od·ic
i·o·dide
i·o·dim·e·try
   pl i·o·dim·e·tries
   or i·o·dom·e·try
   pl i·o·dom·e·tries
i·o·din
   or i·o·dine
i·o·di·nate
i·o·di·na·tion
i·o·dine
   or io·din
i·od·i·nin
i·o·din·o·phil
   or i·o·din·oph·i·lous
i·o·din·o·phil·i·a
i·o·din·o·phil·ic
i·o·din·oph·i·lous
   or i·o·din·o·phil
i·o·dip·a·mide
i·o·dism
i·o·dize
i·o·do·ac·e·tate
i·o·do·a·ce·tic
i·o·do·al·phi·on·ic
i·o·do·ca·sein
i·o·do·chlor·hy·drox·y·quin
i·o·do·der·ma
i·o·do·form

i·o·do·glob·u·lin
i·o·do·gor·go·ic
i·o·do·meth·a·mate
i·o·do·met·ric
i·o·dom·e·try
    pl i·o·dom·e·tries
    or i·o·dim·e·try
    pl i·o·dim·o·tries
i·o·do·pa·no·ic
i·o·do·phe·nol
i·o·do·phil
i·o·do·phile
i·o·do·phil·i·a
i·o·do·phil·ic
i·o·do·phor
i·o·do·phthal·ein
i·o·do·pro·te·in
i·o·dop·sin
i·o·do·pyr·a·cet
i·o·do·ther·a·py
i·o·do·thy·mol
i·o·do·thy·ro·glob·u·lin
i·o·dox·yl
i·o·dum
i·o·gly·cam·ic
i·om·e·ter
i·on
i·on ex·change
i·on ex·chang·er
i·on·ic
i·o·ni·um
i·on·i·za·tion
i·on·ize
i·on·om·e·ter
i·o·none
i·on·o·phose
i·o·no·ther·a·py
i·on·to·pho·re·sis
    pl i·on·to·pho·re·ses
i·on·to·pho·ret·ic
i·o·pa·no·ic
i·o·phen·dy·late
i·o·phen·ox·ic
i·o·pho·bi·a
i·o·py·dol
i·o·py·done
i·o·se·fam·ic
i·o·ta·cism
i·o·thal·a·mate

i·o·tha·lam·ic
i·o·thi·o·u·ra·cil
ip·e·cac
    or ip·e·ca·cu·a·rha
ip·e·ca·cu·a·rha
    or ip·e·cac
ip·o·me·a
ip·o·moe·a
    var of ip·o·me·a
i·prin·dole
i·pro·ni·a·zid
i·pro·nid·a·zole
ip·sa·tion
ip·si·lat·er·al
    or ip·so·lat·er·al
ip·si·lat·er·al·ly
ip·si·ver·sive
ip·so·lat·er·al
    or ip·si·lat·er·al
i·ral·gi·a
i·ras·ci·bil·i·ty
ir·i·dae·mi·a
    var of ir·i·de·mi·a
i·ri·dal
i·ri·dal·gi·a
ir·id·aux·e·sis
ir·id·a·vul·sion
ir·i·dec·tome
ir·i·dec·to·mize
ir·i·dec·to·my
    pl ir·i·dec·to·mies
ir·i·dec·tro·pi·um
ir·i·de·mi·a
ir·i·den·clei·sis
    pl ir·i·den·clei·ses
ir·i·den·tro·pi·um
ir·i·de·re·mi·a
ir·i·des·cence
ir·i·des·cent
i·rid·e·sis
ir·i·di·ag·no·sis
i·rid·i·al
i·rid·i·an
i·rid·ic
ir·i·din
i·rid·i·um
ir·i·di·za·tion
ir·i·do·a·vul·sion
ir·i·do·cap·su·li·tis

ir·i·do·cap·su·lot·o·my
i·rid·o·cele
ir·i·do·cho·roi·di·tis
ir·i·do·col·o·bo·ma
ir·i·do·con·stric·tor
ir·i·do·cor·ne·al
ir·i·do·cy·clec·to·my
    pl ir·i·do·cy·clec·to·mies
ir·i·do·cy·cli·tis
ir·i·do·cy·clo·cho·roi·di·tis
ir·i·do·cys·tec·to·my
    pl ir·i·do·cys·tec·to·mies
i·rid·o·cyte
ir·i·dod·e·sis
ir·i·do·di·ag·no·sis
ir·i·do·di·al·y·sis
    pl ir·i·do·di·al·y·ses
ir·i·do·di·la·tor
ir·i·do·do·ne·sis
    pl ir·i·do·do·ne·ses
ir·i·do·ker·a·ti·tis
ir·i·do·ki·ne·si·a
ir·i·do·ki·ne·sis
ir·i·do·lep·tyn·sis
i·ri·dol·o·gy
ir·i·do·ma·la·ci·a
ir·i·do·me·so·di·al·y·sis
ir·i·do·mo·tor
ir·id·on·co·sis
ir·i·don·cus
ir·i·do·pa·ral·y·sis
ir·i·do·pa·re·sis
ir·i·dop·a·thy
ir·i·do·per·i·pha·ki·tis
ir·i·do·plat·i·num
ir·i·do·ple·gi·a
ir·i·dop·to·sis
    pl ir·i·dop·to·ses
ir·i·do·pu·pil·lar·y
ir·i·dor·rhex·is
    pl ir·i·do·rhex·es
    or ir·i·dor·rhex·is
ir·i·dor·rhex·is
    pl ir·i·do·rhex·es
    or ir·i·do·rhex·is
ir·i·dos·chi·sis
    pl ir·i·dos·chi·ses
ir·i·do·schis·ma

ir·i·do·scle·rot·o·my
   pl ir·i·do·scle·rot·o·mies
ir·i·do·ste·re·sis
ir·i·dot·a·sis
   pl ir·i·dot·a·ses
ir·i·do·tome
ir·i·dot·o·my
ir·i·dot·ro·mos
i·ris
   pl i·ri·des
i·ri·sin
i·ri·tis
ir·i·to·ec·to·my
ir·it·o·my
ir·i·um
i·ron
i·rot·o·my
ir·ra·di·ate
ir·ra·di·a·tion
ir·ra·tion·al
ir·ra·tion·al·i·ty
   pl ir·ra·tion·al·i·ties
ir·ra·tion·al·ly
ir·re·duc·i·bil·i·ty
   pl ir·re·duc·i·bil·i·ties
ir·re·duc·i·ble
ir·reg·u·lar
ir·reg·u·lar·i·ty
   pl ir·reg·u·lar·i·ties
ir·re·me·a·ble
ir·re·me·di·a·ble
ir·re·spir·a·ble
ir·re·sus·ci·ta·ble
ir·re·ver·si·bil·i·ty
ir·re·ver·si·ble
ir·ri·gate
ir·ri·ga·tion
ir·ri·ga·tor
ir·ri·ta·bil·i·ty
   pl ir·ri·ta·bil·i·ties
ir·ri·ta·ble
ir·ri·tant
ir·ri·tate
ir·ri·ta·tion
ir·ri·ta·tive
ir·ru·ma·tion
I·saac gran·ules
i·sa·del·phi·a
I·sam·bert dis·ease

i·sa·tin
is·aux·e·sis
   pl is·aux·e·ses
is·aux·et·ic
is·chae·mi·a
   var of is·che·mi·a
is·chae·mic
   var of is·che·mic
is·che·mi·a
is·che·mic
is·che·sis
is·chi·ad·ic
is·chi·al
is·chi·al·gi·a
is·chi·al·gic
is·chi·at·ic
is·chi·a·ti·tis
is·chi·dro·sis
is·chi·drot·ic
is·chi·ec·to·my
is·chi·o·bul·bar
is·chi·o·bul·bo·sus
is·chi·o·cap·su·lar
is·chi·o·cav·er·no·sus
is·chi·o·cav·er·nous
is·chi·o·cele
is·chi·o·coc·cyg·e·al
is·chi·o·coc·cyg·e·us
   pl is·chi·o·coc·cyg·e·i
is·chi·o·did·y·mus
is·chi·o·dyn·i·a
is·chi·o·fem·o·ral
is·chi·o·fem·o·ral·is
is·chi·o·pu·bi·cus
is·chi·o·pu·bi·ot·o·my
is·chi·o·pu·bis
is·chi·o·rec·tal
is·chi·um
   pl is·chi·a
isch·no·pho·ni·a
is·cho·ga·lac·ti·a
is·cho·ga·lac·tic
is·cho·gy·ri·a
is·cho·me·ni·a
is·chu·ri·a
i·sei·kon·ic
i·se·thi·o·nate
i·se·thi·on·ic
Ish·i·ha·ra test

i·sin·glass
is·land of Lan·ger·hans
is·land of Reil
is·let
i·so·ag·glu·ti·na·tion
i·so·ag·glu·ti·na·tive
i·so·ag·glu·ti·nin
i·so·ag·glu·ti·no·gen
i·so·aj·ma·line
i·so·al·co·hol·ic
i·so·al·lox·a·zine
i·so·am·yl
i·so·am·yl·am·ine
i·so·an·a·phy·lax·is
i·so·an·dros·ter·one
i·so·an·ti·bod·y
   pl i·so·an·ti·bod·ies
i·so·an·ti·gen
i·so·bar
i·so·bar·ic
i·so·bas·tique
i·so·bes·tic
i·so·bor·nyl
i·so·bu·caine
i·so·bu·tyl
i·so·bu·tyr·ic
i·so·ca·lo·ric
i·so·car·box·a·zid
i·so·cel·lo·bi·ose
i·so·cel·lu·lar
i·so·cho·les·ter·ol
i·so·chore
i·so·cho·ric
i·so·chro·mat·ic
i·so·chro·mat·o·phil
i·so·chro·mo·some
i·soch·ro·nal
i·soch·ro·nal·ly
i·soch·ro·ni·a
i·soch·ro·nic
i·soch·ro·nism
i·soch·ro·nous
i·so·cit·ric
i·so·com·ple·ment
i·so·co·ri·a
i·so·cor·tex
   pl i·so·cor·tex·es
   or i·so·cor·ti·ces
i·so·cy·a·nide

199

i·so·cy·clic
i·so·cy·tol·y·sin
i·so·cy·to·sis
i·so·dac·ty·lism
i·so·dac·ty·lous
i·so·di·a·met·ric
i·so·di·a·phere
i·so·dont
i·so·dont·ic
i·so·dose
i·so·do·ses
i·so·dul·ci·tol
i·so·dy·nam·i·a
i·so·dy·nam·ic
i·so·e·lec·tric
i·so·e·lix·ir
i·so·en·er·get·ic
i·so·en·zy·mat·ic
i·so·en·zyme
i·so·en·zy·mic
i·so·eth·a·rine
i·so·feb·ri·fu·gine
is·o·flu·ro·phate
i·so·gam·ete
i·so·ga·met·ic
i·so·gam·e·ty
i·so·gam·ic
    or i·sog·a·mous
i·sog·a·mous
    or i·so·gam·ic
i·sog·a·my
    pl i·sog·a·mies
i·so·ge·ne·ic
i·so·gen·e·sis
    pl i·so·gen·e·ses
i·sog·e·nous
i·so·ger·mine
i·sog·na·thous
i·so·gon·ic
i·sog·o·ny
    pl i·sog·o·nies
i·so·graft
i·so·haem·ag·glu·ti·nin
    var of i·so·hem·ag·glu·ti·
    nin
i·so·hae·mol·y·sin
    var of i·so·he·mol·y·sin
i·so·hae·mol·y·sis
    var of i·so·he·mol·y·sis

i·so·hae·mo·lyt·ic
    var of i·so·he·mo·lyt·ic
is·o·hem·ag·glu·ti·na·tion
i·so·hem·ag·glu·ti·nin
i·so·he·mol·y·sin
i·so·he·mol·y·sis
    pl i·so·he·mol·y·ses
i·so·he·mo·lyt·ic
i·so·hy·dric
i·so·hy·per·cy·to·sis
i·so·hy·po·cy·to·sis
i·so·i·co·ni·a
    or i·so·i·ko·ni·a
i·so·i·con·ic
    or i·so·i·kon·ic
i·so·i·ko·ni·a
    or i·so·i·con·i·a
i·so·i·kon·ic
    or i·so·i·con·ic
i·so·im·mu·ni·za·tion
i·so·i·on·ic
i·so·lac·tose
i·so·late
i·so·lat·er·al
i·so·la·tion
i·so·lec·i·thal
i·so·leu·cine
i·so·leu·cyl
i·so·log
    or i·so·logue
i·sol·o·gous
i·so·logue
    or i·so·log
i·so·ly·ser·gic
i·sol·y·sin
i·sol·y·sis
i·so·mal·tose
i·so·mer
i·som·er·ase
i·so·mer·ic
i·som·er·ide
i·som·er·ism
i·som·er·i·za·tion
i·som·er·ize
i·som·er·ous
i·so·meth·a·done
i·so·me·thep·tene
i·so·met·ric
    or i·so·met·ri·cal

i·so·met·ri·cal
    or i·so·met·ric
i·so·met·rics
i·so·me·tro·pi·a
i·som·e·try
i·so·morph
i·so·mor·phic
i·so·mor·phism
i·so·mor·phous
i·so·ni·a·zid
i·so·nic·o·tin·ic
i·so·nic·o·tin·o·yl·hy·dra·
    zine
    or i·so·nic·o·tin·yl·hy·dra·
    zine
i·so·nic·o·tin·yl·hy·dra·zine
    or i·so·nic·o·tin·o·yl·hy·dra·
    zine
i·so·nip·e·caine
i·so·ni·trile
i·so·os·mot·ic
i·so·path·ic
i·sop·a·thy
    pl i·sop·a·thies
i·so·phane
i·so·phen·ic
i·so·pho·ri·a
i·so·pi·a
i·so·plas·tic
i·so·pre·cip·i·tin
i·so·pren·a·line
i·so·prene
i·so·pren·oid
i·so·pro·pa·mide
i·so·pro·pa·nol
i·so·pro·pyl
i·so·pro·pyl·a·ce·tic
i·so·pro·pyl·ar·te·re·nol
i·so·pro·te·re·nol
i·sop·ter
i·sop·ters
i·so·pyk·no·sis
i·so·quin·o·line
i·so·rau·wol·fine
i·so·ri·bo·fla·vin
i·sor·rhe·a
i·so·scope
i·so·ser·ine
i·so·sex·u·al

i·sos·mot·ic
i·so·sor·bide
i·sos·po·ra
i·so·spore
i·so·spor·ro·sis
i·so·spo·rous
i·so·spo·ry
    pl i·so·spo·ries
i·so·ster
    or i·so·stere
i·so·stere
    or i·so·ster
i·so·ster·ic
i·so·ster·ism
i·sos·the·nu·ri·a
i·so·tel
i·so·ther·a·py
i·so·therm
i·so·ther·mal
i·so·ther·mic
i·so·thi·o·cy·a·nate
i·so·tone
i·so·ton·i·a
i·so·ton·ic

i·so·ton·i·cal·ly
i·so·to·nic·i·ty
    pl i·so·to·nic·i·ties
i·so·tope
i·so·top·ic
i·so·trop·ic
i·sot·ro·pous
i·sot·ro·py
i·so·typ·i·cal
i·so·va·ler·ic
i·so·vol·u·met·ric
i·so·vo·lu·mic
i·sox·su·prine
i·so·zyme
i·so·zy·mic
is·pa·ghul
is·sue
isth·mec·to·my
    pl isth·mec·to·mies
isth·mi·an
isth·mic
isth·mo·pa·ral·y·sis
isth·mo·ple·gi·a
isth·mus

isth·mus of the fau·ces
i·su·ri·a
it·a·con·ic
itch
itch·i·ness
itch·ing
itch·y
i·ter
it·er·a·tion
i·ter·o·par·i·ty
ith·y·lor·do·sis
ith·y·o·ky·pho·sis
I·to-Reen·stier·na test
Ive·mark syn·drome
I·vy meth·od
I·wa·noff cysts
Ix·o·des
ix·o·di·a·sis
ix·od·ic
ix·od·id
Ix·od·i·dae
ix·o·doid
Ix·o·doi·de·a
ix·y·o·my·e·li·tis

J

J disk
J point
jaag·siek·te
    or jaag·ziek·te
    or jag·siek·te
    or jag·xiek·te
jaag·ziek·te
    or jaag·siek·te
    or jag·siek·te
    or jag·xiek·te
jab·o·ran·di
Ja·bou·lay
Jac·coud ar·thri·tis

jack·screw
Jack·son mem·brane
Jack·son-
    Bab·cock op·er·a·tion
Jack·so·ni·an con·vul·sion
Ja·co·be·us op·er·a·tion
Ja·cob·sohn re·flex
Ja·cob·son car·ti·lage,
    nerve, or·gan,
    tur·bi·nal
Jac·quet e·ryth·e·ma
jac·ta·tion
jac·ti·tate

jac·ti·ta·tion
jac·u·lif·er·ous
Jad·as·sohn dis·ease
Jad·as·sohn-Lew·an·dow·
    sky law
Jad·as·sohn-Ti·éche
    ne·vus
Jae·ger test
Jaf·fé test
Jaf·fé-
    Lich·ten·stein dis·ease
jag·sickte
    or jaag·siek·te

or jaag-ziek-te
or jag-xiek-te
jag-xiek-te
  or jag-siek-te
  or jaag-siek-te
  or jaag-ziek-te
jake leg
Jakob-Creutz-feldt
  dis-ease
jal-ap
jal-a-pin
Ja-mai-ca gin-ger
ja-mais vu
jam-bul
James-i-an
James-Lange the-o-ry
James-town weed
  or jimp-son
  or jim-son-weed
  or jimp-son-weed
Ja-net dis-ease
Jane-way le-sions
jan-i-ceps
Jan-sen op-er-a-tion
Jan-sky clas-si-fi-ca-tion
Jan-us-green
Ja-nu-si-an
ja-ra-ra-ca
Ja-risch-Herx-hei-mer
  re-ac-tion
Jat-ro-pha
jat-ro-phic
jaun-dice
jaun-diced
Ja-vel wa-ter
  or Ja-velle wa-ter
Ja-velle wa-ter
  or Ja-vel wa-ter
ja-vell-i-za-tion
jaw
jaw-bone
jaw-line
Ja-wor-ski cor-pus-cles
jec-o-rin
jec-o-rize
Jed-dah ul-cer
Jegh-ers-Peutz syn-drome
je-ju-nal

je-ju-nec-to-my
  pl je-ju-nec-to-mies
je-ju-ni-tis
je-ju-no-cae-cos-to-my
  var of je-ju-no-ce-cos-
    to-my
je-ju-no-ce-cos-to-my
je-ju-no-co-los-to-my
  pl je-ju-no-co-los-to-mies
je-ju-no-gas-tric
je-ju-no-il-e-i-tis
  pl je-ju-no-il-e-it-i-des
je-ju-no-il-e-os-to-my
  pl je-ju-no-il-e-os-to-mies
je-ju-no-il-e-um
je-ju-no-je-ju-nos-to-my
  pl je-ju-no-je-ju-nos-to-mies
je-ju-nor-rha-phy
je-ju-nos-to-my
  pl je-ju-nos-to-mies
je-ju-not-o-my
  pl je-ju-not-o-mies
je-ju-num
  pl je-ju-na
Jel-li-nek sign
jel-ly fish
Je-na Nom-i-na An-a-
  tom-i-ca
Jen-dras-sik ma-neu-ver
Jen-ner stain
Jen-ne-ri-an vac-ci-na-tion
Jen-sen meth-od
jerk
jerk-y
jer-vine
Jes-u-its bal-sam
jet lag
Jew-ett op-er-a-tion
Jez-ler-Ta-ka-ta test
jig-ger
jimp-son
  or jimp-son-weed
  or jim-son-weed
  or James-town weed
jimp-son-weed
  or jimp-son
  or jim-son-weed
  or James-town weed

jim-son-weed
  or James-town weed
  or jimp-son-weed
  or jimp-son
Jirgl re-ac-tion
Job syn-drome
Jo-bert fos-sa
jock itch
Jof-froy re-flex
Joh-ne ba-cil-lus
joh-nin
joint
Jol-ly bo-dies
Jones po-si-tion
Jor-ge Lo-bo blas-to-
  my-co-sis
Jo-seph syn-drome
joule
Joule e-quiv-a-lent
Ju-det op-er-a-tion
ju-ga
ju-gal
ju-gal point
  or ju-ga-le
ju-ga-le
  or ju-gal point
jug-u-lar
jug-u-lum
  pl jug-u-la
ju-gum
  pl ju-gums
  or ju-ga
Jukes u-nit
ju-men-tous
jump-ers
jump-ing French-men of
  Maine
junc-tion
junc-tion-al
junc-tu-ra
  pl junc-tu-rae
junc-ture
Jung-i-an
Jüng-ling dis-ease
jun-i-per oil
ju-ni-per-tar oil
Ju-nip-er-us
Ju-ni-us-Kuhnt dis-ease
jur-ris-pru-dence

ju·ry-mast
Jus·ter re·flex
jus·to ma·jor
jus·to mi·nor
jute

ju·ve·nile
jux·ta·ar·tic·u·lar
jux·ta·cor·ti·cal
jux·ta·glo·mer·u·lar
jux·ta·pap·il·lar·y

jux·ta·pose
jux·ta·po·si·tion
jux·ta·py·lo·ric
jux·ta·res·ti·form
jux·ta·spi·nal

K

Ka·der op·er·a·tion
Ka·der-Senn op·er·a·tion
Kaes-Bekh·ter·ev lay·er
Kaf·fir pox
Kahl·den tu·mor
Kah·ler dis·ease
Kahn re·ac·tion, test
kai·no·pho·bi·a
Kai·ser·ling meth·od
kak·er·ga·si·a
kak·i·dro·sis
    pl kak·i·dro·ses
kak·or·raph·i·o·pho·bi·a
kak·os·mi·a
ka·la a·zar
ka·la·fun·gin
ka·le·mi·a
ka·li·e·mi·a
ka·lig·e·nous
ka·lim·e·ter
ka·li·o·pe·ni·a
ka·li·o·pe·nic
Kal·i·scher dis·ease
ka·li·um
ka·li·u·re·sis
ka·li·u·ret·ic
kal·lak
kal·li·din
kal·li·din·o·gen
kal·li·kre·in
kal·li·krei·no·gen

ka·ma·la
    or ka·me·la
    or ka·mi·la
ka·me·la
    or ka·ma·la
    or ka·mi·la
ka·mi·la
    or ka·me·la
    or ka·ma·la
Kam·mer·er-Bat·tle
    in·ci·sion
ka·na·my·cin
Kan·a·vel op·er·a·tion
Kan·da·har sore
Kan·din·sky com·plex
kan·gri
Kan·ner syn·drome
ka·o·lin
    or ka·o·line
ka·o·line
    or ka·o·lin
ka·o·li·no·sis
    pl ka·o·lin·o·sis·es
    or ka·o·lin·o·ses
Ka·po·si dis·ease
kap·pa
ka·ra·ya
    or ka·ra·ya gum
ka·ra·ya gum
    or ka·ra·ya

Karr meth·od
Kar·ta·gen·er syn·drome
kar·y·en·chy·ma
    pl kar·y·en·chy·mas
    or kar·y·en·chy·ma·ta
kar·y·o·blast
kar·y·o·chrome
kar·y·oc·la·sis
    pl kar·y·oc·la·ses
    or kar·y·ok·la·sis
    pl kar·y·ok·la·ses
kar·y·o·clas·tic
    or kar·y·o·klas·tic
kar·y·o·cyte
kar·y·o·gam·ic
kar·y·og·a·my
    pl kar·y·og·a·mies
kar·y·o·gen·e·sis
kar·y·o·ki·ne·sis
    pl kar·y·o·ki·ne·ses
kar·y·o·ki·net·ic
kar·y·ok·la·sis
    pl kar·y·ok·la·ses
    or kar·y·oc·la·sis
    pl kar·y·oc·la·ses
kar·y·o·klas·tic
    or kar·y·o·clas·tic
kar·y·o·lo·bic
kar·y·ol·o·gy
    pl kar·y·ol·o·gies
kar·y·o·lymph

kar·y·ol·y·sis
pl kar·y·ol·y·ses
kar·y·o·lyt·ic
kar·y·o·meg·a·ly
kar·y·o·mere
kar·y·om·e·try
kar·y·o·mi·cro·so·ma
kar·y·o·mi·cro·some
kar·y·o·mi·tome
kar·y·o·mi·to·sis
pl kar·y·o·mi·to·ses
kar·y·o·mor·phism
kar·y·on
kar·y·o·phage
kar·y·o·plasm
or kar·y·o·plas·ma
kar·y·o·plas·ma
or kar·y·o·plasm
kar·y·o·plas·mat·ic
or kar·y·o·plas·mic
kar·y·o·plas·mic
or kar·y·o·plas·mat·ic
kar·y·o·pyk·no·sis
kar·yo·pyk·not·ic
kar·y·or·rhec·tic
kar·y·or·rhex·is
pl kar·y·or·rhex·es
kar·y·o·some
kar·y·os·ta·sis
pl kar·y·os·ta·ses
kar·y·o·the·ca
kar·y·o·type
kar·y·o·typ·ic
or kar·y·o·typ·i·cal
kar·y·o·typ·i·cal
or kar·y·o·typ·ic
Kas·a·bach-Mer·ritt
syn·drome
ka·sai
Ka·shi·da ther·mic sign
Kash·in-Beck dis·ease
Kast syn·drome
kat
or khat
or quat
ka·tab·o·lism
var of ca·tab·o·lism
kat·a·chro·ma·sis
pl kat·a·chro·ma·ses

kat·a·did·y·mus
kat·a·pla·si·a
or cat·a·pla·si·a
kat·a·ther·mom·e·ter
kat·a·to·ni·a
or cat·a·to·ni·a
or cat·a·to·ny
Kat·a·ya·ma
ka·thar·sis
or ca·thar·sis
ka·thar·tic
or ca·thar·tic
ka·thep·sin
var of ca·thep·sin
kath·i·so·pho·bia
kath·ode
var of cath·ode
ka·thod·ic
var of ca·thod·ic
kat·i·on
or cat·i·on
Katz-Wach·tel sign
kat·zen·jam·mer
Kauff·mann tet·ra·thi·o·
nate broth me·di·um
kau·ri
ka·va
or ka·va·ka·va
ka·va·ka·va
or ka·va
Kay-Gra·ham
pas·teur·i·za·tion
test
Kay·ser-Flei·scher ring
ked
Ke·da·ni fe·ver
Keen point
kef
or kif
kef·ir
Kehr op·er·a·tion
Kehr·er re·flex
Keith node
Keith-Wag·e·ner-
Bar·ker clas·si·fi·ca·tion
ke·lis
Kell blood group sys·tem
Kel·ler op·er·a·tion

kel·lin
var of khel·lin
Kel·ling test
Kel·ly-Pat·er·son syn·
drome
ke·loid
ke·loi·dal
ke·lo·ma
pl ke·lo·mas
or ke·lo·ma·ta
ke·lo·so·mus
kelp
Kel·vin scale
Kemp·ner rice di·et
Ken·ny meth·od, treat·
ment
ken·o·pho·bi·a
ken·o·tox·in
Kent men·tal test
Ken·ya tick ty·phus
keph·a·lin
var of ceph·a·lin
Ker·an·del sign
ker·a·phyl·lo·cele
ker·a·sin
ker·a·tal·gi·a
ker·a·tec·ta·si·a
ker·a·tec·to·my
pl ker·a·tec·to·mies
ke·rat·ic
ker·a·tin
or cer·a·tin
ker·a·ti·nase
ker·a·tin·i·za·tion
ker·a·tin·ize
ke·rat·i·no·cyte
ke·rat·i·no·phil·ic
ke·ra·ti·nous
ké·ra·tite en ban·de·lette
ker·a·tit·ic
ker·a·ti·tis
pl ker·a·ti·ti·des
ker·a·to·ac·an·tho·ma
pl ker·a·to·ac·an·tho·mas
or ker·a·to·ac·an·tho·ma·ta
ker·a·to·cele
ker·a·to·cen·te·sis
pl ker·a·to·cen·te·ses

ker·a·to·chro·ma·to·sis
  pl ker·a·to·chro·ma·to·ses
ker·a·to·con·junc·ti·vi·tis
ker·a·to·co·nus
ker·a·to·der·ma
ker·a·to·der·mat·o·cele
ke·ra·to·der·mi·a
ker·a·to·gen·e·sis
  pl ker·a·to·gen·e·ses
ker·a·tog·e·nous
ker·a·to·glo·bus
ker·a·to·hae·mi·a
  var of ker·a·to·he·mi·a
ker·a·to·hel·co·sis
  pl ker·a·to·hel·co·ses
ker·a·to·he·mi·a
ker·a·to·hy·a·lin
ker·a·toid
ker·a·to·i·rid·o·scope
ker·a·to·i·ri·tis
ker·a·to·lep·tyn·sis
ker·a·to·leu·ko·ma
  pl ker·a·to·leu·ko·mas
  or ker·a·to·leu·ko·ma·ta
ker·a·tol·y·sis
  pl ker·a·tol·y·ses
ker·a·to·lyt·ic
ker·a·to·ma
  pl ker·a·to·mas
  or ker·a·to·ma·ta
ker·a·to·ma·la·ci·a
ker·a·tome
ker·a·to·meg·a·ly
ker·a·tom·e·ter
ker·a·tom·e·try
ker·a·to·my·co·sis
  pl ker·a·to·my·co·ses
ker·a·to·nyx·is
  pl ker·a·to·nyx·es
ker·a·to·top·a·thy
ker·a·to·plas·tic
ker·a·to·plas·ty
  pl ker·a·to·plas·ties
ker·a·to·rhex·is
  pl ker·a·to·rhex·es
ker·a·to·scle·ri·tis
ker·a·to·scope
ker·a·tos·co·py
  pl ker·a·tos·co·pies

ker·a·tose
  or cer·a·tose
ker·a·to·sis
  pl ker·a·to·ses
ker·a·to·sul·fate
ker·a·to·sul·fa·tu·ri·a
ker·a·tot·ic
ker·a·tot·o·my
  pl ker·a·tot·o·mies
ker·a·to·to·rus
ke·rau·no·pho·bi·a
Kerck·ring folds
ke·rec·to·my
ke·ri·on cel·si
Ker·lines
ker·mes
kern·echt·rot
ker·nic·ter·us
Ker·nig sign
Ker·no·han syn·drome
Ker·no·han-Wolt·man
  syn·drome
ker·so·sene
  or ker·o·sine
ker·o·sine
  or ker·o·sene
ke·tal
ke·ta·mine
ke·tene
ke·tip·ra·mine
ke·to
ke·to·ac·i·do·sis
  pl ke·to·ac·i·do·ses
ke·to·ac·i·du·ri·a
ke·to·a·dip·ic
ke·to·bem·i·done
ke·to·cho·lan·ic
ke·to·gen·e·sis
  pl ke·to·gen·e·ses
ke·to·gen·ic
ke·to·glu·ta·rate
ke·to·glu·tar·ic
ke·to·hep·tose
ke·to·hex·ose
ke·to·hy·drox·y·es·trin
ke·tol
ke·tol·y·sis
  pl ke·tol·y·ses
ke·to·lyt·ic

ke·to·nae·mi·a
  var of ke·to·ne·mi·a
ke·tone
ke·to·ne·mi·a
ke·to·ne·mic
ke·to·nic
ke·to·nu·ri·a
ke·to·pro·pi·on·ic
ke·to·re·duc·tase
ke·tose
ke·to·side
ke·to·sis
  pl ke·to·ses
ke·to·ste·roid
ke·to·su·ri·a
ke·tot·ic
ke·tox·ime
key·way
khat
  or kat
  or quat
khel·lin
khel·li·nin
  or chel·lin·in
khel·lol·glu·co·side
Kidd blood group sys·
  tem
kid·ney
Kien·boČk at·ro·phy
kie·sel·guhr
Kies·sel·bach ar·e·a
kif
  or kef
Kil·li·an op·er·a·tion
kil·o·cal·o·rie
ki·lo·cy·cle
kil·o·gram
kil·o·gram-me·ter
ki·lo·hertz
kil·o·joule
kil·o·li·ter
ki·lom·e·ter
kil·o·nem
kil·o·u·nit
kil·o·volt
kil·o·watt
kil·u·rane
Kim·mel·stiel-Wil·son
  syn·drome

kin·aes·the·si·a
  var of kin·es·the·si·a
kin·aes·the·sis
  var of kin·es·the·sis
kin·aes·the·si·om·e·ter
  var of kin·es·the·si·om·
  e·ter
kin·aes·thet·ic
  var of kin·es·thet·ic
kin·ase
kin·e·ma·di·ag·ra·phy
kin·e·mat·ic
  or kin·e·mat·i·cal
kin·e·mat·i·cal
  or kin·e·mat·ic
kin·e·mat·i·cal·ly
kin·e·mat·ics
  or cin·e·mat·ics
kin·e·mat·o·graph
  or cin·e·mat·o·graph
kin·e·plas·tic
kin·e·plas·ty
  pl kin·e·plas·ties
  or cin·e·plas·ty
  pl cin·e·plas·ties
kin·e·ra·di·o·ther·a·py
kin·e·sal·gi·a
kin·e·scope
kin·e·si·a
ki·ne·si·aes·the·si·om·e·ter
  var of ki·ne·si·es·the·si·om·
  e·ter
ki·ne·si·al·gi·a
ki·ne·si·at·rics
ki·ne·sics
ki·ne·si·es·the·si·om·e·ter
ki·ne·si·gen·ic
kin·e·sim·e·ter
  or ki·ne·si·om·e·ter
ki·ne·si·o·log·ic
  or ki·ne·si·o·log·i·cal
ki·ne·si·o·log·i·cal
  or ki·ne·si·o·log·ic
ki·ne·si·ol·o·gy
  pl ki·ne·si·ol·o·gies
ki·ne·si·om·e·ter
  or kin·e·sim·e·ter
ki·ne·si·o·neu·ro·sis

ki·ne·sis
  pl ki·ne·ses
  or ci·ne·sis
ki·ne·si·ther·a·py
  pl ki·ne·si·ther·a·pies
ki·ne·so·pho·bia
kin·es·the·si·a
kin·es·the·si·om·e·ter
kin·es·the·sis
  pl kin·es·the·ses
kin·es·thet·ic
ki·net·ic
ki·net·i·cist
ki·net·ics
ki·ne·tin
ki·ne·tism
ki·net·o·car·di·o·gram
ki·net·o·car·di·og·ra·phy
ki·ne·to·chore
ki·ne·to·gen·ic
ki·ne·to·graph
ki·ne·to·graph·ic
ki·ne·to·nu·cle·us
  pl ki·ne·to·nu·cle·us·es
  or ki·ne·to·nu·cle·i
ki·ne·to·plasm
ki·ne·to·plast
  or ci·ne·to·plast
ki·ne·to·plas·tic
kin·e·to·sis
  pl kin·e·to·ses
ki·ne·to·some
ki·ne·to·ther·a·py
king's e·vil
Kings·bur·y test
ki·nin
ki·no·cil·i·um
ki·nin·o·gen
ki·nin·o·gen·ic
Kin·ney law
Kin·ni·er-Wil·son sign
ki·no
ki·no·cen·trum
  pl ki·no·cen·trums
  or ki·no·cen·tra
kin·o·mere
kin·o·plasm
  or kin·o·plas·ma

kin·o·plas·ma
  or kin·o·plasm
kin·o·sphere
kin·o·tox·in
kin·ship
Kin·youn stain
ki·ot·o·my
  pl ki·ot·o·mies
Kir·chner di·ver·tic·u·lum
Kirk-Bent·ley meth·od
Kir·mis·sion op·er·a·tion
Kirsch·ner trac·tion
Kisch re·flex
Kiss·ing dis·ease
ki·ta·sa·my·cin
ki·tol
Kjel·dahl flask
Kjel·dahl meth·od
kjel·dahl·i·za·tion
kjel·dahl·ize
Klatsch prep·ar·a·tion
Klebs-Löff·ler ba·cil·lus
Kleb·si·el·la
klee·blatt·schä·del de·
  form·i·ty syn·drome
Kleine-Lev·in syn·drome
klein·re·gel
Klem·per·er tu·ber·cu·lin
klep·to·lag·ni·a
klep·to·ma·ni·a
klep·to·ma·ni·ac
klep·to·pho·bi·a
  or clep·to·pho·bi·a
Klieg eyes
Kline re·ac·tion, test
Kline·fel·ter syn·drome
Kline·fel·ter-Rei·fen·stein·
  Al·bright syn·drome
Klip·pel-Feil syn·drome
Klip·pel-Tré·nau·nay-
  Web·er syn·drome
Klip·pel-Weil sign
klis·e·om·e·ter
  or clis·e·om·e·ter
Klump·ke pa·ral·y·sis
knee
knee-cap
knee-jerk
knee·pan

knee·sprung
Kne·mi·do·kop·tes
Knies sign
knife
pl knives
knock
knock-knee
Knoop hard·ness
Knop test
Knopf treat·ment
knuck·le
knuck·le·bone
Ko·belt cyst
Ko·bert test
Koch ba·cil·lus
Koch phe·nom·e·non
Koch pos·tu·lates
Koch·er ma·neu·ver
Koch·er-De·bré-
   Sé·mé·laigne syn·
   drome
Koch-McMeekin meth·od
Koch-Weeks ba·cil·lus
Koeb·ner phe·nom·e·non
Koep·pe nod·ules
Koer·ber-Sa·lus-
   Elsch·nig syn·drome
Köh·ler dis·ease
Köhl·mei·er-
   De·gos dis·ease
koi·lo·cy·to·sis
koi·lo·cy·tot·ic
koi·lo·nych·i·a
koi·lor·rha·chic
koi·lo·ster·ni·a
koi·no·trop·ic
koi·not·ro·py
ko·juc
ko·la nut
   or co·la nut
ko·la tree
Kol·mer test
ko·ly·pep·tic
Kom·mer·ell di·ver·tic·
   u·lum
Kon·do·lé·on op·er·a·tion
Kö·nig dis·ease
ko·nim·e·ter
   or co·nim·om·e·ter

ko·ni·o·cor·tex
   pl ko·ni·o·cor·ti·ces
ko·ni·ol·o·gy
   pl ko·ni·ol·o·gies
   or co·ni·ol·o·gy
   pl co·ni·ol·o·gies
ko·ni·o·sis
   or co·ni·o·sis
ko·nom·e·ter
ko·phe·mi·a
Kop·lik spots
kop·ro·ste·a·rin
Korff fi·bers
Kor·ner-Shil·ling·ford
   meth·od
ko·ro
ko·ros·co·py
Ko·rot·kov meth·od
Kor·sa·koff syn·drome
   or Kor·sa·kov syn·drome
Kor·sa·kov syn·drome
   or Kor·sa·koff syn·drome
ko·sin
ko·so
   or ko·so
   or kous·so
Koss koi·lo·cy·to·tic
   a·typ·i·a
Kos·sel test
Kos·so
   or ko·so
   or kous·so
kou·miss
   or ku·miss
   or ku·mys
   or ku·myss
Kous·so
   or ko·so
   or kos·so
Ko·zhev·ni·kow ep·i·
   lep·sy
Krab·be dis·ease
Kraep·e·lin clas·si·fi·ca·
   tion
Krae·pe·lin·in·an
Kraep·e·lin-Mo·rel
   dis·ease
krait
kra·me·ri·a

Kra·mer-Tis·dall meth·od
Kras·ke op·er·a·tion
kra·tom·e·ter
krau·ro·sis
   pl krau·ro·ses
krau·rot·ic
Kraus fe·tal cells
Krau·se cor·pus·cle
Krau·se end-bulb
Krause mem·brane
Krause-Wolfe graft
kre·a·tin
kre·at·i·nine
Krebs cy·cle
Krebs-Hen·se·leit cy·cle
kre·o·tox·in
   or cre·o·tox·in
kre·o·tox·ism
   or cre·o·tox·ism
Kretsch·mer type
Kre·sig sign
Krom·pech·er tumor
Krö·nig fields
Kru·ken·berg tu·mor
kry·mo·ther·a·py
kryp·ton
ku·bis·a·ga·ri
Kufs dis·ease
Ku·gel ar·te·ry
Ku·gel·berg-
   Wel·an·der syn·drome
Kuhnt-Ju·ni·us dis·ease
Kult·schitz·ky car·ci·
   no·ma
ku·miss
   or kou·miss
   or ku·mys
   or ku·myss
Kum·lin·ge dis·ease
Kum̈·mell dis·ease
ku·mys
   or kou·miss
   or ku·miss
   or ku·myss
ku·myss
   or ku·miss
   or kou·miss
   or ku·mys

Kun·drat lym·pho·
   sar·co·ma
Kun·kel test
Kupf·fer cells
kur·chi
Kur·lov bod·ies
ku·ru
Kus·kok·wim dis·ease
Kuss-Ghon fo·cus
Kuss·maul res·pi·ra·tion
Kuss·maul-Mai·er
   dis·ease
kus·so
Kveim an·ti·gen
kwa·shi·or·kor

Kwi·leck·i meth·od
ky·a·nop·si·a
Kya·sa·nur for·est dis·
   ease
ky·es·te·in
ky·ma·tism
ky·mo·gram
ky·mo·graph
   or cy·mo·graph
ky·mo·graph·ic
ky·mog·ra·phy
   pl ky·mog·ra·phies
ky·no·ceph·a·lus
ky·no·pho·bi·a
kyn·u·ren·ic

ky·nure·nine
ky·pho·ra·chit·ic
ky·pho·ra·chi·tis
ky·phos
ky·pho·sco·li·o·ra·chit·ic
ky·pho·sco·li·o·ra·chi·tis
ky·pho·sco·li·o·sis
   pl ky·pho·sco·li·o·ses
ky·pho·sco·li·ot·ic
ky·pho·sis
   pl ky·pho·ses
ky·phot·ic
Kyrle dis·ease
kyr·tor·rhach·ic

L

la grippe
La Roque sign
Lab·ar·raque so·lu·tion
lab·da·cism
la·bel
la·bi·a ma·jo·ra
la·bi·a mi·no·ra
la·bi·al
la·bi·al·ism
la·bi·al·ly
La·bi·a·tae
la·bile
la·bil·i·ty
   pl la·bil·i·ties
la·bi·o·al·ve·o·lar
la·bi·o·cer·vi·cal
la·bi·o·cho·re·a
la·bi·o·den·tal
la·bi·o·gin·gi·val
la·bi·o·glos·so·la·ryn·ge·al
la·bi·o·glos·so·pha·ryn·ge·
   al

la·bi·o·graph
la·bi·o·men·tal
la·bi·o·na·sal
la·bi·o·pal·a·tine
la·bi·o·plas·ty
   pl la·bi·o·plas·ties
la·bi·o·scro·tal
la·bi·o·ver·sion
la·bi·um
   pl la·bi·a
la·bor
lab·o·ra·to·ty
La·borde meth·od
lab·ro·cyte
la·brum
lab·y·rinth
lab·y·rin·thec·to·my
   pl lab·y·rin·thec·to·mies
lab·y·rin·thine
lab·y·rin·thi·tis
lab·y·rin·thot·o·my
   pl lab·y·rin·thot·o·mies

lab·y·rin·thus
   pl lab·y·rin·thi
lac
   pl lac·ta
lac-case
lac·er·ate
lac·er·a·tion
lac·er·o·con·dy·lar
la·cer·tus fi·bro·sus
Lach·e·sis mu·tus
lach·ry·mal
   or lac·ri·mal
lach·ry·ma·tion
   or lac·ri·ma·tion
lach·ry·mo·tor
   or lac·ri·mo·tor
la·cin·i·ate
lac·ri·ma
   pl lac·ri·mae
lac·ri·mal
   or lach·ry·mal
lac·ri·ma·le

ac·ri·ma·tion
  or lach·ry·ma·tion
ac·ri·ma·tor
  or lach·ry·ma·tor
ac·ri·ma·to·ry
  pl lac·ri·ma·to·ries
ac·ri·mo·max·il·lar·y
ac·ri·mo·na·sal
ac·ri·mot·o·my
  pl lac·ri·mot·o·mies
ac·tac·i·de·mi·a
  var of lac·tac·i·de·mi·a
ac·tac·i·de·mi·a
ac·tac·i·du·ri·a
ac·ta·gogue
ac·tal·bu·min
ac·tam
ac·tam·ic
ac·tam·ide
ac·tar·o·vi·o·lin
ac·tase
ac·tate
ac·ta·tion
ac·ta·tion·al
ac·ta·tion·al·ly
ac·te·al
ac·tes·cence
ac·tes·cent
ac·tic
ac·ti·ce·mi·a
ac·tide
ac·tif·er·ous
ac·ti·fuge
ac·tig·e·nous
ac·tig·er·ous
ac·tim
ac·tin
ac·ti·su·gi·um
ac·tiv·o·rous
ac·to·bac·il·la·ce·ae
ac·to·ba·cil·lic
ac·to·ba·cil·lus
  pl lac·to·ba·cil·li
ac·to·ba·cil·lus ca·sei
  fac·tor
ac·to·cele
ac·to·crit
ac·to·fla·vin
ac·to·gen

lac·to·gen·e·sis
  pl lac·to·gen·e·ses
lac·to·gen·ic
lac·to·glob·u·lin
lac·tom·e·ter
lac·tone
lac·ton·ic
lac·to·per·ox·i·dase
lac·to·phos·phate
lac·to·pro·te·in
lac·tor·rhe·a
lac·tor·rhoe·a
  var of lac·tor·rhe·a
lac·to·sa·zone
lac·tose
lac·to·su·ri·a
lac·to·o·syl cer·a·mi·do·sis
lac·to·ther·a·py
lac·to·tox·in
lac·to·veg·e·tar·i·an
lac·to·vo·veg·e·tar·i·an
lac·tu·car·i·um
lac·tu·lose
lac·tyl
la·cu·na
  pl la·cu·nas
  or la·cu·nae
la·cu·nal
  or la·cu·nar
la·cu·nar
  or la·cu·nal
la·cu·nas of Mor·ga·gni
la·cu·nu·la
  pl la·cu·nu·las
  or la·cu·nu·lae
la·cu·nule
la·cus
Ladd-Frank·lin the·o·ry
lad·re·rie
Laehr-Hen·ne·berg hard
  pal·ate re·flex
Laen·nec cir·rho·sis
lae·ve
La·fo·ra bod·ies
lag
la·ge·na
  pl la·ge·nae
la·ge·ni·form
lag·nei·a

lag·neu·o·ma·ni·a
lag·oph·thal·mi·a
lag·oph·thal·mic
lag·oph·thal·mos
  or lag·oph·thal·mus
lag·oph·thal·mus
  or lag·oph·thal·mos
La·grange op·er·a·tion
Laid·law stain
Laid·low meth·od
lake
lak·y
la·li·a·try
lal·i·o·pho·bi·a
lal·la·tion
lal·og·no·sis
la·lo·pa·thol·o·gy
la·lop·a·thy
  pl la·lop·a·thies
lal·o·pho·bi·a
lal·o·pho·mi·a·trist
lal·o·ple·gi·a
lal·or·rhe·a
lal·or·rhoe·a
  var of lal·or·rhe·a
La·marck·i·an
La·marck·ism
lamb·da
lamb·da·cism
lamb·doid
  or lamb·doi·dal
lamb·doi·dal
  or lamb·doid
lam·bert
Lam·bert law
Lam·bl ex·cres·cen·ces
Lam·bli·a
lam·bli·a·sis
lame
la·mel·la
  pl la·mel·las
  or la·mel·lae
la·mel·lar
La·mi·a·ce·ae
lam·i·na
  pl lam·i·nas
  or lam·i·nae
lam·ina cri·bro·sa
  pl lam·i·nae cri·bro·sae

lam·i·na pro·pri·a
  pl lam·i·nae pro·pri·ae
lam·i·na·gram
  or lam·i·no·gram
lam·i·na·graph
  or lam·i·no·graph
lam·i·nag·ra·phy
lam·i·nar
lam·i·nar·i·a
lam·i·nate
lam·i·na·tion
lam·i·nec·to·my
  pl lam·i·nec·to·mies
lam·i·ni·tis
lam·i·no·gram
  or lam·i·na·gram
lam·i·no·graph
  or lam·i·na·graph
lam·i·not·o·my
  pl lam·i·not·o·mies
lam·pro·phon·ic
lam·proph·o·ny
La·mus me·gis·tus
la·na
la·nat·o·side
Lan·cas·ter ad·vance·ment
lance
Lance·field group
Lan·ce·reaux di·a·be·tes
lan·cet
lan·ci·nate
Lan·ci·si sign
Lan·dau po·si·tion
Lan·dis-Gib·bon test
land·mark
Lan·dolt ring
Lan·dou·zy dis·ease
Lan·dou·zy-Dé·je·rine
  dys·tro·phy
Lan·dou·zy-Gras·set law
Lan·dry pa·ral·y·sis
Lan·dry-Guil·lain-Bar·ré
  syn·drome
Land·stei·ner clas·si·fi·ca·
  tion
Land·ström mus·cle
Lane dis·ease
Lang·don Down a·nom·a·
  ly

Lange test
Lan·gen·beck op·er·a·tion
Lan·gen·dorf pre·par·a·
  tion
Lan·ger lines
lan·ger·han·si·an ad·e·no·
  ma
Lang·hans cell
lan·guor
lan·i·a·ry
Lan·ne·longue op·er·a·tion
lan·o·lin
  or lan·o·line
lan·o·line
  or lan·o·lin
la·nos·ter·ol
Lan·sing vi·rus
Lan·ter·mann in·ci·sure
lan·tha·nic
lan·tha·nide
lan·tha·non
lan·tha·num
lan·thi·o·nine
lan·tho·pine
la·nu·gi·nous
la·nu·go
lan·u·lous
la·pac·tic
lap·a·ror·rha·phy
  pl lap·a·ror·rha·phies
lap·a·ro·scope
lap·a·ros·co·py
lap·a·rot·o·my
  pl lap·a·rot·o·mies
lap·a·ro·tra·che·lot·o·my
lap·in·i·za·tion
lap·in·ize
lap·is
lap·pa
lap·sus
  pl lap·sus
lar·bish
lar·da·ce·in
lar·da·ceous
large in·tes·tine
lark·spur
La·roy·enne op·er·a·tion
Lar·rey sign

Lar·sen-Jo·han·sson
  dis·ease
lar·va
  pl lar·vas
  or lar·vae
lar·va·cide
  or lar·vi·cide
lar·va mi·grans
  pl lar·vae mi·gran·tes
lar·val
lar·vate
  or lar·vat·ed
lar·vat·ed
  or lar·vate
lar·vi·cide
  or lar·va·cide
lar·yn·gal·gi·a
la·ryn·ge·al
la·ryn·ge·al·ly
lar·yn·gec·to·mee
lar·yn·gec·to·mize
lar·yn·gec·to·my
  pl lar·yn·gec·to·mies
lar·yn·gem·phrax·is
lar·yn·gis·mal
lar·yn·gis·mus
  pl lar·yn·gis·mi
lar·yn·gis·mus stri·du·lus
  pl lar·yn·gis·mi stri·du·li
lar·yn·git·ic
lar·yn·gi·tis
  pl lar·yn·git·i·des
la·ryn·go·cele
la·ryn·go·cen·te·sis
la·ryn·go·fis·sure
la·ryn·go·gram
la·ryn·go·graph
lar·yn·gog·ra·phy
la·ryn·go·log·ic
lar·yn·gol·o·gist
lar·yn·gol·o·gy
  pl lar·yn·gol·o·gies
lar·yn·gom·e·try
la·ryn·go·pa·ral·y·sis
  pl la·ryn·go·pa·ral·y·ses
lar·yn·gop·a·thy
  pl lar·yn·gop·a·thies
la·ryn·go·phan·tom
la·ryn·go·pha·ryn·ge·al

la·ryn·go·phar·yn·gec·to·my
pl la·ryn·go·phar·yn·gec·to·mies

lar·yn·go·pha·ryn·ge·us

la·ryn·go·phar·yn·gi·tis
pl la·ryn·go·phar·yn·git·i·des

la·ryn·go·phar·ynx
pl la·ryn·go·phar·ynx·es
or la·ryn·go·phar·yn·ges

lar·yn·goph·o·ny

la·ryn·go·plas·ty
pl la·ryn·go·plas·ties

la·ryn·go·ple·gi·a

la·ryn·go·pto·sis

la·ryn·go·rhi·nol·o·gy
pl la·ryn·go·rhi·nol·o·gies

la·ryn·gor·rha·gi·a

lar·yn·gor·rha·phy

la·ryn·gor·rhe·a

la·ryn·gor·rhoe·a
var of la·ryn·gor·rhe·a

la·ryn·go·scle·ro·ma
pl la·ryn·go·scle·ro·mas
or la·ryn·go·scle·ro·ma·ta

la·ryn·go·scope

la·ryn·go·scop·ic

lar·yn·gos·co·pist

lar·yn·gos·co·py
pl lar·yn·gos·co·pies

la·ryn·go·spasm

lar·yn·gos·ta·sis

la·ryn·go·ste·no·sis
pl la·ryn·go·ste·no·ses

lar·yn·gos·to·my
pl lar·yn·gos·to·mies

la·ryn·go·stro·bo·scope

la·ryn·go·stro·bos·co·py

la·ryn·go·tome

lar·yn·got·o·my
pl lar·yn·got·o·mies

la·ryn·go·tra·che·al

la·ryn·go·tra·che·i·tis

la·ryn·go·tra·che·o·bron·chi·tis
pl la·ryn·go·tra·che·o·bron·chit·i·des

la·ryn·go·tra·che·os·co·py

la·ryn·go·tra·che·ot·o·my
pl la·ryn·go·tra·che·ot·o·mies

la·ryn·go·xe·ro·sis
pl la·ryn·go·xe·ro·ses

lar·ynx
pl la·rynx·es
or la·ryn·ges

las·civ·i·a

las·civ·i·ous

La·sègue law

la·ser

Lash·met and New·burgh test

Las·kow·ski meth·od

Las·saign test

Las·sar paste

las·si·tude

la·ta

la·tah

la·ten·cy
pl la·ten·cies

la·tent

la·ten·ti·a·tion

lat·er·ad

lat·er·al

la·ter·al·i·ty
pl lat·er·al·i·ties

lat·er·al·i·za·tion

lat·er·al·ize

lat·er·i·tious

lat·er·i·ver·sion

lat·er·o·ab·dom·i·nal

lat·er·o·duc·tion

lat·er·o·flex·ion

lat·er·o·mar·gin·al

lat·er·o·pul·sion

lat·er·o·tor·sion

lat·er·o·ver·sion

la·tex

lath·y·rism

lath·y·rit·ic

lath·y·ro·gen·ic

la·tis·si·mo·con·dy·lar·is

la·tis·si·mus dor·si
pl la·tis·si·mi dor·si

la·tro·dect·ism

Lat·ro·dec·tus

lat·tice

la·tus

laud·a·ble

lau·dan·i·dine

lau·da·nine

lau·dan·o·sine

lau·da·num

laugh·ing gas

Laugh·len test

Lau·rence-Moon-Bie·dl syn·drome

lau·ric

lau·rus

lau·ryl

Lauth vi·o·let

la·vage

la·va·tion

la·va·tion·al

lav·en·der

La·ve·ran bod·ies

Lav·er·a·ni·a

Lav·ren·ti·ev phe·nom·e·non

Law pro·jec·tion

lax·a·tion

lax·a·tive

lax·a·tive·ly

lax·a·tor

lax·i·ty

lay·er

lay·er of Lang·hans

laz·ar

laz·a·ret

laz·a·ret·to

laz·a·rine

Laz·a·row meth·od

Le Fort op·er·a·tion

leach

lead

Lead-bet·ter pro·ce·dure

Leake and Guy meth·od

Le·ber dis·ease

lec·a·nop·a·gus

lec·a·no·so·ma·top·a·gus

Le·cat gulf

le·che de he·gue·rón

lech·o·py·ra

lec·i·thal
or lec·i·thic

lec·ith·al·bu·min

lec·i·thic
or lec·i·thal
lec·i·thin
lec·i·thi·nase
lec·i·tho·blast
lec·i·thoid
lec·i·tho·pro·te·in
lec·i·tho·vi·tel·lin
lec·tin
Led·der·hose dis·ease
Led·er·er a·cute a·ne·mi·a
Lee test
leech
Lee-White meth·od
left-eyed
left-foot·ed
left-hand·ed
leg
Le·gal dis·ease
leg·as·the·ni·a
Legg-Cal·vé-Per·thes dis·ease
leg·ged
Legg-Per·thes dis·ease
Le·gion·naire dis·ease
leg·ume
le·gu·min
Lei·boff and Kahn meth·od
Leich·ten·stern phe·nom·e·non
Leif·son meth·od
Leigh syn·drome
Lei·ner disease
lei·o·der·ma·tous
lei·o·der·mi·a
lei·o·my·o·fi·bro·ma
pl lei·o·my·o·fi·bro·mas
or lei·o·my·o·fi·bro·ma·ta
lei·o·my·o·ma
pl lei·o·my·o·mas
or lei·o·my·o·ma·ta
lei·o·my·o·sar·co·ma
pl lei·o·my·o·sar·co·mas
or lei·o·my·o·sar·co·ma·ta
lei·ot·ri·chous
lei·po·me·ri·a
or li·po·me·ri·a
Leish·man stain

Leish·man-Don·o·van bod·ies
Leish·ma·ni·a
leish·ma·ni·a·sis
pl leish·ma·ni·a·ses
or leish·ma·ni·o·sis
pl leish·ma·ni·o·ses
leish·man·in
leish·ma·ni·o·sis
pl leish·ma·ni·o·ses
or leish·ma·ni·a·sis
pl leish·ma·ni·a·ses
le·ma
Lem·bert su·ture
lem·mo·blast
lem·mo·blas·tic
lem·mo·blas·to·ma
pl lem·mo·blas·to·mas
or lem·mo·blas·to·ma·ta
lem·mo·cyte
lem·mo·cy·to·ma
pl lem·mo·cy·to·mas
or lem·mo·cy·to·ma·ta
lem·nis·cal
lem·nis·cus
pl lem·nis·ci
le·mo·pa·ral·y·sis
le·mo·ste·no·sis
Lem·pert op·er·a·tion
Len·drum in·clu·sion-bod·y stain
Len·hartz di·et
len·i·ceps
len·i·quin·sin
len·i·tive
Len·nox syn·drome
lens
len·som·e·ter
len·te
len·tec·to·mize
len·tec·to·my
len·ti·co·nus
len·tic·u·la
pl len·tic·u·las
or len·tic·u·lae
len·tic·u·lar
len·tic·u·late
len·tic·u·lo-stri·ate
len·tic·u·lo-tha·lam·ic

len·ti·form
len·tig·i·nes le·pro·sae
len·tig·i·no·sis
len·ti·glo·bus
len·ti·go
pl len·tig·i·nes
le·on·ti·a·sis
pl le·on·ti·a·ses
le·on·ti·a·sis os·se·a
lep·er
le·pid·ic
lep·i·dine
lep·i·do·ma
pl lep·i·do·mas
or lep·i·do·ma·ta
Lep·i·dop·ter·a
lep·i·dop·ter·an
lep·i·do·sis
pl lep·i·do·ses
lep·o·thrix
pl lep·o·thrix·es
or le·pot·ri·ches
lep·ra
lep·re·chaun·ism
lep·rid
lep·ro·lin
lep·ro·log·ic
lep·rol·o·gist
lep·rol·o·gy
pl lep·rol·o·gies
lep·ro·ma
pl lep·ro·mas
or lep·ro·ma·ta
lep·rom·a·tous
lep·ro·min
lep·ro·pho·bi·a
lep·ro·sar·i·um
pl lep·ro·sar·i·ums
or lep·ro·sar·i·a
lep·ro·ser·y
lep·ro·stat·ic
lep·ro·sy
pl lep·ro·sies
lep·rot·ic
lep·rous
lep·tan·dra
lep·ta·zol
lep·to·ce·pha·li·a

lep·to·ce·phal·ic
or lep·to·ceph·a·lous
lep·to·ceph·a·lous
or lep·to·ce·phal·ic
lep·to·ceph·a·lus
pl lep·to·ceph·a·li
lep·to·chro·mat·ic
lep·to·cyte
lep·to·cyt·ic
lep·to·cy·to·sis
lep·to·dac·ty·lous
lep·to·dac·ty·ly
lep·to·don·tous
lep·to·men·in·ge·al
lep·to·me·nin·ges
lep·to·me·nin·gi·o·ma
pl lep·to·me·nin·gi·o·mas
or lep·to·me·nin·gi·o·ma·ta
lep·to·men·in·gi·tis
pl lep·to·men·in·git·i·des
lep·to·men·in·gop·a·thy
pl lep·to·men·in·gop·a·thies
lep·to·me·ninx
pl lep·to·me·nin·ges
lep·to·mi·cro·gnath·i·a
Lep·to·mi·cru·rus
lep·to·mo·nad
lep·to·mo·nas
lep·ton
lep·to·pel·lic
lep·to·pho·ni·a
lep·to·phon·ic
lep·to·pro·so·pi·a
lep·to·pro·sop·ic
or lep·to·pro·so·pous
lep·to·pro·so·pous
or lep·to·pro·sop·ic
lep·tor·rhine
lep·to·scope
lep·to·spi·ra
pl lep·to·spi·ra
or lep·to·spi·ras
or lep·to·spi·rae
lep·to·spi·ral
lep·to·spire
lep·to·spi·rol·y·sin
lep·to·spi·ro·sis
pl lep·to·spi·ro·ses
lep·to·tene

Lep·to·thrix
lep·to·tri·chal
Lep·to·trich·i·a
lep·to·tri·co·sis
pl lep·to·tri·co·ses
lep·tus
pl lep·tus·es
or lep·ti
le·re·sis
Lé·ri dis·ease
Le·riche op·er·a·tion
Ler·man-Means scratch
Ler·mo·yez syn·drome
les·bi·an
les·bi·an·ism
Lesch-Ny·han dis·ease
Lesch·ke meth·od
le·sion
le·thal
le·thal·i·ty
pl le·thal·i·ties
le·thal·ly
le·thar·gic
leth·ar·gy
pl leth·ar·gies
le·the
Let·o·noff and Rein·hold meth·od
Let·ter·er-Si·we dis·ease
leu·cae·mi·a
var of leu·ke·mi·a
leu·cae·thi·op
leu·ce·mi·a
var of leu·ke·mi·a
leu·cic
leu·cine
leu·ci·nur·i·a
leu·co·blast
var of leu·ko·blast
leu·co·ci·din
leu·co·cyte
var of leu·ko·cyte
leu·co·cy·thae·mi·a
var of leu·co·cy·the·mi·a
leu·co·cy·thae·mic
var of leu·co·cy·the·mic
leu·co·cy·the·mi·a
leu·co·cy·the·mic

leu·co·cyt·ic
var of leu·ko·cy·tic
leu·co·cy·to·blast
var of leu·ko·cy·to·blast
leu·co·cy·to·poi·e·sis
var of leu·ko·cy·to·poi·e·sis
leu·co·cy·to·sis
var of leu·ko·cy·to·sis
leu·co·cy·tot·ic
var of leu·ko·cy·to·tic
leu·co·der·ma
var of leu·ko·der·ma
leu·co·en·ceph·a·li·tis
var of leu·ko·en·ceph·a·li·tis
leu·co·fla·vin
leu·co·lac·to·fla·vin
leu·co·ma
var of leu·ko·ma
leu·co·ma·i·nae·mi·a
var of leu·co·ma·i·ne·mi·a
leu·co·maine
leu·co·ma·i·ne·mi·a
Leu·co·nos·toc
leu·co·pe·ni·a
var of leu·ko·pe·ni·a
leu·co·poi·e·sis
var of leu·ko·poi·e·sis
leu·co·poi·et·ic
var of leu·ko·poi·et·ic
leu·co·pro·te·ase
leu·co·ri·bo·fla·vin
leu·cor·rhe·a
var of leu·kor·rhe·a
leu·cor·rhe·al
var of leu·kor·rhe·al
leu·cor·rhoe·a
var of leu·kor·rhe·a
leu·cor·rhoe·al
var of leu·kor·rhe·al
leu·co·sin
leu·co·sis
var of leu·ko·sis
leu·co·vor·in
leu·cyl
Leu·det sign
leu·kae·mi·a
var of leu·ke·mi·a

213

leu·kae·mic
var of leu·ke·mic
leu·kae·mid
var of leu·ke·mid
leu·kae·moid
var of leu·ke·moid
leuk·a·nae·mi·a
var of leuk·a·ne·mi·a
leuk·a·ne·mi·a
leu·ka·phe·re·sis
leu·kas·mus
leu·ke·mi·a
leu·ke·mic
leu·ke·mid
leu·ke·mo·gen
leu·ke·mo·gen·e·sis
pl leu·ke·mo·gen·e·ses
leu·ke·mo·gen·ic
leu·ke·moid
leu·ker·gy
leu·kin
leu·ko·ag·glu·tin·in
leu·ko·ba·sic
leu·ko·blast
leu·ko·blas·to·sis
pl leu·ko·blas·to·ses
leu·ko·ci·din
leu·ko·cyte
leu·ko·cy·thae·mi·a
var of leu·ko·cy·the·mi·a
leu·ko·cy·the·mi·a
leu·ko·cyt·ic
leu·ko·cy·to·blast
leu·ko·cy·to·gen·e·sis
pl leu·ko·cy·to·gen·e·ses
leu·ko·cy·tol·y·sin
leu·ko·cy·tol·y·sis
pl leu·ko·cy·tol·y·ses
leu·ko·cy·to·lit·ic
leu·ko·cy·to·ma
pl leu·ko·cy·to·mas
or leu·ko·cy·to·ma·ta
leu·ko·cy·tom·e·ter
leu·ko·cy·to·pe·ni·a
leu·ko·cy·to·pla·ni·a
leu·ko·cy·to·poi·e·sis
pl leu·ko·cy·to·poi·e·ses
leu·ko·cy·to·poi·et·ic

leu·ko·cy·to·sis
pl leu·ko·cy·to·ses
leu·ko·cy·to·tax·is
leu·ko·cy·to·tot·ic
leu·ko·cy·to·tox·in
leu·ko·cy·tu·ri·a
leu·ko·der·ma
leu·ko·der·mi·a
leu·ko·der·mic
leu·ko·dys·tro·phy
pl leu·ko·dys·tro·phies
leu·ko·e·de·ma
leu·ko·en·ceph·a·li·tis
pl leu·ko·en·ceph·a·lit·i·des
leu·ko·en·ceph·a·lop·a·thy
pl leu·ko·en·ceph·a·lop·a·
thies
leu·ko·e·ryth·ro·blas·tic
leu·ko·e·ryth·ro·blas·to·sis
leu·ko·ker·a·to·sis
leu·ko·ko·ri·a
leu·ko·krau·ro·sis
leu·ko·lym·pho·sar·co·ma
pl leu·ko·lym·pho·sar·co·
mas
or leu·ko·lym·pho·sar·co·
ma·ta
leu·kol·y·sin
leu·kol·y·sis
pl leu·kol·y·ses
leu·ko·ma
pl leu·ko·mas
or leu·ko·ma·ta
leu·kom·a·toid
leu·kom·a·tous
leu·ko·my·e·li·tis
leu·ko·my·e·lop·a·thy
leu·ko·my·o·ma
pl leu·ko·my·o·mas
or leu·ko·my·o·ma·ta
leu·kon
leu·ko·ne·cro·sis
leu·ko·nych·i·a
leu·ko·ny·chit·ic
leu·ko·path·i·a
leu·kop·a·thy
pl leu·kop·a·thies
leu·ko·pe·de·sis
pl leu·ko·pe·de·sis

leu·ko·pe·ni·a
leu·ko·pe·nic
leu·ko·phe·re·sis
leu·ko·phleg·ma·si·a
leu·koph·thal·mous
leu·ko·pla·ki·a
leu·ko·pla·ki·al
leu·ko·pla·si·a
leu·ko·plas·tid
leu·ko·poi·e·sis
pl leu·ko·poi·e·ses
leu·ko·poi·et·ic
leu·ko·pro·te·ase
leu·kop·sin
leu·kor·rha·gi·a
leu·kor·rhe·a
leu·kor·rhe·al
leu·kor·rhoe·a
var of leu·kor·rhe·a
leu·kor·rhoe·al
var of leu·kor·rhe·al
leu·ko·sar·co·ma
pl leu·ko·sar·co·mas
or leu·ko·sar·co·ma·ta
leu·ko·sar·co·ma·to·sis
pl leu·ko·sar·co·ma·to·ses
leu·ko·sis
pl leu·ko·ses
leu·ko·tax·ine
leu·ko·tax·is
leu·ko·tome
leu·kot·o·my
pl leu·kot·o·mies
leu·ko·tox·ic
leu·ko·tox·in
leu·ko·trich·i·a
leu·kot·ri·chous
leu·ko·u·ro·bil·in
leu·kous
leu·ko·vi·rus
leu·ro·cris·tine
Lev·a·di·ti meth·od
lev·al·lor·phan
lev·am·fet·a·mine
lev·an
lev·ar·te·re·nol
le·va·tor
pl le·va·tors
or le·va·to·res

lev·a·to·res cos·tar·um
lev·el
le·ver
Lé·vi syn·drome
le·vid·u·lin·ose
lev·i·gate
lev·i·ga·tion
Lé·vi-Lo·rain dis·ease
Le·vin tube
Le·vine clenched-fist sign
Lev·in·son test
lev·i·ta·tion
le·vo·car·di·a
le·vo·car·di·o·gram
le·vo·cli·na·tion
le·vo·con·dy·lism
le·vo·cy·clo·ver·sion
le·vo·do·pa
le·vo·duc·tion
le·vo·fu·rae·ta·done
le·vo·gram
le·vo·gy·rate
    or le·vo·gyre
le·vo·gy·ra·tion
le·vo·gyre
    or le·vo·gy·rate
le·vo·gy·rous
le·vo·me·pro·ma·zine
le·vo·nor·de·frin
le·vo·pho·bi·a
le·vo·pro·pox·y·phene
le·vo·ro·ta·ry
    or le·vo·ro·ta·to·ry
le·vo·ro·ta·tion
le·vo·ro·ta·to·ry
    or le·vo·ro·ta·ry
lev·or·phan·ol
le·vo·tar·tar·ic
le·vo·thy·rox·ine
le·vo·tor·sion
le·vo·ver·sion
lev·u·lin
lev·u·lin·ic
lev·u·lo·sae·mi·a
    var of lev·u·lo·se·mi·a
lev·u·lo·san
lev·u·lose
lev·u·lo·se·mi·a
lev·u·lo·su·ri·a

lev·u·rid
Le·vy test
Le·vy-Pal·mer meth·od
Lé·vy-Rous·sy syn·drome
Lew·is dis·ease
lew·is·ite
Ley·den bat·ter·y
Ley·den-Mö·bi·us dys·
    tro·phy
Ley·dig cell
ley·dig·ar·che
Lher·mitte sign
lib·er·a·tion
li·bid·i·nal
li·bid·i·nal·ly
li·bid·i·ni·za·tion
li·bid·i·nize
li·bid·i·nous
li·bid·i·nous·ly
li·bi·do
Lib·man-Sacks en·do·car·
    di·tis
li·bra
    pl li·brae
li·cense
li·cen·ti·ate
li·chen
li·chen pla·nus
li·chen·i·fi·ca·ti·o gi·gan·
    te·a
li·chen·i·fi·ca·tion
li·chen·i·form·in
li·chen·in
li·chen·i·za·tion
li·chen·oid
li·chen·ous
Licht·heim syn·drome
lic·o·rice
    or liq·uo·rice
lid
li·do·caine
li·do·fla·zine
Lie·ben test
Lie·ber·kühn crypt, gland
Lie·ber·mann-Bur·chard
    re·ac·tion
Lie·big test
li·en
li·en·al

li·en·cu·lus
    pl li·en·cu·li
li·e·ni·tis
li·e·no·cele
li·e·nog·ra·phy
    pl li·e·nog·ra·phies
li·e·no·ma·la·ci·a
li·e·no·med·ul·la·ry
li·e·no·my·e·log·e·nous
li·e·no·my·e·lo·ma·la·ci·a
li·e·nop·a·thy
    pl li·e·nop·a·thies
li·e·no·re·nal
li·e·no·tox·in
li·en·ter·ic
li·en·ter·y
    pl li·en·ter·ies
li·e·nun·cu·lus
    pl li·e·nun·cu·li
Liep·mann a·prax·i·a
Lie·se·gang ring
life
    pl lives
life-sup·port sys·tem
lig·a·ment
lig·a·ment of Coo·per
lig·a·ment of Treitz
lig·a·ment of Wins·low
lig·a·ment of Zinn
lig·a·men·ta
lig·a·men·tal
lig·a·men·ta·ry
lig·a·men·to·pex·y
    pl lig·a·men·to·pex·ies
lig·a·men·tous
lig·a·men·tum
    pl lig·a·men·ta
lig·a·men·tum fla·vum
    pl lig·a·men·ta fla·vi·a
lig·a·men·tum nu·chae
    pl lig·a·men·ta nu·chae
lig·and
li·gase
li·gate
li·ga·tion
lig·a·ture
Lig·et sign
light-a·dap·ted
light·head·ed

Li·gnac-de To·ni-Fan·co·ni syn·drome

Li·gnac-Fan·co·ni syn·drome

lig·ne·ous

lig·ni·fi·ca·tion

lig·nin

lig·no·caine

lig·no·cel·lu·lose

lig·no·cel·lu·lo·sic

lig·no·cer·ic

lig·num
  pl lig·nums
  or lig·na

lig·ro·in

lig·u·la
  pl lig·u·las
  or lig·u·lae

lig·ule

Lil·i·en·thal op·er·a·tion

limb

lim·ber·neck

lim·bi

lim·bic

lim·bus
  pl lim·bus·es
  or lim·bi

li·men
  pl lim·i·na

li·mes
  pl li·mi·tes

lim·in·al

lim·i·nom·e·ter

lim·it

lim·i·tans

lim·i·troph·ic

Lim·na·tis

lim·nol·o·gy

lim·o·nene

li·mo·nite

li·moph·thi·sis
  pl li·moph·thi·ses

limp

lin·al·o·ol

lin·a·mar·in

li·nar·i·a

lin·co·my·cin

linc·tus

lin·dane

Lin·dau dis·ease

Lind·bergh flask

Lin·der·strom-Lang meth·od

Lin·der·strom-Lang-Dus·pi·va meth·od

Lin·der·strom-Lang-En·gel meth·od

Lin·der·strom-Lang-Glick meth·od

Lin·der·strom-Lang-Hol·ter meth·od

Lin·der·strom-Lang-Lanz meth·od

Lin·der·strom-Lang-Weil-Hol·ter meth·od

line of Gen·na·ri

lin·ea
  pl lin·e·ae

lin·e·a al·ba
  pl lin·e·ae al·bae

lin·e·ae al·bi·can·tes

lin·e·al

lin·e·ar

lin·gua
  pl lin·guae

lin·gual

lin·gual·ly

Lin·gua·tu·la

lin·guat·u·lo·sis
  pl lin·guat·u·lo·ses

lin·gui·form

lin·gu·la
  pl lin·gu·lae

lin·gu·lec·to·my

lin·guo-clu·sion

lin·guo-dis·tal

lin·guo-gin·gi·val

lin·guo-pap·il·li·tis

lin·guo-ver·sion

lin·i·ment

li·nin

li·ni·tis

link·age

link·ed

Lin·og·na·thus

lin·ole·ic

lin·o·le·nic

li·no·lic

lin·o·no·pho·bi·a

lin·seed

lin·tin

li·o·thy·ro·nine

li·o·trix

lip

li·pa

lip·ac·i·de·ma

lip·ac·i·du·ria

li·pae·mi·a
  var of li·pe·mi·a

lip·a·ro·trich·i·a

lip·a·rous

li·pase

lip·a·su·ria

li·pec·to·my
  pl li·pec·to·mies

lip·e·de·ma

li·pe·mi·a

lip·fan·o·gen

lip·id
  or lip·ide

lip·i·dae·mi·a
  var of lip·i·de·mi·a

lip·ide
  or lip·id

lip·i·de·mi·a

lip·id·ic

lip·i·dol·y·sis

lip·i·do·sis
  pl lip·i·do·ses

lip·i·du·ri·a

lip·o·ar·thri·tis

lip·o·at·ro·phy

li·po·blast

lip·o·blas·tic

lip·o·blas·to·ma
  pl lip·o·blas·to·mas
  or lip·o·blas·to·ma·ta

lip·o·blas·to·sis

lip·o·ca·ic

lip·o·cal·ci·no·gran·u·lo·ma·to·sis

lip·o·car·di·ac

lip·o·cat·a·bol·ic

lip·o·cele

lip·o·cere

lip·o·chon·dro·dys·tro·phy

pl lip·o·chon·dro·dys·tro·phies

lip·o·chon·dro·ma
  pl lip·o·chon·dro·mas
  or lip·o·chon·dro·ma·ta

li·po·chrome

lip·o·cyte

lip·o·di·er·e·sis

lip·o·dys·tro·phi·a

lip·o·dys·tro·phy
  pl lip·o·dys·tro·phies

lip·o·fi·bro·ma
  pl lip·o·fi·bro·mas
  or lip·o·fi·bro·ma·ta

lip·o·fi·bro·myx·o·ma
  pl lip·o·fi·bro·myx·o·mas
  or lip·o·fi·bro·myx·o·ma·ta

lip·o·fi·bro·sar·co·ma
  pl lip·o·fi·bro·sar·co·mas
  or lip·o·fi·bro·sar·co·ma·ta

li·po·fus·cin

lip·o·gen·e·sis
  pl lip·o·gen·e·ses

lip·o·gen·ic
  or li·pog·e·nous

li·pog·e·nous
  or lip·o·gen·ic

lip·o·gran·u·lo·ma
  pl lip·o·gran·u·lo·mas
  or lip·o·gran·u·lo·ma·ta

lip·o·gran·u·lo·ma·to·sis

lip·o·hae·mar·thro·sis
  pl lip·o·hae·mar·thro·ses
  var of lip·o·he·mar·thro·sis

lip·o·he·mar·thro·sis
  pl lip·o·he·mar·thro·ses

li·po·ic

lip·oid
  or lip·oi·dal

lip·oi·dae·mi·a
  var of lip·oi·de·mi·a

lip·oi·dal
  or lip·oid

lip·oi·de·mi·a

li·poid·ic

lip·oi·do·sis
  pl lip·oi·do·ses

lip·oi·du·ri·a

li·pol·y·sis
  pl li·pol·y·ses

lip·o·lyt·ic

li·po·ma
  pl li·po·mas
  or li·po·ma·ta

li·pom·a·toid

li·po·ma·to·sis
  pl li·po·ma·to·ses

li·pom·a·tous

lip·o·mel·a·not·ic

li·po·me·nin·go·cele

li·po·me·ri·a
  or lei·po·me·ri·a

lip·o·me·tab·o·lism

li·pom·pha·lus

lip·o·my·e·lo·me·nin·go·cele

lip·o·my·o·hae·man·gi·o·ma
  pl lip·o·my·o·hae·man·gi·o·mas
  or lip·o·my·o·hae·man·gi·o·ma·ta
  var of lip·o·my·o·he·man·gi·o·ma

lip·o·my·o·he·man·gi·o·ma
  pl lip·o·my·o·he·man·gi·o·mas
  or lip·o·my·o·he·man·gi·o·ma·ta

lip·o·my·o·ma
  pl lip·o·my·o·mas
  or lip·o·my·o·ma·ta

lip·o·my·o·sar·co·ma
  pl lip·o·my·o·sar·co·mas
  or lip·o·my·o·sar·co·ma·ta

lip·o·myx·o·ma
  pl lip·o·myx·o·mas
  or lip·o·myx·o·ma·ta

lip·o·myx·o·sar·co·ma
  pl lip·o·myx·o·sar·co·mas
  or lip·o·myx·o·sar·co·ma·ta

Lip·o·nys·sus

li·po·pe·ni·a

lip·o·pep·tid

lip·o·pep·tide

li·po·phage

li·po·pha·gi·a

li·po·pha·gic

lip·o·pha·gy

li·po·phan·er·o·sis
  pl li·po·phan·e·ro·ses

lip·o·phil

lip·o·phile
  or lip·o·phil·ic

lip·o·phil·i·a

lip·o·phil·ic
  or lip·o·phile

lip·o·phore

li·po·phre·ni·a

lip·o·plas·tic

lip·o·pol·y·sac·cha·ride

lip·o·pro·te·in

lip·o·rho·din

lip·o·sar·co·ma
  pl lip·o·sar·co·mas
  or lip·o·sar·co·ma·ta

lip·o·sar·co·ma·tous

li·po·sis
  pl li·po·ses

lip·o·si·tol

lip·o·sol·u·ble

li·pos·to·my

li·po·thy·mi·a
  or li·poth·y·my

li·po·thy·mi·al

li·poth·y·my
  or li·po·thy·mi·a

lip·o·tro·phic
  or lip·o·trop·ic

li·pot·ro·phy

lip·o·tro·pi·a

lip·o·trop·ic
  or lip·o·tro·phic

lip·o·tro·pism

li·pot·ro·py

lip·o·vac·cine

lip·o·vi·tel·lin

lip·o·xan·thin

li·pox·e·nous

li·pox·e·ny
  pl li·pox·e·nies

li·pox·i·dase

li·pox·y·gen·ase

lip·pa

Lip·pes loop

lip·ping

217

lip·pi·tude
lip·pi·tu·do
Lip·schütz bod·y
li·pu·ri·a
liq·ue·fa·cient
liq·ue·fac·tion
liq·ue·fac·tive
liq·ue·fy
li·ques·cent
liq·uid
liq·uo·gel
li·quor
li·quor am·ni·i
liq·uo·rice
   or lic·o·rice
Lis·franc am·pu·ta·tion
lisp
Lis·sau·er tract
Lis·sen·ceph·a·la
lis·sen·ce·pha·li·a
   or lis·sen·ceph·a·ly
lis·sen·ce·phal·ic
   or lis·sen·ceph·a·lous
lis·sen·ceph·a·lous
   or lis·sen·ce·phal·ic
lis·sen·ceph·a·ly
   pl lis·sen·ceph·a·lies
   or lis·sen·ce·pha·li·a
Lis·ter·el·la
lis·ter·el·lo·sis
   pl lis·ter·el·lo·ses
   or lis·te·ri·o·sis
   pl lis·te·ri·o·ses
Lis·te·ri·a
lis·te·ri·o·sis
   pl lis·te·ri·o·ses
   or lis·ter·el·lo·sis
   pl lis·ter·el·lo·ses
lis·ter·ism
lis·ter·ize
Lis·ting law
li·ter
li·thae·mi·a
   var of li·the·mi·a
li·thae·mic
   var of li·the·mic
lith·a·gogue
lith·arge
li·thec·ta·sy

li·thec·to·my
   pl li·thec·to·mies
li·the·mi·a
li·the·mic
lith·i·a
li·thi·a·sic
li·thi·a·sis
   pl li·thi·a·ses
lith·ic
lith·i·co·sis
lith·i·um
lith·o·cho·lic
lith·o·clast
lith·o·cys·to·to·my
lith·o·di·al·y·sis
   pl lith·o·di·al·y·ses
lith·o·fel·lic
lith·o·gen·e·sis
   pl lith·o·gen·e·ses
lith·o·gen·et·ic
li·thog·e·nous
li·thog·e·ny
lith·oid
   or li·thoi·dal
li·thoi·dal
   or lith·oid
lith·o·kel·y·pho·pe·di·on
lith·o·kel·y·phos
lith·o·labe
li·thol·a·pax·y
   pl li·thol·a·pax·ies
li·thol·o·gy
   pl li·thol·o·gies
lith·ol·y·sis
lith·o·ne·phri·tis
   pl lith·o·ne·phrit·i·des
lith·o·ne·phrot·o·my
   pl lith·o·ne·phrot·o·mies
lith·on·trip·tic
   or lith·o·trip·tic
lith·o·pe·di·on
lith·o·phone
lith·o·scope
li·tho·sis
lith·o·tome
li·thot·o·mist
li·thot·o·mize
li·thot·o·my
   pl li·thot·o·mies

lith·o·trip·sy
   pl lith·o·trip·sies
lith·o·trip·tic
   or lith·on·trip·tic
lith·o·trip·to·scope
lith·o·trite
lith·o·trit·ic
li·thot·ri·tist
li·thot·ri·ty
   pl li·thot·ri·ties
lith·ous
lith·u·re·sis
li·thu·ri·a
lit·mus
li·tre
   var of li·ter
Lit·ten sign
lit·ter
Lit·tle dis·ease
Litt·man ox·gall me·
   di·um
lit·to·ral
Lit·tré gland
lit·tri·tis
Litz·mann ob·liq·ui·ty
live-born
li·ve·do
liv·e·doid
liv·er
liv·er·wort
liv·e·tin
liv·id
li·vid·i·ty
   pl li·vid·i·ties
Li·vi·e·ra·to sign
li·vor
lix·iv·i·a·tion
Liz·ars op·er·a·tion
Lju·bin·sky stain
Lo·a
lo·a·i·a·sis
   pl lo·a·i·a·ses
   or lo·i·a·sis
   pl lo·i·a·ses
lo·bar
lo·bate
   or lo·bat·ed
lo·bat·ed
   or lo·bate

lobe
lo·bec·to·my
  pl lo·bec·to·mies
lo·be·li·a
lo·be·line
lo·bi
lo·bi·tis
lo·bo·cyte
lo·bo·po·di·um
  pl lo·bo·po·di·a
lo·bot·o·mize
lo·bot·o·my
  pl lo·bot·o·mies
Lob·stein dis·ease
lob·u·lar
lob·u·late
  or lob·u·lat·ed
lob·u·lat·ed
  or lob·u·late
lob·u·la·tion
lob·ule
lob·u·li
lob·u·lose
lob·u·lus
  pl lob·u·li
lo·bus
  pl lo·bi
lo·cal
lo·cal·i·za·tion
lo·cal·ize
lo·cal·iz·er
lo·cal·ly
lo·chi·a
  pl lo·chi·a
lo·chi·a al·ba
lo·chi·al
lo·chi·o·col·pos
lo·chi·o·cyte
lo·chi·o·me·tra
lo·chi·o·me·tri·tis
lo·chi·or·rha·gi·a
lo·chi·or·rhe·a
lo·chi·or·rhoe·a
  var of lo·chi·or·rhe·a
lo·chi·os·che·sis
  pl lo·chi·os·che·ses
lo·cho·me·tri·tis
lo·cho·per·i·to·ni·tis
Locke so·lu·tion

Locke-Rin·ger so·lu·tion
lock·jaw
Lock·wood sign
lo·co
  pl lo·cos
  or lo·coes
lo·coed
lo·co·ism
lo·co·mo·tion
lo·co·mo·tive
lo·co·mo·tor
  or lo·co·mo·to·ry
lo·co·mo·to·ry
  or lo·co·mo·tor
loc·u·lar
loc·u·late
  or loc·u·lat·ed
loc·u·lat·ed
  or loc·u·late
loc·u·la·tion
loc·u·lus
  pl loc·u·li
lo·cum ten·ens
  pl lo·cum ten·en·tes
lo·cum·ten·en·cy
  pl lo·cum·ten·en·cies
lo·cus
  pl lo·ci
Loeb de·cid·u·al re·ac·tion
Loef·fler syn·drome
Lo·ele meth·od
Loe·wen·thal tract
Loe·wi sign
löf·fle·ri·a
log·a·dec·to·my
log·ag·no·si·a
log·ag·no·sis
log·a·graph·i·a
log·am·ne·si·a
lo·ga·nin
log·a·pha·si·a
log·as·the·ni·a
log·o·clo·ni·a
log·o·ko·pho·sis
log·o·ma·ni·a
log·o·neu·ro·sis
log·o·pae·di·a
  var of log·o·pe·di·a

log·o·pae·dics
  var of log·o·pe·dics
log·op·a·thy
  pl log·op·a·thies
log·o·pe·di·a
log·o·pe·dics
log·o·pha·si·a
log·o·ple·gi·a
log·or·rhe·a
log·or·rhe·ic
log·or·rhoe·a
  var of log·or·rhe·a
log·o·spasm
log·o·ther·a·py
log·wood
Loh·mann re·ac·tion
lo·i·a·sis
  pl lo·i·a·ses
  or lo·a·i·a·sis
  pl lo·a·i·a·ses
loin
lol·ism
lo·mo·fun·gin
Londe at·ro·phy
long bone
Long co·ef·fi·cient
lon·gev·i·ty
lon·gi·lin·e·al
lon·gi·ma·nous
lon·gi·ped·ate
lon·gis·si·mus dor·si
lon·gi·tu·di·nal
lon·gi·tu·di·na·lis
lon·gi·typ·i·cal
lon·gus
Loo·ney and Dy·er meth·od
loop of Hen·le
Loo·ser zones
loph·o·dont
Lo·phoph·o·ra
lo·phoph·o·rine
lo·phot·ri·chate
  or lo·phot·ri·chous
lo·phot·ri·chous
  or lo·phot·ri·chate
lo·quac·i·ty
Lo·rain-Lé·vi syn·drome
lor·do·sco·li·o·sis

lor·do·sis
  pl lor·do·ses
lor·dot·ic
Lo·renz meth·od
lo·ri·ca
Lo·ri·ga dis·ease
lo·ris
Lo·ris·i·dae
Lor·rain Smith stain
Los·sen op·er·a·tion
Lo·theis·sen op·er·a·tion
lo·ti·o
lo·tion
Lou·is-Bar syn·drome
loupe
louse
  pl lice
lousy
lov·age
Lo·vén re·flex
Lo·vi·bond u·nit
Lö·wen·stein-Jen·sen me·di·um
Low·er tu·ber·cle
Low·ry-Lo·pez-Bes·sey meth·od
Low·sley op·er·a·tion
lox·a
lox·i·a
lox·ic
Lox·os·ce·les
lox·os·ce·lism
lox·ot·ic
lox·ot·o·my
loz·enge
Lu·barsch cry·stals
Lu·barsch-Pick-syn·drome
lu·can·thone
Lu·cas-Cham·pion·nière dis·ease
lu·cen·cy
lu·cent
Lu·ci·a·ni tri·ad
lu·cid
lu·cid·i·ty
  pl lu·cid·i·ties
lu·ci·dum

lu·cif·er·ase
lu·cif·er·in
lu·cif·u·gal
Lu·cil·i·a
Lu·cio lep·ro·sy
lu·cip·e·tal
lück·en·schä·del
lu·dic
Lud·wig an·gi·na
Lu·er sy·ringe
lu·es
  pl lu·es
lu·et·ic
lu·e·tin
Lu·gol so·lu·tion
Lu·kens test
lum·ba·go
lum·bar
lum·bar·i·za·tion
lum·bo·co·los·to·my
  pl lum·bo·co·los·to·mies
lum·bo·co·lot·o·my
lum·bo·cos·tal
lum·bo·dor·sal
lum·bo·dy·ni·a
lum·bo·in·gui·nal
lum·bo·is·chi·al
lum·bo·sa·cral
lum·bo·ver·te·bral
lum·bri·cal
lum·bri·ca·lis
  pl lum·bri·ca·les
lum·bri·cide
lum·bri·coid
lum·bri·co·sis
lum·bri·cus
lum·bus
  pl lum·bi
lu·men
  pl lu·mens
  or lu·mi·na
lu·me·nal
  or lu·mi·nal
lu·mi·chrome
lu·mi·fla·vin
lu·mi·nal
  or lu·me·nal
lu·mi·nance
lu·mi·nesce

lu·mi·nes·cence
lu·mi·nes·cent
lu·mi·nif·er·ous
lu·mi·nol
lu·mi·nous
lu·mi·rho·dop·sin
lu·mis·ter·ol
lump
lump·ec·to·my
lu·na·cy
  pl lu·na·cies
lu·nar
lu·nare
  pl lu·nar·i·a
lu·nate
lu·na·tic
lu·na·to·ma·la·ci·a
lu·na·tum
  pl lu·na·ta
lu·nel·la
lung
lung·mo·tor
lung·worm
lu·nu·la
  pl lu·nu·lae
lu·nule
lu·pa·nine
lu·pi·form
lu·pin
  or lu·pine
lu·pine
  or lu·pin
lu·pi·no·sis
lu·poid
lu·pu·lin
lu·pu·lus
lu·pus
lu·pus er·y·the·ma·to·sus
lu·pus per·ni·o
lu·pus vul·gar·is
Lusch·ka bur·sa
Lust phe·nom·enon
lu·sus
lu·sus na·tu·rae
lute
lu·te·al
lu·te·ci·um
  or lu·te·ti·um
lu·te·in

lu·te·in·ic
lu·te·in·i·za·tion
lu·te·in·ize
lu·te·in·o·ma
  pl lu·te·in·o·mas
  or lu·te·in·o·ma·ta
Lu·tem·bach·er com·plex
lu·te·o·blas·to·ma
  pl lu·te·o·blas·to·mas
  or lu·te·o·blas·to·ma·ta
lu·te·o·hor·mone
lu·te·o·lin
lu·te·o·ma
  pl lu·te·o·mas
  or lu·te·o·ma·ta
lu·te·o·tro·phic
  or lu·te·o·trop·ic
lu·te·o·tro·phin
  or lu·te·o·tro·pin
lu·te·o·tro·pic
  or lu·te·o·tro·phic
lu·te·o·tro·pin
  or lu·te·o·tro·phin
lu·te·ti·um
  or lu·te·ci·um
Lu·ther·an blood group
lu·tu·trin
Lutz-Splen·do·re-
  Al·mei·da dis·ease
lux
  pl lux
  or lux·es
lux·ate
lux·a·tion
lux·u·ri·ant
lux·us
Luys bod·y le·sion
ly·ase
ly·can·thrope
ly·can·throp·ic
ly·can·thro·py
  pl ly·can·thro·pies
ly·cine
ly·co·ma·ni·a
ly·co·pene
Ly·co·per·don
ly·co·per·don·o·sis
  pl ly·co·per·don·o·sis·es
  or ly·co·per·don·o·ses

ly·co·po·di·um
ly·co·pus
ly·co·rex·i·a
ly·di·my·cin
lye
Ly·ell syn·drome
ly·go·phil·i·a
ly·ing-in
  pl ly·ings-in
  or ly·ing-ins
Lym·nae·a
lymph
lym·pha
lymph·ad·e·nec·ta·sis
lymph·ad·e·nec·to·my
  pl lymph·ad·e·nec·to·mies
lymph·a·de·ni·a
lymph·ad·e·ni·tis
lym·phad·e·no·cele
lym·phad·e·no·gram
lymph·ad·e·nog·ra·phy
lym·phad·e·noid
lymph·ad·e·no·ma
  pl lymph·ad·e·no·mas
  or lymph·ad·e·no·ma·ta
lymph·ad·e·no·ma·to·sis
  pl lymph·ad·e·no·ma·to·ses
lymph·ad·e·nop·a·thy
  pl lymph·ad·e·nop·a·thies
lymph·ad·e·no·sis
  pl lymph·ad·e·no·ses
lymph·ad·e·not·o·my
lym·pha·gogue
lym·phan·gi·al
lym·phan·gi·ec·ta·si·a
lym·phan·gi·ec·ta·sis
lym·phan·gi·ec·tat·ic
lym·phan·gi·ec·to·des
lym·phan·gi·ec·to·my
  pl lym·phan·gi·ec·to·mies
lym·phan·gi·i·tis
lym·phan·gi·o·en·do·the·
  li·al
lym·phan·gi·o·en·do·the·
  li·o·ma
  pl lym·phan·gi·o·en·do·the·
  li·o·mas
  or lym·phan·gi·o·en·do·the·
  li·o·ma·ta

lym·phan·gi·o·fi·bro·ma
  pl lym·phan·gi·o·fi·bro·mas
  or lym·phan·gi·o·fi·bro·
  ma·ta
lym·phan·gi·o·gram
lym·phan·gi·og·ra·phy
  pl lym·phan·gi·og·ra·phies
lym·phan·gi·ol·o·gy
lym·phan·gi·o·ma
  pl lym·phan·gi·o·mas
  or lym·phan·gi·o·ma·ta
lym·phan·gi·o·ma·tous
lym·phan·gi·o·phle·bi·tis
lym·phan·gi·o·plas·ty
  pl lym·phan·gi·o·plas·ties
lym·phan·gi·o·sar·co·ma
  pl lym·phan·gi·o·sar·co·
  mas
  or lym·phan·gi·o·sar·co·
  ma·ta
lym·phan·gi·ot·o·my
  pl lym·phan·gi·ot·o·mies
lym·phan·git·ic
lym·phan·gi·tis
  pl lym·phan·gi·ti·des
lym·phat·ic
lym·phat·i·cos·to·my
lym·pha·tism
lym·pha·ti·tis
lym·phat·o·cele
lym·pha·tol·y·sis
lym·phec·ta·si·a
lymph·e·de·ma
lym·phe·mi·a
lym·phen·te·ri·tis
lymph·no·di·tis
lym·pho·blast
lym·pho·blas·tic
lym·pho·blas·to·ma
  pl lym·pho·blas·to·mas
  or lym·pho·blas·to·ma·ta
lym·pho·blas·to·ma·to·sis
lym·pho·blas·to·sis
lym·pho·chlo·ro·ma
  pl lym·pho·chlo·ro·mas
  or lym·pho·chlo·ro·ma·ta
lym·pho·cyte
lym·pho·cyt·ic

221

lym·pho·cy·thae·mi·a
var of lym·pho·cy·the·mi·a
lym·pho·cy·the·mi·a
lym·pho·cy·to·blast
lym·pho·cy·toid
lym·pho·cy·to·ma
pl lym·pho·cy·to·mas
or lym·pho·cy·to·ma·ta
lym·pho·cy·to·pe·ni·a
lym·pho·cy·toph·thi·sis
lym·pho·cy·to·poi·e·sis
pl lym·pho·cy·to·poi·e·ses
lym·pho·cy·to·sis
pl lym·pho·cy·to·ses
lym·pho·cy·tot·ic
lym·pho·der·mi·a
lym·pho·duct
lymph·oe·de·ma
var of lymph·e·de·ma
lym·pho·ep·i·the·li·o·ma
pl lym·pho·ep·i·the·li·o·mas
or lym·pho·ep·i·the·li·o·ma·ta
lym·pho·ep·i·the·li·o·ma·tous
lym·pho·gen·ic
or lym·phog·e·nous
lym·phog·e·nous
or lym·pho·gen·ic
lym·pho·glan·du·la
pl lym·pho·glan·du·lae
lym·pho·go·ni·a
lym·pho·gram
lym·pho·gran·u·lo·ma
pl lym·pho·gran·u·lo·mas
or lym·pho·gran·u·lo·ma·ta
lym·pho·gran·u·lo·ma in·gui·na·le
lym·pho·gran·u·lo·ma ve·ne·re·um
lym·pho·gran·u·lo·ma·to·sis
pl lym·pho·gran·u·lo·ma·to·ses
lym·pho·gran·u·lo·ma·tous
lym·pho·graph·ic
lym·phog·ra·phy
pl lym·phog·ra·phies
lym·pho·his·ti·o·cyt·ic

lym·phoid
lym·phoi·dec·to·my
lym·phoi·do·cyte
lym·pho·ken·tric
lym·pho·kine
lym·pho·ki·ne·sis
lym·phol·o·gy
lym·pho·ma
pl lym·pho·mas
or lym·pho·ma·ta
lym·pho·ma·toid
lym·pho·ma·to·sis
pl lym·pho·ma·to·ses
lym·pho·ma·tous
lym·pho·mon·o·cyte
lym·pho·mon·o·cy·to·sis
pl lym·pho·mon·o·cy·to·ses
lym·pho·no·dus
pl lym·pho·no·di
lym·pho·path·i·a ve·ne·re·um
lym·pho·pa·thy
lym·pho·pe·ni·a
lym·pho·plas·mi·a
lym·pho·poi·e·sis
pl lym·pho·poi·e·ses
lym·pho·poi·et·ic
lym·pho·pro·lif·er·a·tive
lym·pho·pro·te·ase
lym·pho·re·tic·u·lar
lym·pho·re·tic·u·lo·ma
pl lym·pho·re·tic·u·lo·mas
or lym·pho·re·tic·u·lo·ma·ta
lym·pho·re·tic·u·lo·sis
pl lym·pho·re·tic·u·lo·ses
lym·phor·rhage
lym·phor·rhe·a
lym·phor·rhoe·a
var of lym·phor·rhe·a
lym·phor·rhoid
lym·pho·sar·co·ma
pl lym·pho·sar·co·mas
or lym·pho·sar·co·ma·ta
lym·pho·sar·co·ma·to·sis
pl lym·pho·sar·co·ma·to·ses
lym·pho·sar·co·ma·tous
lym·pho·sta·sis
lym·pho·tax·is
lymph·u·ri·a

lymph·vas·cu·lar
lyn·es·tre·nol
ly·o·chrome
ly·o·en·zyme
ly·o·gel
ly·o·gly·co·gen
Ly·on hy·poth·e·sis
ly·o·phil
or ly·o·phile
ly·o·phile
or ly·o·phil
ly·o·philed
ly·o·phil·ic
ly·oph·i·li·za·tion
ly·oph·i·lize
ly·oph·i·liz·er
ly·o·phobe
or ly·o·pho·bic
ly·o·pho·bic
or ly·o·phobe
ly·o·sol
ly·o·sorp·tion
ly·o·trope
ly·o·trop·ic
ly·pe·ma·ni·a
ly·po·thy·mi·a
ly·pres·sin
ly·ra
or lyre
ly·ra Da·vi·dis
lyre
or ly·ra
ly·sate
lyse
or lyze
ly·se·mi·a
ly·ser·gic ac·id di·eth·yl·am·ide
ly·ser·gide
Lys·holm grid
ly·sig·e·nous
ly·sim·e·ter
ly·sin
ly·sine
ly·sin·o·gen
ly·sis
pl ly·ses
ly·so·ceph·a·lin
ly·so·chrome

ly·so·gen
ly·so·gen·e·sis
   pl ly·so·gen·e·ses
ly·so·gen·ic
ly·so·ge·nic·i·ty
   pl ly·so·ge·nic·i·ties
ly·sog·e·ni·za·tion
ly·sog·e·nize
ly·sog·e·ny
   pl ly·sog·e·nies
ly·so·ki·nase

ly·so·lec·i·thin
ly·so·so·mal
ly·so·som·al·ly
ly·so·some
ly·so·staph·in
ly·so·type
ly·so·zyme
ly·so·zy·mu·ri·a
lys·sa
lys·sic

lys·soid
lys·so·pho·bi·a
ly·syl
ly·te·ri·an
lyt·ic
Lyt·ta ves·i·ca·to·ri·a
lyx·o·fla·vin
lyx·ose
lyze
   or lyse

M

ma huang
Ma·ca·ca
ma·ca·cus
Mac·al·lis·ter mus·cle
ma·caque
Mac·Cal·lum patch
Mac·chi·a·vel·lo stain
Mac·Cor·mac re·flex
mac·er·ate
mac·er·a·tion
mac·er·a·tive
Mac·ew·en sign
Mach num·ber
Ma·cha·do-
   Guer·rei·ro re·ac·tion
Mache u·nit
Mach·o·ver test
ma·ci·es
Mac·kee-Herr·mann-
   Ba·ker-Sulz·ber·ger
   meth·od
Mack·en·rodt lig·a·ment
Mac·ken·zie am·pu·ta·tion
Mac·Lean test
Mac·leod syn·drome
Mac·Neal tet·ra·chrome
   stain

Mac·ra·can·tho·rhyn·chus
mac·ra·cu·si·a
mac·ren·ce·phal·ic
   or mac·ren·ceph·a·lous
mac·ren·ceph·a·lous
   or mac·ren·ce·phal·ic
mac·ren·ceph·a·ly
   pl mac·ren·ceph·a·lies
mac·ro·am·y·lase
mac·ro·am·y·la·se·mi·a
mac·ro·bac·te·ri·um
mac·ro·bi·o·ta
mac·ro·bi·ot·ics
mac·ro·blast
mac·ro·ble·phar·i·a
mac·ro·bra·chi·a
mac·ro·car·di·us
mac·ro·ce·pha·li·a
mac·ro·ce·phal·ic
   or mac·ro·ceph·a·lous
mac·ro·ceph·a·lous
   or mac·ro·ce·phal·ic
mac·ro·ceph·a·lus
   pl mac·ro·ceph·a·li
mac·ro·ceph·a·ly
   pl mac·ro·ceph·a·lies
mac·ro·chei·li·a

mac·ro·chei·ri·a
mac·ro·nid·i·um
   pl mac·ro·co·nid·i·a
mac·ro·cra·ni·a
mac·ro·cyst
mac·ro·cyte
mac·ro·cyt·ic
mac·ro·cy·to·sis
   pl mac·ro·cy·to·ses
mac·ro·dac·tyl·i·a
mac·ro·dac·ty·lism
mac·ro·dac·ty·ly
   pl mac·ro·dac·ty·lies
mac·ro·dont
mac·ro·don·ti·a
   or mac·ro·don·tism
mac·ro·don·tism
   or mac·ro·don·ti·a
mac·ro·fol·lic·u·lar
mac·ro·gam·ate
mac·ro·gam·ete
mac·ro·ga·me·to·cyte
ma·crog·a·my
mac·ro·gen·i·to·so·mi·a
ma·crog·li·a
ma·crog·li·al
mac·ro·glob·u·lin

mac·ro·glob·u·li·nae·mi·a
var of mac·ro·glob·u·li·
ne·mi·a
mac·ro·glob·u·li·ne·mi·a
mac·ro·glob·u·li·ne·mic
mac·ro·glos·si·a
mac·ro·gna·thi·a
mac·ro·gnath·ic
mac·rog·na·thism
mac·ro·gy·ri·a
mac·ro·lide
mac·ro·lym·pho·cyte
mac·ro·mas·ti·a
mac·ro·ma·zi·a
mac·ro·me·li·a
ma·crom·e·lus
pl ma·crom·e·li
ma·crom·e·ly
mac·ro·mere
mac·ro·mer·o·zo·ite
mac·ro·meth·od
mac·ro·mo·lec·u·lar
mac·ro·mol·e·cule
mac·ro·mon·o·cyte
mac·ro·my·e·lo·blast
mac·ro·nor·mo·blast
mac·ro·nor·mo·cyte
mac·ro·nu·cle·us
pl mac·ro·nu·cle·us·es
or mac·ro·nu·cle·i
mac·ro·nych·i·a
mac·ro·phage
mac·ro·phag·ic
ma·croph·a·gy
mac·ro·po·di·a
mac·rop·o·dy
mac·ro·pol·y·cyte
mac·ro·pro·so·pi·a
mac·ro·pro·so·pus
mac·ro·pro·so·py
ma·crop·si·a
or mac·rop·sy
mac·rop·sy
pl mac·rop·sies
or ma·crop·si·a
mac·ro·scop·ic
or mac·ro·scop·i·cal
mac·ro·scop·i·cal
or mac·ro·scop·ic

mac·ro·scop·i·cal·ly
mac·ros·mat·ic
mac·ro·so·mi·a
mac·ro·spore
mac·ro·spo·ric
mac·ro·sto·mi·a
ma·cro·ti·a
Ma·cruz in·dex
mac·u·la
pl mac·u·las
or mac·u·lae
mac·u·la a·cu·sti·ca
pl mac·u·lae a·cu·sti·cae
mac·u·la lu·te·a
pl mac·u·lae lu·te·ae
mac·u·lar
mac·u·late
or mac·u·lat·ed
mac·u·lat·ed
or mac·u·late
mac·u·la·tion
mac·ule
mac·u·lo·an·es·thet·ic
mac·u·lo·pap·u·lar
mac·u·lo·pap·ule
mad·a·ro·sis
pl mad·a·ro·ses
mad·a·rot·ic
mad·a·rous
Mad·dox rod
Mad·e·lung de·for·mi·ty
mad·i·dans
mad·ness
ma·du·ra foot
Mad·u·rel·la
mad·u·ro·my·co·sis
pl mad·u·ro·my·co·ses
mae·le·nic
ma·fe·nide
Maf·fu·cci syn·drome
mag·al·drate
ma·gen·bla·se
Ma·gen·die for·a·men
ma·gen·stras·se
ma·gen·ta
mag·got
mag·is·ter·y
pl mag·is·ter·ies

mag·is·tral
mag·ma
Mag·nan sign
mag·ne·si·a
mag·ne·site
mag·ne·si·um
mag·net
mag·net·ic
mag·ne·tism
mag·ne·ti·za·tion
mag·ne·tize
mag·ne·to·car·di·o·gram
mag·ne·to·car·di·o·graph
mag·ne·to·car·di·o·graph·ic
mag·ne·to·car·di·og·ra·phy
pl mag·ne·to·car·di·og·ra·
phies
mag·ne·to·e·lec·tric·i·ty
mag·ne·to·graph
mag·ne·to·in·duc·tion
mag·ne·tom·e·ter
mag·ne·ton
mag·ne·to·op·tic
mag·ne·to·stric·tion
mag·ne·to·ther·a·py
mag·ne·tron
mag·ni·fi·ca·tion
mag·ni·fy
mag·no·cel·lu·lar
mag·num
Mag·nus-de Kleijn
re·flex·es
Ma·haim fi·bers
maid·en·head
ma·ieu·si·o·ma·ni·a
ma·ieu·si·o·pho·bi·a
ma·ieu·tic
ma·ieu·tics
ma·ieu·tol·o·gist
maim
Mai·mon·i·de·an
main en grif·fe
main en lor·gnette
Main syn·drome
Mais·sat band
Ma·joc·chi dis·ease
ma·jor

Ma·jor·ström meth·od
Make·ham law
mal
mal de ca·de·ras
mal del pin·to
mal de mer
Mal·a·bar itch
mal·ab·sorp·tion
mal·a·chite
ma·la·ci·a
mal·a·co·pla·ki·a
  or mal·a·ko·pla·ki·a
mal·a·cot·ic
mal·ad·ap·ta·tion
mal·adap·tive
ma·la·die bleu
mal·ad·just·ed
mal·ad·jus·tive
mal·ad·just·ment
mal·a·dy
  pl mal·a·dies
ma·laise
mal·a·ko·pla·ki·a
  or mal·a·co·pla·ki·a
mal·a·lign·ment
mal·an·ders
  or mal·len·ders
ma·lar
ma·lar·i·a
ma·lar·i·ae ma·lar·i·a
ma·lar·i·al
  or ma·lar·i·an
ma·lar·i·an
  or ma·lar·i·al
ma·lar·i·ol·o·gist
ma·lar·i·ol·o·gy
  pl ma·lar·i·ol·o·gies
ma·lar·i·o·ther·a·py
  pl ma·lar·i·o·ther·a·pies
ma·la·ri·ous
mal·ar·tic·u·la·tion
Mal·as·se·zi·a
mal·as·sim·i·la·tion
ma·late
mal·a·thi·on
mal·ax·ate
mal·ax·a·tion
mal·de·vel·op·ment

mal·di·ges·tion
male
male Tur·ner syn·drome
ma·lease
  var of ma·laise
ma·le·ate
ma·le·ic
mal·e·rup·tion
male-ster·ile
mal·eth·a·mer
mal·for·ma·tion
mal·formed
mal·func·tion
Mal·gaigne am·pu·ta·tion
Ma·li·bu dis·ease
mal·ic
ma·lig·nan·cy
  pl ma·lig·nan·cies
ma·lig·nant
ma·lig·nant·ly
ma·lig·ni·ty
  pl ma·lig·ni·ties
ma·lin·ger
ma·lin·ger·er
Mall for·mu·la
mal·le·a·bil·i·ty
mal·le·a·ble
mal·le·a·tion
mal·le·in
mal·le·in·i·za·tion
mal·len·ders
  or mal·an·ders
mal·le·o·in·cu·dal
mal·le·o·lar
mal·le·o·lus
  pl mal·le·o·li
Mal·le·o·my·ces
mal·le·o·my·rin·go·plas·ty
mal·le·ot·o·my
  pl mal·le·ot·o·mies
mal·let
mal·le·us
  pl mal·le·i
Mal·loph·a·ga
Mal·lo·ry bod·ies
Mal·lo·ry-Weiss
  syn·drome
mal·low

Mal·loy-Ev·e·lyn meth·od
mal·nour·ish
mal·nour·ished
mal·nour·ish·ment
mal·nu·tri·tion
mal·oc·clu·sion
ma·lo·lac·tic
mal·o·nate
ma·lo·nic
mal·o·nyl
mal·o·nyl·u·re·a
mal·pigh·i·an pyr·a·mid
mal·po·si·tion
mal·pos·ture
mal·prac·tice
mal·prac·ti·tion·er
mal·prax·is
  pl mal·prax·es
mal·pre·sen·ta·tion
mal·re·duc·tion
mal·ro·ta·tion
malt
Mal·ta fe·ver
malt·ase
Mal·thu·si·an
Mal·thu·si·an·ism
mal·to·bi·ose
malt·ose
malt·os·u·ri·a
mal·um
  pl mal·a
mal·un·ion
mal·u·ni·ted
ma·man·pi·an
mam·ba
mam·e·lon
ma·mil·la
  pl ma·mil·lae
mam·il·lar·y
mam·il·lat·ed
mam·il·la·tion
ma·mil·li·form
ma·mil·li·plas·ty
ma·mil·li·tis
mam·ma
  pl mam·mae
mam·mal
mam·mal·gi·a

Mam·ma·li·a
mam·ma·li·an
mam·ma·plas·ty
  pl mam·ma·plas·ties
mam·ma·ry
mam·mec·to·my
  pl mam·mec·to·mies
mam·mi·form
mam·mil·la
  pl mam·mil·lae
  var of ma·mil·la
Mam·mil·lar·i·a
mam·mil·lar·y
  var of mam·il·lar·y
mam·mil·late
  or mam·mil·lat·ed
  var of mam·il·lat·ed
mam·mil·lat·ed
  or mam·mil·late
  var of mam·il·lat·ed
mam·mil·la·tion
  var of mam·il·la·tion
mam·mil·li·form
  var of mam·il·li·form
mam·mil·li·plas·ty
  pl mam·mil·li·plas·ties
mam·mil·li·tis
mam·mil·lo·in·fun·dib·u·lar
mam·mil·lo·teg·men·tal
mam·mil·lo·tha·lam·ic
mam·mi·pla·si·a
  var of mam·mo·pla·si·a
mam·mi·tis
  pl mam·mi·ti·des
mam·mo·gen
mam·mo·gen·ic
mam·mo·gen·i·cal·ly
mam·mo·gram
mam·mo·graph·ic
mam·mog·ra·phy
  pl mam·mog·ra·phies
mam·mo·pla·si·a
mam·mo·plas·ty
  pl mam·mo·plas·ties
mam·mose
mam·mot·o·my
  pl mam·mot·o·mies
mam·mo·tro·phic

mam·mo·tro·phin
mam·mo·tro·pic
mam·mo·tro·pin
mam·pir·ra
man
man·cha·da
man·chette
Man·chu·ri·an fe·ver
man·ci·nism
Man·cke-Som·mer test
man·del·ate
Man·del·baum re·ac·tion
man·del·ic
man·di·ble
man·dib·u·la
  pl man·dib·u·lae
man·dib·u·lar
man·dib·u·late
man·dib·u·lec·to·my
man·dib·u·lo·fa·cial
man·dib·u·lo·glos·sus
man·dib·u·lo·mar·gi·na·lis
Man·dl op·er·a·tion
man·drel
man·dril
  var of man·drel
man·drill
Man·dril·lus
man·drin
man·du·cate
man·du·ca·tion
man·du·ca·to·ry
ma·neu·ver
man·ga·bey
man·ga·nese
man·gan·ic
man·ga·nous
mange
man·gy
ma·ni·a
ma·ni·ac
ma·ni·a·cal
ma·ni·a·cal·ly
man·i·cal·ly
man·ic-de·pres·sive
man·i·kin
man·i·ple
man·i·plies
  var of man·y·plies

ma·nip·u·la·ble
ma·nip·u·late
ma·nip·u·la·tion
ma·nip·u·la·tive
ma·nip·u·la·tive·ly
ma·nip·u·la·tor
ma·nip·u·la·to·ry
Mann pal·sy
Mann-Boll·man fis·tu·la
Mann-William·son ul·cer
man·na
man·nan
man·ner·ism
man·ni·kin
  var of man·i·kin
man·ni·tan
man·nite
man·ni·tol
man·non·ic
man·no·sac·char·ic
man·no·san
man·nose
man·nu·ron·ic
ma·nom·e·ter
man·o·met·ric
  or man·o·met·ri·cal
man·o·met·ri·cal
  or man·o·met·ric
man·o·met·ri·cal·ly
ma·nom·e·try
  pl ma·nom·e·tries
man·o·scope
Man·son·el·la
Man·so·ni·a
Man·son dis·ease
man·tle
Man·toux test
ma·nu·bri·al
ma·nu·bri·um
  pl ma·nu·bri·ums
  or ma·nu·bri·a
ma·nu·bri·um ster·ni
man·u·duc·tion
man·u·dy·na·mom·e·ter
ma·nus
  pl ma·nus
man·u·stu·pra·tion
man·y·plies
Ma·ran·ta

ma·ran·tic
ma·ras·ma
ma·ras·mic
ma·ras·mus
mar·ble
mar·ble·i·za·tion
Mar·burg vi·rus
marc
marche à pe·tit pas
Mar·che·sa·ni syn·drome
Mar·chi glob·ules
Mar·chi·a·fa·va-Bi·gna·mi
    syn·drome
Mar·chi·a·fa·va-Mi·che·li
    syn·drome
Marck·wald op·er·a·tion
mar·cor
Mar·cus Gunn phe·nom·e·
    non
mard el bich·a
Mar·ek dis·ease
Mar·esch stain
Ma·rey law
Mar·fan syn·drome
mar·ga·ri·to·ma
    pl mar·ga·ri·to·mas
    or mar·ga·ri·to·ma·ta
Mar·gar·o·pus an·nu·la·tus
mar·gin
mar·gin·al
mar·gin·ate
mar·gin·a·tion
mar·gin·o·plas·ty
    pl mar·gin·o·plas·ties
mar·go
    pl mar·gi·nes
Ma·rie a·tax·i·a
Ma·rie-Bam·ber·ger
    dis·ease
Ma·rie-Foix re·trac·tion
    sign
Ma·rie-Strüm·pell
    ar·thri·tis
Ma·rie-Tooth dis·ease
mar·i·hua·na
    or mar·i·jua·na
mar·i·jua·na
    or mar·i·hua·na
Ma·rin A·mat syn·drome

Ma·ri·nes·co hand
Ma·ri·nes·co-Sjö·gren-
    Gar·land syn·drome
Ma·ri·otte blind spot
Mar·jo·lin ul·cer
mark
mark·er
mar·mo·rate
    or mar·mo·rat·ed
mar·mo·rat·ed
    or mar·mo·rate
mar·mo·ra·tion
mar·mo·ri·za·tion
mar·mo·set
Ma·ro·teaux-La·my
    syn·drome
mar·row
mar·row·bone
Mar·schal·ko plas·ma cell
Mar·seilles fe·ver
Marsh test
Mar·shall Hall meth·od
Mar·shall vein
Mar·ston de·cep·tion test
mar·su·pi·al
mar·su·pi·al·i·za·tion
mar·su·pi·al·ize
mar·su·pi·um
    pl mar·su·pi·a
Mar·ti·not·ti cells
Mar·to·rell syn·drome
Mar·we·del op·er·a·tion
mas·cu·line
mas·cu·line·ly
mas·cu·line·ness
mas·cu·lin·i·ty
    pl mas·cu·lin·i·ties
mas·cu·lin·i·za·tion
mas·cu·lin·ize
mas·cu·lin·o·ma
    pl mas·cu·lin·o·mas
    or mas·cu·lin·o·ma·ta
mas·cu·lin·o·vo·blas·to·ma
    pl mas·cu·lin·o·vo·blas·to·
    mas
    or mas·cu·lin·o·vo·blas·to·
    ma·ta
ma·ser
mask

mas·o·chism
mas·o·chist
mas·o·chis·tic
mas·o·chis·ti·cal·ly
Ma·son in·ci·sion
mas·que bi·liaire
mass
mas·sa
    pl mas·sae
mas·sage
mas·se·ter
mas·se·ter·ic
mas·seur
mas·seuse
Mas·son bod·y
mas·so·ther·a·pist
mas·so·ther·a·py
    pl mas·so·ther·a·pies
mast·ad·e·ni·tis
mast·ad·e·no·ma
    pl mast·ad·e·no·mas
    or mast·ad·e·no·ma·ta
mas·tal·gi·a
mas·ta·tro·phi·a
mas·tat·ro·phy
mas·taux·y
mast·ec·chy·mo·sis
mas·tec·to·my
    pl mas·tec·to·mies
Mas·ter two-step test
mast·hel·co·sis
mas·tic
    or mas·tich
    or mas·ti·che
mas·ti·cate
mas·ti·ca·tion
mas·ti·ca·tor
mas·ti·ca·to·ry
mas·tich
    or mas·tic
    or mas·ti·che
mas·ti·che
    or mas·tich
    or mas·tic
Mas·ti·goph·o·ra
mas·ti·goph·o·ran
mas·ti·goph·o·rous
mas·ti·gote
mas·tit·ic

mas·ti·tis
   pl mas·ti·ti·des
mas·to·car·ci·no·ma
   pl mas·to·car·ci·no·mas
   or mas·to·car·ci·no·ma·ta
mas·to·cyte
mas·to·cy·to·ma
   pl mas·to·cy·to·mas
   or mas·to·cy·to·ma·ta
mas·to·cy·to·sis
mas·to·dyn·i·a
mas·toid
mas·toi·dal
   or mas·toi·de·al
   or mas·toi·de·an
mas·toid·al·gi·a
mas·toi·de·al
   or mas·toi·dal
   or mas·toi·de·an
mas·toi·de·an
   or mas·toi·dal
   or mas·toi·de·al
mas·toid·ec·to·my
   pl mas·toid·ec·to·mies
mas·toi·de·o·cen·te·sis
mas·toid·i·tis
   pl mas·toid·i·ti·des
mas·toid·ot·o·my
   pl mas·toid·ot·o·mies
mas·ton·cus
mas·to·oc·cip·i·tal
mas·to·pa·ri·e·tal
mas·top·a·thy
   pl mas·top·a·thies
mas·to·pex·y
   pl mas·to·pex·ies
mas·to·pla·si·a
mas·to·plas·ti·a
mas·to·plas·ty
   pl mas·to·plas·ties
mas·to·pto·sis
mas·tor·rha·gi·a
mas·to·scir·rhus
   pl mas·to·scir·rhi
mas·to·squa·mous
mas·tos·to·my
mas·tot·o·my
   pl mas·tot·o·mies
mas·tous

mas·tur·bate
mas·tur·ba·tion
mas·tur·ba·tor
mas·tur·ba·tory
ma·su·ri·um
Mat·as op·er·a·tion
match
mate
ma·te·ri·a al·ba
ma·te·ria med·i·ca
ma·te·ri·al
ma·te·ri·es
ma·ter·nal
ma·ter·ni·ty
   pl ma·ter·ni·ties
ma·ti·co
mat·ing
ma·tri·cal
mat·ri·car·i·a
   pl mat·ri·car·i·a
   or mat·ri·car·i·as
ma·tri·cid·al
ma·tri·cide
ma·trix
   pl ma·trix·es
   or ma·tri·ces
matt
matte
mat·ter
mat·u·rate
mat·u·ra·tion
mat·u·ra·tion·al
ma·tur·a·tive
ma·ture
ma·tu·ri·ty
   pl ma·tu·ri·ties
ma·tu·ti·nal
ma·tu·ti·nal·ly
Mau·chart lig·a·ments
Mau·me·né test
Mau·noir hy·dro·cele
Mau·rer dots
max·il·la
   pl max·il·las
   or max·il·lae
max·il·lar·y
max·il·lo·fa·cial
max·il·lo·fron·ta·le
max·il·lo·lac·ri·mal

max·il·lo·man·dib·u·lar
max·il·lo·pal·a·tal
   or max·il·lo·pal·a·tine
max·il·lo·pal·a·tine
   or max·il·lo·pal·a·tal
max·il·lot·o·my
max·il·lo·tur·bi·nal
max·i·mal
max·i·mal·ly
max·i·mum
   pl max·i·mums
   or max·i·ma
May·er re·flex
May-Grün·wald stain
May-Heg·glin a·nom·a·ly
may·hem
Ma·yo op·er·a·tion
Ma·yo-Rob·son in·ci·sion
ma·za
ma·zal·gi·a
maze
maz·ic
ma·zo·ca·coth·e·sis
ma·zo·dyn·i·a
ma·zo·i·tis
ma·zol·y·sis
ma·zop·a·thy
ma·zo·pex·y
ma·zo·pla·si·a
Maz·za·mar·ra itch
Maz·zi·ni test
Maz·zo·ni cor·pus·cle
Mc·Ar·dle syn·drome
Mc·Bur·ney point
Mc·Call fes·toon
Mc·Car·thy re·flex
Mc·Cune-Al·bright
   syn·drome
Mc·Ell·roy test
Mc·Gill op·er·a·tion
Mc·Gun·kin meth·od
Mc·In·tosh test
Mc·Lean for·mu·la
Mc·Mee·kin meth·od
Mc·Mur·ray sign
mean
mea·sle
mea·sles
mea·sly

me·a·tal
me·a·ti·tis
me·a·tor·rha·phy
me·a·tos·co·py
me·a·tot·o·my
  pl me·a·tot·o·mies
me·a·tus
  pl me·a·tus·es
  or me·a·tus
me·bev·er·ine
me·bu·ta·mate
mec·a·mine
mec·a·myl·a·mine
me·chan·i·cal
me·chan·i·cal·ly
me·chan·ics
mech·a·nism
mech·a·no·chem·i·cal
mech·a·no·chem·is·try
  pl mech·a·no·chem·is·tries
mech·a·no·re·cep·tion
mech·a·no·re·cep·tive
mech·a·no·re·cep·tor
mech·a·no·ther·a·pist
mech·a·no·ther·a·py
  pl mech·a·no·ther·a·pies
mech·lor·eth·a·mine
me·cism
Me·cis·to·cir·rus
Meck·el car·ti·lage
Meck·el cav·i·ty
Meck·el di·ver·tic·u·lum
Meck·el gan·gli·on
mec·li·zine
mec·lo·qua·lon
mec·lo·qua·lone
me·com·e·ter
me·co·nal·gi·a
mec·o·nate
mec·o·neu·ro·path·i·a
me·con·ic
me·co·ni·or·rhe·a
me·co·ni·um
me·cys·ta·sis
mec·y·stat·ic
me·daz·e·pam
me·di·ad
me·di·al
me·di·a·lec·i·thal

me·di·a·lis
me·di·al·ly
me·di·an
me·di·as·ti·nal
me·di·as·ti·ni·tis
  pl me·di·as·ti·ni·ti·des
me·di·as·ti·no·gram
me·di·as·ti·nog·ra·phy
me·di·as·ti·no·per·i·car·di·tis
  pl me·di·as·ti·no·per·i·car·di·ti·des
me·di·as·tin·o·scope
me·di·as·ti·nos·co·py
  pl me·di·as·ti·nos·co·pies
me·di·as·ti·not·o·my
  pl me·di·as·ti·not·o·mies
me·di·as·ti·num
  pl me·di·as·ti·na
me·di·ate
me·di·a·tion
me·di·a·tion·al
me·di·a·tor
med·ic
med·i·ca·ble
Med·ic·aid
med·i·cal
med·i·ca·ment
med·i·ca·men·to·sus
med·i·ca·men·tous
med·i·cant
Med·i·care
med·i·cate
med·i·ca·tion
med·i·ca·tive
med·i·ca·tor
me·dic·i·na·ble
me·dic·i·nal
me·dic·i·nal·ly
med·i·cine
med·i·co·chi·rur·gi·cal
med·i·co·le·gal
med·i·co·psy·chol·o·gy
  pl med·i·co·psy·chol·o·gies
med·i·co·sta·tis·tic
med·i·co·sur·gi·cal
med·i·cus
Med·in dis·ease
Me·di·na worm

me·di·o·car·pal
me·di·o·cen·tric
me·di·o·dor·sal
me·di·o·fron·tal
me·di·o·lat·er·al
me·di·o·ne·cro·sis
  pl me·di·o·ne·cro·ses
me·di·o·plan·tar
me·di·o·su·pe·ri·or
me·di·o·tar·sal
Med·i·ter·ra·ne·an a·ne·mi·a
me·di·um
  pl me·di·ums
  or me·di·a
me·di·us
  pl me·di·i
med·ro·ges·tone
me·drox·y·pro·ges·ter·one
med·ry·sone
me·dul·la
  pl me·dul·las
  or me·dul·lae
me·dul·la ob·lon·ga·ta
  pl me·dul·la ob·lon·ga·tas
  or me·dul·lae ob·lon·ga·tae
med·ul·lar
  or med·ul·lar·y
med·ul·lar·in
med·ul·lar·y
  or med·ul·lar
med·ul·lat·ed
med·ul·la·tion
me·dul·lin
me·dul·li·spi·nal
me·dul·li·za·tion
me·dul·lo·a·dre·nal
me·dul·lo·blast
med·ul·lo·blas·to·ma
  pl med·ul·lo·blas·to·mas
  or med·ul·lo·blas·to·ma·ta
med·ul·lo·ep·i·the·li·o·ma
  pl med·ul·lo·ep·i·the·li·o·mas
  or med·ul·lo·ep·i·the·li·o·ma·ta
Med·u·na meth·od
Meek·rin-Eh·lers-Dan·los syn·drome

Mees lines
mef·e·nam·ic
me·fen·o·rex
me·fex·a·mide
mef·ru·side
meg·a·blad·der
meg·a·cae·cum
  var of meg·a·ce·cum
meg·a·car·di·a
meg·a·car·y·o·cyte
  var of meg·a·kar·y·o·cyte
meg·a·ce·cum
meg·a·ce·phal·ic
  or meg·a·ceph·a·lous
meg·a·ceph·a·lous
  or meg·a·ce·phal·ic
meg·a·ceph·a·ly
  pl meg·a·ceph·a·lies
meg·a·coc·cus
  pl meg·a·coc·ci
meg·a·co·lon
meg·a·co·ni·al
meg·a·cy·cle
meg·a·death
meg·a·dont
meg·a·don·tism
meg·a·don·ty
  pl meg·a·don·ties
meg·a·du·o·de·num
meg·a·dyne
meg·a·e·soph·a·gus
  pl meg·a·e·soph·a·gi
meg·a·far·ad
meg·a·gam·ete
meg·a·ga·me·to·phyte
meg·a·gna·thus
meg·a·kar·y·o·blast
meg·a·kar·y·o·blas·to·ma
  pl meg·a·kar·y·o·blas·to·
  mas
  or meg·a·kar·y·o·blas·to·
  ma·ta
meg·a·kar·y·o·cyte
meg·a·kar·y·o·cyt·ic
meg·a·kar·y·o·cy·to·pe·ni·a
meg·a·kar·y·o·cy·to·sis
meg·a·kar·y·oph·thi·sis
meg·a·lec·i·thal
meg·a·len·ceph·a·ly

meg·a·ler·y·the·ma
me·gal·gi·a
meg·a·lo·blast
meg·a·lo·blas·tic
meg·a·lo·blas·toid
meg·a·lo·car·di·a
meg·a·lo·ce·phal·ic
  or meg·a·lo·ceph·a·lous
meg·a·lo·ceph·a·lous
  or meg·a·lo·ce·phal·ic
meg·a·lo·ceph·a·ly
  pl meg·a·lo·ceph·a·lies
meg·a·loc·er·us
meg·a·lo·chei·ri·a
meg·a·lo·chei·rous
meg·a·lo·cor·ne·a
meg·a·lo·cys·tic
meg·a·lo·cyte
meg·a·lo·cyt·ic
meg·a·lo·cy·to·sis
meg·a·lo·dac·ty·ly
meg·a·lo·don·ti·a
meg·a·lo·en·ter·on
me·ga·lo·e·soph·a·gus
meg·a·lo·gas·tri·a
meg·a·lo·glos·si·a
meg·a·lo·he·pat·i·a
meg·a·lo·kar·y·o·blast
meg·a·lo·kar·y·o·cyte
meg·a·lo·ma·ni·a
meg·a·lo·ma·ni·ac
  or meg·a·lo·ma·ni·a·cal
meg·a·lo·ma·ni·a·cal
  or meg·a·lo·man·ic
meg·a·lo·ma·ni·a·cal·ly
meg·a·lo·man·ic
meg·a·lo·mas·ti·a
meg·a·lo·me·li·a
meg·a·lon·y·cho·sis
meg·a·lo·pe·nis
meg·a·loph·thal·mos
  or meg·a·loph·thal·mus
meg·a·loph·thal·mus
  or meg·a·loph·thal·mos
meg·a·lo·pi·a
meg·a·lo·po·di·a
meg·a·lop·si·a
meg·a·lo·splanch·nic

meg·a·lo·sple·ni·a
meg·a·lo·spore
me·ga·lo·syn·dac·ty·ly
meg·a·lo·u·re·ter
meg·a·mer·o·zo·ite
meg·a·nu·cle·us
meg·a·oe·soph·a·gus
  var of meg·a·e·soph·a·gus
meg·a·phone
mega·pros·o·pous
meg·a·rec·tum
meg·a·sig·moid
meg·a·spore
meg·a·spor·ic
meg·a·spo·ro·gen·e·sis
  pl meg·a·spo·ro·gen·e·ses
meg·a·u·re·ter
meg·a·vi·ta·min
meg·a·volt
me·ges·trol
me·glu·mine
meg·ohm
meg·oph·thal·mos
meg·oph·thal·mus
me·grim
Meh·lis gland
Mei·bo·mi·an gland
mei·bo·mi·a·ni·tis
mei·bo·mi·tis
Meige dis·ease
Meigs syn·drome
Mei·ni·cke test
mei·o·lec·i·thal
  or mi·o·lec·i·thal
mei·o·sis
  pl mei·o·ses
mei·ot·ic
mei·ot·i·cal·ly
Mei·row·sky phe·nom·e·
  non
Meiss·ner cor·pus·cle
mel
me·lae·na
  var of me·le·na
me·lae·nic
  var of me·le·nic
me·lag·ra
me·lal·gi·a
mel·a·mine

mel·an·cho·li·a
  pl mel·an·cho·li·as
  or mel·an·cho·li·ae
mel·an·cho·li·ac
mel·an·chol·ic
mel·an·chol·i·cal·ly
mel·an·chol·y
  pl mel·an·chol·ies
mel·a·ne·mia
mé·lan·geur
Me·la·ni·a
me·lan·ic
mel·a·ni·dro·sis
mel·a·nif·er·ous
mel·a·nin
mel·a·nism
mel·a·nis·tic
mel·a·ni·za·tion
mel·a·nize
mel·a·no·am·e·lo·blas·to·ma
  pl mel·a·no·am·e·lo·blas·to·mas
  or mel·a·no·am·e·lo·blas·to·ma·ta
me·la·no·blast
me·la·no·blas·tic
me·la·no·blas·to·ma
  pl me·la·no·blas·to·mas
  or me·la·no·blas·to·ma·ta
mel·a·no·car·ci·no·ma
  pl mel·a·no·car·ci·no·mas
  or mel·a·no·car·ci·no·ma·ta
mel·a·noch·roi
me·la·no·chro·ic
mel·a·noch·ro·ous
mel·a·noc·o·mous
me·la·no·cyte
me·la·no·cyte-stim·u·lat·ing hor·mone
mel·a·no·cy·to·ma
  pl mel·a·no·cy·to·mas
  or mel·a·no·cy·to·ma·ta
mel·a·no·cy·to·sis
me·la·no·derm
me·la·no·der·ma
mel·a·no·der·ma·ti·tis
mel·a·no·der·mi·a
me·la·no·der·mic

mel·a·no·ep·i·the·li·o·ma
  pl mel·a·no·epi·the·li·o·mas
  or mel·a·no·epi·the·li·o·ma·ta
mel·a·no·floc·cu·la·tion
me·lan·o·gen
mel·a·no·gen·e·sis
  pl mel·a·no·gen·e·ses
mel·a·no·ge·net·ic
mel·a·no·gen·ic
mel·a·no·glos·si·a
mel·a·noid
mel·a·no·leu·ko·der·ma
mel·a·no·leu·ko·der·ma col·li
mel·a·no·ma
  pl mel·a·no·mas
  or mel·a·no·ma·ta
mel·a·no·ma·to·sis
  pl mel·a·no·ma·to·ses
mel·a·no·nych·i·a
mel·a·no·phage
mel·a·no·phore
mel·a·no·phor·ic
mel·a·no·pla·ki·a
mel·a·no·pro·te·in
mel·a·nor·rha·gi·a
mel·a·nor·rhe·a
mel·a·nor·rhoe·a
  var of mel·a·nor·rhe·a
mel·a·no·sar·co·ma
  pl mel·a·no·sar·co·mas
  or mel·a·no·sar·co·ma·ta
mel·a·no·sis
  pl mel·a·no·ses
mel·a·no·some
mel·a·not·ic
mel·a·no·trich·i·a lin·guae
mel·a·not·ri·chous
mel·a·nous
mel·a·nu·ri·a
mel·a·nu·ric
me·lar·sen
me·lar·so·prol
me·las·ma
me·las·mic
mel·a·to·nin
me·le·na
Me·le·ney ul·cer

mel·en·ges·trol
me·le·nic
mel·e·tin
me·lez·i·tose
mel·i·bi·ase
mel·i·bi·ose
mel·i·lo·tox·in
mel·in
mel·i·oi·do·sis
  pl mel·i·oi·do·ses
Me·lis·sa
me·lis·sic
me·lis·so·pho·bi·a
me·lis·syl
mel·i·ten·sis
me·li·tis
mel·i·top·ty·a·lism
mel·i·tose
mel·i·tox·in
mel·i·tra·cen
mel·i·tri·ose
mel·i·tu·ri·a
Mel·kers·son-Ro·sen·thal syn·drome
mel·lit·ic
mel·li·tu·ri·a
  var of mel·i·tu·ri·a
mel·o·di·dy·mi·a
mel·o·did·y·mus
me·lo·ma·ni·a
mel·o·ma·ni·ac
me·lom·e·lus
Me·loph·a·gus
mel·o·plas·ty
  pl mel·o·plas·ties
mel·o·rhe·os·to·sis
me·los·chi·sis
me·lo·ti·a
mel·o·trid·y·mus
me·lo·tus
mel·pha·lan
Melt·zer meth·od
mem·ber
mem·bra·na
  pl mem·bra·nae
mem·bra·na·ceous
mem·bra·nal
mem·bra·nate
mem·brane

mem·bra·ni·form
mem·bra·no·car·ti·lag·
  i·nous
mem·bra·no·cra·ni·um
mem·bra·noid
mem·bra·nous
mem·bra·nous·ly
mem·brum
  pl mem·bra
mem·o·ry
  pl mem·o·ries
men·ac·me
men·a·di·ol
men·a·di·one
men·a·gogue
me·naph·thene
me·naph·thone
men·ar·che
men·ar·che·al
  or men·ar·chi·al
men·ar·chi·al
  or men·ar·che·al
men·a·zon
Men·del laws
Men·de·lé·ev law
Men·de·li·an ra·tio
Men·de·li·an·ism
Men·de·li·an·ist
men·del·ism
men·del·ist
men·del·ize
Men·del·son syn·drome
men·el·lip·sis
Mé·ne·trier dis·ease
Men·go vi·rus
men·hi·dro·sis
  or men·i·dro·sis
men·i·dro·sis
  or men·hi·dro·sis
Mé·nière dis·ease
men·in·ge·al
me·nin·ge·or·rha·phy
me·nin·gi·o·blas·to·ma
  pl me·nin·gi·o·blas·to·mas
  or me·nin·gi·o·blas·to·ma·ta
me·nin·gi·o·fi·bro·blas·
  to·ma
  pl me·nin·gi·o·fi·bro·blas·
    to·mas

or me·nin·gi·o·fi·bro·blas·
  to·ma·ta
me·nin·gi·o·ma
  pl me·nin·gi·o·mas
  or me·nin·gi·o·ma·ta
me·nin·gi·o·ma-en·plaque
me·nin·gi·o·ma·to·sis
me·nin·gi·o·sar·co·ma
  pl me·nin·gi·o·sar·co·mas
  or me·nin·gi·o·sar·co·ma·ta
me·nin·gi·o·the·li·o·ma
  pl me·nin·gi·o·the·li·o·mas
  or me·nin·gi·o·the·li·o·ma·ta
me·nin·gism
  or men·in·gis·mus
men·in·gis·mus
  pl men·in·gis·mi
  or men·in·gism
men·in·git·ic
men·in·gi·tis
  pl men·in·gi·ti·des
men·in·git·o·pho·bi·a
me·nin·go·ar·te·ri·tis
me·nin·go·cele
me·nin·go·ceph·a·li·tis
me·nin·go·cer·e·bral
me·nin·go·cer·e·bri·tis
me·nin·go·coc·cae·mi·a
  var of me·nin·go·coc·ce·
    mi·a
me·nin·go·coc·cal
  or me·nin·go·coc·cic
me·nin·go·coc·ce·mi·a
me·nin·go·coc·cic
  or me·nin·go·coc·cal
me·nin·go·coc·cus
  pl me·nin·go·coc·ci
me·nin·go·coele
  var of me·nin·go·cele
me·nin·go·cor·ti·cal
me·nin·go·cyte
me·nin·go·en·ceph·a·lit·ic
me·nin·go·en·ceph·a·li·tis
  pl me·nin·go·en·ceph·a·li·
    ti·des
me·nin·go·en·ceph·a·lo·
  my·e·lo·
    ra·dic·u·lo·neu·ri·tis

me·nin·go·en·ceph·a·lop·
  a·thy
men·in·go·ma·la·ci·a
me·nin·go·my·e·li·tis
me·nin·go·my·e·lo·cele
men·in·go-
  os·te·o·phle·bi·tis
men·in·gop·a·thy
  pl men·in·gop·a·thies
me·nin·go·ra·chid·i·an
me·nin·go·ra·dic·u·lar
men·in·go·ra·dic·u·li·tis
me·nin·gor·rha·gi·a
men·in·gor·rhe·a
men·in·go·sis
me·nin·go·the·li·al
me·nin·go·the·li·o·ma
  pl me·nin·go·the·li·o·mas
  or me·nin·go·the·li·o·ma·ta
me·nin·go·the·li·om·a·tous
me·nin·go·the·li·um
me·nin·go·vas·cu·lar
men·in·gu·ri·a
me·ninx
  pl me·nin·ges
men·is·cec·to·my
  pl men·is·cec·to·mies
me·nis·ci tac·tus
men·is·ci·tis
me·nis·co·cyte
me·nis·co·cy·to·sis
  pl me·nis·co·cy·to·ses
me·nis·cus
  pl me·nis·cus·es
  or me·nis·ci
Men·kes syn·drome
me·noc·tone
men·o·lip·sis
men·o·me·tror·rha·gi·a
men·o·pau·sal
men·o·pause
men·o·pau·sic
men·o·pha·ni·a
men·o·pla·ni·a
Men·o·pon
men·or·rha·gi·a
men·or·rha·gic
men·or·rhal·gi·a

men·or·rhe·a
me·nos·che·sis
men·o·sta·si·a
me·nos·ta·sis
men·o·stax·is
  pl men·o·tax·es
men·o·tro·pins
men·o·xe·ni·a
mens
men·ses
men·stru·al
men·stru·ant
men·stru·ate
men·stru·a·tion
men·stru·ous
men·stru·um
  pl men·stru·ums
  or men·stru·a
men·su·al
men·su·ra·tion
men·tag·ra
men·tal
men·tal·is
  pl men·tal·es
men·tal·i·ty
  pl men·tal·i·ties
men·tal·ly
men·ta·tion
Men·tha
Men·tha·ce·ae
men·thane
men·thol
men·thol·a·ted
men·thyl
men·ti·cide
men·to·an·te·ri·or
men·to·hy·oid
men·ton
men·to·pa·ri·e·tal
men·to·pos·te·ri·or
men·tu·lo·ma·ni·a
men·tum
  pl men·ta
mep·a·crine
mep·a·zine
me·pen·zo·late
me·per·i·dine
me·phen·e·sin

meph·en·ox·a·lone
me·phen·ter·mine
me·phen·y·to·in
me·phit·ic
  or me·phit·i·cal
me·phit·i·cal
  or me·phit·ic
meph·o·bar·bi·tal
me·piv·a·caine
me·pred·ni·sone
mep·ryl·caine
me·pyr·a·mine
me·pyr·a·pone
meq·ui·dox
me·ral·gi·a
mer·al·lu·ride
mer·a·lo·pi·a
mer·am·au·ro·sis
mer·bro·min
mer·cap·tal
mer·cap·tan
mer·cap·tide
mer·cap·to·a·ce·tic
mer·cap·tol
mer·cap·tole
mer·cap·to·mer·in
mer·cap·to·pu·rine
mer·cap·tu·ric
Mer·cier bar
mer·co·cre·sols
mer·cu·mat·i·lin
mer·cu·ri·al
mer·cu·ri·al·ism
mer·cu·ri·al·i·za·tion
mer·cu·ri·al·ize
mer·cu·ric
mer·cu·ro·phyl·line
mer·cu·rous
mer·cu·ry
  pl mer·cu·ries
mer·er·ga·si·a
mer·er·gas·tic
mer·eth·ox·yl·line
me·rid·i·an
me·rid·i·a·ni bul·bi oc·u·li
me·rid·i·a·nus
  pl me·rid·i·a·ni
me·rid·ic

me·rid·i·o·nal
mer·in·tho·pho·bi·a
mer·i·sis
  pl mer·i·ses
mer·i·so·prol
mer·i·spore
me·ris·tic
me·ris·ti·cal·ly
Mer·kel cor·pus·cle, disc
Mer·kel-
  Ran·vier cor·pus·cle
mer·o·a·cra·ni·a
mer·o·blas·tic
mer·o·blas·ti·cal·ly
mer·o·crine
me·roc·ri·nous
mer·o·en·ceph·a·ly
mer·o·gen·e·sis
  pl mer·o·gen·e·ses
mer·o·ge·net·ic
  or mer·o·gen·ic
mer·o·gen·ic
  or mer·o·ge·net·ic
mer·o·gon
  or mer·o·gone
mer·o·gone
  or mer·o·gon
mer·o·gon·ic
  or me·rog·o·nous
me·rog·o·nous
  or mer·o·gon·ic
me·rog·o·ny
  pl me·rog·o·nies
mer·o·me·li·a
mer·o·mi·cro·so·mi·a
mer·o·my·o·sin
me·ro·pi·a
mer·o·ra·chis·chi·sis
me·ros·mi·a
mer·o·som·a·tous
mer·o·some
me·rot·o·my
  pl me·rot·o·mies
mer·o·zo·ite
mer·sal·yl
Me·ru·li·us
mer·ru·tu
mer·y·cism

Merz·bach·er- Pel·i·zae·us
  dis·ease
me·sad
  or me·si·ad
me·sal
  var of me·si·al
me·sal·ly
  var of me·si·al·ly
mes·a·me·boid
mes·an·gi·al
mes·an·gi·um
mes·a·or·ti·tis
mes·a·ra·ic
mes·ar·te·ri·tis
me·sat·i·ceph·al·ic
  or me·sat·i·ceph·a·lous
me·sat·i·ceph·a·lous
  or me·sat·i·ceph·al·ic
me·sat·i·ceph·a·ly
me·sat·i·pel·lic
me·sat·i·pel·ly
  pl me·sat·i·pel·lies
me·sat·i·pel·vic
mes·ax·on
mes·cal
mes·ca·line
mes·ca·lism
mes·ec·to·derm
mes·ec·to·der·mal
  or mes·ec·to·der·mic
mes·ec·to·der·mic
  or mes·ec·to·der·mal
mes·en·ce·phal·ic
mes·en·ceph·a·li·tis
mes·en·ceph·a·lon
mes·en·ceph·a·lot·o·my
me·sen·chy·ma
mes·en·chy·mal
mes·en·chy·ma·tous
mes·en·chyme
mes·en·chy·mo·ma
  pl mes·en·chy·mo·mas
  or mes·en·chy·mo·ma·ta
mes·en·ter·ec·to·my
mes·en·ter·ic
mes·en·ter·i·co·mes·o·co·lic
mes·en·ter·i·o·lum
  pl mes·en·ter·i·o·la
mes·en·ter·i·o·pex·y

mes·en·ter·i·or·rha·phy
mes·en·ter·i·pli·ca·tion
mes·en·ter·i·tis
mes·en·te·ri·um
  pl mes·en·te·ri·a
mes·en·ter·on
  pl mes·en·ter·a
mes·en·ter·y
  pl mes·en·ter·ies
mes·en·to·derm
mes·en·tor·rha·phy
mesh·work
me·si·ad
  or me·sad
me·si·al
me·si·al·ly
me·si·o·buc·cal
me·si·o·buc·co·oc·clu·sal
me·si·o·cer·vi·cal
me·si·oc·clu·sal
me·si·o·clu·sion
  or me·si·o·oc·clu·sion
me·si·o·dens
me·si·o·dis·tal
me·si·o·gres·sion
me·si·o·in·ci·sal
me·si·o·la·bi·al
me·si·o·lin·gual
me·si·o·lin·guo·oc·clu·sal
me·si·on
me·si·o·oc·clu·sal
me·si·o·oc·clu·sion
  or me·si·o·clu·sion
me·si·o·ver·sion
me·sit·y·lene
mes·mer·ism
mes·mer·ist
mes·mer·i·za·tion
mes·mer·ize
mes·mer·iz·er
me·so·ap·pen·di·ce·al
mes·o·ap·pen·di·ci·tis
mes·o·ap·pen·dix
  pl mes·o·ap·pen·dix·es
  or mes·o·ap·pen·di·ces
mes·o·bi·lane
mes·o·bil·i·fus·cin
mes·o·bil·i·leu·kan

mes·o·bil·i·rho·din
mes·o·bil·i·ru·bin
mes·o·bil·i·ru·bin·o·gen
mes·o·bil·i·vi·o·lin
mes·o·blast
mes·o·blas·te·ma
  pl mes·o·blas·te·mas
  or mes·o·blas·te·ma·ta
mes·o·blas·tem·ic
mes·o·blas·tic
mes·o·bran·chi·al
mes·o·bron·chi·tis
mes·o·car·di·a
mes·o·car·di·um
mes·o·carp
mes·o·ce·cum
  pl mes·o·ce·ca
mes·o·ce·phal·ic
mes·o·ceph·a·lon
mes·o·ceph·a·ly
  pl mes·o·ceph·a·lies
mes·o·cne·mic
mes·o·co·lic
mes·o·co·lon
mes·o·co·lo·pex·y
mes·o·co·lo·pli·ca·tion
mes·o·conch
  or mes·o·conch·ic
mes·o·conch·ic
  or mes·o·conch
mes·o·cord
mes·o·cra·ni·al
mes·o·derm
mes·o·der·mal
  or mes·o·der·mic
mes·o·der·mic
  or mes·o·der·mal
mes·o·di·a·stol·ic
mes·o·dont
mes·o·don·ty
  pl mes·o·don·ties
mes·o·du·o·de·num
  pl mes·o·du·o·de·nums
  or mes·o·du·o·de·na
mes·o·ep·i·did·y·mus
mes·o·e·soph·a·gus
  pl mes·o·e·soph·a·gi
mes·o·gas·ter
mes·o·gas·tric

mes·o·gas·tri·um
   pl mes·o·gas·tri·a
mes·o·gle·a
me·sog·li·a
mes·o·gloe·a
   var of mes·o·gle·a
mes·o·glu·te·us
mes·o·gnath·ic
   or me·sog·na·thous
mes·o·gna·thi·on
me·sog·na·thous
   or mes·o·gnath·ic
me·sog·na·thy
   pl me·sog·na·thies
mes·o·il·e·um
mes·o·i·no·si·tol
mes·o·je·ju·num
mes·o·lec·i·thal
mes·o·lym·pho·cyte
mes·o·mere
mes·o·mer·ic
me·som·er·ism
mes·o·me·tri·al
   or mes·o·met·ric
mes·o·met·ric
   or mes·o·me·tri·al
mes·o·me·tri·um
   pl mes·o·me·tri·a
mes·o·morph
mes·o·mor·phic
mes·o·mor·phism
mes·o·mor·phy
   pl mes·o·mor·phies
mes·on
mes·o·neph·ric
mes·o·neph·roid
mes·o·ne·phro·ma
   pl mes·o·ne·phro·mas
   or mes·o·ne·phro·ma·ta
mes·o·neph·ron
   pl mes·o·neph·ra
   or mes·o·neph·ros
   pl mes·o·neph·roi
mes·o·neph·ros
   pl mes·o·neph·roi
   or mes·o·neph·ron
   pl mes·o·neph·ra
mes·o·on·to·morph
mes·o·pex·y

mes·o·phile
mes·o·phil·ic
   or me·soph·i·lous
me·soph·i·lous
   or mes·o·phil·ic
mes·o·phle·bi·tis
mes·o·phrag·ma
mes·o·phrag·mal
me·soph·ry·on
   pl me·soph·ry·a
mes·o·pic
mes·o·por·phy·rin
mes·o·pro·sop·ic
mes·o·pro·so·py
   pl mes·o·pro·so·pies
mes·o·pul·mo·num
me·sor·chi·um
   pl me·sor·chi·a
mes·o·rec·tum
mes·o·rhi·nal
   or mes·or·rhi·nal
mes·o·rhine
   or mes·or·rhine
   or mes·or·rhin·ic
mes·o·rid·a·zine
mes·o·rop·ter
mes·or·rha·phy
mes·or·rhi·nal
   or mes·o·rhi·nal
mes·or·rhine
   or mes·or·rhin·ic
   or mes·o·rhine
mes·or·rhin·ic
   or mes·or·rhine
   or mes·o·rhine
mes·o·sal·pin·ge·al
mes·o·sal·pinx
   pl mes·o·sal·pin·ges
mes·o·seme
mes·o·sig·moid
mes·o·sig·moi·do·pex·y
mes·o·some
mes·o·ster·num
   pl mes·o·ster·na
mes·o·tar·tar·ic
mes·o·ten·din·e·um
mes·o·ten·don
mes·o·the·li·al

mes·o·the·li·o·ma
   pl mes·o·the·li·o·mas
   or mes·o·the·li·o·ma·ta
mes·o·the·li·um
   pl mes·o·the·li·a
mes·o·tho·ri·um
me·sot·o·my
mes·o·tron
mes·o·var·i·an
mes·o·var·i·um
   pl mes·o·var·i·a
Me·so·zo·a
me·so·zo·an
mes·sen·ger RNA
mes·ter·o·lone
mes·tra·nol
mes·u·prine
mes·yl·ate
met·a
me·tab·a·sis
   pl me·tab·a·ses
met·a·bi·o·sis
   pl met·a·bi·o·ses
met·a·bi·ot·ic
met·a·bi·ot·i·cal·ly
met·a·bi·sul·fite
met·a·bol·ic
   or met·a·bol·i·cal
met·a·bol·i·cal
   or met·a·bol·ic
met·a·bol·i·cal·ly
me·tab·o·lim·e·ter
me·tab·o·lism
me·tab·o·lite
me·tab·o·li·za·bil·i·ty
   pl me·tab·o·li·za·bil·i·ties
me·tab·o·liz·a·ble
me·tab·o·lize
met·a·bol·o·gy
me·tab·o·lous
met·a·brom·sa·lan
met·a·bu·teth·a·min
met·a·bu·tox·y·caine
met·a·car·pal
met·a·car·pec·to·my
meta·car·po·pha·lan·ge·al
met·a·cen·tric
met·a·cer·car·i·a
   pl met·a·cer·car·i·ae

met·a·cer·car·i·al
met·a·chro·ma·si·a
   or met·a·chro·ma·sy
met·a·chro·ma·sy
   pl met·a·chro·ma·sy
   or met·a·chro·ma·si·a
met·a·chro·mat·ic
met·a·chro·ma·tism
met·a·chro·mo·phil
met·a·chro·sis
   pl met·a·chro·ses
met·a·coele
met·a·cone
met·a·co·nid
met·a·co·nule
met·a·cre·sol
met·a·cy·e·sis
met·a·di·hy·drox·y·ben·
  zene
met·a·dra·sis
met·a·drom·ic
met·a·fa·cial
met·a·fil·tra·tion
met·a·gen·e·sis
   pl met·a·gen·e·ses
met·a·ge·net·ic
met·a·ge·net·i·cal·ly
met·a·gen·ic
Met·a·gon·i·mus
met·a·gran·u·lo·cyte
met·a·kar·y·o·cyte
met·a·ken·trin
met·al
met·al·bu·min
me·tal·lic
me·tal·lo·en·zyme
met·al·loid
   or met·al·loi·dal
met·al·loi·dal
   or met·al·loid
me·tal·lo·phil·i·a
me·tal·lo·pho·bi·a
met·al·lo·por·phy·rin
me·tal·lo·pro·te·in
met·al·lur·gy
me·ta·lol
me·tal·o·phil
met·a·mer
met·a·mere

met·a·mer·ic
met·a·mer·i·cal·ly
me·tam·er·ism
met·a·mor·phic
met·a·mor·phop·si·a
met·a·mor·phose
met·a·mor·pho·sis
   pl met·a·mor·pho·ses
met·a·my·e·lo·cyte
met·a·neph·ric
   or met·a·neph·ri·tic
met·a·neph·rine
met·a·neph·rit·ic
   or met·a·neph·ric
met·a·neph·ro·gen·ic
met·a·neph·ron
   pl met·a·neph·ra
   or met·a·neph·ros
   pl met·a·neph·roi
met·a·neph·ros
   pl met·a·neph·roi
   or met·a·neph·ron
   pl met·a·neph·ra
met·a·neu·tro·phil
met·a·phase
met·a·phos·pho·ric
me·taph·y·se·al
met·a·phys·i·al
me·taph·y·sis
   pl me·taph·y·ses
me·taph·y·si·tis
met·a·pla·si·a
met·a·pla·sis
met·a·plasm
met·a·plas·tic
met·a·pneu·mon·ic
met·a·poph·y·sis
   pl met·a·poph·y·ses
met·a·pro·te·in
met·a·pro·ter·e·nol
met·a·psy·chol·o·gy
met·a·ram·i·nol
met·a·rho·dop·sin
met·ar·te·ri·ole
met·a·ru·bri·cyte
met·a·sta·ble
me·tas·ta·sis
   pl me·tas·ta·ses
me·tas·ta·size

met·a·stat·ic
met·a·stat·i·cal·ly
met·a·ster·num
Met·a·stron·gy·lus
met·a·tar·sal
met·a·tar·sal·gi·a
met·a·tar·sal·ly
met·a·tar·sec·to·my
met·a·tar·so·pha·lan·ge·al
met·a·tar·sus
met·a·thal·a·mus
me·tath·e·sis
   pl me·tath·e·ses
met·a·thet·ic
met·a·troph·ic
me·tat·ro·phy
   pl me·tat·ro·phies
me·tax·a·lone
Met·a·zo·a
met·a·zo·al
met·a·zo·an
met·a·zo·on
Metch·ni·koff the·o·ry
me·te·cious
met·em·pir·ic
met·en·ce·phal·ic
met·en·ceph·a·lon
me·te·or·ic
me·te·or·ism
me·te·or·o·graph
me·te·or·ol·o·gy
me·te·or·o·path·o·log·ic
me·te·o·rot·ro·pism
me·ter
me·ter·an·gle
met·es·trum
   or met·es·trus
met·es·trous
met·es·trus
   or met·es·trum
met·for·min
meth·a·cho·line
meth·ac·ry·late
meth·a·cy·cline
meth·a·done
met·hae·mo·glo·bi·nae·
  mi·a
   var of met·he·mo·glo·bi·
  ne·mi·a

meth·hae·mo·glo·bi·nu·ri·a
var of met·he·mo·glo·bi·
nu·ri·a
meth·al·le·nes·tril
meth·al·li·bure
meth·al·thi·a·zide
meth·am·phet·a·mine
meth·a·nal
meth·an·dri·ol
meth·an·dro·sten·o·lone
meth·ane
meth·ane·sul·fo·nate
meth·a·no·ic
meth·a·nol
meth·an·the·line
meth·a·pyr·i·lene
meth·a·qua·lone
meth·ar·bi·tal
meth·a·zol·a·mide
meth·dil·a·zine
met·hem·al·bu·min
met·hem·al·bu·mi·ne·mi·a
met·heme
me·he·mo·glo·bin
met·he·mo·glo·bi·ne·mi·a
met·he·mo·glo·bi·nu·ri·a
me·the·na·mine
meth·ene
me·the·no·lone
meth·e·nyl
meth·et·o·in
meth·i·cil·lin
meth·im·a·zole
meth·ine
or meth·yne
me·thi·o·dal
me·thi·o·nine
me·thi·o·nyl
me·this·a·zone
me·thix·ene
meth·o·car·ba·mol
meth·od
meth·o·dol·o·gy
meth·o·hex·i·tal
meth·o·in
meth·o·ma·ni·a
me·tho·ni·um
meth·o·pho·line
meth·o·pro·ma·zine

meth·o·pyr·a·pone
meth·o·trex·ate
meth·o·tri·mep·ra·zine
me·thox·a·mine
me·thox·sa·len
me·thox·y·chlor
me·thox·y·flu·rane
me·thox·y·phen·a·mine
meth·sco·pol·a·mine
meth·sux·i·mide
meth·y·clo·thi·a·zide
meth·yl
meth·yl·a·cet·y·lene
meth·yl·al
meth·yl·am·ine
meth·yl·a·mi·no·hep·tane
meth·yl·am·phet·a·mine
meth·yl·ase
meth·yl·ate
meth·yl·a·tion
meth·yl·at·ro·pine
meth·yl·ben·zene
meth·yl·benz·e·tho·ni·um
meth·yl·ben·zo·yl·ec·
go·nine
meth·yl·car·bi·nol
meth·yl·cel·lu·lose
meth·yl·cho·lan·threne
meth·yl·do·pa
meth·yl·do·pate
meth·yl·ene
meth·yl·en·o·phil
meth·yl·e·noph·i·lous
meth·y·lep·si·a
meth·yl·er·go·no·vine
meth·yl·eth·yl·a·ce·tic
meth·yl·glu·ca·mine
meth·yl·gly·ox·al
meth·yl·hex·a·mine
meth·yl·hex·ane·a·mine
meth·yl·ma·lon·ic
meth·yl·ma·ni·a
meth·yl·mer·cap·tan
meth·yl·meth·ane
meth·yl·mor·phine
meth·yl·par·a·ben
meth·yl·par·a·fy·nol
meth·yl·phen·i·date
meth·yl·phe·no·bar·bi·tal

meth·yl·phe·no·bar·bi·tone
meth·yl·phe·nol
meth·yl·pred·nis·o·lone
meth·yl·pu·rine
meth·yl·ro·san·i·line
meth·yl·sul·fo·nal
meth·yl·tes·tos·ter·one
meth·yl·thi·o·nine
meth·yl·thi·o·u·ra·cil
meth·yl·trans·fer·ase
meth·yne
or meth·ine
meth·y·pry·lon
meth·y·ser·gide
meth·y·sis
me·ti·a·pine
met·my·o·glo·bin
met·o·clo·pram·ide
me·toe·cious
var of me·te·cious
met·oes·trous
var of met·es·trous
met·oes·trum
var of met·es·trus
met·oes·trus
var of met·es·trus
me·to·la·zone
me·top·a·gus
me·top·ic
met·o·pim·a·zine
me·to·pi·on
met·o·pism
me·to·pi·um
met·o·pon
met·o·pop·a·gus
met·o·qui·zine
met·o·ser·pate
me·tox·e·nous
me·tox·e·ny
me·tra
pl me·trae
me·trae·mi·a
var of me·tre·mi·a
me·tral·gi·a
met·ra·pec·tic
met·ra·to·ni·a
me·tra·tro·phi·a
me·traux·e

237

me·tre
var of me·ter
me·trec·ta·si·a
me·trec·to·pi·a
me·trec·to·py
me·tre·mi·a
me·treu·ryn·ter
me·treu·ry·sis
me·tri·a
met·ric
or met·ri·cal
met·ri·cal
or met·ric
met·ri·cal·ly
met·ri·o·ce·phal·ic
me·trit·ic
me·tri·tis
me·tro·cele
me·tro·clyst
me·tro·col·po·cele
me·tro·cys·to·sis
pl me·tro·cys·to·sis·es
or me·tro·cys·to·ses
me·tro·cyte
me·tro·dy·na·mom·e·ter
me·tro·dyn·i·a
me·tro·ec·ta·si·a
me·tro·en·do·me·tri·tis
me·trog·ra·phy
pl me·trog·ra·phies
me·tro·leu·kor·rhe·a
me·trol·o·gy
me·tro·lym·phan·gi·tis
me·tro·ma·la·ci·a
met·ro·ni·da·zole
met·ro·nome
me·tro·pa·ral·y·sis
pl me·tro·pa·ral·y·ses
me·tro·path·i·a hem·or·
rhag·i·ca
me·tro·path·ic
me·trop·a·thy
pl me·trop·a·thies
me·tro·per·i·to·ni·tis
me·tro·pex·i·a
me·tro·pex·y
me·tro·phle·bi·tis
me·tro·plas·ty

me·trop·to·sis
pl me·trop·to·ses
me·tror·rha·gi·a
me·tror·rha·gic
me·tror·rhe·a
me·tror·rhex·is
pl me·tror·rhex·es
me·tro·sal·pin·gi·tis
me·tro·sal·pin·gog·ra·phy
pl me·tro·sal·pin·gog·
ra·phies
me·tro·scope
me·tro·stax·is
me·tro·ste·no·sis
pl me·tro·ste·no·ses
me·tro·tome
me·trot·o·my
me·try·per·ci·ne·sis
me·try·per·e·mi·a
me·try·per·es·the·si·a
me·try·per·tro·phi·a
Mett meth·od
me·tu·re·dep·a
me·tyr·a·pone
Meu·len·gracht di·et
Meuse fe·ver
mev·a·lon·ic
Mey·er loop
Mey·er·hof cycle
Mey·er-O·ver·ton the·o·ry
Mey·nert bun·dle
Mey·net no·dos·i·ties
mho
Mi·an·a fe·ver
or Mi·an·eh fe·ver
Mi·an·eh fe·ver
or Mi·an·a fe·ver
mi·an·ser·in
mi·asm
or mi·as·ma
mi·as·ma
pl mi·as·mas
or mi·as·ma·ta
or mi·asm
mi·as·mal
mi·as·mat·ic
mi·as·mic
Mi·bel·li dis·ease

mi·ca
mi·ca·ceous
mi·cel·la
pl mi·cel·lae
or mi·celle
mi·cel·lar
mi·celle
or mi·cel·la
Mi·chae·lis con·stant
Mi·chae·lis-Gut·mann
bod·ies
Mi·chai·low test
Mi·chel flecks
Mi·chel·i syn·drome
mi·cra·cous·tic
mi·cren·ceph·a·lon
pl mi·cren·ceph·a·la
mi·cren·ceph·a·lous
mi·cren·ceph·a·ly
pl mi·cren·ceph·a·lies
mi·cro·ab·scess
mi·cro·ab·sorp·tion
mi·cro·aer·o·phile
or mi·cro·aer·o·phil·ic
or mi·cro·aer·oph·i·lous
mi·cro·aer·o·phil·ic
or mi·cro·aer·o·phile
or mi·cro·aer·oph·i·lous
mi·cro·aer·oph·i·lous
or mi·cro·aer·o·phile
or mi·cro·aer·o·phil·ic
mi·cro·aer·o·to·nom·e·ter
mi·cro·a·nal·y·sis
pl mi·cro·a·nal·y·ses
mi·cro·an·al·yst
mi·cro·an·a·lyt·ic
or mi·cro·an·a·lyt·i·cal
mi·cro·an·a·lyt·i·cal
or mi·cro·an·a·lyt·ic
mi·cro·a·na·tom·i·cal
mi·cro·a·nat·o·mist
mi·cro·a·nat·o·my
pl mi·cro·a·nat·o·mies
mi·cro·an·eu·rysm
mi·cro·an·gi·op·a·thy
mi·cro·ar·te·ri·o·gram
mi·gro·ar·te·ri·o·graph·ic
mi·cro·ar·te·ri·og·ra·phy

238

mi·cro·au·di·phone
Mi·cro·bac·te·ri·um
   pl Mi·cro·bac·te·ri·a
mi·cro·bal·ance
mi·crobe
mi·cro·bi·al
   or mi·cro·bic
   or mi·cro·bi·an
mi·cro·bi·an
   or mi·cro·bic
mi·cro·bic
   or mi·cro·bi·al
   or mi·cro·bi·an
mi·cro·bi·ci·dal
mi·cro·bi·cide
mi·crob·in·ert
mi·cro·bi·o·log·ic
   or mi·cro·bi·o·log·i·cal
mi·cro·bi·o·log·i·cal
   or mi·cro·bi·o·log·ic
mi·cro·bi·o·log·i·cal·ly
mi·cro·bi·ol·o·gist
mi·cro·bi·ol·o·gy
   pl mi·cro·bi·ol·o·gies
mi·cro·bi·on
   pl mi·cro·bi·a
mi·cro·bi·o·pho·bi·a
mi·cro·bi·o·sis
   pl mi·cr·bi·o·ses
mi·cro·bi·o·ta
mi·cro·bi·ot·ic
mi·cro·bism
mi·cro·blast
mi·cro·ble·phar·i·a
mi·cro·bleph·a·rism
mi·cro·bleph·a·ron
mi·cro·body
   pl mi·cro·bod·ies
mi·cro·bra·chi·a
mi·cro·bra·chi·us
mi·cro·brach·y·ce·pha·li·a
mi·cro·brach·y·ceph·a·ly
mi·cro·bu·ret
   or mi·cro·bu·rette
mi·cro·bu·rette
   or mi·cro·bu·ret
mi·cro·cal·cu·lus
   pl mi·cro·cal·cu·li

mi·cro·cal·o·rie
mi·cro·cap·sule
mi·cro·car·di·a
mi·cro·car·di·us
mi·cro·cav·i·ta·tion
mi·cro·cen·trum
   pl mi·cro·cen·trums
   or mi·cro·cen·tra
mi·cro·ce·phal·ic
   or mi·cro·ceph·a·lous
mi·cro·ceph·a·lism
mi·cro·ceph·a·lous
   or *mi·cro·ce·phal·ic*
mi·cro·ceph·a·lus
   or mi·cro·ceph·a·li
mi·cro·ceph·a·ly
mi·cro·chei·li·a
mi·cro·chei·ri·a
mi·cro·chem·i·cal
mi·cro·chem·is·try
   pl mi·cro·chem·is·tries
mi·cro·cin·e·mat·o·graph·ic
mi·cro·cin·e·ma·tog·ra·phy
   pl mi·cro·cin·e·ma·tog·ra·phies
   or mi·cro·kin·e·ma·tog·ra·phy
   pl mi·cro·kin·e·ma·tog·ra·phies
mi·cro·cir·cu·la·tion
mi·cro·cir·cu·la·to·ry
Mi·cro·coc·ca·ce·ae
mi·cro·coc·cal
mi·cro·coc·cin
mi·cro·coc·cus
   pl mi·cro·coc·ci
mi·cro·co·lon
mi·cro·col·o·ny
mi·cro·co·nid·i·um
   pl mi·cro·co·nid·i·a
mi·cro·co·ri·a
mi·cro·cor·ne·a
mi·cro·cos·mic
mi·cro·cou·lomb
mi·cro·cous·tic
mi·cro·crys·tal·line

mi·cro·crys·tal·lin·i·ty
   pl mi·cro·crys·tal·lin·i·ties
mi·cro·cul·tur·al
mi·cro·cul·ture
mi·cro·cu·rie
mi·cro·curie-hour
mi·cro·cyst
mi·cro·cys·tic
mi·cro·cy·tase
mi·cro·cyte
mi·cro·cy·thae·mi·a
   var of mi·cro·cy·the·mi·a
mi·cro·cy·the·mi·a
mi·cro·cy·the·mic
mi·cro·cyt·ic
mi·cro·cy·to·sis
   pl mi·cro·cy·to·ses
mi·cro·dac·tyl·i·a
   or mi·cro·dac·ty·ly
mi·cro·dac·ty·lous
mi·cro·dac·ty·ly
   pl mi·cro·dac·ty·lies
   or mi·cro·dac·tyl·i·a
mi·cro·de·ter·mi·na·tion
mi·cro·dis·sec·tion
mi·cro·dont
mi·cro·don·ti·a
mi·cro·dont·ism
mi·cro·drep·a·no·cyt·ic
mi·cro·drep·a·no·cy·to·sis
   pl mi·cro·drep·a·no·cy·to·ses
mi·cro·e·lec·tro·pho·re·sis
mi·cro·e·lec·tro·pho·ret·ic
   or mi·cro·e·lec·tro·pho·ret·i·cal
mi·cro·e·lec·tro·pho·ret·i·cal
   or mi·cro·e·lec·tro·pho·ret·ic
mi·cro·e·lec·tro·pho·ret·i·cal·ly
mi·cro·en·cap·su·late
mi·cro·en·cap·su·la·tion
mi·cro·en·ceph·a·ly
   pl mi·cro·en·ceph·a·lies
mi·cro·e·ryth·ro·cyte
mi·cro·far·ad

mi·cro·fau·na
mi·cro·fi·bril
mi·cro·fi·bril·lar
mi·cro·fi·bro·ad·e·no·ma
    pl mi·cro·fi·bro·ad·e·no·
      mas
    or mi·cro·fi·bro·ade·no·
      ma·ta
mi·cro·fil·a·ment
mi·cro·fil·a·rae·mi·a
    var of mi·cro·fil·a·re·mi·a
mi·cro·fil·a·re·mi·a
mi·cro·fi·lar·i·a
    pl mi·cro·fi·lar·i·ae
mi·cro·fi·lar·i·al
mi·cro·flo·ra
mi·cro·fol·lic·u·lar
mi·cro·frac·ture
mi·cro·gam·ete
mi·cro·ga·me·to·cyte
mi·crog·a·my
mi·cro·gas·tri·a
mi·cro·gen·e·sis
mi·cro·ge·ni·a
mi·cro·gen·i·tal·ism
mi·crog·li·a
mi·crog·li·al
mi·crog·li·o·cyte
mi·crog·li·o·ma
    pl mi·crog·li·o·mas
    or mi·crog·li·o·ma·ta
mi·crog·li·o·ma·to·sis
mi·cro·glos·si·a
mi·cro·gna·thi·a
mi·cro·gnath·ic
mi·crog·na·thous
mi·cro·go·nio·scope
mi·cro·gram
mi·cro·graph
mi·cro·graph·i·a
mi·cro·graph·ic
mi·crog·ra·phy
    pl mi·crog·ra·phies
mi·cro·gy·ri·a
mi·cro·gy·rus
mi·cro·hertz
mi·crohm
mi·cro·in·cin·er·a·tion
mi·cro·in·farct

mi·cro·in·jec·tion
mi·cro·in·jec·tor
mi·cro·in·va·sion
mi·cro·ker·a·tome
mi·cro·kin·e·ma·tog·ra·phy
    pl mi·cro·kin·e·ma·tog·ra·
      phies
    or mi·cro·cin·e·ma·tog·
      ra·phy
    pl mi·cro·cin·e·ma·tog·ra·
      phies
mi·cro·len·ti·a
mi·cro·le·sion
mi·cro·leu·ko·blast
mi·cro·li·ter
mi·cro·lith
mi·cro·li·thi·a·sis
    pl mi·cro·li·thi·a·ses
mi·cro·log·ic
    or mi·cro·log·i·cal
mi·cro·log·i·cal
    or mi·cro·log·ic
mi·crol·o·gist
mi·crol·o·gy
    pl mi·crol·o·gies
mi·cro·ma·ni·a
mi·cro·ma·nip·u·la·tion
mi·cro·ma·nip·u·la·tor
mi·cro·ma·nom·e·ter
mi·cro·mas·ti·a
mi·cro·ma·zi·a
mi·cro·me·li·a
mi·cro·mel·ic
mi·crom·e·lus
    pl mi·crom·e·li
mi·crom·e·ly
mic·ro·mere
mi·crom·e·ter
mi·cro·meth·od
mi·crom·e·try
mi·cro·mi·cron
mi·cro·mil
mi·cro·mil·li·me·ter
mi·cro·mo·le·cu·lar
mi·cro·mor·pho·log·ic
    or mi·cro·mor·pho·log·i·cal
mi·cro·mor·pho·log·i·cal
    or mi·cro·mor·pho·log·ic
mi·cro·mor·pho·log·i·cal·ly

mi·cro·mor·phol·o·gy
    pl mi·cro·mor·phol·o·gies
mi·cro·mo·to·scope
mi·cro·my·e·li·a
mi·cro·my·e·lo·blast
mi·cro·my·e·lo·lym·pho·
    cyte
mi·cron
    pl mi·crons
    or mi·cra
mi·cro·nee·dle
mi·cron·e·mous
mi·cro·nod·u·lar
mi·cro·nod·u·la·tion
mi·cro·nu·cle·us
    pl mi·cro·nu·cle·us·es
    or mi·cro·nu·cle·i
mi·cro·nu·tri·ent
mi·cro·nych·i·a
mi·cro·or·chism
mi·cro·or·gan·ic
mi·cro·or·gan·ism
mi·cro·pap·u·lar
mi·cro·par·a·site
mi·cro·pa·thol·o·gy
mi·cro·pe·nis
    pl mi·cro·pe·nis·es
    or mi·cro·pe·nes
mi·cro·phage
mi·cro·pha·ki·a
mi·cro·phal·lus
    pl mi·cro·phal·lus·es
    or mi·cro·phal·li
mi·cro·pho·bi·a
mi·cro·phone
mi·cro·pho·ni·a
mi·cro·pho·no·graph
mi·cro·pho·no·scope
mi·croph·o·ny
mi·cro·pho·to·graph
mi·cro·pho·tog·ra·pher
mi·cro·pho·tog·raph·ic
mi·cro·pho·tog·ra·phy
    pl mi·cro·pho·tog·ra·phies
mi·cro·pho·tom·e·ter
mi·croph·thal·mi·a
mi·croph·thal·mic
mi·croph·thal·mos
    pl mi·croph·thal·mi

240

or mi·croph·thal·mus
pl mi·croph·thal·moi
mi·croph·thal·mus
pl mi·croph·thal·moi
or mi·croph·thal·mos
pl mi·croph·thal·mi
mi·cro·phys·i·cal
mi·cro·phys·i·cal·ly
mi·cro·phys·ics
mi·cro·phyte
mi·cro·pi·a
mi·cro·pi·pet
or mi·cro·pi·pette
mi·cro·pi·pette
or mi·cro·pi·pet
mi·cro·ple·thys·mo·gram
mi·cro·ple·thys·mo·graph
mi·cro·pleth·ys·mog·ra·phy
mi·cro·po·di·a
mi·crop·o·dy
mi·cro·po·lar·i·scope
mi·cro·probe
mi·cro·pro·jec·tion
mi·cro·pro·so·pia
mi·cro·pro·so·pus
mi·cro·pros·o·py
mi·crop·si·a
or mi·crop·sy
mi·crop·sy
pl mi·crop·sies
or mi·crop·si·a
mi·cro·psy·chi·a
mi·crop·tic
mi·cro·punc·ture
mi·cro·pus
mi·cro·pyk·nom·e·ter
mi·cro·py·lar
mi·cro·pyle
mi·cro·ra·di·o·graph
mi·cro·ra·di·o·graph·ic
mi·cro·ra·di·og·ra·phy
pl mi·cro·ra·di·og·ra·phies
mi·cro·re·frac·tom·e·ter
mi·cro·res·pi·rom·e·ter
mi·cro·res·pi·ro·met·ric
mi·cror·rhi·ni·a
mi·cro·ruth·er·ford
mi·cro·scel·ous

mi·cro·scope
mi·cro·scop·ic
or mi·cro·scop·i·cal
mi·cro·scop·i·cal
or mi·cro·scop·ic
mi·cro·scop·i·cal·ly
mi·cros·co·pist
mi·cros·co·py
pl mi·cros·co·pies
mi·cro·sec·ond
mi·cro·seme
mi·cros·mat·ic
mi·cro·som·al
mi·cro·some
mi·cro·so·mi·a
mi·cro·spec·trog·ra·phy
mi·cro·spec·tro·pho·tom·e·ter
mi·cro·spec·tro·pho·to·met·ric
or mi·cro·spec·tro·pho·to·met·ri·cal
mi·cro·spec·tro·pho·to·met·ri·cal
or mi·cro·spec·tro·pho·to·met·ric
mi·cro·spec·tro·pho·to·met·ri·cal·ly
mi·cro·spec·tro·pho·tom·e·try
pl mi·cro·spec·tro·pho·tom·e·tries
mi·cro·spec·tro·scope
mi·cro·sphe·ro·cyte
mi·cro·sphe·ro·cy·to·sis
mi·cro·sphyg·mi·a
mi·cro·sphyg·my
mi·cro·sphyx·i·a
mi·cro·splanch·nic
mi·cro·sple·ni·a
mi·cros·po·rid
Mi·cros·po·rid·i·a
Mi·cros·po·ron
mi·cro·spo·ro·sis
pl mi·cro·spo·ro·ses
Mi·cros·po·rum
mi·cro·steth·o·phone
mi·cro·steth·o·scope

mi·cro·sto·mi·a
or mi·cros·to·mus
mi·cros·to·mus
pl mi·cros·to·mi
or mi·cro·sto·mi·a
mi·cro·struc·tur·al
mi·cro·struc·ture
mi·cro·sur·ger·y
pl mi·cro·sur·ger·ies
mi·cro·sur·gi·cal
mi·cro·syr·inge
mi·cro·the·li·a
mi·cro·therm
mi·cro·ti·a
mi·cro·ti·tri·met·ric
mi·cro·ti·trim·e·try
mi·cro·tome
mi·cro·tom·ic
or mi·cro·tom·i·cal
mi·cro·tom·i·cal
or mi·cro·tom·ic
mi·crot·o·my
pl mi·crot·o·mies
mi·cro·to·nom·e·ter
mi·cro·to·pos·co·py
mi·cro·trau·ma
mi·cro·tu·bu·lar
mi·cro·tu·bule
Mi·cro·tus
mi·cro·u·nit
mi·cro·vas·cu·lar
mi·cro·vas·cu·la·ture
mi·cro·vil·lar
mi·cro·vil·lous
mi·cro·vil·lus
pl mi·cro·vil·li
mi·cro·volt
mi·cro·wave
mi·crox·y·cyte
mi·crox·y·phil
mi·cro·zo·on
pl mi·cro·zo·a
mi·cro·zo·o·sper·mi·a
mi·crur·gic
or mi·crur·gi·cal
mi·crur·gi·cal
or mi·crur·gic
mi·crur·gist

241

mi·crur·gy
   pl mi·crur·gies
Mi·cru·roi·des
Mi·cru·rus
mic·tion
mic·tu·rate
mic·tu·ri·tion
mi·da·flur
mid·ax·il·la
mid·ax·il·lar·y
mid·bod·y
mid·brain
mid·car·pal
mid·cla·vic·u·lar
Mid·dle·brook-Du·bos
   test
mid·dor·sal
mid·ep·i·gas·tric
mid·fron·tal
midge
midg·et
mid·gut
mid·head
mid·line
mid·pain
mid·pal·mar
mid·plane
mid·rang·er
mid·riff
mid·sag·it·tal
mid·sec·tion
mid·ster·nal
mid·tar·sal
mid·ven·tral
mid·ves·i·cal
mid·wife
mid·wife·ry
   pl mid·wife·ries
Mie·scher tubes
mi·graine
mi·grai·noid
mi·grain·ous
mi·grant
mi·grate
mi·gra·tion
mi·gra·tion·al
mi·grat·or
mi·gra·to·ry

mi·kron
   pl mi·krons
   or mi·kra
   var of mi·cron
Mik·u·licz cell
mil·am·me·ter
mil·dew
Miles op·er·a·tion
mile·stones
Mil·i·an ear sign
mil·i·ar·i·a
mil·i·ar·y
mi·lieu
   pl mi·lieus
   or mi·lieux
mil·i·per·tine
mil·i·um
   pl mil·i·a
milk
Milk·man syn·drome
Mil·lar asth·ma
Mil·lard-Gub·ler syn·
   drome
mil·le·pede
   var of mil·li·pede
Mil·ler-Ab·bott tube
mil·let
mil·li·am·me·ter
mil·i·am·pere
mil·li·bar
mil·li·cu·rie
mil·li·e·quiv·a·lent
mil·li·gram
Mil·li·kan rays
mil·li·li·ter
mil·li·me·ter
mil·li·met·ric
mil·li·mi·cro·cu·rie
mil·li·mi·cro·gram
mil·li·mi·cron
mil·li·mi·cro·sec·ond
mil·li·mol
mil·li·mol·ar
mil·li·mo·lar·i·ty
   pl mil·li·mo·lar·i·ties
mil·li·mole
Mil·lin·gen op·er·a·tion
mil·li·os·mol

mil·li·os·mole
mil·li·pede
mil·li·roent·gen
mil·li·ruth·er·ford
mil·li·sec·ond
mil·li·u·nit
mil·li·volt
mil·li·volt·me·ter
Mil·lon re·a·gent
Mi·lov·i·dov meth·od
mil·phae
mil·pho·sis
Mil·roy dis·ease
milz·brand
mim·bane
mi·me·sis
   pl mi·me·ses
mi·met·ic
mim·ma·tion
mim·ic
mim·ic·ry
   pl mim·ic·ries
mim·ma·tion
Min·a·ma·ta dis·ease
mind
mind-ex·pand·ing
min·er·al
min·er·al·i·za·tion
min·er·al·o·cor·ti·coid
min·im
min·i·mal
min·i·mum
   pl min·i·ma
min·i·pig
min·is·ter
Min·kow·ski-Chauf·fard
   he·mol·yt·ic jaun·
   dice
Min·ne·so·ta Mul·ti·pha·
   sic Per·son·al·i·ty In·
   ven·to·ry
mi·nom·e·ter
mi·nor
Mi·nor dis·ease
Mi·not-Mur·phy di·et
mi·o·car·di·a
mi·o·did·y·mus
mi·o·lec·i·thal
   or mei·o·lec·i·thal

mi·o·pus
mi·o·sis
   pl mi·o·ses
mi·ot·ic
mi·ra·cid·i·um
   pl mi·ra·cid·i·a
mir·a·cil D
mi·rage
Mi·rault op·er·a·tion
mire
mir·ror
mir·ya·chit
mis·an·dry
   pl mis·an·dries
mis·an·thrope
mis·an·throp·ic
   or mis·an·throp·i·cal
mis·an·throp·i·cal
   or mis·an·throp·ic
mis·an·throp·i·cal·ly
mis·an·thro·py
   pl mis·an·thro·pies
mis·car·riage
mis·car·ry
mis·ce
mis·ce·ge·na·tion
mis·ci·ble
mis·ci·bil·i·ty
   pl mis·ci·bil·i·ties
mis·ci·ble
mis·di·ag·nose
mis·di·ag·no·sis
   pl mis·di·ag·no·ses
mi·so·cai·ne·a
mi·sog·a·mist
mi·sog·a·my
   pl mi·sog·a·mies
mi·sog·y·nic
   or mi·sog·y·nous
mi·sog·y·nist
mi·sog·y·nis·tic
mi·sog·y·nous
   or mi·sog·y·nic
mi·sog·y·ny
   pl mi·sog·y·nies
mi·sol·o·gy
   pl mi·sol·o·gies
mis·o·ne·ism
mis·o·ne·ist

mis·o·ne·is·tic
mis·o·pe·di·a
mis·o·pe·dist
mis·o·psy·chi·a
mis·sence
Mitch·ell dis·ease
mite
mith·ra·my·cin
mith·ri·date
mith·ri·da·tism
mi·ti·ci·dal
mi·ti·cide
mit·i·gate
mit·i·ga·tion
mit·i·ga·tive
mi·tis
mi·to·chon·dri·al
mi·to·chon·dri·on
   pl mi·to·chon·dri·a
mi·to·cro·min
mi·to·gen
mi·to·gen·e·sis
   pl mi·to·gen·e·ses
mi·to·ge·net·ic
mi·to·gen·ic
mi·to·ge·nic·i·ty
   pl mi·to·ge·nic·i·ties
mi·to·gil·lin
mi·to·mal·cin
mi·tome
mi·to·my·cin
mi·to·qui·none
mi·to·sis
   pl mi·to·ses
mi·to·some
mi·to·spore
mi·to·tane
mi·tot·ic
mi·tot·i·cal·ly
mi·tral
mi·tral·i·za·tion
mi·troid
Mit·su·da re·ac·tion
mit·tel·schmerz
Mit·ten·dorf dot
mix·o·sco·pi·a
mix·o·scop·ic
mix·ture
Mi·ya·ga·wa·nel·la

M'Nagh·ten rule
mne·mas·the·ni·a
mne·me
mne·mic
mne·mo·der·mi·a
mne·mon·ic
   or mne·mon·i·cal
mne·mon·i·cal
   or mne·mon·ic
mne·mon·i·cal·ly
mne·mon·ics
mne·mo·tech·nics
mne·mo·tech·ny
mo·bile
mo·bil·i·ty
   pl mo·bil·i·ties
mo·bi·li·za·tion
mo·bi·lize
Mö·bi·us dis·ease
Mö·bi·us-Ley·den dys·
   tro·phy
moc·ca·sin
mo·dal
mod·a·line
mo·dal·i·ty
   pl mo·dal·i·ties
mode
mod·er·ate
mod·er·a·tor
mod·i·fi·er
mo·di·o·lus
   pl mo·di·o·li
mod·u·la·tion
mod·u·la·tor
mod·u·lus
mo·dus
Moel·ler flu·id
Moel·ler-Bar·low dis·ease
Mo·ë·na a·nom·a·ly
mo·gi·graph·i·a
mog·i·la·li·a
mog·i·pho·ni·a
Mohr salt
Mohs scale
moi·e·ty
   pl moi·e·ties
mol
mo·lal

mo·lal·i·ty
pl mo·lal·i·ties
mo·lar
mo·lar·i·form
mo·lar·i·ty
pl mo·lar·i·ties
mold
moldy
mole
mo·lec·to·my
mo·lec·u·lar
mo·lec·u·lar·ly
mol·e·cule
mol·i·la·li·a
mo·li·men
pl mo·lim·i·na
mo·lin·a·zone
mo·lin·done
Mo·lisch test
Moll glands
Mol·la·ret men·in·gi·tis
Mol·ler, Mc·In·tosh, and
  Van Slyke test
mol·li·ti·es
mol·lusc
var of mol·lusk
Mol·lus·ca
mol·lus·can
or mol·lus·kan
mol·lus·coid
mol·lus·cous
mol·lus·cum
pl mol·lus·ca
mol·lus·cum con·ta·gi·
  o·sum
pl mol·lus·ca con·ta·gi·o·sa
mol·lusk
mol·lus·kan
or mol·lus·can
Mo·lo·ney test
molt
mo·lyb·date
mo·lyb·de·no·sis
mo·lyb·de·num
mo·lyb·dic
mo·lyb·do·phos·phate
mo·lyb·dous
mo·lys·mo·pho·bi·a
mo·ment

mo·men·tum
pl mo·men·tums
or mo·men·ta
mo·nad
Mon·ad·i·dae
Mon·a·kow bun·dle
Mo·nal·di drain·age
mon·al·kyl·a·mine
mon·am·ide
mon·am·ine
mon·ar·thric
mon·ar·thri·tis
pl mon·ar·thri·ti·des
mon·ar·tic·u·lar
Mo·nas
pl Mon·a·des
mon·as·ter
mon·ath·e·to·sis
pl mon·ath·e·to·ses
mon·a·tom·ic
mon·au·ral
mon·au·ral·ly
mon·ax·on·ic
Mön·cke·berg ar·te·ri·o·
  scle·ro·sis
Mon·dor dis·ease
mon·e·cious
var of mon·oe·cious
mo·nen·sin
Mo·ne·ra
mon·es·thet·ic
mon·es·trous
mon·e·tite
Mon·ge dis·ease
mon·gol
mon·go·li·an
mon·go·li·an·ism
or mon·gol·ism
mon·gol·ism
or mon·go·li·an·ism
mon·gol·oid
Mon·i·e·zi·a
mo·nil·e·thrix
pl mo·nil·e·tri·ches
or mo·nil·i·thrix
pl mo·nil·i·tri·ches
Mo·nil·i·a
pl Mo·nil·i·as
or Mo·nil·i·a

mo·nil·i·al
Mo·nil·i·a·les
mon·i·li·a·sis
pl mon·i·li·a·ses
mo·nil·i·form
Mo·nil·i·for·mis
mo·nil·i·form·ly
mo·nil·i·id
mo·nil·i·thrix
pl mo·nil·i·tri·ches
or mo·nil·e·thrix
pl mo·nil·e·tri·ches
mo·nism
mo·nis·tic
mon·i·tor
Mo·niz sign
mon·key
monks·hood
Mon·ne·ret pulse
mono
mon·o·ac·id
mon·o·ac·id·ic
mon·o·am·ide
mon·o·am·ine
var of mon·am·ine
mon·o·am·i·ner·gic
mon·o·am·ni·ot·ic
mon·o·ar·tic·u·lar
mon·o·az·o
mon·o·bal·lism
mon·o·ba·sic
mon·o·ben·zone
mon·o·blast
mon·o·blep·si·a
mon·o·blep·sis
mon·o·bra·chi·us
mon·o·bro·mat·ed
mon·o·car·box·yl·ic
mon·o·car·di·an
mon·o·car·di·o·gram
mon·o·cel·lu·lar
mon·o·ceph·a·lus
pl mon·o·ceph·a·li
mon·o·chlo·ro·phe·nol
mon·o·chord
mon·o·cho·re·a
mon·o·cho·ri·on·ic
mon·o·chro·ic
mon·o·chro·ma·si·a

mon·o·chro·ma·sy
  pl mon·o·chro·ma·sies
  or mon·o·chro·ma·tism
mon·o·chro·mat
mon·o·chro·mate
mon·o·chro·mat·ic
mon·o·chro·mat·i·cal·ly
mon·o·chro·ma·tism
  or mon·o·chro·ma·sy
mon·o·chro·mat·o·phil
mon·o·chro·ma·tor
mon·o·chro·mic
mon·o·clin·ic
mon·o·clo·nal
mon·o·coc·cus
  pl mon·o·coc·ci
mon·o·con·tam·i·nate
mon·o·con·tam·i·na·tion
mon·o·cot·y·le·do·nous
mon·o·cra·ni·us
mon·o·crot·ic
mo·noc·u·lar
mo·noc·u·lar·ly
mo·noc·u·lus
  pl mo·noc·u·li
mon·o·cy·e·sis
mon·o·cys·tic
mon·o·cyte
mon·o·cyt·ic
mon·o·cy·toid
mon·o·cy·to·ma
  pl mon·o·cy·to·mas
  or mon·o·cy·to·ma·ta
mon·o·cy·to·pe·ni·a
mon·o·cy·to·sis
  pl mon·o·cy·to·ses
mon·o·dac·ty·lism
  or mon·o·dac·ty·ly
mon·o·dac·ty·ly
  pl mon·o·dac·ty·lies
  or mon·o·dac·ty·lism
mon·o·der·mo·ma
mon·o·di·plo·pi·a
mon·oe·cious
mon·o·en·er·get·ic
mon·o·es·ter
mon·o·eth·a·nol·a·mine
mon·o·fac·to·ri·al
mon·o·fil·a·ment

mon·o·func·tion·al
mo·nog·a·my
  pl mo·nog·a·mies
mon·o·gas·tic
mon·o·gen·e·sis
  pl mon·o·gen·e·ses
mon·o·ge·net·ic
mon·o·gen·ic
mon·o·gen·i·cal·ly
mo·nog·e·nous
mon·o·ger·mi·nal
mo·nog·o·nous
mo·nog·o·ny
mon·o·graph
mon·o·graph·ic
mon·o·hy·brid
mon·o·hy·drate
mon·o·hy·drat·ed
mon·o·hy·dric
mon·o·hy·drol
mon·o·i·de·ism
mon·o·i·de·is·tic
mon·o·i·o·do·a·ce·tic
mon·o·i·o·do·ty·ro·sine
mon·o·ke·tone
mon·o·lay·er
mon·o·lep·sis
mon·o·lob·u·lar
mon·o·loc·u·lar
mon·o·ma·ni·a
mon·o·ma·ni·ac
mon·o·mas·ti·gote
mon·o·mel·ic
mon·o·mer
mon·o·mer·ic
mon·o·me·tal·lic
mon·o·mo·lec·u·lar
mon·o·mo·lec·u·lar·ly
mon·o·mo·ri·a
mon·o·mor·phic
  or mon·o·mor·phous
mon·o·mor·phism
mon·o·mor·phous
  or mon·o·mor·phic
mon·om·pha·lus
  pl mon·om·pha·li
mon·o·my·o·ple·gi·a
mon·o·my·o·si·tis
mon·o·neph·rous

mon·o·neu·ral
mon·o·neu·ri·tis
  pl mon·o·neu·ri·tis·es
  or mon·o·neu·ri·ti·des
mon·o·neu·rop·a·thy
mon·o·nu·cle·ar
mon·o·nu·cle·ate
mon·o·nu·cle·o·sis
  pl mon·o·nu·cle·o·ses
mon·o·nu·cle·o·tide
mon·o·pa·re·sis
  pl mon·o·pa·re·ses
mon·o·par·es·the·si·a
mon·op·a·thy
mon·o·pha·gi·a
mo·noph·a·gism
mon·o·pha·si·a
mon·o·pha·sic
mon·o·phe·nol
mon·o·pho·bi·a
mon·o·phos·phate
mon·oph·thal·mi·a
mon·oph·thal·mic
mon·oph·thal·mus
mon·o·phy·let·ic
mon·o·phy·le·tism
  or mon·o·phy·le·ty
mon·o·phy·le·ty
  pl mon·o·phy·le·ties
  or mon·o·phy·le·tism
mon·o·phy·o·dont
mon·o·ple·gi·a
mon·o·ple·gic
mon·o·ploid
mon·o·po·di·a
mon·o·po·lar
mon·ops
mo·nop·si·a
mon·o·psy·cho·sis
mon·o·pty·chi·al
mon·o·pus
mon·o·py·ram·i·dal
mon·or·chid
mon·or·chid·ism
  or mon·or·chism
mon·or·chis
  pl mon·or·chi·des
mon·or·chism
  or mon·or·chid·ism

mon·or·rhi·nous
mon·o·sac·cha·ride
mon·o·scel·ous
mon·ose
mon·o·so·di·um
mon·o·sex·u·al
mon·o·sex·u·al·i·ty
   pl mon·o·sex·u·al·i·ties
mon·o·so·di·um glu·
   ta·mate
mon·o·som·a·tous
mon·o·some
mon·o·so·mic
mon·o·so·mus
mon·o·so·my
mon·o·spasm
Mon·o·spo·ri·um
mon·o·ste·a·rin
mon·os·tot·ic
mon·o·stra·tal
mon·o·sub·sti·tut·ed
mon·o·sub·sti·tu·tion
mon·o·symp·to·mat·ic
mon·o·sy·nap·tic
mon·o·sy·nap·ti·cal·ly
mon·o·ter·pene
mon·o·ther·mi·a
mo·not·ic
mo·not·o·cous
Mon·o·tre·ma·ta
mon·o·treme
mon·o·trich·ic
   or mo·not·ri·chous
   or mo·not·ri·chate
mo·not·ri·chate
   or mon·o·trich·ic
   or mo·not·ri·chous
mo·not·ri·chous
   or mon·o·trich·ic
   or mo·not·ri·chate
mon·o·trop·ic
mon·o·typ·ic
mon·o·va·lent
mon·o·vu·lar
mon·o·xen·ic
mon·nox·e·nous
mon·ox·ide
mon·o·zy·got·ic

Mon·ro for·a·men
mons
   pl mon·tes
mons pu·bis
mons ven·er·is
Mon·sel salt
Mon·son curve
mon·ster
mon·stri·cide
mon·strip·a·ra
mon·stro·cel·lu·lar
mon·stros·i·ty
   pl mon·stros·i·ties
mon·strous
Mon·teg·gi·a frac·ture
Mon·te·ne·gro test
Mon·te·zu·ma re·venge
Mont·gom·er·y glands
mon·tic·u·lus
mont·mo·ril·lon·ite
Moon mo·lars
moon-blind
moon-blind·ness
Moore syn·drome
Moor·en ul·cer
Moo·ser bod·ies
mo·rale
mor·a·men·ti·a
mo·ran·tel
Mo·rax-Ax·en·feld
   con·junc·ti·vi·tis
Mo·rax·el·la lac·u·na·ta
mor·bid
mor·bid·i·ty
   pl mor·bid·i·ties
mor·bid·ly
mor·bif·ic
mor·bil·li
mor·bil·li·form
mor·bus
   pl mor·bi
mor·cel·la·tion
mor·da·cious
mor·dant
Mo·rel syn·drome
Mo·rel-Krae·pe·lin
   dis·ease

Mo·rel-Moore syn·
   drome
Mor·ga·gni crypt
Mor·ga·gni-Ad·ams-
   Stokes syn·drome
Mor·ga·gni·an cyst
Mor·ga·gni-Stew·art-
   Mo·rel syn·drome
Mor·ga·gni-Stokes-
   Ad·ams syn·drome
Morgan ba·cil·lus
morgue
mo·ri·a
mor·i·bund
mor·i·bun·di·ty
   pl mor·i·bun·di·ties
Mor·i·son pouch
Mor·i·son-Tal·ma
   op·er·a·tion
Mör·ner test
Mo·ro re·flex
mo·ron
mo·ron·ic
mo·ron·ism
mo·ron·i·ty
   pl mo·ron·i·ties
mo·ro·sis
mor·phal·lax·is
   pl mor·phal·lax·es
mor·phe·a
   pl mor·phe·ae
mor·pheme
mor·phe·mic
mor·phe·mi·cal·ly
mor·phi·a
mor·phine
mor·phin·ic
mor·phin·ism
mor·phin·ize
mor·phi·no·ma·ni·a
   or mor·phi·o·ma·ni·a
mor·phi·no·ma·ni·ac
   or mor·phi·o·ma·ni·ac
mor·phi·o·ma·ni·a
   or mor·phi·no·ma·ni·a
mor·phi·o·ma·ni·ac
   or mor·phi·no·ma·ni·ac
mor·pho·bi·o·met·ric

mor·pho·bi·om·e·try
mor·phoc·a
  pl mor·phoe·ac
  var of mor·phe·a
mor·pho·gen·e·sis
  pl mor·pho·gen·e·ses
mor·pho·ge·net·ic
mor·pho·ge·net·i·cal·ly
mor·pho·gen·ic
mor·phog·e·ny
mor·pho·graph·ic
mor·phog·ra·phy
  pl mor·phog·ra·phies
mor·pho·line
mor·pho·log·ic
  or mor·pho·log·i·cal
mor·pho·log·i·cal
  or mor·pho·log·ic
mor·pho·log·i·cal·ly
mor·phol·o·gist
mor·phol·o·gy
  pl mor·phol·o·gies
mor·phom·e·try
  pl mor·phom·e·tries
mor·pho·phys·i·o·log·i·cal
mor·pho·phys·i·ol·o·gy
  pl mor·pho·phys·i·ol·o·gies
mor·pho·sis
  pl mor·pho·ses
mor·phot·ic
mor·phous
Mor·qui·o-Brails·ford
  dis·ease
Mor·qui·o syn·drome
Mor·ris meth·od
mors
mor·sal
mor·sus
mor·tal
mor·tal·i·ty
  pl mor·tal·i·ties
mor·tal·ly
mor·tar
mor·ti·fi·ca·tion
mor·ti·fy
Mor·ton toe
mor·tu·ar·y
  pl mor·tu·ar·ies

mor·u·la
  pl mor·u·lae
mor·u·lar
mor·u·la·tion
Mor·van dis·ease
mor·vin
mo·sa·ic
mo·sa·i·cism
Mosch·co·witz dis·ease
Mo·sen·thal test
mos·qui·to
  pl mos·qui·tos
  or mos·qui·toes
Moss groups
Moss·man fe·ver
Mo·tais op·er·a·tion
moth·er
mo·tile
mo·til·i·ty
  pl mo·til·i·ties
mo·tion
mo·ti·vate
mo·ti·va·tion
mo·ti·va·tion·al
mo·ti·va·tion·al·ly
mo·tive
mo·to·neu·ron
  or mo·to·neu·rone
mo·to·neu·rone
  or mo·to·neu·ron
mo·to·neu·ro·ni·tis
mo·tor
mo·to·ri·al
mo·to·ri·um
  pl mo·to·ri·a
Mott law
mot·tle
mouches vo·lantes
mou·lage
mould
  var of mold
mould·y
  var of mold·y
moult
  var of molt
mound
mound·ing
moun·tant

mount·ing
mouse
  pl mice
mouse·pox
mouth
mouth·piece
mouth-to-mouth
mouth·wash
mouve·ment de ma·nège
move·a·ble
move·ment
mox·a
mox·i·bus·tion
Mox·on pa·ra·ple·gi·a
Moy·a·noy·a syn·drome
Moy·ni·han symp·tom
  com·plex
Mo·zam·bique ul·cer
mu·cate
Much gran·u·les
Mu·cha-Ha·ber·mann
  dis·ease
mu·cic
mu·ci·car·mine
mu·cif·er·ous
mu·cif·ic
mu·ci·fi·ca·tion
mu·ci·form
mu·ci·fy
mu·ci·gen
mu·cig·e·nous
mu·ci·lage
mu·ci·lag·i·nous
mu·ci·la·go
  pl mu·ci·lag·i·nes
mu·cin
mu·ci·nase
mu·ci·no·blast
mu·cin·o·gen
mu·ci·noid
mu·ci·no·lyt·ic
mu·ci·no·sis
  pl mu·ci·no·ses
mu·ci·nous
mu·cip·a·rous
mu·co·al·bu·mi·nous
mu·co·buc·cal
mu·co·cele

mu·co·co·li·tis
mu·co·col·pos
mu·co·cu·ta·ne·ous
mu·co·derm
mu·co·en·ter·i·tis
  pl mu·co·en·ter·i·tis·es
  or mu·co·en·ter·i·ti·des
mu·co·ep·i·der·moid
mu·co·gin·gi·val
mu·co·glob·u·lin
mu·co·hem·or·rhag·ic
mu·coid
mu·co·i·tin
mu·co·i·tin·sul·fu·ric
mu·co·lyt·ic
mu·co·mem·bra·nous
mu·co·me·tri·a
mu·co·peri·os·te·al
mu·co·peri·os·te·um
  pl mu·co·peri·os·te·a
mu·co·pol·y·sac·cha·ride
mu·co·pol·y·sac·cha·ri·
  do·sis
mu·co·po·ly·sac·cha·ri·
  du·ri·a
mu·co·pro·te·in
mu·co·pu·ru·lent
mu·co·pus
Mu·cor
Mu·co·ra·ce·ae
Mu·co·ra·les
mu·cor·my·co·sis
  pl mu·cor·my·co·ses
mu·co·sa
  pl mu·co·sas
  or mu·co·sae
mu·so·cal
  or mu·co·cal
mu·co·sal·pinx
mu·co·san·guin·e·ous
mu·co·se·rous
mu·co·sin
mu·co·sis
mu·co·si·tis
mu·cos·i·ty
  pl mu·cos·i·ties
mu·co·stat·ic
mu·cous

mu·co·vis·ci·do·sis
  pl mu·co·vis·ci·do·ses
mu·cro
  pl mu·cros
  or mu·cro·nes
mu·cro·nate
  or mu·cro·nat·ed
mu·cro·nat·ed
  or mu·cro·nate
mu·cu·lent
Mu·cu·na
mu·cus
Muel·ler spots
Muel·le·ri·us
mu·guet
mu·laire
mu·lat·to
  pl mu·lat·tos
  or mu·lat·toes
Mules op·er·a·tion
mu·li·e·bri·a
mu·li·eb·ri·ty
  pl mu·li·eb·ri·ties
mull
Müll·er duct, flu·id,
  mus·cle
Mül·le·ri·an
Mül·le·ri·an duct
mult·an·gu·lar
mult·an·gu·lum
  pl mult·an·gu·la
mul·ti·ar·tic·u·lar
mul·ti·cap·su·lar
mul·ti·cel·lu·lar
mul·ti·cel·lu·lar·i·ty
  pl mul·ti·cel·lu·lar·i·ties
mul·ti·cen·tric
mul·ti·cen·tri·cal·ly
mul·ti·cen·tric·i·ty
  pl mul·ti·cen·tric·i·ties
Mul·ti·ceps
mul·ti·cip·i·tal
mul·ti·clo·nal
mul·ti·cos·tate
mul·ti·cus·pid
mul·ti·cus·pi·date
mu·ti·cys·tic

mul·ti·den·tate
mu·ti·dig·i·tate
mul·ti·fac·et·ed
mul·ti·fac·to·ri·al
mul·ti·fa·mil·ial
mul·ti·fe·ta·tion
mul·ti·fid
mul·ti·fid·ly
mul·tif·i·dus
  pl mul·tif·i·di
mul·ti·flag·el·late
mul·ti·fo·cal
mul·ti·form
mul·ti·gan·gli·o·nate
mul·ti·glan·du·lar
mul·ti·grav·i·da
  pl mul·ti·grav·i·das
  or mul·ti·grav·i·dae
mul·ti·gra·vid·i·ty
mul·ti·hem·a·tin·ic
mul·ti·in·fec·tion
mul·ti·lay·ered
mul·ti·lo·bar
mul·ti·lo·bate
mul·ti·lobed
mul·ti·lob·u·lar
mul·ti·loc·u·lar
mul·ti·loc·u·lat·ed
mul·ti·mam·mae
mul·ti·nod·u·lar
mul·ti·nu·cle·ar
  or mul·ti·nu·cle·ate
  or mul·ti·nu·cle·at·ed
mul·ti·nu·cle·ate
  or mul·ti·nu·cle·ar
  or mul·ti·nu·cle·at·ed
mul·ti·nu·cle·at·ed
  or mul·ti·nu·cle·ar
  or mul·ti·nu·cle·ated
mul·tip·a·ra
  pl mul·tip·a·ras
  or mul·tip·a·rae
mul·ti·par·i·ty
  pl mul·ti·par·i·ties
mul·tip·a·rous
mul·ti·par·tite
mul·ti·pen·nate
mul·ti·pha·sic

mul·ti·ple
mul·ti·plex
mul·ti·plic·i·ty
mul·ti·po·lar
mul·ti·pol·y·poid
mul·ti·re·sis·tance
mul·ti·re·sis·tant
mul·ti·sen·so·ry
mul·ti·sep·tate
mul·ti·syn·ap·tic
mul·ti·sys·tem
mul·ti·ter·mi·nal
mul·ti·va·lence
mul·ti·va·lent
mul·ti·vi·ta·min
mum·mi·fi·ca·tion
mum·mi·fy
mumps
Mun·chau·sen syn·
  drome
Münch·mey·er dis·ease
mun·dif·i·cant
mu·ral
mu·ram·ic
mu·ram·i·dase
mu·re·in
mu·rex·ide
mu·rex·ine
mu·ri·ate
mu·ri·at·ed
mu·ri·at·ic
mu·rine
mur·mur
Mur·phy but·ton
Mur·phy-Sturm lym·
  pho·sar·co·ma
mur·rain
Mur·ray Val·ley en·ceph·
  a·li·tis
mur·ri·na
Mus
Mus·ca
mus·cae vol·i·tan·tes
mus·ca·rine
mus·ca·rin·ic
mus·ca·rin·ism
mus·ci·cide
Mus·ci·dae

mus·cle
mus·cle-bound
mus·cled
mus·cu·lar
mus·cu·la·ris
ms·cu·lar·i·ty
  pl mus·cu·lar·i·ties
mus·cu·lar·ly
mus·cu·la·tion
mus·cu·la·ture
mus·cu·li
mus·cu·lo·ap·o·neu·rot·ic
mus·cu·lo·cu·ta·ne·ous
mus·cu·lo·fas·ci·al
mus·cu·lo·fi·brous
mus·cu·lo·mem·bra·nous
mus·cu·lo·phren·ic
mus·cu·lo·skel·e·tal
mus·cu·lo·spi·ral
mus·cu·lo·ten·di·nous
mus·cu·lo·trop·ic
mus·cu·lo·tu·bal
mus·cu·lus
  pl mus·cu·li
mush·room
mu·si·co·ma·ni·a
mu·si·co·ther·a·py
  pl mu·si·co·ther·a·pies
mus·si·ta·tion
mus·tard
mus·tine
mu·ta·cism
mu·ta·fa·cient
mu·ta·gen
mu·ta·gen·e·sis
  pl mu·ta·gen·e·ses
mu·ta·gen·ic
mu·ta·gen·i·cal·ly
mu·ta·gen·ic·i·ty
  pl mu·ta·ge·nic·i·ties
mu·tant
mu·ta·ro·tase
mu·ta·ro·ta·tion
mu·tase
mu·tate
mu·ta·tion
mu·ta·tion·al
mu·ta·tion·al·ly

mu·ta·tor
mute
mu·ti·late
mu·ti·la·tion
mu·ti·la·tor
mut·ism
mu·ton
mu·tu·al·ism
mu·tu·al·ist
muz·zle
my·al·gi·a
my·al·gic
my·as·the·ni·a
my·as·the·ni·a grav·is
my·as·then·ic
my·a·to·ni·a
my·at·ro·phy
my·ce·li·al
my·ce·li·oid
my·ce·li·um
  pl my·ce·li·a
my·cete
my·ce·tes
my·ce·the·mi·a
my·ce·tism
my·ce·tis·mus
  pl my·ce·tis·mi
my·ce·to·gen·ic
my·ce·tog·e·nous
my·ce·toid
my·ce·to·ma
  pl my·ce·to·mas
  or my·ce·to·ma·ta
My·ce·to·zo·a
my·ce·to·zo·an
my·co·an·gi·o·neu·ro·sis
My·co·bac·te·ri·a·ce·ae
my·co·bac·te·ri·al
my·co·bac·te·ri·o·sis
  pl my·co·bac·te·ri·o·ses
My·co·bac·te·ri·um
  pl My·co·bac·te·ri·a
my·co·cide
my·co·ci·din
My·co·der·ma
my·co·der·ma·ti·tis
my·co·der·ma·toid
  or my·co·der·ma·tous

249

my·co·der·ma·tous
  or my·co·der·ma·toid
my·coid
my·col·ic
my·co·log·ic
  or my·co·log·i·cal
my·co·log·i·cal
  or my·co·log·ic
my·co·log·i·cal·ly
my·col·o·gist
my·col·o·gy
  pl my·col·o·gies
my·co·my·cin
my·co·myr·in·gi·tis
my·coph·o·gous
my·coph·thal·mi·a
My·co·plas·ma
  pl My·co·plas·mas
  or My·co·plas·ma·ta
my·co·plas·mal
My·co·plas·ma·ta·ce·ae
my·cose
my·co·sis
  pl my·co·ses
my·co·sis fun·goi·des
my·co·stat·ic
my·cos·ter·ol
my·co·sub·ti·lin
my·cot·ic
my·cot·i·za·tion
my·co·tox·ic
my·co·tox·ic·i·ty
  pl my·co·tox·ic·i·ties
my·co·tox·i·co·sis
  pl my·co·tox·i·co·ses
myc·co·tox·in
myc·ter·o·pho·ni·a
my·de·sis
my·dri·a·sis
  pl my·dri·a·ses
myd·ri·at·ic
my·ec·to·my
  pl my·ec·to·mies
my·ec·to·pi·a
my·ec·to·py
my·e·lae·mi·a
  var of my·e·le·mi·a
my·e·lal·gia
my·el·ap·o·plex·y

my·el·la·te·li·a
my·el·at·ro·phy
  pl my·el·at·ro·phies
my·e·le·mi·a
my·el·en·ce·phal·ic
my·el·en·ceph·a·lon
  pl my·el·en·ceph·a·la
my·el·ic
my·e·lin
my·e·li·nat·ed
my·e·lin·ic
my·e·lin·a·tion
  or my·e·lin·i·za·tion
my·e·lin·ic
my·e·lin·i·za·tion
  or my·e·lin·a·tion
my·e·li·noc·la·sis
  pl my·e·li·noc·la·ses
my·e·lin·o·gen·e·sis
  pl my·e·lin·o·gen·e·ses
my·e·li·nol·y·sis
  pl my·e·li·nol·y·ses
my·e·li·nop·a·thy
my·e·li·no·sis
  pl my·e·li·no·sis·es
  or my·e·li·no·ses
my·e·lit·ic
my·e·li·tis
  pl my·e·li·ti·des
my·e·lo·blast
my·e·lo·blas·te·mi·a
my·e·lo·blas·tic
my·e·lo·blas·to·ma
  pl my·e·lo·blas·to·mas
  or my·e·lo·blas·to·ma·ta
my·e·lo·blas·to·sis
  pl my·e·lo·blas·to·ses
my·e·lo·cele
my·e·lo·chlo·ro·ma
my·e·lo·cyst
my·e·lo·cys·to·cele
my·e·lo·cys·tog·ra·phy
my·e·lo·cyte
my·e·lo·cy·thae·mi·a
  var of my·e·lo·cy·the·mi·a
my·e·lo·cy·the·mi·a
my·e·lo·cyt·ic
my·e·lo·cy·to·ma
  pl my·e·lo·cy·to·mas

  or my·e·lo·cy·to·ma·ta
my·e·lo·cy·to·sis
  pl my·e·lo·cy·to·ses
my·e·lo·dys·pla·si·a
my·e·lo·en·ceph·a·li·tis
  pl my·e·lo·en·ceph·a·li·ti·des
my·e·lo·fi·bro·sis
  pl my·e·lo·fi·bro·ses
my·e·lo·fi·brot·ic
my·e·lo·gen·e·sis
  pl my·e·lo·gen·e·ses
my·e·lo·gen·ic
  of my·e·log·e·nous
my·e·log·e·nous
  or my·e·lo·gen·ic
my·e·lo·gone
my·e·lo·gram
my·e·lo·graph·ic
my·e·lo·graph·i·cal·ly
my·e·log·ra·phy
  pl my·e·log·ra·phies
my·e·loid
my·e·loi·do·sis
my·e·lo·ken·tric
my·e·lo·li·po·ma
  pl my·e·lo·li·po·mas
  or my·e·lo·li·po·ma·ta
my·e·lo·lym·phan·gi·o·ma
my·e·lo·lym·pho·cyte
my·e·lol·y·sis
my·e·lo·ma
  pl my·e·lo·mas
  or my·e·lo·ma·ta
my·e·lo·ma·la·ci·a
my·e·lo·my·to·sis
  pl my·e·lo·ma·to·ses
my·e·lo·ma·tous
my·e·lo·men·i·a
my·e·lo·men·in·gi·tis
  pl my·e·lo·men·in·gi·ti·des
my·e·lo·me·nin·go·cele
my·e·lo·mere
my·e·lo·mon·o·cyte
my·e·lo·mon·o·cyt·ic
my·e·lon
my·e·lo·neu·ri·tis
  pl my·e·lo·neu·ri·tis·es
  or my·e·lo·neu·ri·ti·des

250

my·e·lon·ic
my·e·lo·pa·ral·y·sis
  pl my·e·lo·pa·ral·y·ses
my·e·lo·path·ic
my·e·lop·a·thy
  pl my·e·lop·a·thies
my·e·lop·e·tal
my·e·lo·phthis·ic
my·e·lo·phthi·sis
  pl my·e·lo·phthi·ses
my·e·lo·plaque
my·e·lo·plast
my·e·lo·plax
  pl my·e·lo·plax·es
  or my·e·lo·pla·ces
my·e·lo·plax·ic
my·e·lo·ple·gi·a
my·e·lo·poi·e·sis
  pl my·e·lo·poi·e·ses
my·e·lo·poi·e·tic
my·e·lo·pore
my·e·lo·pro·lif·er·a·tive
my·e·lo·ra·dic·u·li·tis
my·e·lo·ra·dic·u·lo·dys·
  pla·sia
my·e·lo·ra·dic·u·lop·a·thy
  pl my·e·lo·ra·dic·u·lop·
    a·thies
my·e·lor·rha·gi·a
my·e·lo·sar·co·ma
  pl my·e·lo·sar·co·mas
  or my·e·lo·sar·co·ma·ta
my·e·los·chi·sis
  pl my·e·los·chi·sis·es
  or my·e·los·chi·ses
my·e·lo·scin·to·gram
my·e·lo·scin·tog·ra·phy
my·e·lo·scle·ro·sis
my·e·lo·scle·rot·ic
my·e·lo·sis
  pl my·e·lo·ses
my·e·lo·spon·gi·um
  pl my·e·lo·spon·gi·a
my·e·lo·sy·rin·go·cele
my·e·lot·o·my
my·e·lo·tox·ic
my·e·lo·tox·in
my·en·ta·sis
my·en·ter·ic

my·en·ter·on
My·er meth·od
My·ers and War·dell
  meth·od
My·er·son re·flex
my·es·the·si·a
my·i·a·sis
  pl my·i·a·ses
my·i·o·de·op·si·a
my·i·o·des·op·si·a
my·i·o·sis
my·la·ceph·a·lus
my·lo·hy·oid
my·lo·hy·oi·de·an
my·lo·hy·oi·de·us
  pl my·lo·hy·oi·de·i
my·lo·pha·ryn·ge·al
my·o·al·bu·min
my·o·ar·chi·tec·ton·ic
my·o·at·ro·phy
my·o·blast
my·o·blas·tic
my·o·blas·to·ma
  pl my·o·blas·to·mas
  or my·o·blas·to·ma·ta
my·o·bra·di·a
my·o·car·di·al
my·o·car·di·o·graph
my·o·car·di·op·a·thy
  pl my·o·car·di·op·a·thies
my·o·car·di·tis
my·o·car·di·um
  pl my·o·car·di·a
my·o·car·do·sis
  pl my·o·car·do·ses
my·o·cele
my·o·cel·lu·li·tis
my·o·cep·tor
my·o·cer·o·sis
my·o·clo·ni·a
my·o·clon·ic
my·o·clo·nus
my·o·coel
  or my·o·coele
my·o·coele
  or my·o·coel
my·o·com·ma
  pl my·o·com·mas
  or my·o·com·ma·ta

my·o·cyte
my·o·cy·tol·y·sis
my·o·cy·to·ma
my·o·de·mi·a
my·o·dy·nam·ics
my·o·dys·to·ni·a
  or my·o·dys·to·ny
my·o·dys·to·ny
  pl my·o·dys·to·nies
  or my·o·dys·to·ni·a
my·o·dys·tro·phy
  pl my·o·dys·tro·phies
my·o·e·de·ma
  pl my·o·e·de·mas
  or my·o·e·de·ma·ta
my·o·e·las·tic
my·o·e·lec·tric
  or my·o·e·lec·tri·cal
my·o·e·lec·tri·cal
  or my·o·e·lec·tric
my·o·e·lec·tri·cal·ly
my·o·en·do·car·di·tis
my·o·ep·i·the·li·al
my·o·ep·i·the·li·o·ma
  pl my·o·ep·i·the·li·o·mas
  or my·o·epi·the·li·o·ma·ta
my·o·ep·i·the·li·um
my·o·fas·ci·al
my·o·fas·ci·tis
my·o·fi·bril
  or my·o·fi·bril·la
my·o·fi·bril·la
  or my·o·fi·bril
my·o·fi·bro·ma
  pl my·o·fi·bro·mas
  or my·o·fi·bro·ma·ta
my·o·fi·bro·sar·co·ma
  pl my·o·fi·bro·sar·co·mas
  or my·o·fi·bro·sar·co·ma·ta
my·o·fi·bro·sis
  pl my·o·fi·bro·ses
my·o·fi·bro·si·tis
my·o·fil·a·ment
my·o·ge·lo·sis
my·o·gen
my·o·gen·ic
my·o·ge·nic·i·ty
  pl my·o·ge·nic·i·ties
my·og·e·nous

my·og·li·a
my·o·glo·bin
my·o·glo·bi·nu·ri·a
my·o·glo·bu·lin
my·og·na·thus
my·o·gram
my·o·graph
my·o·graph·ic
my·o·graph·i·cal·ly
my·og·ra·phy
  pl my·og·ra·phies
my·o·haem·a·tin
  var of my·o·hem·a·tin
my·o·hae·mo·glo·bin
  var of my·o·hem·o·glo·bin
myo·hae·mo·glo·bi·nu·ria
  var of my·o·he·mo·glo·bi·
    nu·ri·a
my·o·hem·a·tin
my·o·he·mo·glo·bin
my·o·he·mo·glo·bi·nu·ri·a
my·oid
my·oi·des
my·o·i·no·si·tol
my·o·ki·nase
my·o·kin·e·sim·e·ter
my·o·ki·ne·si·o·gram
my·o·ki·ne·si·og·ra·phy
my·o·ki·net·ic
my·o·ky·mi·a
my·o·lei·ot·ic
my·o·lem·ma
  pl my·o·lem·mas
  or my·o·lem·ma·ta
my·o·li·po·ma
  pl my·o·li·po·mas
  or my·o·li·po·ma·ta
my·o·lo·gi·a
my·o·log·ic
  or my·o·log·i·cal
my·o·log·i·cal
  or my·o·log·ic
my·ol·o·gy
  pl my·ol·o·gies
my·ol·y·sis
my·o·ma
  pl my·o·mas
  or my·o·ma·ta
my·o·ma·la·ci·a

my·o·ma·to·sis
my·o·ma·tous
my·o·mec·to·my
  pl my·o·mec·to·mies
my·ome dar·to·ique
my·o·me·lan·o·sis
my·o·mere
my·o·mer·ic
my·o·me·ter
my·o·me·tri·al
my·o·me·tri·tis
my·o·me·tri·um
my·o·ne·cro·sis
my·o·ne·ma
  or my·o·neme
my·o·neme
  or my·o·ne·ma
my·o·neu·ral
my·o·neu·ral·gi·a
my·o·pal·mus
my·o·pa·ral·y·sis
  pl my·o·pa·ral·y·ses
my·o·pa·re·sis
  pl my·o·pa·re·ses
my·o·path·i·a
my·o·path·ic
my·op·a·thy
  pl my·op·a·thies
my·ope
my·o·per·i·car·di·tis
  pl my·o·per·i·car·di·ti·des
my·o·pha·gi·a
my·o·pi·a
my·op·ic
my·op·i·cal·ly
my·o·plasm
my·o·plas·ty
  pl my·o·plas·ties
my·o·por·tho·sis
my·o·psy·chop·a·thy
my·o·psy·cho·sis
  pl my·o·psy·cho·ses
my·o·rhyth·mi·a
my·o·rhyth·mic
my·or·rha·phy
  pl my·or·rha·phies
my·or·rhex·is
my·o·san

my·o·sar·co·ma
  pl my·o·sar·co·mas
  or my·o·sar·co·ma·ta
my·o·schwan·no·ma
  pl my·o·schwan·no·mas
  or my·o·schwan·no·ma·ta
my·o·scle·ro·sis
  pl my·o·scle·ro·sis
my·o·sep·tum
  pl my·o·sep·ta
my·o·sin
my·o·sin·o·gen
my·o·sis
  pl my·o·ses
  var of mi·o·sis
my·o·sit·ic
my·o·si·tis
my·o·spasm
my·o·tac·tic
my·o·su·ture
my·o·syn·o·vi·tis
my·o·tac·tic
my·ot·a·sis
my·o·tat·ic
my·o·ten·di·nous
my·o·ten·o·si·tis
my·o·te·not·o·my
  pl my·o·te·not·o·mies
my·ot·ic
  var of mi·ot·ic
my·o·tome
my·ot·o·my
  pl my·ot·o·mies
my·o·to·ni·a
my·o·ton·ic
my·o·to·noid
my·ot·o·nus
my·o·tro·phic
my·ot·ro·phy
  pl my·ot·ro·phies
my·o·tu·bule
myr·cene
myr·ci·a
myr·i·a·gram
myr·i·a·li·ter
myr·i·a·me·ter
myr·i·cyl
my·rin·ga

myr·in·gec·to·my
   pl myr·in·gec·to·mies
myr·in·gi·tis
my·rin·go·dec·to·my
   pl my·rin·go·dec·to·mies
my·rin·go·my·co·sis
   pl my·rin·go·my·co·ses
my·rin·go·plas·tic
my·rin·go·plas·ty
   pl my·rin·go·plas·ties
my·rin·go·tome
myr·in·got·o·my
   pl myr·in·got·o·mies
my·rinx
myr·i·o·pod
my·ris·tic
my·ris·ti·ca
my·ris·tin
myr·me·si·a
my·ro·si·nase
myrrh
My·so·line
my·so·phil·i·a
my·so·pho·bi·a
my·so·pho·bic
my·ta·cism
myth·o·ma·ni·a
myth·o·ma·ni·ac
myth·o·pho·bi·a
myt·i·lo·tox·in
myt·i·lo·tox·ism
my·u·rous
myx·ad·e·ni·tis
myx·ad·e·no·ma
   pl myx·ad·e·no·mas
   or myx·ad·e·no·ma·ta
myx·as·the·ni·a

myx·e·de·ma
   pl myx·e·de·mas
   or myx·e·de·ma·ta
myx·e·de·ma·toid
myx·e·de·ma·tous
myx·id·i·o·cy
   pl myx·id·i·o·cies
myx·i·o·sis
myx·o·ad·e·no·ma
   pl myx·o·ad·e·no·mas
   or myx·o·ad·e·no·ma·ta
myx·o·chon·dro·fi·bro·
   sar·co·ma
   pl myx·o·chon·dro·fi·bro·
     sar·co·mas
   or myx·o·chon·dro·fi·bro·
     sar·co·ma·ta
myx·o·chon·dro·ma
   pl myx·o·chon·dro·mas
   or myx·o·chon·dro·ma·ta
myx·o·chon·dro·sar·co·ma
   pl myx·o·chon·dro·sar·
     co·mas
   or myx·o·chon·dro·sar·
     co·mata
myx·o·cyte
myx·oe·de·ma
   var of myx·e·de·ma
myx·oe·de·ma·tous
   var of myx·e·de·ma·tous
myx·o·fi·bro·ma
   pl myx·o·fi·bro·mas
   or myx·o·fi·bro·ma·ta
myx·o·fi·bro·sar·co·ma
   pl myx·o·fi·bro·sar·co·mas
   or myx·o·fi·bro·sar·co·
     ma·ta

myx·o·gli·o·ma
   pl myx·o·gli·o·mas
   or myx·o·gli·o·ma·ta
myx·oid
myx·o·li·po·ma
   pl myx·o·li·po·mas
   or myx·o·li·po·ma·ta
myx·o·lip·o·sar·co·ma
   pl myx·o·lip·o·sar·co·mas
   or myx·o·lip·o·sar·co·ma·ta
myx·o·ma
   pl myx·o·mas
   or myx·o·ma·ta
myx·o·ma·to·sis
   pl myx·o·ma·to·ses
myx·om·a·tous
myx·o·my·cete
Myx·o·my·ce·tes
myx·o·my·ce·tous
myx·o·my·o·ma
myx·o·neu·ro·ma
   pl myx·o·neu·ro·mas
   or myx·o·neu·ro·ma·ta
myx·o·ple·o·mor·phic
myx·o·poi·e·sis
myx·or·rhe·a
myx·or·rhoe·a
   var of myx·or·rhe·a
myx·o·sar·co·ma
   pl myx·o·sar·co·mas
   or myx·o·sar·co·ma·ta
myx·o·sar·com·a·tous
myx·o·spore
Myx·o·spo·rid·i·a
myx·o·vi·ral
myx·o·vi·rus
My·zo·my·ia

N

Na·bo·thi·an

na·cre·ous

  or na·crous

na·crous

  or na·cre·ous

Nad·i re·a·gent

nad·ide

Nae·ge·le o·bliq·ui·ty

Nae·ge·li test

nae·paine

nae·vo·car·ci·no·ma

  pl nae·vo·car·ci·no·mas

  or nae·vo·car·ci·no·ma·ta

  var of ne·vo·car·ci·no·ma

nae·void

  var of ne·void

nae·vo·mel·a·no·ma

  pl nae·vo·mel·a·no·mas

  or nae·vo·mel·a·no·ma·ta

  var of ne·vo·mel·a·no·ma

nae·vose

  var of ne·vose

nae·vo·xan·tho·en·do·the·li·o·ma

  pl nae·vo·xan·tho·en·do·the·li·o·mas

  or nae·vo·xan·tho·en·do·the·li·o·ma·ta

  var of ne·vo·xan·tho·en·do·the·li·o·ma

nae·vus

  pl nae·vi

  var of ne·vus

naf·cil·lin

Naff·zi·ger op·er·a·tion

naf·ox·i·dine

Na·ga sore

na·ga·na

Na·gel test

Na·geotte-Ba·bin·ski syn·drome

Na·gler re·ac·tion

nail

Nai·man test

na·ive

Na·ja

Naj·jar ri·bo·fla·vin meth·od

na·ked

nal·bu·phine

nal·i·dix·ic

nal·mex·one

nal·or·phine

nal·ox·one

nam·ox·y·rate

nan·dro·lone

na·nism

na·nit·ic

na·no·ceph·a·lus

na·no·ceph·a·ly

na·no·cor·mi·a

na·no·cor·mus

na·no·cu·rie

na·no·gram

na·noid

na·nom·e·lus

na·no·me·ter

nan·oph·thal·mi·a

nan·oph·thal·mos

  or nan·oph·thal·mus

nan·oph·thal·mus

  or nan·oph·thal·mos

Na·no·phy·e·tus sal·min·co·la

na·no·sec·ond

na·no·so·ma

na·no·so·mi·a

na·no·so·mus

na·nous

na·nu·ka·ya·mi

na·nus

na·palm

na·pe

na·pel·line

na·pex

na·phaz·o·line

naph·tha

naph·tha·lene

naph·tha·lene a·ce·tic

naph·tha·qui·none

  or naph·tho·qui·none

naph·thene

naph·thi·on·ic

naph·thol

naph·tho·qui·none

  or naph·tha·qui·none

naph·thyl

naph·thyl·thi·o·u·re·a

na·pi·form

nap·ra·path

na·prap·a·thy

  pl na·prap·a·thies

nap·sy·late

nar·ce·ine

Nar·ath op·er·a·tion

nar·cism

nar·cis·sine

nar·cis·sism

nar·cis·sist

nar·cis·sis·tic

naï·cis·sis·ti·cal·ly

nar·co·an·aes·the·si·a

  var of nar·co·an·es·the·si·a

nar·co·a·nal·y·sis

  pl nar·co·a·nal·y·ses

nar·co·an·es·the·si·a

nar·co·di·ag·no·sis

  pl nar·co·di·ag·no·ses

nar·co·hyp·ni·a

nar·co·hyp·no·sis

  pl nar·co·hyp·no·ses

nar·co·lep·sy

  pl nar·co·lep·sies

nar·co·lep·tic

nar·co·ma

  pl nar·co·mas

  or nar·co·ma·ta

nar·co·ma·ni·a

nar·co·ma·ni·ac

nar·com·a·tous

nar·co·pep·si·a

nar·cose

  or nar·cous

nar·co·sis

  pl nar·co·ses

nar·co·spasm

nar·co·syn·the·sis

  pl nar·co·syn·the·ses

nar·co·ther·a·py

  pl nar·co·ther·a·pies

nar·cot·ic

nar·cot·i·cal·ly

nar·cot·i·cism

nar·cot·i·co·ac·rid

nar·cot·i·co·ir·ri·tant

nar·co·tine

nar·co·tism
nar·co·ti·za·tion
nar·co·tize
nar·cous
  or nar·cose
nar·i·al
na·ris
  pl na·res
na·sal
na·sa·lis
na·scent
na·si·o·al·ve·o·lar
na·si·on
na·si·tis
Nas·myth mem·brane
na·so·al·ve·o·lar
na·so·an·tral
na·so·bas·i·lar
na·so·breg·mat·ic
na·so·cil·i·ar·y
na·so·fa·cial
na·so·fron·tal
na·so·gas·tric
na·so·gen·i·tal
na·so·la·bi·al
na·so·la·bi·a·lis
na·so·lac·ri·mal
  or na·so·lach·ry·mal
na·so·lach·ry·mal
  or na·so·lac·ri·mal
na·so·lat·er·al
na·so·ma·lar
na·so·max·il·lar·y
na·so·me·di·al
na·so·me·di·an
na·so·men·tal
na·so·oc·cip·i·tal
na·so·o·ral
na·so·or·bit·al
na·so·pal·a·tal
  or na·so·pal·a·tine
na·so·pal·a·tine
  or na·so·pal·a·tal
na·so·pal·pe·bral
na·so·pha·ryn·ge·al
na·so·phar·yn·gi·tis
  pl na·so·phar·yn·gi·ti·des
na·so·pha·ryn·go·scope
na·so·pha·ryn·go·scop·ic

na·so·phar·yn·gos·co·py
na·so·phar·ynx
  pl na·so·phar·ynx·es
  or na·so·pha·ryn·ges
na·so·scope
na·sos·co·py
na·so·si·nu·i·tes
  or na·so·si·nus·i·tis
na·so·si·nus·i·tis
  or na·so·si·nu·i·tes
na·so·spi·na·le
na·so·tra·che·al
na·so·tur·bi·nal
na·sus
  pl na·si
na·tal
na·tal·i·ty
  pl na·tal·i·ties
na·tant
na·tes
na·ti·mor·tal·i·ty
na·tive
na·trae·mi·a
  var of na·tre·mi·a
na·tre·mi·a
na·tri·um
na·tri·u·re·sis
  or na·tru·re·sis
na·tri·u·ret·ic
na·tron
na·tru·re·sis
  or na·tri·u·re·sis
nat·u·ral
na·tur·o·path
na·tur·o·path·ic
na·tur·op·a·thy
Nau·heim bath
nau·pa·thi·a
nau·se·a
nau·se·ant
nau·se·ate
nau·seous
nau·seous·ly
na·vel
na·vic·u·la
na·vic·u·lar
na·vic·u·la·re
na·vic·u·lar·thri·tis
na·vic·u·lo·cu·boid

na·vic·u·lo·cu·ne·i·form
near·sight·ed
near·sight·ed·ly
near·sight·ed·ness
ne·ar·thro·sis
  pl ne·ar·thro·ses
ne·ben·kern
neb·ra·my·cin
neb·u·la
  pl neb·u·las
  or neb·u·lae
neb·u·lar
neb·u·li·za·tion
neb·u·lize
neb·u·liz·er
Ne·ca·tor
ne·ca·to·ri·a·sis
neck
nec·rec·to·my
nec·ro·bac·il·lar·y
nec·ro·bac·il·lo·sis
  pl nec·ro·bac·il·lo·ses
Nec·ro·bac·te·ri·um
nec·ro·bi·o·sis
  pl nec·ro·bi·o·ses
nec·ro·bi·ot·ic
nec·ro·cy·to·sis
nec·ro·cy·to·tox·in
nec·ro·gen·ic
  or ne·crog·e·nous
ne·crog·e·nous
  or nec·ro·gen·ic
nec·ro·log·ic
  or nec·ro·log·i·cal
nec·ro·log·i·cal
  or nec·ro·log·ic
ne·crol·o·gist
ne·crol·o·gy
  pl ne·crol·o·gies
ne·crol·y·sis
nec·ro·ma·ni·a
nec·ro·mi·me·sis
nec·ro·pha·gi·a
  or ne·croph·a·gy
nec·ro·pha·gic
ne·croph·a·gous
ne·croph·a·gy
  pl ne·croph·a·gies
  or nec·ro·pha·gi·a

nec·ro·phile
nec·ro·phil·i·a
nec·ro·phil·ic
ne·croph·i·lism
ne·croph·i·lous
ne·croph·i·ly
nec·ro·pho·bi·a
nec·ro·pho·bic
ne·cro·pneu·mo·ni·a
nec·rop·sy
  pl nec·rop·sies
nec·rop·sy
ne·crose
nec·ro·sin
ne·cro·sis
  pl ne·cro·ses
ne·cro·sper·mi·a
ne·crot·ic
nec·ro·tize
ne·crot·o·my
  pl ne·crot·o·mies
nec·ro·tox·in
nec·ro·zo·o·sper·mi·a
nec·tar·e·ous
nec·ta·ry
nee·dle
nee·dling
Neel·sen meth·od
ne·en·ceph·a·lon
  pl ne·en·ceph·a·la
ne·frens
  pl ne·fren·des
Nef·tel dis·ease
neg·a·tive
neg·a·ti·vism
neg·a·tiv·is·tic
neg·a·tron
neg·li·gence
Ne·gri body
Neg·ri-Ja·cod syn·drome
Ne·gro sign
ne·groid
Neill-Moo·ser bod·ies
Neis·ser coc·cus
Neis·se·ri·a
Ne·la·ton fi·bers
Nel·son test
nem
nem·a·line

nem·a·thel·minth
Nem·a·thel·min·thes
ne·ma·ti·cid·al
  or ne·ma·to·cid·al
ne·ma·ti·cide
  or ne·ma·to·cide
ne·ma·to·cid·al
  or ne·ma·ti·cid·al
ne·ma·to·cide
  or ne·ma·ti·cide
Nem·a·to·da
nem·a·tode
ne·ma·to·di·a·sis
  pl ne·ma·to·di·a·ses
Nem·a·to·di·rus
nem·a·toid
  or nem·a·toi·de·an
nem·a·toi·de·an
  or nem·a·toid
nem·a·to·log·i·cal
nem·a·tol·o·gist
nem·a·tol·o·gy
  pl nem·a·tol·o·gies
Nem·a·to·mor·pha
nem·a·to·sper·mi·a
ne·o·an·ti·gen
ne·o·ars·phen·a·mine
ne·o·ar·thro·sis
ne·o·blas·tic
ne·o·cer·e·bel·lar
ne·o·cer·e·bel·lum
  pl ne·o·cer·e·bel·lums
  or ne·o·cer·e·bel·la
ne·o·cin·cho·phen
ne·o·ci·net·ic
ne·o·cor·tex
  pl ne·o·cor·tex·es
  or ne·o·cor·ti·ces
ne·o·cor·ti·cal
ne·o·cys·tos·to·my
ne·o·den·ta·tum
ne·o·dym·i·um
ne·o·en·ceph·a·lon
ne·o·fe·tus
ne·o·for·ma·tion
ne·o-Freud·i·an
ne·og·a·la
ne·o·gen·e·sis
  pl ne·o·gen·e·ses

ne·o·ge·net·ic
  or ne·o·gen·ic
ne·o·gen·ic
  or ne·o·ge·net·ic
ne·o·ger·mi·trine
ne·o·ki·net·ic
ne·o·la·li·a
ne·ol·o·gism
ne·o·mem·brane
ne·o·morph
ne·o·mor·phic
ne·o·mor·phism
ne·o·my·cin
ne·on
ne·o·na·tal
ne·o·na·tal·ly
ne·o·nate
ne·o·na·ti·cide
ne·o·na·tol·o·gist
ne·o·na·tol·o·gy
ne·o·na·to·rum
ne·o·na·tus
  pl ne·o·na·ti
ne·o·pal·li·al
ne·o·pal·li·um
  pl ne·o·pal·li·ums
  or ne·o·pal·li·a
ne·o·pen·tane
ne·oph·il·ism
ne·o·pho·bi·a
ne·o·pho·bic
ne·o·phre·ni·a
ne·o·pine
ne·o·pla·si·a
ne·o·plasm
ne·o·plas·tic
ne·o·prene
ne·o·sen·si·bil·i·ty
ne·o·stig·mine
ne·o·stri·a·tum
  pl ne·o·stri·a·tums
  or ne·o·stri·a·ta
ne·o·tei·ni·a
  or ne·ote·ny
ne·o·ten·ic
ne·ot·e·ny
  pl ne·ot·e·nies
  or ne·o·tei·ni·a

e·o·thal·a·mus
  pl ne·o·thal·a·mi
e·o·u·ni·tar·i·an
e·o·vas·cu·lar
e·o·vas·cu·lar·i·za·tion
e·o·vas·cu·la·ture
eph·a·lism
eph·a·list
eph·a·lis·tic
eph·e·lom·e·ter
eph·e·lo·met·ric
eph·e·lo·met·ri·cal·ly
eph·e·lom·e·try
  pl neph·e·lom·e·tries
e·phe·lo·pi·a
e·phral·gi·a
e·phral·gic
eph·rec·ta·si·a
e·phrec·to·mize
e·phrec·to·my
  pl ne·phrec·to·mies
eph·rel·co·sis
eph·ric
e·phrid·i·al
e·phrid·i·um
  pl ne·phrid·i·a
e·phrit·ic
e·phri·tis
  pl ne·phri·tis·es
  or ne·phri·ti·des
eph·ri·to·gen·ic
eph·ro·ab·dom·i·nal
eph·ro·blas·to·ma
  pl neph·ro·blas·to·mas
  or neph·ro·blas·to·ma·ta
eph·ro·cal·ci·no·sis
  pl neph·ro·cal·ci·no·ses
eph·ro·cap·sec·to·my
eph·ro·cap·su·lec·to·my
eph·ro·cap·su·lot·o·my
eph·ro·car·ci·no·ma
  pl neph·ro·car·ci·no·mas
  or neph·ro·car·ci·no·ma·ta
eph·ro·car·di·ac
eph·ro·cele
eph·ro·coele
eph·ro·co·lic
eph·ro·col·o·pex·y
eph·ro·co·lop·to·sis

neph·ro·cyst·an·as·to·mo·
  sis
neph·ro·cys·ti·tis
neph·ro·cyte
neph·ro·dys·tro·phy
neph·ro·gen·e·sis
neph·ro·gen·ic
  or ne·phrog·e·nous
ne·phrog·e·nous
  or ne·phro·gen·ic
neph·ro·gram
neph·ro·graph·ic
ne·phrog·ra·phy
neph·roid
neph·ro·lith
neph·ro·li·thi·a·sis
  pl neph·ro·li·thi·a·ses
neph·ro·lith·ic
neph·ro·li·thot·o·my
  pl neph·ro·li·thot·o·mies
ne·phrol·o·gist
ne·phrol·o·gy
  pl ne·phrol·o·gies
ne·phrol·y·sin
ne·phrol·y·sine
ne·phrol·y·sis
neph·ro·lyt·ic
ne·phro·ma
  pl ne·phro·mas
  or ne·phro·ma·ta
neph·ro·meg·a·ly
neph·ro·mere
neph·ron
  or neph·rone
neph·rone
  or neph·ron
neph·ro·noph·thi·sis
neph·ro·path·ic
ne·phrop·a·thy
  pl ne·phrop·a·thies
neph·ro·pex·y
  pl neph·ro·pex·ies
neph·ro·poi·e·tin
neph·rop·to·si·a
neph·rop·to·sis
  pl neph·rop·to·ses
neph·ro·py·e·li·tis
neph·ro·py·e·lo·plas·ty
neph·ro·py·o·sis

neph·ror·rha·gi·a
neph·ror·rha·phy
  pl neph·ror·rha·phies
neph·ros
  pl neph·roi
neph·ro·scle·ro·sis
  pl neph·ro·scle·ro·ses
neph·ro·sid·er·o·sis
ne·phro·sis
  pl ne·phro·ses
ne·phro·so·ne·phri·tis
ne·phros·to·gram
neph·ro·stom
  or neph·ro·stome
  or ne·phros·to·ma
ne·phros·to·ma
  pl neph·ro·sto·ma·ta
  or neph·ro·stom
  or neph·ro·stome
neph·ro·sto·mal
neph·ro·stome
  or neph·ro·stom
  or ne·phros·to·ma
neph·ro·sto·mic
ne·phros·to·my
ne·phrot·ic
neph·ro·tome
neph·ro·to·mo·gram
neph·ro·to·mog·ra·phy
ne·phrot·o·my
  pl ne·phrot·o·mies
neph·ro·tox·ic
neph·ro·tox·i·ci·ty
  pl neph·ro·tox·ic·i·ties
neph·ro·tox·in
neph·ro·trop·ic
neph·ro·tu·ber·cu·lo·sis
neph·ro·u·re·ter·al
neph·ro·u·re·ter·ec·to·my
nep·i·ol·o·gy
nep·tu·ni·um
ne·ral
Ne·ri sign
Nernst lamp
ner·o·li oil
ner·va·tion
nerve of Lan·ci·si
nerve of Wris·berg
ner·vi

ner·vi·mo·tor
ner·von
ner·vone
ner·von·ic
ner·vo·sism
ner·vos·i·ty
ner·vous
ner·vous·ly
ner·vous·ness
ner·vus
   pl ner·vi
ner·vus ter·mi·nal·is
ne·sid·i·ec·to·my
ne·sid·i·o·blast
ne·sid·i·o·blas·to·ma
   pl ne·sid·i·o·blas·to·mas
   or ne·sid·i·o·blas·to·ma·ta
ne·sid·i·o·blas·to·sis
ness·ler·i·za·tion
ness·ler·ize
Ness·ler re·a·gent, so·lu·tion
nes·tei·a
nes·ti·at·ri·a
nes·ti·os·to·my
nes·tis
nes·ti·ther·a·py
nes·to·ther·a·py
nests of Gol·gi-Holm·gren
neth·a·lide
Neth·er·ton syn·drome
ne·tran·eu·rysm
net·work
Neu·ber tubes
Neu·berg es·ter
Neu·feld nail
Neu·hau·ser sign
Neu·mann cells
neu·rad
neu·ral
neu·ral·gi·a
neu·ral·gic
neu·ral·gi·form
neu·ral·ly
neur·a·min·ic
neur·a·min·i·dase
neur·a·min·lac·tose
neu·ran·a·gen·e·sis

neur·a·poph·y·sis
   pl neur·a·poph·y·ses
neur·a·prax·i·a
neu·rar·throp·a·thy
neur·as·the·ni·a
neur·as·then·ic
neur·as·then·i·cal·ly
neu·ra·tro·phi·a
neu·ra·troph·ic
neur·ax·is
   pl neur·ax·es
neur·ax·i·tis
neur·ax·on
   or neur·ax·one
neur·ax·one
   or neur·ax·on
neur·ec·ta·si·a
neu·rec·ta·sis
neu·rec·to·my
   pl neu·rec·to·mies
neur·ec·to·pi·a
neu·rec·to·py
neur·en·ter·ic
neur·ep·i·the·li·um
neu·rer·gic
neur·ex·er·e·sis
neu·ri·a·sis
neu·ri·a·try
neu·ri·dine
neu·ri·lem·a
   or neu·ri·lem·ma
   or neu·ro·lem·ma
neu·ri·lem·ma
   or neu·ri·lem·a
   or neu·ro·lem·ma
neu·ri·lem·mal
   or neu·ri·lem·mat·ic
   or neu·ri·lem·ma·tous
neu·ri·lem·mat·ic
   or neu·ri·lem·mal
   or neu·ri·lem·ma·tous
neu·ri·lem·ma·tous
   or neu·ri·lem·mat·ic
   or neu·ri·lem·mal
neu·ri·lem·mi·tis
neu·ri·lem·mo·ma
   pl neu·ri·lem·mo·mas
   or neu·ri·lem·mo·ma·ta
   or neu·ri·le·mo·ma

neu·ri·lem·mo·sar·co·ma
   pl neu·ri·lem·mo·sar·co·mas
   or neu·ri·lem·mo·sar·co·ma·ta
neu·ri·le·mo·ma
   pl neu·ri·le·mo·mas
   or neu·ri·le·mo·ma·ta
   or neu·ri·lem·mo·ma
neu·ril·i·ty
   pl neu·ril·i·ties
neu·rin
   or neu·rine
neu·rine
   or neu·rin
neu·ri·no·ma
   pl neu·ri·no·mas
   or neu·ri·no·ma·ta
neu·ri·no·ma·to·sis
neu·rit
neu·rite
neu·rit·ic
neu·ri·tis
   pl neu·ri·tis·es
   or neu·ri·ti·des
neu·ro·ac·tive
neu·ro·a·bi·ot·ro·phy
neu·ro·a·nae·mi·a
   var of neu·ro·a·ne·mi·a
neu·ra·nae·mic
   var of neu·ro·a·ne·mic
neu·ro·a·nas·to·mo·sis
neu·ro·a·nat·o·mist
neu·ro·a·nat·o·my
   pl neu·ro·a·nat·o·mies
neu·ro·a·ne·mi·a
neu·ro·a·ne·mic
neu·ro·ar·thri·tism
neu·ro·ar·throp·a·thy
neu·ro·as·the·ni·a
neu·ro·as·tro·cy·to·ma
   pl neu·ro·as·tro·cy·to·mas
   or neu·ro·as·tro·cy·to·ma·ta
neu·ro·ax·no·al
neu·ro·bar·ton·el·lo·sis
neu·ro·bi·o·log·i·cal
neu·ro·bi·ol·o·gist
neu·ro·bi·ol·o·gy
   pl neu·ro·bi·ol·o·gies

neu·ro·bi·o·tax·is
pl neu·ro·bi·o·tax·es
neu·ro·blast
neu·ro·blas·tic
neu·ro·blas·to·ma
pl neu·ro·blas·to·mas
or neu·ro·blas·to·ma·ta
neu·ro·blas·to·ma·to·sis
neu·ro·bru·cel·lo·sis
neu·ro·cal·o·rim·e·ter
neu·ro·ca·nal
neu·ro·car·di·ac
neu·ro·cele
var of neu·ro·coele
neu·ro·cen·trum
pl neu·ro·cen·trums
or neu·ro·cen·tra
neu·ro·chem·i·cal
neu·ro·chem·ist
neu·ro·chem·is·try
pl neu·ro·chem·is·tries
neu·ro·chord
neu·ro·cho·ri·o·ret·i·ni·tis
neu·ro·cho·roi·di·tis
neu·ro·cir·cu·la·to·ry
neu·ro·cla·dism
neu·ro·clon·ic
neu·ro·coele
neu·ro·cra·ni·um
pl neu·ro·cra·ni·ums
or neu·ro·cra·ni·a
neu·ro·crine
neu·ro·crin·ism
neu·ro·cu·ta·ne·ous
neu·ro·cyte
neu·ro·cy·tol·y·sin
neu·ro·cy·tol·y·sis
neu·ro·cy·to·ma
pl neu·ro·cy·to·mas
or neu·ro·cy·to·ma·ta
neu·ro·de·a·tro·phi·a
neu·ro·den·drite
or neu·ro·den·dron
neu·ro·den·dron
or neu·ro·den·drite
neu·ro·der·ma·tit·ic
neu·ro·der·ma·ti·tis
pl neu·ro·der·ma·ti·tis·es
or neu·ro·der·ma·ti·ti·des

neu·ro·der·ma·to·sis
neu·ro·der·ma·tro·phi·a
neu·ro·di·as·ta·sis
neu·ro·dy·nam·ic
neu·ro·dyn·i·a
neu·ro·ec·to·derm
neu·ro·ec·to·der·mal
neu·ro·e·lec·tro·ther·a·peu·
tics
neu·ro·en·ceph·a·lo·my·e·
lop·a·thy
neu·ro·en·do·crine
neu·ro·en·do·cri·nol·o·gy
pl neu·ro·en·do·cri·nol·o·
gies
neu·ro·en·ter·ic
neu·ro·ep·i·der·mal
neu·ro·ep·i·the·li·al
neu·ro·ep·i·the·li·o·ma
pl neu·ro·ep·i·the·li·o·mas
or neu·ro·ep·i·the·li·o·ma·ta
neu·ro·ep·i·the·li·um
pl neu·ro·ep·i·the·li·a
neu·ro·fi·bril
neu·ro·fi·bril·la
pl neu·ro·fi·bril·lae
neu·ro·fi·bril·lar
neu·ro·fi·bril·lar·y
neu·ro·fi·bro·ma
pl neu·ro·fi·bro·mas
or neu·ro·fi·bro·ma·ta
neu·ro·fi·bro·ma·to·sis
pl neu·ro·fi·bro·ma·to·ses
neu·ro·fi·bro·myx·o·ma
pl neu·ro·fi·bro·myx·o·mas
or neu·ro·fi·bro·myx·o·ma·
ta
neu·ro·fi·bro·pha·co·ma·to·
sis
neu·ro·fi·bro·sar·co·ma
pl neu·ro·fi·bro·sar·co·mas
or neur·o·fi·bro·sar·co·ma·
ta
neu·ro·fil·a·ment
neu·ro·gan·gli·i·tis
neu·ro·gan·gli·o·ma my·e·
lin·i·cum ve·rum
neu·ro·gan·gli·on·i·tis
neu·ro·gas·tric

neu·ro·gen
neu·ro·gen·e·sis
neu·ro·gen·ic
neu·ro·gen·i·cal·ly
neu·rog·e·nous
neu·rog·e·ny
neu·rog·li·a
neu·rog·li·al
neu·rog·li·ar
neu·rog·li·o·cyte
neu·rog·li·o·cy·to·ma
pl neu·rog·li·o·cy·to·mas
or neu·rog·li·o·cy·to·ma·ta
neu·rog·li·o·ma
pl neu·rog·li·o·mas
or neu·rog·li·o·ma·ta
neu·rog·li·o·sis
pl neu·rog·li·o·ses
neu·ro·gram
neu·ro·gram·mic
neu·ro·graph·ic
neu·rog·ra·phy
pl neu·rog·ra·phies
neu·ro·his·tol·o·gy
neu·ro·hor·mo·nal
neu·ro·hor·mone
neu·ro·hu·mor
neu·ro·hu·mor·al
neu·ro·hyp·nol·o·gy
neu·ro·hy·poph·y·se·al
or neu·ro·hy·poph·y·si·al
neu·ro·hy·poph·y·si·al
or neu·ro·hy·poph·y·se·al
neu·ro·hy·poph·y·sis
pl neu·ro·hy·poph·y·ses
neu·roid
neu·ro·in·duc·tion
neu·ro·in·su·lar
neu·ro·ker·a·tin
neu·ro·kin·in
neu·ro·kyme
neu·ro·lath·y·rism
neu·ro·lem·ma
or neu·ri·lem·a
or neu·ri·lem·ma
neu·ro·lem·mi·tis
neu·ro·lem·mo·ma
neu·ro·lep·rid

259

neu·ro·lep·tan·al·ge·si·a
  or neu·ro·lep·to·an·al·ge·
    si·a
neu·ro·lept·an·al·ge·sic
neu·ro·lep·tic
neu·ro·lep·to·an·al·ge·si·a
  or neu·ro·lep·tan·al·ge·si·a
neu·ro·lep·to·an·es·the·si·a
neu·ro·lo·gi·a
neu·ro·log·ic
  or neu·ro·log·i·cal
neu·ro·log·i·cal
  or neu·ro·log·ic
neu·ro·log·i·cal·ly
neu·rol·o·gist
neu·rol·o·gize
neu·rol·o·gy
  pl neu·rol·o·gies
neu·ro·lu·es
neu·ro·lymph
neu·ro·lym·pho·ma·to·sis
  pl neu·ro·lym·pho·ma·to·
    ses
neu·rol·y·sin
neu·rol·y·sis
  pl neu·rol·y·ses
neu·ro·lyt·ic
neu·ro·ma
  pl neu·ro·mas
  or neu·ro·ma·ta
neu·ro·ma·la·ci·a
neu·rom·a·toid
neu·rom·a·to·sis
neu·rom·a·tous
neu·ro·mech·a·nism
neu·ro·mere
neu·rom·er·ism
neu·rom·er·y
neu·ro·mi·me·sis
neu·ro·mi·met·ic
neu·ro·mo·tor
neu·ro·mus·cu·lar
neu·ro·my·al
neu·ro·my·as·the·ni·a
neu·ro·my·e·li·tis
  pl neu·ro·my·e·li·ti·des
neu·ro·my·ic
neu·ro·my·o·ar·te·ri·al
neu·ro·my·on

neu·ro·my·o·path·ic
neu·ro·my·o·si·tis
neu·ron
  or neu·rone
neu·ro·nal
  or neu·ron·ic
neu·rone
  or neu·ron
neu·ro·ne·vus
neu·ron·ic
  or neu·ro·nal
neu·ron·ism
neu·ro·ni·tis
neu·ro·nog·ra·phy
neu·ro·nop·a·thy
neu·ron·o·phage
neu·ro·no·pha·gi·a
  or neu·ro·noph·a·gy
neu·ro·noph·a·gy
  pl neu·ro·noph·a·gies
  or neu·ro·no·pha·gi·a
neu·ro·oph·thal·mol·o·gy
neu·ro·op·tic
neu·ro·pa·pil·li·tis
neu·ro·pa·ral·y·sis
neu·ro·par·a·lyt·ic
neu·ro·path
neu·ro·path·ic
neu·ro·path·i·cal·ly
neu·rop·a·thist
neu·ro·path·o·gen·e·sis
neu·ro·path·o·gen·ic·i·ty
neu·ro·path·o·log·ic
neu·ro·pa·thol·o·gist
neu·ro·pa·thol·o·gy
neu·rop·a·thy
neu·ro·phar·ma·co·log·ic
  or neu·ro·phar·ma·co·log·
    i·cal
neu·ro·phar·ma·co·log·i·cal
  or neu·ro·phar·ma·co·log·ic
neu·ro·phar·ma·col·o·gist
neu·ro·phar·ma·col·o·gy
neu·ro·phile
  or neu·ro·phil·ic
neu·ro·phil·ic
  or neu·ro·phile
neu·ro·phleg·mon
neu·ro·pho·ni·a

neu·ro·phre·ni·a
neu·roph·thal·mo·log·ic
neu·roph·thal·mol·o·gist
neu·roph·thal·mol·o·gy
neu·roph·thi·sis
neu·ro·phys·i·o·log·ic
  or neu·ro·phys·i·o·log·i·cal
neu·ro·phys·i·o·log·i·cal
  or neu·ro·phys·i·o·log·ic
neu·ro·phys·i·ol·o·gist
neu·ro·phys·i·ol·o·gy
  pl neu·ro·phys·i·ol·o·gies
neu·ro·pil
  or neu·ro·pile
neu·ro·pi·lar
neu·ro·pile
  or neu·ro·pil
neu·ro·pi·tu·i·tar·y
neu·ro·plasm
neu·ro·plas·mat·ic
  or neu·ro·plas·mic
neu·ro·plas·mic
  or neu·ro·plas·mat·ic
neu·ro·plas·ty
neu·ro·ple·gic
neu·ro·po·di·um
  pl neu·ro·po·di·a
neu·ro·pore
neu·ro·po·ten·tial
neu·ro·psy·chi·at·ric
neu·ro·psy·chi·at·ri·cal·ly
neu·ro·psy·chi·a·trist
neu·ro·psy·chi·a·try
  pl neu·ro·psy·chi·a·tries
neu·ro·psy·chic
  or neu·ro·psy·chi·cal
neu·ro·psy·chi·cal
  or neu·ro·psy·chic
neu·ro·psy·cho·log·i·cal
neu·ro·psy·chol·o·gist
neu·ro·psy·chol·o·gy
  pl neu·ro·psy·chol·o·gies
neu·ro·psy·cho·path·ic
neu·ro·psy·chop·a·thy
neu·ro·psy·cho·sis
neur·op·ti·co·my·e·li·tis
neu·ro·ra·di·o·log·ic
neu·ro·ra·di·ol·o·gy
neu·ro·rec·i·dive

260

neu·ro·re·cur·rence
neu·ro·re·lapse
neu·ro·ret·i·ni·tis
  pl neu·ro·ret·i·ni·ti·des
neu·ro·ret·i·nop·a·thy
neu·ro·roent·gen·og·ra·phy
neu·ro·roent·ge·nol·o·gy
neu·ror·rha·py
neu·ror·rhex·is
neu·ror·rhyc·tes hy·dro·
  pho·bi·ae
neu·ro·sal
neu·ro·sar·co·klei·sis
neu·ro·sar·co·ma
  pl neu·ro·sar·co·mas
  or neu·ro·sar·co·ma·ta
neu·ro·sci·ence
neu·ro·sci·en·tist
neu·ro·scle·ro·sis
neu·ro·se·cre·tion
neu·ro·se·cre·to·ry
neu·ro·sen·so·ry
neu·ro·sis
  pl neu·ro·ses
neu·ro·sism
neu·ro·skel·e·tal
neu·ro·ske·le·ton
neu·ro·some
neu·ro·spasm
neu·ro·splanch·nic
neu·ro·spon·gi·o·ma
  pl neu·ro·spon·gi·o·mas
  or neu·ro·spon·gi·o·ma·ta
neu·ro·spon·gi·um
  pl neu·ro·spon·gi·a
Neu·ros·po·ra
neu·ro·ste·a·ric
neu·ro·sthe·ni·a
neu·ro·sthen·ic
neu·ro·sur·geon
neu·ro·sur·ger·y
  pl neu·ro·sur·ger·ies
neu·ro·sur·gi·cal
neu·ro·su·ture
neu·ro·syph·i·lid
neu·ro·syph·i·lis
neu·ro·ten·di·nal
neu·ro·ten·di·nous
neu·ro·the·ci·tis

neu·ro·ther·a·py
neu·rot·ic
neu·rot·i·ca
neu·rot·i·cal·ly
neu·rot·i·cism
neu·ro·ti·za·tion
neu·ro·tize
neu·rot·me·sis
neu·rot·o·gen·ic
neu·ro·tol·o·gy
neu·ro·tome
neu·rot·o·my
  pl neu·rot·o·mies
neu·ro·ton·ic
neu·rot·o·ny
neu·ro·tox·ic
neu·ro·tox·ic·i·ty
  pl neu·ro·tox·ic·i·ties
neu·ro·tox·in
neu·ro·trans·mit·ter
neu·ro·trau·ma
neu·ro·trip·sy
neu·ro·troph·ic
neu·rot·ro·phy
neu·ro·trop·ic
neu·rot·ro·pism
neu·ro·tu·bule
neu·ro·vac·cine
neu·ro·var·i·co·sis
neu·ro·vas·cu·lar
neu·ro·veg·e·ta·tive
neu·ro·vis·cer·al
neu·ru·la
  pl neu·ru·las
  or neu·ru·lae
neu·ru·lar
neu·ru·la·tion
Neus·ser gran·u·les
neu·tral
neu·tral·i·za·tion
neu·tral·ize
neu·tri·no
neu·tro·clu·sion
neu·tro·cyte
neu·tro·cyt·ic
neu·tron
neu·tro·oc·clu·sion
neu·tro·pe·ni·a
neu·tro·pe·nic

neu·tro·phil
neu·tro·phile
neu·tro·phil·i·a
neu·tro·phil·ic
neu·tro·phil·in
  or neu·tro·phil·ine
neu·tro·phil·line
  or neu·tro·phil·in
ne·vi·form
ne·vo·car·ci·no·ma
  pl ne·vo·car·ci·no·mas
  or ne·vo·car·ci·no·ma·ta
ne·void
ne·vo·mel·a·no·ma
  pl ne·vo·mel·a·no·mas
  or ne·vo·mel·a·no·ma·ta
ne·vose
ne·vo·xan·tho·en·do·the·li·
  o·ma
  pl ne·vo·xan·tho·en·do·the·
    li·o·mas
  or ne·vo·xan·tho·en·do·the·
    li·o·ma·ta
ne·vus
  pl ne·vi
new·born
New·burgh test
New·cas·tle dis·ease
New·com·er meth·od
new·ton
New·to·ni·an
nex·us
  pl nex·uses
  or nex·us
Nez·e·lof syn·drome
n'ga·na
  var of na·ga·na
ni·a·cin
ni·a·cin·a·mide
ni·a·cin·am·i·do·sis
ni·al·a·mide
nic·co·lum
niche
nick·el
Nick·er·son-Kveim test
nick·ing
ni·clo·sa·mide
Nic·ol prism
Nic·co·la op·er·a·tion

Ni·co·las-Fa·vre dis·ease
Ni·co·las-Kult·schitz·ky
  cells
Ni·co·ti·an·a
nic·o·tin·a·mide
ni·co·tin·a·mide-ad·e·nine
  di·nu·cle·o·tide
nic·o·tin·a·mide-ad·e·nine
  di·nu·cle·o·tide phos·
  phate
nic·o·tin·ate
nic·o·tine
nic·o·tin·ic
nic·o·tin·ism
nic·o·tin·ize
nic·o·tin·ur·ic
nic·o·tin·yl
ni·cou·ma·lone
nic·tate
nic·ta·tion
nic·ti·tate
nic·ti·ta·tion
ni·dal
ni·da·tion
ni·dus
  pl ni·dus·es
  or ni·di
Niel·sen meth·od
Nie·mann-Pick dis·
  ease
Nie·wen·glow·ski rays
ni·fu·ri·mide
ni·fur·mer·one
ni·fur·ox·ime
Ni·ger·i·an ty·phus
night·blind
night·blind·ness
night·mare
night·shade
ni·gra
ni·gral
ni·gran·i·line
ni·gri·cans
ni·gri·ti·es
ni·gro·re·tic·u·lar
ni·gro·ru·bral
ni·gro·sin
  or ni·gro·sine

ni·gro·sine
  or ni·gro·sin
ni·gro·stri·a·tal
ni·hil·ism
nik·eth·a·mide
Ni·kol·sky sign
Nile blue
ni·met·ti
Nin·hy·drin
Nin·hy·drin Schiff re·ac·
  tion
ni·o·bi·um
niph·a·blep·si·a
niph·o·typh·lo·sis
nip·i·ol·o·gy
nip·pers
nip·ple
ni·rid·a·zole
ni·sin
ni·so·bam·ate
Nissl bod·ies, gran·ules,
  sub·stance
ni·sus
  pl ni·sus
nit
Nit·a·buch mem·brane
ni·ter
ni·ton
ni·trate
ni·tra·tion
ni·tra·ze·pam
ni·tre
  var of ni·ter
ni·tric
ni·tri·da·tion
ni·tride
ni·tri·fi·ca·tion
ni·tri·fi·er
ni·tri·fy
ni·trile
ni·trite
ni·tri·toid
ni·tri·tu·ri·a
ni·tro·ben·zene
ni·tro·cel·lu·lose
ni·tro·cel·lu·los·ic
ni·tro·dan
ni·tro·fu·ran

ni·tro·fu·ran·to·in
ni·tro·fu·ra·zone
ni·tro·gen
ni·tro·ge·nase
ni·tro·gen·i·za·tion
ni·tro·ge·nize
ni·tro·gen-nar·co·sis
ni·trog·e·nous
ni·tro·glyc·er·in
  or ni·tro·glyc·er·ine
ni·tro·glyc·er·ine
  or ni·tro·glyc·er·in
ni·tro·hy·dro·chlo·ric
ni·tro·man·nite
ni·tro·man·ni·tol
ni·tro·mer·sol
ni·trom·e·ter
ni·tro·met·ric
ni·tro·mu·ri·at·ic
ni·tron
ni·tro·prus·side
ni·tro·sa·mine
  or ni·tro·so·a·mine
ni·tro·sate
ni·tro·sa·tion
ni·tro·so·a·mine
  or ni·tro·sa·mine
ni·tro·syl
ni·trous
ni·trox·yl
ni·tryl
no·as·the·ni·a
no·bel·i·um
No·ble pos·ture
No·car·di·a
no·car·di·al
no·car·di·o·sis
  pl no·car·di·o·ses
no·ci·as·so·ci·a·tion
no·ci·cep·tive
no·ci·cep·tor
no·ci·fen·sor
noci·in·flu·ence
no·ci·per·cep·tion
no·ci·per·cep·tive
noc·tal·bu·mi·nu·ri·a
noc·tam·bu·la·tion
noc·tam·bule

noc·tam·bu·lic
or noc·tam·bu·lis·tic
noc·tam·bu·lism
noc·tam·bu·list
noc·tam·bu·lis·tic
or noc·tam·bu·lic
noc·ti·pho·bi·a
Noc·tu·i·dae
noc·tu·ri·a
noc·tur·nal
noc·tur·nal·ly
noc·u·ous
noc·u·ous·ly
no·dal
no·dal·ly
node of Ran·vier
no·di
no·dose
or no·dous
no·dos·i·ty
pl no·dos·i·ties
no·dous
or no·dose
nod·u·lar
nod·u·late
nod·u·la·tion
nod·ule
nod·u·li
nod·u·lose
or nod·u·lous
nod·u·lous
or nod·u·lose
nod·u·lus
pl nod·u·li
no·dus
pl no·di
no·e·gen·e·sis
no·e·ma·tach·o·graph
no·e·ma·ta·chom·e·ter
no·e·mat·ic
no·e·sis
no·et·ic
no·gal·a·my·cin
no·ma
no·mad·ic
no·men·cla·ture
Nom·i·na An·a·tom·i·ca
nom·i·nal

nom·o·gram
nom·o·graph
nom·o·thet·ic
nom·o·top·ic
no·na
non·ab·sorb·a·ble
non·ac·cess
non·ad·di·tive
non·ad·di·tiv·i·ty
pl non·ad·di·tiv·i·ties
non·ad·her·ent
non·al·le·lic
no·nan
non·a·que·ous
non·chro·maf·fin
non·chro·mo·som·al
non·com·mu·ni·cat·ing
non com·pos men·tis
non·con·duc·tor
non·con·ges·tive
non·con·trac·tile
non·con·trib·u·to·ry
non·cross·o·ver
Non·de·cid·u·a·ta
non·de·form·ing
non·di·a·bet·ic
non·di·rec·tive
non·dis·junc·tion
non·dis·junc·tion·al
non·di·vid·ing
non·dom·i·nant
non·e·lec·tro·lyte
non·en·cap·su·lat·ed
non·en·dem·ic
non·en·zy·mat·ic
or non·en·zy·mic
or non·en·zyme
non·en·zy·mat·i·cal·ly
non·en·zyme
or non·en·zy·mat·ic
or non·en·zy·mic
non·en·zy·mic
or non·en·zyme
or non·en·zy·mat·ic
non·e·quil·i·bra·to·ry
non·fat
non·flu·ent
non·func·tion·al

non·gran·u·lar
non·hi·ber·nat·ing
non·his·tone
non·i·den·ti·cal
no·ni·grav·i·da
non·in·fect·ed
non·in·fec·tious
non·in·flam·ma·to·ry
non·in·sec·ti·cid·al
non·i·on·ic
no·nip·a·ra
non·la·mel·lar
non·lip·id
non·lu·et·ic
non·ma·lig·nant
non·med·ul·lat·ed
non·mo·tile
non·mus·cu·lar
mon·my·e·li·nat·ed
Non·ne dis·ease
Non·ne-A·pelt test
Non·ne-Ma·rie syn·drome
Non·ne-Mil·roy-Meige
    syn·drome
non·ne·o·plas·tic
non·nu·cle·at·ed
non·o·paque
non·ose
non·os·te·o·gen·ic
non·ov·u·la·to·ry
non·ox·y·nol
non·par·a·lyt·ic
non·par·a·sit·ic
non·par·a·sit·i·cal·ly
non·par·ous
non·path·o·gen
non·path·o·gen·ic
non·path·og·no·mon·ic
non·per·sis·tent
non·pig·ment·ed
non·preg·nant
non·pre·scrip·tion
non·pro·pri·e·tar·y
non·pro·te·in
non·pro·te·in·a·ceous
non·psy·chot·ic
non·pu·ru·lent
non·py·o·gen·ic

263

non·re·com·bi·nant
non·re·frac·tive
non·re·pro·duc·tive
non·re·straint
non·se·cre·tor
non·sed·i·ment·a·ble
non·seg·ment·ed
non·sep·tate
non·sex·u·al
non·spe·cif·ic
non·spo·rog·e·nous
non·strep·to·coc·cal
non·ste·roid
non·ste·roi·dal
non·stri·at·ed
non·sup·pu·ra·tive
non·sur·gi·cal
non·sym·bol·ic
non·tar·get
non·throm·bo·cy·to·pe·nic
non·throm·bo·pe·nic
non·tox·ic
non·trop·i·cal
non·un·ion
non·vec·tor
non·ve·ne·re·al
non·vi·a·ble
non·vi·su·al·i·za·tion
non·yl
no·o·klo·pi·a
no·o·log·i·cal
no·ol·o·gy
   pl no·ol·o·gies
Noon pol·len u·nit
no·o·psy·che
nor·a·cy·meth·a·dol
nor·a·dren·a·lin
   or nor·a·dren·a·line
nor·a·dren·a·line
   or nor·adren·a·lin
nor·bi·o·tin
nor·bol·eth·one
Nor·dau dis·ease
Nor·dau·ism
nor·de·frin
nor·e·phed·rine
nor·ep·i·neph·rine
nor·eth·an·dro·lone

nor·eth·in·drone
nor·e·thy·no·drel
nor·flu·rane
nor·ges·trel
nor·leu·cine
nor·leu·cyl
norm
nor·ma
   pl nor·mae
nor·mal
nor·mal·cy
   pl nor·mal·cies
nor·mal·i·ty
   pl nor·mal·i·ties
nor·mal·i·za·tion
nor·mal·ize
nor·mal·iz·er
nor·mer·gy
   pl nor·mer·gies
nor·mét·a·neph·rine
nor·mo·blast
nor·mo·blas·tic
nor·mo·blas·to·sis
nor·mo·cal·cae·mi·a
   var of nor·mo·cal·ce·mi·a
nor·mo·cal·cae·mic
   var of nor·mo·cal·ce·mic
nor·mo·cal·ce·mi·a
nor·mo·cal·ce·mic
nor·mo·chro·ma·si·a
nor·mo·chro·mat·ic
nor·mo·chro·mi·a
nor·mo·chro·mic
nor·mo·cyte
nor·mo·cyt·ic
nor·mo·cy·to·sis
nor·mo·gly·ce·mi·a
nor·mo·ka·le·mi·a
nor·mo·ka·le·mic
nor·mo·re·flex·i·a
nor·mo·sper·mic
nor·mo·ten·sion
nor·mo·ten·sive
nor·mo·ther·mi·a
nor·mo·ther·mic
nor·mo·to·ni·a
nor·mo·ton·ic
nor·mo·to·pi·a

nor·mo·vo·le·mi·a
Nor·rie dis·ease
nor·trip·ty·line
nor·val·ine
Nor·we·gian itch
nos·ca·pine
nose
nose·bleed
No·se·ma
no·se·ma·to·sis
no·sen·ceph·a·lus
nose·piece
nos·er·es·the·si·a
nos·och·tho·nog·ra·phy
nos·o·co·mi·al
nos·o·gen·e·sis
nos·o·ge·net·ic
nos·o·ge·o·graph·ic
   or no·so·ge·o·graph·i·cal
no·so·ge·o·graph·i·cal
   or no·so·ge·o·graph·ic
no·so·ge·og·ra·phy
   pl no·so·ge·og·ra·phies
nos·o·graph·ic
no·sog·ra·phy
   pl no·sog·ra·phies
nos·o·log·ic
   or nos·o·log·i·cal
no·so·log·i·cal
   or no·so·log·ic
no·so·log·i·cal·ly
no·sol·o·gist
no·sol·o·gy
   pl no·sol·o·gies
nos·o·ma·ni·a
no·som·e·try
no·so·my·co·sis
no·son·o·my
nos·o·par·a·site
nos·o·phil·i·a
nos·o·pho·bi·a
nos·o·phyte
no·so·poi·et·ic
Nos·o·psyl·lus
nos·o·tax·y
nos·tal·gi·a
nos·tal·gic

nos·tal·gi·cal·ly
nos·to·ma·ni·a
nos·top·a·thy
nos·to·pho·bi·a
nos·tras
nos·trate
nos·tril
nos·trum
no·tal
no·tal·gi·a
no·tan·ce·pha·li·a
no·tan·en·ce·pha·li·a
no·ta·tion
notch
note-blind·ness
No·te·chis
no·ten·ceph·a·lo·cele
no·en·ceph·a·lus
Noth·na·gel di·sease
no·ti·fi·a·ble
no·to·chord
no·to·chord·al
No·to·ed·res
no·to·ed·ric
no·to·gen·e·sis
no·tom·e·lus
Nou·ga·ret blind·ness
no·vo·bi·o·cin
no·vo·caine
nox·a
   pl nox·ae
nox·ious
nox·ious·ness
nu·bile
nu·bil·i·ty
   pl nu·bil·i·ties
nu·cel·lus
nu·cha
   pl nu·chae
nu·chal
Nuck ca·nal
nu·cle·ar
nu·cle·ase
ne·cle·ate
   or nu·cle·at·ed
nu·cle·at·ed
   or nu·cle·ate
nu·cle·a·tion

nu·cle·i
nu·cle·ic
nu·cle·ide
nu·cle·i·form
nu·cle·in
nu·cle·in·ase
nu·cle·in·ic
nu·cle·o·cap·sid
nu·cle·o·chy·le·ma
nu·cle·o·chyme
nu·cle·o·cy·to·plas·mic
nu·cle·of·u·gal
nu·cle·o·his·tone
nu·cle·o·hy·a·lo·plasm
nu·cle·oid
ne·cle·o·lar
ne·cle·ole
nu·cle·o·li·form
nu·cle·o·lin
ne·cle·o·loid
nu·cle·o·lo·ne·ma
nu·cle·o·lus
   pl nu·cle·o·li
nu·cle·o·mi·cro·so·ma
nu·cle·o·mi·cro·some
nu·cle·on
nu·cle·on·ic
nu·cle·on·ics
nu·cle·op·e·tal
Nu·cle·oph·a·ga
nu·cle·o·phil·ic
nu·cle·o·phil·i·cal·ly
nu·cle·o·plasm
nu·cle·o·plas·mat·ic
   or nu·cle·o·plas·mic
nu·cle·o·plas·mic
   or nu·cle·o·plas·mat·ic
nu·cle·o·pro·te·id
nu·cle·o·pro·te·in
nu·cle·o·re·tic·u·lum
nu·cle·o·si·dase
nu·cle·o·side
nu·cle·o·spin·dle
nu·cle·o·ti·dase
nu·cle·o·tide
nu·cle·o·tid·yl
nu·cle·o·tox·ic
nu·cle·o·tox·in

nu·cle·us
   pl nu·cle·us·es
   or nu·cle·i
nu·cle·us dor·sa·lis
   pl nu·clei dor·sa·les
nu·cle·us of Pan·der
nu·cle·us pul·po·sus
   pl nu·clei pul·po·si
nu·clide
nu·clid·ic
Nu·el space
Nuhn glands
nul·li·grav·i·da
   pl nul·li·gra·vi·das
   or nul·li·gra·vi·dae
nul·lip·a·ra
   pl nul·lip·a·ras
   or nul·lip·a·rae
nul·li·par·i·ty
nul·lip·a·rous
nul·li·some
nul·li·so·mic
numb
num·ber
numb·ness
nu·mer·al
nu·mer·i·cal
num·mi·form
num·mu·lar
num·mu·la·tion
nun·na·tion
nurse
nur·se·ry
   pl nur·se·ries
nurs·ling
nu·ta·tion
nu·ta·tion·al
nut·gall
nu·tri·ent
nu·tri·lite
nu·tri·ment
nu·tri·tion
nu·tri·tion·al
nu·tri·tion·al·ly
nu·tri·tion·ist
nu·tri·tious
nu·tri·tious·ly
nu·tri·tive

nu·tri·tive·ly
nu·tri·to·ry
Nut·tal·li·a
nut·tal·li·a·sis
   pl nut·tal·li·a·ses
   or nut·tal·li·o·sis
   pl nut·tal·li·o·ses
nut·tal·li·o·sis
   pl nut·tal·li·o·ses
   or nut·tal·li·a·sis
   pl nut·tal·li·a·ses
nux vom·i·ca
   pl nux vom·i·ca
ny·a·loi·de·o·cap·su·lar
nyc·tal·gi·a
nyc·ta·lope
nyc·ta·lo·pi·a
nyc·ta·lop·ic
nyc·ta·pho·ni·a

nyc·ter·ine
nyc·ter·o·hem·er·al
nyc·to·hem·er·al
nyc·to·phil·i·a
nyc·to·pho·bi·a
nyc·to·pho·ni·a
nyc·to·typh·lo·sis
nyc·tu·ri·a
Ny·lan·der test
ny·li·drin
ny·lon
nymph
nym·pha
   pl nym·phae
nym·phec·to·my
nym·phi·tis
nym·pho·ca·run·cu·lar

nym·pho·lep·sy
   pl nym·pho·lep·sies
nym·pho·lept
nym·pho·lep·tic
nym·pho·ma·ni·a
nym·pho·ma·ni·ac
nym·pho·ma·ni·a·cal
nym·phon·cus
nym·phot·o·my
nys·tag·mic
nys·tag·mi·form
nys·tag·mog·ra·phy
nys·tag·moid
nys·tag·mus
nys·ta·tin
Nys·ten law
nyx·is
   pl nyx·es

O

oat-cell
oath of Hip·poc·ra·tes
ob·cae·ca·tion
   var of ob·ce·ca·tion
ob·ce·ca·tion
ob·dor·mi·tion
ob·duc·tion
o·be·li·ac
   or o·be·li·al
o·be·li·al
   or o·be·li·ac
o·be·li·on
   pl o·be·li·a
O·ber op·er·a·tion
O·ber·may·er test
O·ber·stei·ner lay·er

O·ber·stei·ner-Red·lich
   ar·e·a
o·bese
o·be·si·ty
   pl o·be·si·ties
o·bex
ob·fus·cate
ob·fus·ca·tion
ob·fus·ca·to·ry
ob·ject
ob·jec·tive
ob·jec·tive·ly
ob·late
ob·li·gate
ob·lig·a·tor·i·ly
ob·lig·a·to·ry
ob·ligue

o·bliq·ui·ty
   pl o·bliq·ui·ties
o·bli·quus
o·blit·er·ate
o·blit·er·a·tion
o·blit·er·a·tive
ob·lon·ga·ta
   pl ob·lon·ga·tas
   or ob·lon·ga·tae
ob·lon·gat·al
ob·mu·tes·cence
ob·nu·bi·la·tion
ob·ses·sion
ob·ses·sion·al
ob·ses·sive
ob·ses·sive-com·pul·sive
ob·ses·sive·ly
ob·ses·sive·ness

ob·so·les·cence
ob·so·les·cent
ob·stet·ric
or ob·stet·ri·cal
ob·stet·ri·cal
or ob·stet·ric
ob·stet·ri·cal·ly
ob·ste·tri·cian
ob·stet·rics
ob·sti·na·cy
pl ob·sti·na·cies
ob·sti·pate
ob·sti·pa·tion
ob·struct
ob·struct·ed
ob·struc·tion
ob·struc·tive
ob·struc·tive·ness
ob·stru·ent
ob·tund
ob·tun·da·tion
ob·tun·dent
ob·tu·rate
ob·tu·ra·tion
ob·tu·ra·tor
ob·tuse
ob·tu·sion
oc·cip·i·tal
oc·cip·i·ta·lis
oc·cip·i·tal·i·za·tion
oc·cip·i·tal·ize
oc·cip·i·tal·ly
oc·cip·i·to·an·te·ri·or
oc·cip·i·to·ax·i·al
oc·cip·i·to·cer·vi·cal
oc·cip·i·to·fron·tal
oc·cip·i·to·fron·ta·lis
oc·cip·i·to·lae·vo·an·te·ri·or
oc·cip·i·to·lae·vo·pos·te·ri·or
oc·cip·i·to·mas·toid
oc·cip·i·to·men·tal
oc·cip·i·to·pa·ri·e·tal
oc·cip·i·to·pon·tine
oc·cip·i·to·pos·te·ri·or
oc·cip·i·to·scap·u·lar·is
oc·cip·i·to·tem·po·ral
oc·cip·i·to·tha·lam·ic

oc·ci·put
pl oc·ci·puts
or oc·cip·i·ta
oc·clude
oc·clu·sal
oc·clu·si·o
oc·clu·sion
oc·clu·sive
oc·clu·som·e·ter
oc·cult
oc·cu·pa·tion
oc·cu·pa·tion·al
oc·cu·pa·tion·al·ly
o·cel·lar
o·cel·lus
pl o·cel·li
och·le·sis
och·lo·pho·bi·a
och·ra·tox·in
o·chrom·e·ter
o·chro·no·sis
pl o·chro·no·ses
o·chro·not·ic
Ochs·ner-Ma·hor·ner test
oc·i·mene
oc·ta·ben·zone
oc·tad
oc·ta·de·ca·di·e·no·ic
oc·ta·dec·a·no·ic
oc·ta·dec·e·no·ic
oc·ta·meth·yl·py·ro·phos·phor·am·ide
oc·tan
oc·tane
oc·ta·no·ic
oc·ta·pep·tide
oc·ta·ploid
oc·ta·ploi·dy
oc·tar·i·us
oc·ta·va·lent
oc·tene
oc·ti·grav·i·da
oc·tip·a·ra
oc·to·drine
oc·to·ge·nar·i·an
oc·to·pine
oc·to·roon
oc·tose
oc·tox·y·nol

oc·tyl
oc·tyl·ene
oc·u·lar
oc·u·len·tum
oc·u·li mar·ma·ry·go·des
oc·u·list
oc·u·lo·au·ric·u·lo·ver·te·bral
oc·u·lo·car·di·ac
oc·u·lo·ceph·a·lo·gy·ric
oc·u·lo·cer·e·bro·re·nal
oc·u·lo·cu·ta·ne·ous
oc·u·lo·den·to·dig·i·tal
oc·u·lo·fa·cial
oc·u·lo·gas·tric
oc·u·lo·glan·du·lar
oc·u·lo·gy·ral
oc·u·lo·gy·ra·tion
oc·u·lo·gy·ral
or oc·u·lo·gy·ric
oc·u·lo·gy·ric
or oc·u·lo·gy·ral
oc·u·lo·mo·tor
oc·u·lo·mo·to·ri·us
oc·u·lo·my·co·sis
pl oc·u·lo·my·co·ses
oc·u·lo·na·sal
oc·u·lo·o·to·cu·ta·ne·ous
oc·u·lo·pha·ryn·ge·al
oc·u·lo·phren·i·co·re·cur·rent
oc·u·lo·pu·pil·lar·y
oc·u·lo·sen·so·ry
oc·u·lo·zy·go·mat·ic
oc·u·lus
pl oc·u·li
o·cy·o·din·ic
o·dax·es·mus
Od·di sphinc·ter
od·ic
o·don·tal·gi·a
o·don·tal·gic
o·don·tec·to·my
pl o·don·tec·to·mies
o·don·tex·e·sis
o·don·thy·a·lus
o·don·ti·a·sis
pl o·don·ti·a·ses
o·don·tic

o·don·ti·noid
o·don·ti·tis
pl o·don·ti·ti·des
o·don·to·am·e·lo·sar·co·ma
pl o·don·to·am·e·lo·sar·co·mas
or o·don·to·am·e·lo·sar·co·ma·ta
o·don·to·at·lan·tal
o·don·to·blast
o·don·to·blas·tic
o·don·to·blas·to·ma
pl o·don·to·blas·to·mas
or o·don·to·blas·to·ma·ta
o·don·to·cele
o·don·to·cla·sis
o·don·to·clast
o·don·to·gen·e·sis
o·don·to·gen·ic
o·don·tog·e·ny
o·don·to·graph
o·don·to·graph·ic
o·don·tog·ra·phy
pl o·don·tog·ra·phies
o·don·toid
o·don·to·log·i·cal
o·don·tol·o·gist
o·don·tol·o·gy
pl o·don·tol·o·gies
o·don·to·lox·i·a
o·don·tol·ox·y
o·don·tol·y·sis
o·don·to·ma
pl o·don·to·mas
or o·don·to·ma·ta
o·don·top·a·thy
o·don·to·pho·bi·a
o·don·to·plas·ty
o·don·to·pri·sis
o·don·to·scope
o·don·to·sis
pl o·don·to·ses
o·don·tot·o·my
pl o·don·tot·o·mies
o·dor
o·dor·ant
o·do·ra·tion
o·dor·if·er·ous
o·dor·if·er·ous·ly

o·dor·if·er·ous·ness
o·dor·im·e·ter
o·dor·im·e·try
pl o·dor·im·e·tries
o·dor·i·phore
o·dor·ous
o·dyn·a·cou·sis
o·dyn·a·cu·sis
o·dyn·o·me·ter
o·dyn·o·pha·gi·a
o·dyn·o·pho·bi·a
o·dy·nu·ri·a
oe·coid
var of e·coid
oe·de·ma
var of e·de·ma
oe·di·pal
Oed·i·pe·an
oed·i·pism
Oe·di·pus
pl oe·di·pus·es
oe·nol·o·gy
pl oe·nol·o·gies
var of e·nol·o·gy
Oer·tel treat·ment
oe·soph·a·ge·al
var of e·soph·a·ge·al
oe·soph·a·gos·to·mi·a·sis
Oe·soph·a·gos·to·mum
oe·soph·a·gus
var of e·soph·a·gus
oes·tra·di·ol
var of es·tra·di·ol
oes·tral
var of es·tral
oes·trid
Oes·tri·dae
oes·trin
var of es·trin
oes·tri·ol
var of es·tri·ol
oes·tro·gen
var of es·tro·gen
oes·tro·gen·ic
var of es·tro·gen·ic
oes·trone
var of es·trone
oes·trous
var of es·trous

oes·tru·al
var of es·tru·al
oes·trum
var of es·trus
oes·trus
var of es·trus
of·fal
of·fi·cial
of·fi·ci·nal
of·fi·ci·nal·ly
off·spring
Og·ston-Luc op·er·a·tion
O·gu·chi dis·ease
O·ha·ra dis·ease
Ohl·mach·er fix·a·tive so·lu·tion
Ohm law
ohm-am·me·ter
ohm·me·ter
o·id·i·o·my·cin
o·id·i·o·my·co·sis
pl o·id·i·o·my·co·ses
O·id·i·um
pl O·id·i·a
oi·ki·o·ma·ni·a
oi·kol·o·gy
oi·ko·ma·ni·a
oi·ko·pho·bi·a
oi·ko·site
oil
oil·y
oi·no·ma·ni·a
oint·ment
O·ka·mo·to meth·od
Ok·kels meth·od
ol·a·mine
o·le·ag·i·nous
o·le·an·der
o·le·an·do·my·cin
o·le·ate
o·lec·ra·nal
o·le·cra·nar·thri·tis
o·le·cra·nar·throc·a·ce
o·le·cra·nar·throp·a·thy
o·lec·ra·noid
o·lec·ra·non
o·lef·i·ant
o·le·fin
or o·le·fine

o·le·fine
  or o·le·fin
o·le·fin·ic
o·le·ic
o·le·in
o·le·o·gran·u·lo·ma
  pl o·le·o·gran·u·lo·mas
  or o·le·o·gran·u·lo·ma·ta
o·leo·mar·ga·rine
o·le·om·e·ter
o·le·op·tene
o·le·o·res·in
o·le·o·sac·cha·rum
  pl o·le·o·sac·cha·ra
o·le·o·ther·a·py
o·le·o·tho·rax
  pl o·le·o·tho·rax·es
  or o·le·o·tho·ra·ces
o·le·o·vi·ta·min
o·le·um
  pl o·le·a
o·le·yl
ol·fact
ol·fac·tion
ol·fac·to·hy·po·tha·lam·ic
ol·fac·tol·o·gy
  pl ol·fac·tol·o·gies
ol·fac·tom·e·ter
ol·fac·to·met·ric
ol·fac·to·met·ri·cal·ly
ol·fac·tom·e·try
  pl ol·fac·tom·e·tries
ol·fac·to·ry
ol·fac·tron·ics
o·lib·a·num
ol·i·gae·mi·a
  var of ol·i·ge·mi·a
ol·i·ge·mi·a
ol·i·ge·mic
ol·i·ger·ga·si·a
ol·ig·hy·dri·a
ol·i·gid·ic
ol·i·go·am·ni·os
ol·i·go·blast
ol·i·go·blen·ni·a
o·li·go·car·di·a
ol·i·go·cho·li·a
ol·i·go·chro·ma·si·a
ol·i·go·chro·me·mi·a

ol·i·go·chy·li·a
o·li·go·cys·tic
ol·i·go·cy·thae·mi·a
  var of ol·i·go·cy·the·mi·a
ol·i·go·cy·thae·mic
  var of o·li·go·cy·the·mic
ol·i·go·cy·the·mi·a
ol·i·go·cy·the·mic
ol·i·go·dac·ry·a
ol·i·go·dac·tyl·i·a
ol·i·go·dac·tyl·ism
  or ol·i·go·dac·ty·ly
o·li·go·dac·ty·ly
  pl o·li·go·dac·ty·lies
  or o·li·go·dac·tyl·ism
o·li·go·den·dri·a
ol·i·go·den·dro·blas·to·ma
  pl ol·i·go·den·dro·blas·to·
      mas
  or ol·i·go·den·dro·blas·to·
      ma·ta
ol·i·go·den·dro·cyte
ol·i·go·den·dro·cy·to·ma
  pl ol·i·go·den·dro·cy·to·mas
  or ol·i·go·den·dro·cy·to·ma·
      ta
ol·i·go·den·drog·li·a
ol·i·go·den·drog·li·al
ol·i·go·den·dro·gli·o·ma
  pl ol·i·go·den·dro·gli·o·mas
  or ol·i·go·den·dro·gli·o·ma·
      ta
ol·i·go·den·drog·li·o·ma·to·
      sis
ol·i·go·den·dro·ma
  pl ol·i·go·den·dro·mas
  or ol·i·go·den·dro·ma·ta
o·li·go·dip·si·a
ol·i·go·don·ti·a
ol·i·go·dy·nam·ic
ol·i·go·el·e·ment
ol·i·go·en·ceph·a·ly
ol·i·go·ga·lac·ti·a
ol·i·go·gene
ol·i·go·gen·ic
ol·i·go·gen·ics
ol·i·gog·li·a
ol·i·go·graph·i·a
o·li·go·he·mi·a

ol·i·go·hid·ri·a
ol·i·go·hy·dram·ni·os
ol·i·go·hy·dri·a
ol·i·go·hy·dru·ri·a
ol·i·go·la·li·a
ol·i·go·lec·i·thal
ol·i·go·lo·gi·a
ol·i·go·ma·ni·a
ol·i·go·me·lus
ol·i·go·men·or·rhe·a
ol·i·go·men·or·rhoe·a
  var of ol·i·go·men·or·rhe·a
ol·i·go·mer
ol·i·go·mer·ic
ol·i·go·mer·iza·tion
ol·i·go·mor·phic
ol·i·go·my·cin
ol·i·go·nu·cle·o·tide
ol·i·go·pha·si·a
ol·i·go·phos·pha·tu·ri·a
ol·i·go·phre·ni·a
ol·i·go·phren·ic
o·li·go·plas·mi·a
ol·i·gop·ne·a
ol·i·gop·noe·a
  var of ol·i·gop·ne·a
ol·i·go·psy·chi·a
ol·i·go·pty·a·lism
ol·i·go·py·rene
ol·i·go·ri·a
ol·i·go·sac·cha·ride
ol·i·go·si·al·i·a
ol·i·go·sper·mat·ic
ol·i·go·sper·mi·a
ol·i·go·trich·i·a
o·li·go·tro·phi·a
o·li·got·ro·phy
ol·i·go·zo·o·sper·mi·a
ol·i·gu·re·sis
ol·i·gu·ri·a
ol·i·gyd·ri·a
o·lis·ther·o·chro·ma·tin
o·lis·ther·o·zone
o·li·va
o·li·var·y
ol·ive
Ol·i·ver sign
Ol·i·ver-Car·da·rel·li sign
ol·i·vif·u·gal

269

ol·i·vip·e·tal
ol·i·vo·cer·e·bel·lar
ol·i·vo·pon·to·cer·e·bel·lar
ol·i·vo·spi·nal
Ol·lier dis·ease
ol·o·li·u·qui
ol·o·pho·ni·a
o·ma·ceph·a·lus
o·ma·gra
o·mal·gi·a
o·mar·thral·gi·a
o·mar·thri·tis
o·ma·si·tis
o·ma·sum
  pl o·ma·sa
om·bro·pho·bi·a
o·me·ga
o·men·tal
o·men·tec·to·my
  pl o·men·tec·to·mies
o·men·ti·tis
o·men·to·cele
o·men·to·fix·a·tion
o·men·to·pex·y
  pl o·men·to·pex·ies
o·men·tor·rha·phy
o·men·tot·o·my
o·men·tu·lum
  pl o·men·tu·la
o·men·tum
  pl o·men·tums
  or o·men·ta
o·men·tum·ec·to·my
o·mi·tis
om·ma·tid·i·um
  pl om·ma·tid·i·a
om·ni·fo·cal
om·niv·o·rous
o·mo·cer·vi·ca·lis
o·mo·cla·vic·u·lar
om·o·dyn·i·a
o·mo·hy·oid
o·mo·hy·oi·de·us
  pl o·mo·hy·oi·de·i
o·mo·pha·gi·a
o·mo·ver·te·bral
om·pha·lec·to·my
om·phal·el·co·sis
om·phal·lic

om·pha·li·tis
  pl om·pha·li·ti·des
om·pha·lo·an·gi·op·a·gus
om·pha·lo·cele
om·pha·lo·cho·ri·on
om·pha·lo·cra·ni·o·did·y·
  mus
om·pha·lo·did·y·mus
om·pha·lo·gen·e·sis
om·pha·lo·mes·en·ter·ic
om·pha·lo·mon·o·did·y·
  mus
om·pha·lop·a·gus
om·pha·lo·phle·bi·tis
  pl om·pha·lo·phle·bi·ti·des
om·pha·lo·prop·to·sis
om·phal·or·rha·gi·a
om·pha·lor·rhe·a
om·pha·lor·rhex·is
om·pha·los
  pl om·pha·li
om·pha·lo·site
om·pha·lo·so·tor
om·pha·lo·tax·is
om·phal·o·tome
om·pha·lot·o·my
om·pha·lo·trip·sy
o·nan·ism
o·nan·ist
o·nan·is·tic
On·cho·cer·ca
on·cho·cer·cal
on·cho·cer·ci·a·sis
  pl on·cho·cer·ci·a·ses
on·cho·cer·co·ma
on·cho·cer·co·sis
  pl on·cho·cer·co·sis
on·cho·der·ma·ti·tis
on·cho·sphere
  or on·co·sphere
on·co·cyte
on·co·cy·to·ma
  pl on·co·cy·to·mas
  or on·co·cy·to·ma·ta
on·co·gen·e·sis
  pl on·co·gen·e·ses
on·co·gen·ic
  or on·cog·en·ous

on·co·gen·ic·i·ty
  pl on·co·gen·ic·i·ties
on·cog·en·ous
  or on·co·gen·ic
on·cog·e·ny
  pl on·cog·e·nies
on·co·graph
on·cog·ra·phy
  pl on·cog·ra·phies
on·co·log·ic
  or on·co·log·i·cal
on·co·log·i·cal
  or on·co·log·ic
on·col·o·gist
on·col·o·gy
  pl on·col·o·gies
on·col·y·sis
  pl on·col·y·ses
on·co·lyt·ic
on·co·ma
On·co·me·la·ni·a
on·com·e·ter
on·co·met·ric
on·com·e·try
on·co·sis
on·co·sphere
  or on·cho·sphere
on·co·ther·a·py
on·cot·ic
on·cot·o·my
  pl on·cot·o·mies
on·co·trop·ic
o·nei·ric
o·nei·rism
o·nei·ro·dyn·i·a
o·nei·rog·mus
o·nei·rol·o·gy
o·nei·ron·o·sus
o·nei·ros·co·py
o·ni·o·ma·ni·a
o·ni·o·ma·ni·ac
o·ni·um
on·kin·o·cele
on·ko·cy·to·ma
  pl on·ko·cy·to·mas
  or on·ko·cy·to·ma·ta
on·lay
on·o·ma·tol·o·gy
  pl on·o·ma·tol·o·gies

on·o·mat·o·ma·ni·a
on·o·mat·o·pho·bia
on·o·ma·to·poi·e·sis
  pl on·o·mat·o·poi·e·ses
on·o·mat·o·poi·et·ic
on·set
on·to·a·nal·y·sis
on·to·an·a·lyt·ic
on·to·gen·e·sis
  pl on·to·gen·e·ses
on·to·ge·net·ic
on·to·ge·net·i·cal·ly
on·to·gen·ic
on·to·gen·i·cal·ly
on·tog·e·ny
  pl on·tog·e·nies
on·y·al·ai
on·y·chal·gi·a ner·vo·sa
on·y·cha·tro·phi·a
on·y·chat·ro·phy
on·ych·aux·is
  pl on·ych·aux·es
on·y·chec·to·my
on·y·chex·al·lax·is
o·nych·i·a
on·y·chin
on·y·chi·tis
  pl on·y·chi·ti·des
on·y·choc·la·sis
on·y·cho·cryp·to·sis
on·y·cho·dys·tro·phy
on·y·cho·gen·ic
o·ny·cho·graph
on·y·cho·gry·po·sis
  pl on·y·cho·gry·po·ses
on·y·cho·het·er·o·to·pi·a
on·y·choid
on·y·chol·y·sis
  pl on·y·chol·y·ses
on·y·cho·ma
  pl on·y·cho·mas
  or on·y·cho·ma·ta
on·y·cho·ma·de·sis
on·y·cho·ma·la·ci·a
on·y·cho·my·co·sis
  pl on·y·cho·my·co·ses
on·y·cho·no·sus
on·y·cho·os·te·o·ar·thro·
  dys·pla·si·a

on·y·cho·os·te·o·dys·pla·
  si·a
on·y·cho·pac·i·ty
on·y·cho·path·ic
on·y·chop·a·thy
on·y·cho·pha·gi·a
on·y·choph·a·gist
on·y·choph·a·gy
  pl on·y·choph·a·gies
on·y·chor·rhex·is
  pl on·y·chor·rhex·es
on·y·chor·rhi·za
on·y·cho·schiz·i·a
on·y·cho·sis
  pl on·y·cho·ses
on·y·cho·stro·ma
on·y·chot·il·lo·ma·ni·a
on·y·chot·o·my
on·y·cho·tro·phi·a
on·y·chot·ro·phy
on·yx
on·yx·is
on·yx·i·tis
o·o·blast
o·o·ceph·a·lus
o·o·cy·e·sis
  pl o·o·cy·e·ses
o·o·cyst
o·o·cyte
o·o·gen·e·sis
  pl o·o·gen·e·ses
o·o·ge·net·ic
o·o·ge·ni·al
o·o·go·ni·um
  pl o·o·go·ni·a
o·o·ki·ne·sis
  pl o·o·ki·ne·ses
o·o·ki·nete
o·o·ki·net·ic
o·o·lem·ma
o·o·pho·rec·to·mize
o·o·pho·rec·to·my
  pl o·o·pho·rec·to·mies
o·o·pho·ri·tis
o·oph·o·ro·cae·cal
  var of o·oph·o·ro·ce·cal
o·oph·o·ro·ce·cal
o·oph·o·ro·cys·tec·to·my

  pl o·oph·o·ro·cys·tec·to·
  mies
o·oph·o·ro·cys·to·sis
o·oph·o·ro·cys·tos·to·my
o·oph·o·ro·hys·ter·ec·to·my
o·oph·o·ro·ma
  pl o·oph·o·ro·mas
  or o·oph·o·ro·ma·ta
o·oph·o·ro·ma·la·ci·a
o·oph·o·ro·ma·ni·a
o·oph·o·ron
o·oph·o·ro·path·i·a
o·oph·o·ro·pex·y
o·oph·o·ro·plas·ty
o·oph·o·ro·sal·pin·gec·to·my
o·oph·o·ro·sal·pin·gi·tis
o·oph·o·ros·to·my
o·oph·o·rot·o·my
o·o·phor·rha·phy
o·o·plasm
o·o·plas·mic
o·o·por·phy·rin
o·o·sperm
O·os·po·ra
o·o·spore
o·o·the·ca
  pl o·o·the·cae
o·o·the·cal
o·o·tid
o·o·type
o·pac·i·fi·ca·tion
o·pac·i·fy
o·pac·i·ty
  pl o·pac·i·ties
o·pal·es·cence
o·pal·es·cent
O·pal·ski cells
o·paque
o·pei·do·scope
o·pen-heart
o·pen·ing
op·er·a·bil·i·ty
  pl op·er·a·bil·i·ties
op·er·a·ble
op·er·a·bly
op·er·ant
op·er·ate
op·er·a·tion
op·er·a·tion·al

op·er·a·tive
op·er·a·tive·ly
op·er·a·tor
o·per·cu·lar
o·per·cu·late
   or o·per·cu·lat·ed
o·per·cu·lat·ed
   or o·per·cu·late
o·per·cu·lum
   pl o·per·cu·lums
   or oper·cu·la
op·er·on
o·phi·a·sis
O·phid·i·a
o·phid·i·o·pho·bia
o·phid·ism
O·phi·oph·a·gus
oph·i·o·phobe
oph·ry·i·tis
oph·ry·on
Oph·ry·o·sco·lec·i·dae
oph·ry·o·sis
oph·ryph·thei·ri·a·sis
oph·rys
o·phry·tic
oph·thal·ma·cro·sis
oph·thal·ma·gra
oph·thal·mal·gi·a
oph·thal·mec·chy·mo·sis
oph·thal·mec·to·my
   pl oph·thal·mec·to·mies
oph·thal·men·ceph·a·lon
   pl oph·thal·men·ceph·a·la
oph·thal·mi·a
oph·thal·mi·a ne·o·na·to·
   rum
oph·thal·mi·a·ter
oph·thal·mi·at·rics
oph·thal·mic
oph·thal·mit·ic
oph·thal·mi·tis
oph·thal·mo·blen·nor·rhe·a
oph·thal·mo·blen·nor·
   rhoe·a
   var of oph·thal·mo·blen·
   nor·rhe·a
oph·thal·mo·moc·a·ce
oph·thal·mo·cele

oph·thal·mo·cen·te·sis
oph·thal·mo·co·pi·a
oph·thal·mo·di·as·tim·e·ter
oph·thal·mo·do·ne·sis
oph·thal·mo·dy·na·mom·e·
   ter
oph·thal·mo·dy·na·mom·e·
   try
oph·thal·mo·dyn·i·a
oph·thal·mo·ei·ko·nom·e·
   ter
   var of oph·thal·mo·i·co·
   nom·e·ter
oph·thal·mo·ei·ko·nom·e·
   try
   var of oph·thal·mo·i·co·
   nom·e·try
oph·thal·mo·fun·do·scope
oph·thal·mo·graph
oph·thal·mog·ra·phy
oph·thal·mo·gy·ric
oph·thal·mo·i·co·nom·e·ter
oph·thal·mo·i·co·nom·e·try
oph·thal·mo·ko·pi·a
   var of oph·thal·mo·co·pia
oph·thal·mo·leu·co·scope
   or oph·thal·mo·leu·ko·
   scope
oph·thal·mo·leu·ko·scope
   or oph·thal·mo·leu·co·
   scope
oph·thal·mo·lith
oph·thal·mo·log·ic
   or oph·thal·mo·log·i·cal
oph·thal·mo·log·i·cal
   or oph·thal·mo·log·ic
oph·thal·mol·o·gist
oph·thal·mol·o·gy
   pl oph·thal·mol·o·gies
oph·thal·mo·ma·cro·sis
oph·thal·mo·ma·la·ci·a
oph·thal·mom·e·ter
oph·thal·mom·e·try
   pl oph·thal·mom·e·tries
oph·thal·mo·my·co·sis
   pl oph·thal·mo·my·co·ses
oph·thal·mo·my·i·a·sis
oph·thal·mo·my·ot·o·my

oph·thal·mo·neu·ri·tis
oph·thal·mo·neu·ro·my·e·
   li·tis
oph·thal·mop·a·thy
   pl oph·thal·mop·a·thies
oph·thal·mo·pha·com·e·ter
oph·thal·mo·pha·kom·e·ter
   var of oph·thal·mo·pha·
   com·e·ter
oph·thal·mo·phas·ma·tos·
   co·py
oph·thal·mo·pho·bi·a
oph·thal·moph·thi·sis
oph·thal·mo·phy·ma
oph·thal·mo·plas·tic
oph·thal·mo·plas·ty
oph·thal·mo·ple·gi·a
oph·thal·mo·ple·gic
oph·thal·mop·to·sis
oph·thal·mo·re·ac·tion
oph·thal·mor·rha·gi·a
oph·thal·mor·rhe·a
oph·thal·mor·rhex·is
oph·thal·mor·rhoe·a
   var of oph·thal·mor·rhoe·a
oph·thal·mos
oph·thal·mo·scope
oph·thal·mo·scop·ic
   or oph·thal·mo·scop·i·cal
oph·thal·mo·scop·i·cal
   or oph·thal·mo·scop·ic
oph·thal·mo·scop·i·cal·ly
oph·thal·mos·co·pist
oph·thal·mos·co·py
   pl oph·thal·mos·co·pies
oph·thal·mo·so·nom·e·try
oph·thal·mo·spin·ther·ism
oph·thal·mos·ta·sis
   pl oph·thal·mos·ta·ses
oph·thal·mo·stat
oph·thal·mo·sta·tom·e·ter
oph·thal·mo·sta·tom·e·try
oph·thal·mo·ste·re·sis
oph·thal·mo·syn·chy·sis
oph·thal·mo·to·my
oph·thal·mo·to·nom·e·ter
oph·thal·mo·to·nom·e·try
oph·thal·mo·trope

ph·thal·mo·tro·pom·e·ter
ph·thal·mo·tro·pom·e·try
ph·thal·mo·xe·ro·sis
ph·thal·mus
    pl oph·thal·mi
·pi·ate
·pie par·a·dox
·pi·o·ma·ni·a
·pi·o·ma·ni·ac
·pi·o·pha·gi·a
·pi·oph·a·gism
·pi·oph·a·gy
·pi·o·phile
·pip·ra·mol
·pis·then
·pis·the·nar
·pis·thi·on
    pl o·pis·thi·ons
    or o·pis·thi·a
·pis·tho·cra·ni·on
·pis·thog·na·thism
·pis·tho·neph·ros
·pis·tho·po·rei·a
·pis·thor·chi·a·sis
Op·is·thor·chis
·pis·thot·ic
·pis·thot·o·noid
·pis·thot·o·nos
·pis·thot·o·nus
    var of o·pis·thot·o·nos
·pi·um
p·o·bal·sam
    var of op·o·bal·sa·mum
p·o·bal·sa·mum
p·o·ceph·a·lus
p·o·did·y·mus
·pod·y·mus
Op·pen·heim dis·ease
Op·pen·heim-Ur·bach
    dis·ease
p·pi·la·tion
p·pi·la·tive
p·po·nens
    pl op·po·nen·tes
p·por·tun·ist
p·por·tun·is·tic
p·sig·e·nes

op·sin
op·sin·o·gen
op·si·nog·e·nous
op·si·om·e·ter
op·si·o·no·sis
op·si·u·ri·a
op·so·clo·ni·a
op·so·clo·nus
op·so·ma·ni·a
op·so·ma·ni·ac
op·son·ic
op·so·nin
op·so·ni·za·tion
op·so·nize
op·so·no·cy·to·pha·gic
op·so·no·nom·e·try
op·so·no·ther·a·py
op·tes·the·si·a
op·tic
    or op·ti·cal
op·ti·cal
    or op·tic
op·ti·cian
op·ti·cian·ry
op·ti·co·chi·as·mat·ic
op·ti·co·chi·as·mic
op·ti·co·cil·i·ar·y
op·ti·coele
op·ti·co·fa·cial
op·ti·co·ki·net·ic
op·ti·co·pu·pil·lar·y
op·tics
op·ti·mal
op·tim·e·ter
op·ti·mum
op·to·chi·as·mic
op·to·gram
op·to·ki·net·ic
op·tom·e·ter
op·to·met·ric
    or op·to·met·ri·cal
op·to·met·ri·cal
    or op·to·met·ric
op·tom·e·trist
op·tom·e·try
    pl op·tom·e·tries
op·to·my·om·e·ter
op·to·type

o·ra ser·ra·ta
    pl o·rae ser·ra·tae
o·rad
o·ral
o·ra·le
o·ral·i·ty
    pl o·ral·i·ties
o·ral·ly
o·ral·o·gy
    pl o·ral·o·gies
or·be·li ef·fect
or·bic·u·lar
or·bic·u·lar·e
or·bic·u·lar·is
    pl or·bi·cu·la·res
or·bic·u·lar·i·ty
    pl or·bic·u·lar·i·ties
or·bic·u·lar·ly
or·bic·u·lus
    pl or·bic·u·li
or·bit
or·bi·ta
    pl or·bi·tae
or·bi·tal
or·bi·ta·le
    pl or·bi·ta·li·a
or·bi·ta·lis
or·bi·to·na·sal
or·bi·to·nom·e·ter
or·bi·to·nom·e·try
or·bi·to·sphe·noid
    or or·bi·to·sphe·noi·dal
or·bi·to·sphe·noi·dal
    or or·bi·to·sphe·noid
or·bi·tot·o·my
or·ce·in
or·chec·to·my
    pl or·chec·to·mies
    or or·chi·ec·to·my
    pl or·chi·ec·to·mies
or·che·i·tis
or·ches·tro·ma·ni·a
or·chi·al·gi·a
or·chic
or·chi·dal·gi·a
or·chi·dec·to·my
    pl or·chi·dec·to·mies
or·chi·di·tis

or·chi·dop·a·thy
or·chi·do·pex·y
  pl or·chi·o·pex·ies
  or or·chi·o·pex·y
  pl or·chi·do·pex·ies
or·chi·do·plas·ty
or·chi·dor·rha·phy
or·chi·dot·o·my
or·chi·ec·to·my
  pl or·chi·ec·to·mies
  or or·chec·to·my
  pl or·chec·to·mies
or·chi·en·ceph·a·lo·ma
  pl or·chi·en·ceph·a·lo·mas
  or or·chi·en·ceph·a·lo·ma·ta
or·chi·ep·i·did·y·mi·tis
or·chil
  var of ar·chil
or·chi·o·ca·tab·a·sis
or·chi·o·cele
or·chi·op·a·thy
or·chi·o·pex·y
  pl or·chi·o·pex·ies
  or or·chi·do·pex·y
  pl or·chi·do·pex·ies
or·chi·o·plas·ty
  pl or·chi·o·plas·ties
or·chi·ot·o·my
or·chis
or·chit·ic
or·chi·tis
or·chit·o·my
or·chot·o·my
or·cin
or·cin·ol
or·der
or·der·ly
  pl or·der·lies
or·di·nate
o·rec·tic
o·rex·i·a
o·rex·is
orf
or·gan
or·gan of Cor·ti
or·gan of Ja·cob·son
or·gan·el·la
  or or·gan·elle

or·gan·elle
  or or·gan·el·la
or·gan·ic
or·gan·i·cal·ly
or·gan·i·cism
or·gan·i·cist
or·gan·i·cis·tic
or·gan·ism
or·ga·ni·za·tion
or·ga·nize
or·ga·niz·er
or·ga·no·ax·i·al
or·gan·o·gel
or·gan·o·gen·e·sis
  pl or·gan·o·gen·e·ses
or·gan·o·ge·net·ic
or·gan·o·ge·net·i·cal·ly
or·gan·o·gen·ic
or·ga·nog·e·ny
  pl or·ga·nog·e·nies
or·gan·o·gra·phic
or·ga·nog·ra·phy
  pl or·ga·nog·ra·phies
or·ga·noid
or·ga·no·lep·tic
or·ga·no·lep·ti·cal·ly
or·ga·no·log·ic
  or or·ga·no·log·i·cal
or·ga·no·log·i·cal
  or or·ga·no·log·ic
or·ga·nol·o·gy
  pl or·ga·nol·o·gies
or·gan·o·mer·cu·ri·al
or·gan·o·me·tal·lic
or·ga·non
  pl or·ga·na
or·gan·o·phos·phate
or·gan·o·phos·pho·rus
or·ga·nos·co·py
  pl or·ga·nos·co·pies
or·gan·o·sol
or·ga·no·ther·a·peu·tic
or·ga·no·ther·a·py
  pl or·ga·no·ther·a·pies
or·ga·no·troph·ic
or·ga·no·trop·ic
or·ga·no·trop·i·cal·ly
or·ga·not·ro·pism

or·ga·not·ro·py
  pl or·ga·not·ro·pies
or·gans of Zuck·er·kandl
or·gan·spe·cif·ic
or·ga·num
  pl or·ga·na
or·gasm
or·gas·mic
  or or·gas·tic
or·gas·mo·lep·sy
or·gas·tic
  or or·gas·mic
or·go·tein
o·ri·en·ta·tion
or·i·fice
or·i·fi·cial
o·ri·fi·ci·um
  pl o·ri·fi·ci·a
o·rig·a·num
o·ri·gin
Orms·by meth·od
or·ni·thine
or·ni·thi·ne·mi·a
Or·ni·thod·o·ros
or·ni·tho·sis
  pl or·ni·tho·ses
or·ni·thu·ric
or·ni·thyl
o·ro·an·thral
o·ro·di·ag·no·sis
o·ro·fa·cial
o·ro·lin·gual
o·ro·na·sal
o·ron·o·sus
o·ro·pha·ryn·ge·al
o·ro·phar·ynx
  pl o·ro·phar·ynx·es
  or o·ro·pha·ryn·ges
o·ro·sin
o·ro·so·mu·coid
o·rot·ic
O·ro·ya fe·ver
or·phen·a·drine
or·rho·men·in·gi·tis
or·rhos
or·ris·root
Or·ta·la·ni sign
or·ther·ga·si·a
or·the·sis

or·thet·ics
or·the·tist
or·thi·auch·e·nus
or·thi·o·chor·dus
or·thi·o·cor·y·phus
or·thi·o·don·tus
or·thi·o·me·to·pus
or·thi·o·pis·thi·us
or·thi·o·pis·tho·cra·ni·us
or·thi·o·pro·so·pus
or·thi·op·y·lus
or·thi·or·rhi·nus
or·thi·u·ra·nis·cus
or·tho
or·tho·bo·ric
or·tho·car·di·ac
or·tho·ce·phal·ic
  or or·tho·ceph·a·lous
or·tho·ceph·a·lous
  or or·tho·ce·phal·ic
or·tho·ceph·a·ly
  pl or·tho·ceph·a·lies
or·tho·chlo·ro·phe·nol
or·tho·cho·re·a
or·tho·chro·mat·ic
or·tho·chro·mic
or·tho·cra·si·a
or·tho·cre·sol
or·tho·dac·ty·lous
or·tho·den·tin
or·tho·di·a·gram
or·tho·di·a·graph
or·tho·di·ag·ra·phy
or·tho·dol·i·cho·ceph·a·lous
or·tho·don·ti·a
or·tho·don·tic
or·tho·don·tics
or·tho·don·tist
or·tho·drom·ic
or·tho·gen·e·sis
  pl or·tho·gen·e·ses
or·tho·ge·net·ic
or·tho·ge·net·i·cal·ly
or·tho·gen·ic
or·thog·nath·ic
or·thog·na·thism
or·thog·na·thous
or·thog·o·nal

or·tho·grade
or·tho·hy·drox·y·ben·zo·ic
or·tho·mes·o·ceph·a·lous
or·thom·e·ter
or·tho·mo·lec·u·lar
or·tho·myx·o·vi·rus
or·tho·pae·dic
  var of or·tho·pe·dic
or·tho·pae·dics
  var of or·tho·pe·dics
or·tho·pae·dist
  var of or·tho·pe·dist
or·tho·pe·dic
or·tho·pe·dics
or·tho·pe·dist
or·tho·per·cus·sion
or·tho·phe·nan·thro·line
or·tho·phe·nol·ase
or·tho·phen·yl·phe·nol
or·tho·pho·ri·a
or·tho·phos·phate
or·tho·phos·pho·ric
or·thop·ne·a
or·thop·ne·ic
or·thop·noe·a
  var of or·thop·ne·a
or·thop·noe·ic
  var of or·thop·ne·ic
or·tho·prax·is
or·tho·prax·y
  pl or·tho·prax·ies
or·tho·psy·chi·at·ric
  or or·tho·psy·chi·at·ri·cal
or·tho·psy·chi·at·ri·cal
  or or·tho·psy·chi·at·ric
or·tho·psy·chi·a·trist
or·tho·psy·chi·a·try
  pl or·tho·psy·chi·a·tries
Or·thop·ter·a
or·thop·tic
or·thop·tics
or·thop·tist
or·thop·to·scope
or·tho·roent·gen·og·ra·phy
or·tho·scope
or·tho·scop·ic
or·thos·co·py
or·tho·sis
  pl or·tho·ses

or·tho·stat·ic
or·tho·stat·ism
or·tho·ster·e·o·scope
or·tho·ster·e·o·scop·ic
or·tho·sym·pa·thet·ic
or·tho·tast
or·tho·ter·i·on
or·tho·ther·a·py
or·thot·ic
or·thot·ics
or·tho·tist
or·tho·ton·ic
or·thot·o·nos
or·thot·o·nus
  var of or·thot·o·nos
or·tho·to·pi·a
or·tho·top·ic
or·tho·trop·ic
or·thot·ro·pism
or·tho·volt·age
o·ry·za·min
os
  pl os·sa
  or o·ra
os cal·cis
  pl os·sa cal·cis
os cox·ae
  pl os·sa cox·ae
o·sa·zone
os·che·a
os·che·al
os·che·i·tis
os·che·o·cele
os·che·o·ma
os·che·o·plas·ty
Os·cil·lar·i·a ma·lar·i·ae
os·cil·late
os·cil·la·tion
os·cil·la·tor
os·cil·la·to·ry
os·cil·lo·gram
os·cil·lo·graph
os·cil·lo·graph·ic
os·cil·lo·graph·i·cal·ly
os·cil·log·ra·phy
  pl os·cil·log·ra·phies
os·cil·lom·e·ter
os·cil·lo·met·ric

os·cil·lom·e·try
   pl os·cil·lom·e·tries
os·cil·lop·si·a
os·cil·lo·scope
os·cil·lo·scop·ic
os·cil·lo·scop·i·cal·ly
os·cine
Os·cin·i·dae
Os·ci·nis
os·ci·tan·cy
os·ci·ta·tion
os·cu·la·tion
os·cu·lum
   pl os·cu·la
Os·er·et·sky test
Os·good-Has·kins test
Os·good-Schlat·ter
  dis·ease
O'Shaugh·nes·sy op·er·a·
  tion
Os·ler dis·ease
Os·ler-Lib·man-Sacks
  syn·drome
Os·ler-Ren·du-Web·er
  dis·ease
Os·ler-Va·quez dis·ease
os·mate
os·mat·ic
  or os·mic
os·me·sis
os·mes·the·si·a
os·mic
  or os·mat·ic
os·mics
os·mi·dro·sis
  pl os·mi·dro·ses
os·mi·o·phil
  or os·mi·o·phil·ic
os·mi·o·phil·ic
  or os·mi·o·phil
os·mi·um
os·mo·dys·pho·ri·a
os·mol
os·mol·al
os·mo·lal·i·ty
  pl os·mo·lal·i·ties
os·mo·lar
os·mo·lar·i·ty
  pl os·mo·lar·i·ties

os·mole
os·mol·o·gy
os·mom·e·ter
os·mo·met·ric
os·mom·e·try
  pl os·mom·e·tries
os·mo·no·sol·o·gy
os·mo·phil·ic
os·mo·pho·bi·a
os·mo·phore
os·mo·phor·ic
os·mo·re·cep·tor
os·mo·reg·u·la·tion
os·mo·reg·u·la·tor
os·mo·reg·u·la·to·ry
os·mose
os·mo·sis
  pl os·mo·ses
os·mot·ic
os·mot·i·cal·ly
os·phre·si·ol·o·gy
os·phre·si·om·e·ter
os·phre·sis
os·phret·ic
os·phy·o·my·e·li·tis
os·se·in
os·se·ine
  var of os·se·in
os·se·let
os·se·o·al·bu·min·oid
os·se·o·car·ti·lag·i·nous
os·se·o·fi·brous
os·se·o·lig·a·men·tous
os·se·o·mu·cin
os·se·o·mu·coid
os·se·ous
os·se·ous·ly
os·si·cle
os·sic·u·la au·di·tus
os·sic·u·lar
os·si·cu·lec·to·my
  pl os·si·cu·lec·to·mies
os·si·cu·lot·o·my
  pl os·si·cu·lot·o·mies
os·sic·u·lum
  pl os·sic·u·la
os·sif·er·ous
os·sif·ic
os·si·fi·ca·tion

os·sif·i·ca·to·ry
os·sif·lu·ence
os·sif·lu·ent
os·si·form
os·si·fy
os·tal·gi·a
os·tal·gic
os·tal·gi·tis
os·te·al
os·te·al·gi·a
os·te·al·le·o·sis
os·te·al·loe·o·sis
  var of os·te·al·le·o·sis
os·te·an·a·gen·e·sis
os·te·a·naph·y·sis
os·te·ar·thri·tis
os·te·ar·throt·o·my
os·tec·to·my
  pl os·tec·to·mies
os·tec·to·py
os·te·ec·to·my
os·te·ec·to·pi·a
os·te·in
os·te·ine
  var of os·te·in
os·te·it·ic
os·te·i·tis
  pl os·te·i·ti·des
os·te·i·tis de·for·mans
os·te·i·tis fi·bro·sa
ost·em·bry·on
os·tem·py·e·sis
os·te·o·an·a·gen·e·sis
os·te·o·an·eu·rysm
os·te·o·ar·threc·to·my
os·te·o·ar·thrit·ic
os·te·o·ar·thri·tis
  pl os·te·o·ar·thri·ti·des
os·te·o·ar·throp·a·thy
  pl os·te·o·ar·throp·a·thies
os·te·o·ar·thro·sis
os·te·o·ar·throt·o·my
  pl os·te·o·ar·throt·o·mies
os·te·o·blast
os·te·o·blas·tic
os·te·o·blas·to·ma
  pl os·te·o·blas·to·mas
  or os·te·o·blas·to·ma·ta
os·te·o·camp·si·a

os·te·o·car·ci·no·ma
pl os·te·o·car·ci·no·mas
or os·te·o·car·ci·no·ma·ta
os·te·o·car·ti·lag·i·nous
os·te·o·chon·dral
or os·te·o·chon·drous
os·te·o·chon·dri·tis
os·te·o·chon·dro·dys·pla·
si·a
os·te·o·chon·dro·dys·tro·
phi·a de·for·mans
os·te·o·chon·dro·dys·tro·
phy
os·te·o·chon·dro·ly·sis
os·te·o·chon·dro·ma
pl os·te·o·chon·dro·mas
or os·te·o·chon·dro·ma·ta
os·te·o·chon·dro·ma·to·sis
os·te·o·chon·dro·myx·o·ma
pl os·te·o·chon·dro·myx·o·
mas
or os·te·o·chon·dro·myx·o·
ma·ta
os·te·o·chon·dro·myx·o·
sar·co·ma
pl os·te·o·chon·dro·myx·o·
sar·co·mas
or os·te·o·chon·dro·myx·o·
sar·co·ma·ta
os·te·o·chon·drop·a·thy
pl os·te·o·chon·drop·a·thies
os·te·o·chon·dro·sar·co·ma
pl os·te·o·chon·dro·sar·co·
mas
or os·te·o·chon·dro·sar·co·
ma·ta
os·te·o·chon·dro·sis
pl os·te·o·chon·dro·ses
os·te·o·chon·drot·ic
os·te·o·chon·drous
or os·te·o·chon·dral
os·te·oc·la·sis
os·te·o·clast
os·te·o·clas·tic
os·te·o·clas·to·ma
pl os·te·o·clas·to·mas
or os·te·o·clas·to·ma·ta
os·te·o·com·ma
os·te·o·cope

os·te·o·cop·ic
os·te·o·cra·ni·um
pl os·te·o·cra·ni·ums
or os·te·o·cra·ni·a
os·te·o·cys·to·ma
pl os·te·o·cys·to·mas
or os·te·o·cys·to·ma·ta
os·te·o·cyte
os·te·o·den·tin
or os·te·o·den·tine
os·te·o·den·tine
or os·te·o·den·tin
os·te·o·der·ma·to·plas·tic
os·te·o·der·ma·tous
or os·te·o·der·mous
os·te·o·der·mi·a
os·te·o·der·mous
or os·te·o·der·ma·tous
os·teo·di·as·ta·sis
os·te·o·dyn·i·a
os·te·o·dys·tro·phi·a
os·te·o·dys·tro·phy
pl os·te·o·dys·tro·phies
os·te·o·e·piph·y·sis
os·te·o·fi·bro·chon·dro·ma
pl os·te·o·fi·bro·chon·dro·
mas
or os·te·o·fi·bro·chon·dro·
ma·ta
os·te·o·fi·bro·li·po·ma
pl os·te·o·fi·bro·li·po·mas
or os·te·o·fi·bro·li·po·ma·ta
os·te·o·fi·bro·ma
pl os·te·o·fi·bro·ma
or os·te·o·fi·bro·ma·ta
os·te·o·fi·bro·sar·co·ma
pl os·te·o·fi·bro·sar·co·ma·
ta
or os·te·o·fi·bro·sar·co·mas
os·te·o·fi·bro·sis
pl os·te·o·fi·bro·ses
os·te·o·fi·brous
os·te·o·gen
os·te·o·gen·e·sis
pl os·te·o·gen·e·ses
os·te·o·gen·e·sis im·per·
fec·ta
os·te·o·ge·net·ic
or os·te·o·gen·ic

os·te·o·gen·ic
or os·te·o·ge·net·ic
os·te·og·e·nous
os·te·og·e·ny
os·te·og·ra·phy
pl os·te·og·ra·phies
os·te·o·hal·i·ste·re·sis
os·te·o·hy·per·troph·ic
os·te·oid
os·te·o·lath·y·rism
os·te·o·lip·o·chon·dro·ma
pl os·te·o·lip·o·chon·dro·
mas
or os·te·o·lip·o·chon·dro·
ma·ta
os·te·o·lith
os·te·o·lo·gi·a
os·te·o·log·ic
or os·te·o·log·i·cal
os·te·o·log·i·cal
or os·te·o·log·ic
os·te·o·log·i·cal·ly
os·te·ol·o·gist
os·te·ol·o·gy
pl os·te·ol·o·gies
os·te·ol·y·sis
pl os·te·ol·y·ses
os·te·o·lyt·ic
os·te·o·ma
pl os·te·o·mas
or os·te·o·ma·ta
os·te·o·ma·la·ci·a
os·te·o·ma·la·ci·al
os·te·o·ma·la·cic
os·te·o·ma·toid
os·te·o·ma·to·sis
os·te·o·ma·tous
os·te·o·mere
os·te·o·met·ric
or os·te·o·met·ri·cal
os·te·o·met·ri·cal
or os·te·o·met·ric
os·te·om·e·try
pl os·te·om·e·tries
os·te·o·mu·coid
os·te·o·my·e·lit·ic
os·te·o·my·e·li·tis
pl os·te·o·my·e·li·ti·des
os·te·o·my·e·lo·dys·pla·si·a

os·te·o·myx·o·chon·dro·ma
  pl os·te·o·myx·o·chon·dro·
    mas
  or os·te·o·myx·o·chon·dro·
    ma·ta
os·te·on
os·te·o·ne·cro·sis
  pl os·te·o·ne·cro·ses
os·te·o·ne·phrop·a·thy
os·te·o·neu·ral·gi·a
os·te·o·on·y·cho·dys·tro·
  phi·a
os·te·o·pae·di·on
  var of os·te·o·pe·di·on
os·te·o·path
os·te·o·path·i·a
os·te·o·path·ic
os·te·o·path·i·cal·ly
os·te·op·a·thist
os·te·op·a·thy
  pl os·te·op·a·thies
os·te·o·pe·cil·i·a
os·te·o·pe·di·on
os·te·o·pe·ni·a
os·te·o·per·i·os·te·al
os·te·o·per·i·os·ti·tis
os·te·o·pe·tro·sis
  pl os·te·o·pe·tro·ses
os·te·o·pe·trot·ic
os·te·o·phage
os·te·o·pha·gi·a
os·te·o·oph·o·ny
os·te·o·phle·bi·tis
os·te·o·phore
os·te·o·oph·thi·sis
os·te·o·phy·ma
os·te·o·phyte
os·te·o·phyt·ic
os·te·o·phy·to·sis
os·te·o·plaque
os·te·o·plast
os·te·o·plas·tic
os·te·o·plas·ty
  pl os·te·o·plas·ties
os·te·o·poi·ki·lo·sis
os·te·o·po·ro·sis
  pl os·te·o·po·ro·ses
os·te·o·po·rot·ic
os·te·op·sath·y·ro·sis

pl os·te·op·sath·y·ro·ses
os·te·o·pul·mo·nar·y
os·te·o·ra·di·o·ne·cro·sis
  pl os·te·o·ra·di·o·ne·cro·ses
or·te·or·rha·gi·a
os·te·or·rha·phy
os·te·o·sar·co·ma
  pl os·te·o·sar·co·mas
  or os·te·o·sar·co·ma·ta
os·te·o·sar·co·ma·tous
os·te·o·scle·ro·sis
  pl os·te·o·scle·ro·ses
os·te·o·scle·rot·ic
os·te·o·sis
os·te·o·spon·gi·o·ma
  pl os·te·o·spon·gi·o·mas
  or os·te·o·spon·gi·o·ma·ta
os·te·o·stix·is
os·te·o·su·ture
os·te·o·syn·o·vi·tis
os·te·o·syn·the·sis
  pl os·te·o·syn·the·ses
os·te·o·ta·bes
os·te·o·throm·bo·sis
os·te·o·tome
os·te·o·to·mo·cla·si·a
os·te·o·to·moc·la·sis
os·te·ot·o·my
  pl os·te·ot·o·mies
os·te·o·tribe
os·te·o·trite
os·te·ot·ro·phy
Os·ter·ta·gi·a
os·ti·a
os·ti·al
os·ti·tis
os·ti·um
  pl os·ti·a
os·to·mate
os·to·my
  pl os·to·mies
os·to·sis
os·tre·o·tox·ism
ot·ac·a·ri·a·sis
  pl ot·ac·a·ri·a·ses
ot·a·cous·tic
o·tal·gi·a
o·tal·gic
o·tan·tri·tis

o·tec·to·my
ot·hae·ma·to·ma
  pl ot·hae·ma·to·mas
  or ot·hae·ma·to·ma·ta
  var of ot·he·ma·to·ma
ot·haem·or·rha·gi·a
  var of ot·hem·or·rha·gi·a
ot·haem·or·rhoe·a
  var of ot·hem·or·rhe·a
o·thel·co·sis
ot·he·ma·to·ma
ot·hem·or·rha·gi·a
ot·hem·or·rhe·a
o·tic
o·ti·co·din·i·a
o·tit·ic
o·tit·is
  pl o·ti·ti·des
oti·tis ex·ter·na
oti·tis me·di·a
o·to·ac·a·ri·a·sis
o·to·an·tri·tis
O·to·bi·us
o·to·blen·nor·rhe·a
o·to·blen·nor·rhoe·a
  var of o·to·blen·nor·rhe·a
o·to·ca·tarrh
o·to·ce·phal·ic
o·to·ceph·a·lus
o·to·ceph·a·ly
  pl o·to·ceph·a·lies
o·to·clei·sis
o·to·co·ni·um
  pl o·to·co·ni·a
o·to·cra·ni·um
o·to·cyst
o·to·cys·tic
O·to·dec·tes
oto·dec·tic
o·to·dyn·i·a
o·to·en·ceph·a·li·tis
o·to·gan·gli·on
o·to·gen·ic
  or o·tog·e·nous
o·tog·e·nous
  or o·to·gen·ic
o·tog·ra·phy
o·to·hem·i·neur·as·the·ni·a
o·to·lar·yn·go·log·i·cal

o·to·lar·yn·gol·o·gist
o·to·lar·yn·gol·o·gy
  pl o·to·lar·yn·gol·o·gies
o·to·lith
o·to·lith·ic
o·to·log·ic
  or o·to·log·i·cal
o·to·log·i·cal
  or o·to·log·ic
o·to·log·i·cal·ly
o·tol·o·gist
o·tol·o·gy
  pl o·tol·o·gies
o·to·mu·cor·my·co·sis
o·to·my·as·the·ni·a
o·to·my·co·sis
  pl o·to·my·co·ses
o·to·my·cot·ic
o·to·neu·ral·gi·a
o·to·neur·as·the·ni·a
o·top·a·thy
o·to·pha·ryn·ge·al
o·to·plas·ty
  pl o·to·plas·ties
o·to·pol·y·pus
o·to·py·or·rhe·a
o·to·py·or·rhoe·a
  var of o·to·py·or·rhe·a
o·to·py·o·sis
o·to·rhi·no·lar·yn·gol·o·gy
  pl o·to·rhi·no·lar·yn·gol·o·
    gies
o·to·rhi·nol·o·gy
o·to·rha·gi·a
o·tor·rhe·a
o·tor·rhoe·a
  var of o·tor·rhe·a
o·to·rhi·nol·o·gy
o·to·sal·pinx
  pl o·to·sal·pin·ges
o·to·scle·ro·sis
  pl o·to·scle·ro·ses
o·to·scle·rot·ic
o·to·scope
o·to·scop·ic
o·tos·co·py
  pl o·tos·co·pies
o·to·sis
  pl o·to·ses

o·tos·te·al
o·tos·te·on
o·tot·o·my
  pl o·tot·o·mies
o·to·tox·ic
o·to·tox·ic·i·ty
  pl o·to·tox·ic·i·ties
Ott pre·cip·i·ta·tion test
ot·to
Ot·to dis·ease
oua·bain
Ouch·ter·lo·ny tech·nique
ou·la
ou·loid
ounce
out·flow
out·growth
out·let
out·pa·tient
out·pock·et·ing
out·pouch·ing
out·put
o·val
ov·al·bu·min
o·va·le
o·val·o·cyte
o·val·o·cyt·ic
o·val·o·cy·to·sis
  pl o·val·o·cy·to·ses
o·var·i·al
o·var·i·al·gi·a
o·var·i·an
o·var·i·ec·to·mize
o·var·i·ec·to·my
o·var·i·o·cele
o·var·i·o·cen·te·sis
o·var·i·o·cy·e·sis
o·var·i·o·dys·neu·ri·a
o·var·i·o·gen·ic
o·var·i·o·hys·ter·ec·to·my
  pl o·var·i·o·hys·ter·ec·to·
    mies
o·var·i·o·lyt·ic
o·var·i·on·cus
o·var·i·o·pex·y
o·var·i·or·rhex·is
o·var·i·o·sal·pin·gec·to·my
o·var·i·o·ste·re·sis
o·var·i·os·to·my

o·var·i·o·tes·tis
  pl o·var·i·o·tes·tes
o·var·i·ot·o·my
  pl o·var·i·ot·o·mies
o·var·i·o·tu·bal
o·va·ri·tis
  pl o·va·ri·ti·des
o·var·i·um
  pl o·var·i·a
o·va·ry
  pl o·va·ries
o·va·tes·ti·cu·lar
o·ver·a·chieve
o·ver·a·chiev·er
o·ver·bite
o·ver·com·pen·sate
o·ver·com·pen·sa·tion
o·ver·cor·rec·tion
o·ver·de·pen·den·cy
o·ver·de·ter·mi·na·tion
o·ver·dos·age
o·ver·dose
o·ver·ex·ten·sion
o·ver·flex·ion
o·ver·growth
o·ver·hang
o·ver·hy·dra·tion
o·ver·jet
o·ver·lay
o·ver·ly·ing
o·ver·max·i·mal
o·ver·nu·tri·tion
o·ver·pro·tec·tion
o·ver·rid·ing
o·vert
O·ver·ton the·o·ry
o·ver·ven·ti·la·tion
o·ver·weight
o·vi·cap·sule
o·vi·cid·al
o·vi·cide
o·vi·du·cal
o·vi·duct
o·vi·duc·tal
o·vif·er·ous
o·vi·fi·ca·tion
o·vi·form
o·vi·gen·e·sis
  pl o·vi·gen·e·ses

o·vi·ge·net·ic
o·vig·e·nous
o·vi·germ
o·vig·er·ous
o·vi·na·tion
o·vine
o·vip·a·rous
o·vip·a·rous·ly
o·vip·a·rous·ness
o·vi·pos·it
o·vi·po·si·tion
o·vi·po·si·tion·al
o·vi·pos·i·tor
o·vi·sac
o·vo·cen·ter
o·vo·cyte
o·vo·fla·vin
o·vo·gen·e·sis
   pl o·vo·gen·e·ses
o·vo·glob·u·lin
o·vo·go·ni·um
o·void
o·vo·mu·cin
o·vo·mu·coid
o·vo·plasm
o·vo·plas·mic
o·vo·tes·tic·u·lar
o·vo·tes·tis
   pl o·vo·tes·tes
o·vo·tid
o·vo·vi·tel·lin
o·vo·viv·i·par·i·ty
   pl o·vo·viv·i·par·i·ties
o·vo·vi·vip·a·rous
o·vo·vi·vip·a·rous·ly
o·vo·vi·vip·a·rous·ness
o·vu·lar
o·vu·late
o·vu·la·tion
o·vu·la·tion·al
o·vu·la·to·ry
o·vule
o·vu·log·e·nous
o·vu·lum
   pl o·vu·la
o·vum
   pl o·va
Ow·ren dis·ease
ox·a·cil·lin

ox·al·ac·e·tate
ox·al·a·ce·tic
ox·a·lae·mia
   var of ox·a·le·mi·a
ox·a·late
ox·a·le·mi·a
ox·al·ic
ox·a·lism
ox·a·lo·ac·e·tate
ox·a·lo·a·ce·tic
ox·a·lo·sis
ox·a·lo·suc·cin·ic
ox·al·u·ri·a
ox·al·u·ric
ox·a·lyl
ox·a·lyl·u·re·a
ox·am·ide
ox·am·i·dine
ox·an·a·mide
ox·an·dro·lone
ox·az·e·pam
ox·a·zine
ox·a·zol·i·dine
ox·eth·a·zaine
Ox·ford u·nit
ox·gall
ox·i·dant
ox·i·dase
ox·i·da·sic
ox·i·date
ox·i·da·tion
ox·i·da·tion-re·duc·tion
ox·i·da·tive
ox·i·da·tive·ly
ox·ide
ox·id·ic
ox·i·di·za·tion
ox·i·dize
ox·i·do·re·duc·tase
ox·ime
ox·im·e·ter
ox·i·met·ric
ox·im·e·try
   pl ox·im·e·tries
ox·o·ges·tone
ox·o·i·som·er·ase
ox·o·ni·um
ox·o·phen·ar·sine
ox·o·trem·o·rine

ox·pren·o·lol
ox·tri·phyl·line
ox·y
ox·y·a·can·thine
ox·y·ac·id
ox·y·a·co·a
ox·y·aes·the·si·a
   var of ox·y·es·the·si·a
ox·y·a·koi·a
ox·y·a·phi·a
ox·y·ben·zone
ox·y·bi·o·tin
ox·y·blep·si·a
ox·y·bu·ty·nin
ox·y·cal·o·rim·e·ter
ox·y·ce·phal·ic
   or ox·y·ceph·a·lous
ox·y·ceph·a·lous
   or ox·y·ce·phal·ic
ox·y·ceph·a·ly
   pl ox·y·ceph·a·lies
ox·y·chlo·ride
ox·y·chro·mat·ic
   or ox·y·chro·ma·tin·ic
ox·y·chro·ma·tin
ox·y·chro·ma·tin·ic
   or ox·y·chro·mat·ic
ox·y·ci·ne·si·a
ox·y·ci·ne·sis
ox·y·co·done
ox·y·cor·ti·co·ste·roid
ox·y·dase
   var of ox·i·dase
ox·y·es·the·si·a
ox·y·gen
ox·y·gen·ase
ox·y·gen·ate
ox·y·gen·a·tion
ox·y·gen·a·tor
ox·y·gen·ic
ox·y·gen·ic·i·ty
   pl ox·y·gen·ic·i·ties
ox·y·gen·ize
ox·y·geu·si·a
ox·y·hem·a·tin
ox·y·hem·a·to·por·phy·rin
ox·y·he·mo·glo·bin
ox·y·hy·dro·gen
ox·y·i·o·dide

ox·y·la·li·a
ox·y·mel
ox·y·me·taz·o·line
ox·ym·e·ter
  var of ox·im·e·ter
ox·y·meth·o·lone
ox·ym·e·try
  var of ox·im·e·try
ox·y·mor·phone
ox·y·my·o·glo·bin
ox·y·ner·von
ox·y·ner·von·ic
ox·y·neu·rine
ox·yn·tic
ox·y·opi·a
  or ox·y·o·py
ox·y·op·ter
ox·y·o·py
  pl ox·y·o·pies
  or ox·y·o·pi·a
ox·y·os·mi·a
ox·y·os·phre·si·a
ox·yp·a·thy
ox·y·per·tine
ox·y·phen·bu·ta·zone

ox·y·phen·cy·cli·mine
ox·y·phen·ic
ox·y·phen·i·sa·tin
ox·y·phe·no·ni·um
ox·y·phil
ox·y·phil·i·a
ox·y·phil·ic
  or ox·yph·i·lous
ox·yph·i·lous
  or ox·y·phil·ic
ox·y·pho·ni·a
ox·y·pol·y·gel·a·tin
ox·y·pro·line
ox·y·pu·ri·nol
ox·y·quin·o·line
ox·y·rhine
ox·y·some
Ox·y·spi·ru·ra
ox·y·ste·roid
ox·yt·a·lan
ox·y·tet·ra·cy·cline
ox·y·thi·a·mine
ox·y·to·ci·a
ox·y·to·cic
ox·y·to·cin

ox·y·u·ri·a·sis
  pl ox·y·u·ri·a·ses
ox·y·u·ric
ox·y·u·ri·cide
ox·y·u·rid
Ox·y·u·ri·dae
Ox·y·u·ris
o·zae·na
  var of o·ze·na
o·ze·na
o·zo·chro·ti·a
o·zoch·ro·tous
o·zoe·na
  var of o·ze·na
o·zo·ker·ite
o·zo·na·tor
o·zone
o·zon·ide
o·zo·ni·za·tion
o·zo·nize
o·zo·niz·er
o·zo·nol·y·sis
  pl o·zo·nol·y·ses
o·zo·nom·e·ter
o·zo·sto·mi·a

P

P pul·mo·nale
pab·u·lum
Pac·chi·o·ni·an·bod·y,
  cor·pus·cle
pace·mak·er
pa·chom·e·ter
pach·y·ac·ri·a
pach·y·bleph·a·ron
pach·y·bleph·a·ro·sis
pach·y·ce·pha·li·a
  or pach·y·ceph·a·ly
pach·y·ce·phal·ic
pach·y·ceph·a·lous

pach·y·ceph·a·ly
  pl pach·y·ceph·a·ly
  or pach·y·ac·pha·li·a
pach·y·chei·li·a
  or pach·y·chi·li·a
pach·y·chi·li·a
  or pach·y·chei·li·a
pach·y·chro·mat·ic
pach·y·dac·tyl·i·a
pach·y·dac·ty·ly
pach·y·der·ma
pach·y·der·ma·to·cele
pach·y·der·ma·to·sis

pach·y·der·ma·tous
pach·y·der·mi·a
pach·y·der·mi·al
pach·y·der·mic
pach·y·glos·si·a
pach·y·gy·ri·a
pach·y·haem·a·tous
  var of pach·y·hem·a·**tous**
pach·y·hem·a·tous
pach·y·hy·men·ic
pach·y·lep·to·men·in·gi·tis
  pl pach·y·lep·to·men·
    in·ti·ti·des

pach·y·lo·sis
pach·y·men·in·git·ic
pach·y·men·in·gi·tis
    pl pach·y·men·in·gi·ti·des
pach·y·men·in·gop·a·thy
pach·y·me·ninx
    pl pach·y·me·nin·ges
pach·y·ne·ma
pa·chyn·sis
pa·chyn·tic
pach·y·o·nych·i·a
pach·y·o·ti·a
pach·y·pel·vi·per·i·to·ni·tis
pach·y·per·i·os·to·sis
pach·y·per·i·to·ni·tis
pa·chyp·o·dous
pach·y·rhine
pach·y·rhi·nic
pach·y·sal·pin·go·o·o·the·ci·tis
pach·y·sal·pin·go·o·va·ri·tis
pach·y·tene
pach·y·tes
pa·chyt·ic
pach·y·vag·i·ni·tis
pac·i·fi·er
Pa·ci·ni cor·pus·cle
    or pa·cin·i·an cor·pus·cle
pa·cin·i·an cor·pus·cle
    or Pa·ci·ni cor·pus·cle
pack
pack·er
pad
Padg·ett op·er·a·tion
pae·di·a·tric
    var of pe·di·a·tric
pae·di·at·rics
    var of pe·di·a·trics
pae·do·phil·i·a
    var of pe·do·phil·i·a
Page syn·drome
page·ism
pa·get can·cer
pag·et·oid
pa·go·pha·gi·a
pa·go·plex·i·a

pain
pain·ful
pain·kill·er
pain·kill·ing
pain·less
paired-as·so·ci·ate learn·ing
pa·ja·huel·lo
    or pa·ja·ro·el·lo
pa·ja·ro·el·lo
    or pa·ja·huel·lo
pal·a·dang
pal·a·tal
pal·ate
pa·lat·ic
pa·lat·i·form
pal·a·tine
pal·a·ti·tis
pal·a·to·glos·sal
pal·a·to·glos·sus
    pl pal·a·to·glos·si
pal·a·to·gram
pal·a·to·graph
pal·a·to·graph·ic
pal·a·tog·ra·phy
    pl pal·a·tog·ra·phies
pal·a·to·max·il·lar·y
pal·a·to·my·o·graph
pal·a·to·na·sal
pal·a·top·a·gus par·a·sit·i·cus
pal·a·to·pha·ryn·ge·al
pal·a·to·pha·ryn·ge·us
pal·a·to·plas·ty
    pl pal·a·to·plas·ties
pal·a·to·ple·gi·a
pal·a·to·pter·y·goid
pal·a·tor·rha·phy
    pl pal·a·tor·rha·phies
pal·a·to·sal·pin·ge·us
pal·a·tos·chi·sis
    pl pal·a·tos·chi·si·es
    or pal·a·tos·chi·ses
pal·a·tum
    pl pal·a·ta
pa·le·en·ceph·a·lon
    pl pa·le·en·ceph·a·la
pa·le·o·cer·e·bel·lar

pa·le·o·cer·e·bel·lum
    pl pa·le·o·cer·e·bel·lums
    or pa·le·o·cer·e·bel·la
pa·le·o·cor·tex
    pl pa·le·o·cor·ti·ces
pa·le·o·en·ceph·a·lon
    pl pa·le·o·en·ceph·a·la
pa·le·o·gen·e·sis
pa·le·o·ki·net·ic
pa·le·on·tol·o·gy
pa·le·o·ol·ive
pa·le·o·pal·li·um
    pl pa·le·o·pal·li·ums
    or pa·le·o·pal·li·a
pa·le·o·pa·thol·o·gy
pa·le·o·sen·si·bil·i·ties
pa·le·o·stri·a·tal
pa·le·o·stri·a·tum
    pl pa·le·o·stri·a·ta
pa·le·o·thal·a·mus
    pl pa·le·o·thal·a·mi
pa·li·ki·ne·si·a
pa·li·ki·ne·sis
pal·i·la·li·a
pal·in·dro·mi·a
pal·in·drom·ic
pal·in·drom·i·cal·ly
pal·in·gen·e·sis
pal·in·graph·i·a
pal·i·nop·si·a
pal·in·phra·si·a
pal·i·phra·si·a
pal·ir·rhe·a
pal·ir·rhoe·a
    var of pal·ir·rhe·a
pal·la·di·um
pall·aes·the·si·a
    var of pall·es·the·si·a
pall·an·aes·the·si·a
    var of pall·an·es·the·si·a
pall·an·es·the·si·a
pall·es·the·si·a
pal·li·al
pal·li·ate
pal·li·a·tion
pal·li·a·tive
pal·li·a·tive·ly

pal·li·dal
pal·li·do·hy·po·tha·lam·ic
pal·li·doi·do·sis
pal·li·do·py·ram·i·dal
pal·li·do·re·tic·u·lar
pal·li·do·sub·tha·lam·ic
pal·li·dot·o·my
pal·li·o·pon·tine
pal·li·um
pl pal·li·ums
or pal·li·a
pal·lor
palm
pal·ma
pl pal·mae
pal·mar
pal·mar·is
pl pal·mar·es
pal·mate
pal·ma·ture
pal·mel·lin
pal·mer meth·od
pal·mi·ped
pal·mi·tate
pal·mit·ic
pal·mi·tin
pal·mi·tyl
pal·mod·ic
pal·mo·men·tal
pal·mo·plan·tar
pal·mo·spas·mus
pal·mus
pl pal·mi
pal·pa·ble
pal·pate
pal·pa·tion
pal·pa·to·per·cus·sion
pal·pa·to·ry
pal·pe·bra
pl pal·pe·brae
pal·pe·bral
pal·pe·brate
pal·pe·bra·tion
pal·pe·bri·tis
pal·pi·tate
pal·pi·ta·tion
pal·sied
pal·sy
pl pal·sies

Pal·tauf dwarf·ism
Pal·tauf-Stern·berg
    dis·ease
pa·lu·dal
pal·u·dide
pal·u·dism
pal·lus·tral
Pal-Wei·gert meth·od
pam·a·quin
    or pam·a·quine
pam·a·quine
    or pam·a·quin
pam·o·ate
pam·pin·i·form
Pan
pan·a·ce·a
pan·ac·i·nar
pan·aes·the·si·a
    var of pan·es·the·si·a
pan·ag·glu·ti·na·bil·i·ty
    pl pan·ag·glu·ti·na·bil·i·ties
pan·ag·glu·ti·na·ble
pan·ag·glu·ti·na·tion
pan·ag·glu·ti·nin
pan·an·aes·the·si·a
    var of pan·an·es·the·si·a
pan·an·es·the·si·a
pan·a·ris
pan·a·ri·ti·um
    pl pan·a·ri·ti·a
pan·ar·te·ri·tis
pan·ar·thri·tis
    pl pan·ar·thri·ti·des
pan·at·ro·phy
    pl pan·at·ro·phies
pan·blas·to·trop·ic
pan·car·di·tis
pan·cav·er·no·si·tis
pan·chrome
Pan·coast op·er·a·tion
pan·co·lec·to·my
    pl pan·co·lec·to·mies
pan·col·po·hys·ter·
    ec·to·my
pan·cre·as
    pl pan·cre·a·ta
pan·cre·a·tec·to·mize
pan·cre·a·tec·to·my
    pl pan·cre·a·tec·to·mies

pan·cre·at·ic
pan·cre·at·i·co·du·o·de·nal
pan·cre·at·i·co·du·o·
    de·nec·to·my
pan·cre·at·i·co·du·o·
    de·nos·to·my
pan·cre·at·i·co·en·
    ter·os·to·my
    pl pan·cre·at·i·co·en·
    ter·os·to·mies
pan·cre·at·i·co·gas·
    tros·to·my
    pl pan·cre·at·i·co·gas·
    tros·to·mies
pan·cre·at·i·co·je·
    ju·nos·to·my
    pl pan·cre·at·i·co·
    je·ju·nos·to·mies
pan·cre·at·i·co·li·thot·o·my
pan·cre·at·i·co·splen·ic
pan·cre·a·tin
pan·cre·a·tism
pan·cre·a·ti·tis
    pl pan·cre·a·ti·ti·des
pan·cre·a·to·du·o·de·
    nec·to·my
pan·cre·a·to·du·o·
    de·nos·to·my
pan·cre·a·to·en·ter·os·
    to·my
pan·cre·a·tog·e·nous
pan·cre·a·to·li·pase
pan·cre·at·o·lith
pan·cre·a·to·li·thec·to·my
pan·cre·a·to·li·thot·o·my
    pl pan·cre·a·to·li·thot·
    o·mies
pan·cre·a·tol·y·sis
pan·cre·a·to·lyt·ic
pan·cre·a·tot·o·my
    pl pan·cre·a·tot·o·mies
pan·cre·ec·to·my
pan·cre·li·pase
pan·cre·o·lith
pan·cre·o·li·thot·o·my
pan·cre·ol·y·sis
pan·cre·o·path·i·a
pan·cre·op·a·thy
pan·cre·o·zyme

283

pan·cre·o·zy·min
pan·cu·ro·ni·um
pan·cy·to·pe·ni·a
pan·cy·to·pe·nic
pan·de·mi·a
pan·dem·ic
pan·de·my
pan·dic·u·la·tion
Pan·dy re·a·gent
pan·e·lec·tro·scope
pan·en·ceph·a·li·tis
pan·en·do·scope
pan·en·do·scop·ic
pan·en·dos·co·py
    pl pan·en·dos·co·pies
pan·es·the·si·a
Pa·neth cells
pang
Pang·born test
pan·gen·e·sis
pan·glos·si·a
pan·haem·a·to·pe·ni·a
    var of pan·hem·a·to·pen·i·a
pan·hem·a·to·pe·ni·a
pan·hi·dro·sis
pan·hy·grous
pan·hy·po·go·nad·ism
pan·hy·po·pi·tu·i·ta·rism
pan·hy·po·pi·tu·i·tar·y
pan·hys·ter·ec·to·my
    pl pan·hys·ter·ec·to·mies
pan·hys·ter·o·col·
    pec·to·my
pan·hys·ter·o-
    o·oph·o·rec·to·my
pan·hys·ter·o·sal·
    pin·gec·to·my
    pl pan·hys·ter·o·sal·
    pin·gec·to·mies
pan·hys·ter·o·sal·pin·go-
    o·oph·o·rec·to·my
    pl pan·hys·ter·o·sal·pin·go-
    o·oph·o·rec·to·mies
pan·ic
pan·im·mu·ni·ty
pa·niv·o·rous
pan·leu·co·pe·ni·a
    var of pan·leu·ko·pe·ni·a
pan·leu·ko·pe·ni·a

pan·lob·u·lar
pan·me·tri·tis
pan·mne·si·a
pan·my·e·lop·a·thy
    pl pan·my·e·lop·a·thies
pan·my·e·lo·phthi·sis
    pl pan·my·e·lo·phthi·ses
pan·my·e·lo·sis
pan·my·e·lo·tox·i·co·sis
pan·my·o·si·tis
Pan·ner dis·ease
pan·nic·u·li·tis
pan·nic·u·lus
    pl pan·nic·u·li
pan·nus
    pl pan·ni
pan·o·pho·bi·a
pan·oph·thal·mi·a
pan·oph·thal·mi·tis
pan·op·tic
    or pan·op·ti·cal
pan·op·ti·cal
    or pan·op·tic
pan·os·te·i·tis
pan·o·ti·tis
    pl pan·o·ti·ti·des
pan·phar·ma·con
pan·phle·bi·tis
pan·pho·bi·a
pan·scle·ro·sis
    pl pan·scle·ro·ses
pan·si·nus·i·tis
pan·sper·ma·tism
    or pan·sper·mi·a
pan·sper·mi·a
    or pan·sper·ma·tism
Pan·stron·gy·lus
pan·sys·tol·ic
pant
pan·ta·mor·phi·a
pan·ta·mor·phic
pan·tan·en·ce·pha·li·a
pan·tan·en·ce·phal·ic
pan·tan·en·ceph·a·lus
pan·tan·ky·lo·bleph·a·ron
pan·ta·pho·bi·a
pan·ta·som·a·tous
pan·ta·tro·phi·a
pan·tat·ro·phy

pan·te·the·ine
pan·te·thine
pan·the·nol
pan·ther·a·pist
pan·to·graph
pan·to·ic
pan·to·mime
pan·to·mim·ic
pan·to·pho·bi·a
pan·top·to·sis
pan·to·scop·ic
pan·to·som·a·tous
pan·to·then·ate
pan·to·then·ic
pan·to·then·yl
pan·to·yl-be·ta-al·a·nine
pan·trop·ic
Pa·num ar·e·as
pa·nus
    pl pa·ni
pan·u·ve·i·tis
pan·zo·ot·ic
Pap smear, test
pa·pa·in
Pap·a·nic·o·la·ou test
Pa·pa·ver
pa·pav·er·a·mine
pa·pav·er·ine
pa·paw
pa·pa·ya
pa·pes·cent
Pa·pez cir·cuit
pa·pil·la
    pl pa·pil·lae
pa·pil·la of Va·ter
pap·il·lar
pap·il·lar·y
pap·il·late
    or pap·il·lat·ed
pap·il·lat·ed
    or pap·il·late
pap·il·lec·to·my
    pl pap·il·lec·to·mies
pa·pil·le·de·ma
    pl pa·pil·le·de·mas
    or pa·pil·le·de·ma·ta
pap·il·lif·er·ous
pa·pil·li·form
pap·il·li·tis

pap·il·lo·cys·to·ma
  pl pap·il·lo·cys·to·mas
  or pap·il·lo·cys·to·ma·ta
pa·pil·loe·de·ma
  pl pa·pil·loe·de·mas
  or pa·pil·loe·de·ma·ta
  var of pa·pil·le·de·ma
pap·il·lo·ma
  pl pap·il·lo·mas
  or pap·il·lo·ma·ta
pap·il·lo·mac·u·lar
pap·il·lo·ma·to·sis
  pl pap·il·lo·ma·to·ses
pap·il·lom·a·tous
Pa·pil·lon-Le·fe·vre
  syn·drome
pap·il·lo·ret·i·ni·tis
  pl pap·il·lo·ret·i·ni·ti·des
Pa·pi·o
pa·po·va·vi·rus
pap·pa·ta·ci
Pap·pen·hei·mer bod·ies
pap·pose
  or pap·pous
pap·pous
  or pap·pose
pap·pus
  pl pap·pi
pa·pri·ka
pap·u·la
  pl pap·u·lae
pap·u·lar
pap·u·la·tion
pap·ule
pap·u·lif·er·ous
pap·u·lo·er·y·the·ma·tous
pap·u·lo·ne·crot·ic
pap·u·lo·pus·tu·lar
pap·u·lo·sis
pap·u·lo·squa·mous
pap·u·lo·ve·sic·u·lar
pap·y·ra·ceous
par·a
  pl par·as
  or par·ae
Pa·ra·rub·ber
par·a·a·cet·a·mi·no·phe·nol
par·a·a·mi·no·ben·
  zene·ar·son·ic ac·id
par·a·a·mi·no·ben·zo·ate
par·a·a·mi·no·ben·
  zo·ic ac·id
par·a·a·mi·no·hip·pu·rate
par·a·a·mi·no·hip·
  pu·ric ac·id
par·a·a·mi·no·sa·lic·y·late
par·a·a·mi·no·sal·i·cyl·ic
  ac·id
par·a·am·y·loid
par·a·am·y·loi·do·sis
par·a·an·aes·the·si·a
  var of par·a·an·es·the·si·a
par·a·an·al·ge·si·a
par·a·an·es·the·si·a
par·a·a·or·tic
par·a·ap·pen·di·ci·tis
par·a·ba·sal
par·ab·du·cent
par·a·bi·gem·i·nal
par·a·bi·o·sis
  pl par·a·bi·o·ses
par·a·bi·ot·ic
par·a·bi·ot·i·cal·ly
par·a·blep·si·a
  or par·a·blep·sis
  or par·a·blep·sy
par·a·blep·sis
  pl par·a·blep·ses
  or par·a·blep·si·a
  or par·a·blep·sy
par·a·blep·sy
  pl par·a·blep·sies
  or par·a·blep·si·a
  or par·a·blep·sis
pa·rab·o·loid
pa·ra·bu·li·a
pa·rac·an·tho·ma
  pl pa·rac·an·tho·mas
  or pa·rac·an·tho·ma·ta
pa·rac·an·tho·sis
par·a·ca·ri·nal
par·a·car·mine
par·a·ca·se·in
par·a·ce·cal
par·a·cele
  or par·a·coele
Par·a·cel·si·an
par·a·cen·te·sis
  pl par·a·cen·te·ses
par·a·cen·tral
par·a·ceph·a·lus
par·a·cer·a·to·sis
par·a·chlo·ro·phe·nol
par·a·chol·er·a
par·a·cho·li·a
par·a·chor·dal
par·a·chro·da·li·a
par·a·chro·ma
par·a·chro·ma·tism
par·a·chro·ma·to·blep·si·a
par·a·chro·ma·top·si·a
par·a·chro·ma·to·sis
par·a·chro·mo·phore
par·a·chro·moph·o·rous
par·ac·mas·tic
par·ac·me
par·ac·mic
par·a·coc·cid·i·oi·dal
Par·a·coc·cid·i·oi·des
par·a·coc·cid·i·oi·do·my·
  o·sis
par·a·coele
  or par·a·cele
par·a·co·li·tis
par·a·co·lon
par·a·col·pi·tis
par·a·col·pi·um
par·a·con·dy·lar
par·a·cone
par·a·co·nid
par·a·cu·si·a
  or par·a·cu·sis
par·a·cu·sis
  pl par·a·cu·ses
  or par·a·cu·si·a
par·a·cy·e·sis
par·a·cys·tic
par·a·cys·ti·tis
  pl par·a·cys·ti·ti·des
par·a·cyt·ic
par·a·cys·ti·um
  pl par·a·cys·ti·a
par·ad·e·ni·tis
par·a·den·tal
par·a·den·ti·tis

par·a·den·ti·um
  pl par·a·den·ti·a
par·a·den·to·sis
  pl par·a·den·to·ses
par·a·di·chlo·ro·ben·zene
par·a·did·y·mis
  pl par·a·di·dym·i·des
par·a·dipth·the·ri·al
par·a·diph·the·rit·ic
par·a·dis·tem·per
par·a·dox·i·a sex·u·a·lis
par·a·dox·ic
  or par·a·dox·i·cal
par·a·dox·i·cal
  or par·a·dox·ic
par·a·dox·i·cal sleep
par·a·du·o·de·nal
par·a·dys·en·ter·y
par·a·ep·i·lep·sy
par·a·e·ryth·ro·blast
par·a·e·soph·a·ge·al
par·aes·the·si·a
  var of par·es·the·si·a
par·aes·thet·ic
  var of par·es·thet·ic
par·a·fas·cic·u·lar
par·af·fin
  or par·af·fine
par·af·fine
  or par·af·fin
par·af·fin·o·ma
  pl par·af·fin·o·mas
  or par·af·fin·o·ma·ta
par·a·floc·cu·lus
  pl par·a·floc·cu·li
par·a·fol·lic·u·lar
par·a·form
par·a·for·mal·de·hyde
Par·a·fos·sar·u·lus
par·a·fuch·sin
par·a·gam·ma·cism
  or par·a·gam·ma·cis·mus
par·a·gam·ma·cis·mus
  pl par·a·gam·ma·cis·
    mus·es
  or par·a·gam·ma·cism
par·a·gan·gli·o·ma
  pl par·a·gan·gli·o·mas
  or par·a·gan·gli·o·ma·ta

par·a·gan·gli·on
  pl par·a·gan·gli·ons
  or par·a·gan·gli·a
par·a·gan·gli·o·neu·ro·ma
  pl par·a·gan·gli·
    o·neu·ro·mas
  or par·a·gan·gli·o·neu·
    ro·ma·ta
par·a·gan·gli·on·ic
par·a·gen·i·tal
par·a·gen·i·ta·lis
par·a·geu·si·a
par·a·geu·sic
par·a·geu·sis
par·ag·glu·ti·na·tion
par·a·gle·noi·dal
par·a·glos·sa
  pl par·a·glos·sae
par·a·glos·si·a
pa·rag·na·thus
par·a·gom·pho·sis
par·a·gon·i·mi·a·sis
  pl par·a·gon·i·mi·a·ses
Par·a·gon·i·mus
par·a·gram·ma·tism
par·a·gran·u·lo·ma
par·a·graph·i·a
par·a·graph·ic
par·a·hae·mo·phil·i·a
  var of par·a·he·mo·phil·i·a
par·a·he·mo·phil·i·a
par·a·he·pat·ic
par·a·hep·a·ti·tis
par·a·hex·yl
par·a·hi·a·tal
par·a·hip·po·cam·pal
par·a·hor·mone
  or par·a·hor·mon·ic
par·a·hor·mon·ic
  or par·a·hor·mone
par·a·hy·drox·y·ben·zo·ic
par·a·hyp·no·sis
par·a·in·flu·en·za
par·a·in·flu·en·zal
par·a·ker·a·to·sis
  pl par·a·ker·a·to·ses
par·a·ker·a·tot·ic
par·a·ki·ne·si·a
  or par·a·ki·ne·sis

par·a·ki·ne·sis
  pl par·a·ki·ne·ses
  or par·a·ki·ne·si·a
par·a·ki·net·ic
par·a·lac·tic
par·a·la·li·a
par·a·lamb·da·cism
par·al·bu·min
par·al·de·hyde
par·a·lep·ro·sis
par·a·lep·ro·sy
par·a·lep·sy
par·a·le·re·ma
par·a·le·re·sis
par·a·lex·i·a
pa·ra·lex·ic
par·al·ge·si·a
par·al·ge·sic
par·a·lip·o·pho·bi·a
par·al·lax
par·al·lel·ism
par·al·lel·om·e·ter
par·a·lo·gi·a
par·a·log·i·cal
pa·ral·o·gism
pa·ral·o·gis·tic
par·a·lu·te·in
par·a·ly·sant
  or par·a·ly·zant
pa·ral·y·sis
  pl pa·ral·y·ses
pa·ral·y·sis ag·i·tans
par·a·lys·sa
par·a·lyt·ic
  or par·a·lyt·i·cal
par·a·lyt·i·cal
  or par·a·lyt·ic
par·a·ly·zant
  or par·a·ly·sant
par·a·ly·za·tion
par·a·lyze
par·a·lyz·er
par·a·mag·net·ic
par·a·mag·net·ism
par·a·mam·ma·ry
par·a·ma·ni·a
par·a·mas·ti·tis
  pl par·a·mas·ti·ti·des
par·a·mas·toid

286

par·a·mas·toid·i·tis
Pa·ra·me·ci·um
par·a·me·di·al
par·a·me·di·an
par·a·med·ic
par·a·med·i·cal
par·a·me·ni·a
par·a·men·tal
par·a·mes·o·neph·ric
pa·ram·e·ter
par·a·meth·a·di·one
par·a·meth·a·sone
par·a·me·tri·al
par·a·me·tric
par·a·me·trism
par·a·me·trit·ic
para·me·tri·tis
par·a·me·tri·um
    pl par·a·me·tri·a
par·a·me·trop·a·thy
par·a·mim·i·a
par·a·mi·tome
par·am·ne·si·a
par·am·ne·sis
Par·a·moe·ci·um
    var of Par·a·me·ci·um
par·a·mo·lar
par·a·mor·phine
par·a·mor·phism
Par·am·phis·to·mum
par·a·mu·cin
par·a·mu·si·a
par·a·mu·ta·tion
par·a·my·e·lo·blast
pa·ram·y·loid
pa·ram·y·loi·do·sis
pa·ram·y·lum
par·a·my·oc·lo·nus mul·ti·
    plex
par·a·my·o·sin·o·gen
par·a·my·o·to·ni·a con·gen·
    i·ta
par·a·na·sal
par·a·nee
par·a·ne·mic
par·a·ne·o·plas·tic
par·a·neph·ric
par·a·ne·phri·tis
    pl par·a·ne·phri·ti·des

par·a·neph·ros
    pl par·a·neph·roi
par·a·neu·ral
par·a·neu·tal
pa·ran·gi
par·a·ni·tro·sul·fa·thi·a·zole
par·a·noi·a
par·a·noi·ac
par·a·no·ic
par·a·noid
par·a·noid·ism
par·a·no·mi·a
par·an·tral
par·a·nu·cle·ar
par·a·nu·cle·ate
par·a·nu·cle·in
par·a·nu·cle·o·pro·te·in
par·a·nu·cle·us
    pl par·a·nu·cle·us·es
    or par·a·neu·cle·i
par·a·ny·line
par·a·oc·cip·i·tal
par·a·oe·soph·a·ge·al
    var of par·ae·soph·a·ge·al
par·a·o·ral
par·a·or·tic
par·a·os·ti·al
par·a·ox·on
par·a·pan·cre·at·ic
par·a·pa·re·sis
    pl par·a·pa·re·ses
par·a·pa·ret·ic
par·a·pa·tel·lar
par·a·path·i·a
par·a·pen·zo·late
par·a·per·tus·sis
par·a·pha·ryn·ge·al
par·a·pha·si·a
par·a·pha·sic
par·a·phe·mi·a
par·a·phen·yl·ene·di·am·
    ine
pa·ra·phi·a
par·a·phil·i·a
par·a·phil·i·ac
par·a·phi·mo·sis
    pl par·a·phi·mo·ses
par·a·pho·bi·a

par·a·pho·ni·a
    pl par·a·pho·ni·as
    or par·a·pho·ni·ae
pa·raph·o·ra
par·a·phra·si·a
par·a·phre·ne·sis
par·a·phre·ni·a
par·a·phren·ic
par·a·phre·ni·tis
pa·raph·y·se·al
    or pa·raph·y·si·al
pa·raph·y·si·al
    or pa·raph·y·se·al
pa·raph·y·sis
    pl pa·raph·y·ses
par·a·pla·si·a
par·a·plasm
par·a·plas·tic
par·a·plas·tin
par·a·plec·tic
par·a·ple·gi·a
par·a·ple·gic
par·a·ple·gi·form
par·a·pneu·mo·ni·a
par·ap·o·plex·y
    pl par·ap·o·plex·ies
par·a·prax·i·a
    or par·a·prax·is
par·a·prax·is
    pl par·a·prax·es
    or par·a·prax·i·a
par·a·proc·ti·tis
par·a·proc·ti·um
    pl par·a·proc·ti·a
par·a·pros·ta·ti·tis
par·a·pro·te·in
par·a·pro·te·in·ae·mi·a
    var of par·a·pro·te·in·e·mi·a
par·a·pro·te·in·e·mi·a
par·a·pso·ri·a·sis
    pl par·a·pso·ri·a·ses
par·a·psy·cho·log·i·cal
par·a·psy·chol·o·gist
par·a·psy·chol·o·gy
    pl par·a·psy·chol·o·gies
par·a·pyk·no·mor·phous
par·a·rec·tal
par·a·rho·ta·cism
par·a·ro·san·i·line

par·ar·rhyth·mi·a
par·ar·thri·a
par·a·sa·cral
par·a·sag·it·tal
par·a·sal·pin·gi·tis
Par·as·ca·ris
par·a·scar·la·ti·na
par·a·se·cre·tion
par·a·sel·lar
par·a·sep·tal
par·a·sex·u·al
par·a·sex·u·al·i·ty
   pl par·a·sex·u·al·i·ties
par·a·sig·ma·tism
par·a·si·nus·oi·dal
par·a·si·tae·mi·a
   var of par·a·si·te·mi·a
par·a·site
par·a·si·te·mi·a
par·a·sit·ic
   or par·a·sit·i·cal
par·a·sit·i·cal
   or par·a·sit·ic
par·a·sit·i·cal·ly
par·a·sit·i·ci·dal
par·a·sit·i·cide
par·a·sit·ism
par·a·sit·i·za·tion
par·a·sit·ize
par·a·si·to·gen·ic
par·a·si·to·log·ic
   or par·a·si·to·log·i·cal
par·a·si·to·log·i·cal
   or par·a·si·to·log·ic
par·a·si·tol·o·gist
par·a·si·tol·o·gy
   pl par·a·si·tol·o·gies
par·a·si·to·pho·bi·a
par·a·si·to·sis
   pl par·a·si·to·ses
par·a·si·to·trope
par·a·si·to·trop·ic
par·a·si·tot·ro·pism
par·a·si·tot·ro·py
par·a·small·pox
par·a·some
par·a·spa·di·as
par·a·spasm
par·a·sprue

par·a·ste·a·to·sis
par·a·ster·nal
par·a·ster·nal·ly
par·a·stri·ate
par·a·sym·pa·thet·ic
par·a·sym·pa·thet·i·co·mi·
   met·ic
par·a·sym·path·i·co·to·ni·a
par·a·sym·pa·tho·lyt·ic
par·a·sym·pa·tho·mi·met·ic
par·a·syn·ap·sis
   pl par·a·syn·ap·ses
par·a·syph·i·lis
par·a·syph·i·lit·ic
par·a·sys·to·le
par·a·sys·tol·ic
par·a·tae·ni·al
par·a·tax·i·a
par·a·tax·is
par·a·ten·on
par·a·te·re·si·o·ma·ni·a
par·a·ter·mi·nal
par·a·the·li·o·ma
   pl par·a·the·li·o·mas
   or par·a·the·li·o·ma·ta
par·a·thi·on
par·a·thy·mi·a
par·a·thy·roid
   or par·a·thy·roi·dal
par·a·thy·roi·dal
   or par·a·thy·roid
par·a·thy·roi·dec·to·mized
par·a·thy·roi·dec·to·my
   pl par·a·thy·roi·dec·to·mies
par·a·thy·ro·pri·val
   or par·a·thy·ro·priv·ic
par·a·thy·ro·priv·ic
   or par·a·thy·ro·pri·val
par·a·thy·ro·trop·ic
par·a·thy·ro·tro·pin
par·a·to·ni·a
par·a·ton·sil·lar
par·a·tra·che·al
par·a·tra·cho·ma
par·a·tri·cho·sis
par·a·tri·gem·i·nal
par·a·trip·sis
par·a·troph·ic

pa·rat·ro·phy
   pl pa·rat·ro·phies
par·a·tu·bal
par·a·tu·ber·cu·lin
par·a·tu·ber·cu·lo·sis
   pl par·a·tu·ber·cu·lo·ses
par·a·tu·ber·cu·lous
par·a·typh·li·tis
par·a·ty·phoid
par·a·typ·ic
   or par·a·typ·i·cal
par·a·typ·i·cal
   or par·a·typ·ic
par·a·um·bil·i·cal
par·a·u·re·ter·ic
par·a·u·re·ter·i·tis
par·a·u·re·thral
par·a·u·ter·ine
par·a·vac·cin·i·a
par·a·vag·i·nal
par·a·vag·i·nal·ly
par·a·vag·i·ni·tis
par·a·vas·cu·lar
par·a·ven·tric·u·lar
par·a·ven·tric·u·lo·hy·
   poph·y·se·al
par·a·ver·te·bral
par·a·ver·te·bral·ly
par·a·ves·i·cal
par·a·vi·ta·min·o·sis
   pl par·a·vi·ta·min·o·ses
par·a-Wer·ni·cke en·
   ceph·a·lop·a·thy
par·a·xan·thine
par·ax·i·al
par·ax·i·al·ly
par·ax·on
par·a·zo·on
par·ben·da·zole
Par·dee T wave
par·ec·ta·si·a
   or par·ec·ta·sis
par·ec·ta·sis
   pl par·ec·ta·ses
   or par·ec·ta·si·a
par·e·gor·ic
pa·rei·ra
par·e·le·i·din

a·ren·chy·ma
or pa·ren·chyme
a·ren·chy·mal
or pa·ren·chy·mous
a·ren·chy·mat·ic
or pa·ren·chym·a·tous
ar·en·chym·a·ti·tis
ar·en·chym·a·tous
or pa·ren·chy·mat·ic
a·ren·chy·ma·tous·ly
a·ren·chyme
or pa·ren·chy·ma
a·ren·chy·mous
or pa·ren·chy·mal
ar·ent
a·ren·ter·al
a·ren·ter·al·ly
ar·ep·i·did·y·mis
pl ar·ep·i·did·y·mi·des
ar·ep·i·gas·tric
ar·ep·i·thym·i·a
ar·e·reth·i·sis
ar·er·ga·si·a
a·re·sis
pl pa·re·ses
ar·es·the·si·a
ar·es·thet·ic
ar·eth·ox·y·caine
a·ret·ic
a·ret·i·cal·ly
a·reu·ni·a
ar·fo·cal
ar·gy·line
Ar·ham-Mar·tin band
ar·hi·dro·sis
ar·i·es
pl pa·ri·e·tes
a·ri·e·tal
a·ri·e·to·fron·tal
a·ri·e·to·mas·toid
a·ri·e·to·oc·cip·i·tal
a·ri·e·to·pon·tine
a·ri·e·to·sphe·noid
a·ri·e·to·splanch·nic
a·ri·e·to·squa·mo·sal
a·ri·e·to·tem·po·ral
a·ri·e·to·tem·po·ro·pre·oc·
cip·i·tal
a·ri·e·to·vis·cer·al

Pa·ri·naud syn·drome
par·isth·mi·on
par·i·ty
Park an·eu·rysm
Par·ker flu·id
Parkes Web·er syn·drome
Par·kin·son dis·ease
par·kin·so·ni·an
par·kin·son·ism
Par·num test
par·oc·ci·pi·tal
par·o·don·tal
par·o·don·ti·tis
pl par·o·don·ti·ti·des
par·o·don·ti·um
pl par·o·don·ti·a
par·o·dyn·i·a
pa·role
pa·rol·ee
par·ol·fac·to·ry
par·ol·i·var·y
par·o·mo·my·cin
par·o·ni·ri·a
par·o·nych·i·a
par·o·nych·i·um
pl par·o·nych·i·a
pa·ron·y·cho·my·co·sis
pa·ron·y·cho·sis
par·o·oph·o·ri·tis
par·o·oph·o·ron
par·oph·thal·mi·a
par·oph·thal·mon·cus
par·op·si·a
par·op·sis
par·op·tic
par·o·ra·sis
par·o·rex·i·a
par·os·mi·a
par·os·phre·sis
par·os·te·i·tis
par·os·ti·tis
par·os·to·sis
pa·rot·ic
pa·rot·id
pa·rot·i·dec·to·my
pl pa·rot·i·dec·to·mies
pa·rot·i·di·tis
pl pa·rot·i·di·tis·es
pa·rot·i·do·scle·ro·sis

par·o·tit·ic
par·o·ti·tis
par·ous
par·o·var·i·an
par·o·var·i·ot·o·my
pl par·o·var·i·ot·o·mies
par·o·va·ri·tis
par·o·var·i·um
pl par·o·var·i·a
par·ox·ysm
par·ox·ys·mal
par·ox·ys·mic
Par·rot at·ro·phy
Par·ry dis·ease
pars
pl par·tes
pars ner·vo·sa
par·the·no·gen·e·sis
pl par·the·no·gen·e·ses
par·the·no·ge·net·ic
or par·the·no·gen·ic
par·the·no·ge·net·i·cal·ly
par·the·no·gen·ic
or par·the·no·ge·net·ic
par·ti·cle
par·tic·u·late
par·ti·tion
par·tu·ri·en·cy
par·tu·ri·ent
par·tu·ri·fa·cient
par·tu·ri·om·e·ter
par·tu·ri·tion
par·tus
pa·ru·lis
pl pa·ru·li·des
par·um·bil·i·cal
par·vi·cel·lu·lar
par·vi·loc·u·lar
Par·vo·bac·te·ri·a·ce·ae
par·vule
par·vus et tar·dus pulse
Pas·cal law
pas·cha·chur·da
Pasch·en bod·ies
Pa·schu·tin de·gen·er·a·
tion
pas·sage
Pas·sa·vant bar
pas·si·flo·ra

pas·sion
pas·sion·al
pas·sion·ate
pas·sive
pas·sive-ag·gres·sive
pas·sive-de·pen·dent
pas·siv·ism
pas·siv·ist
paste
pas·tern
Pas·teur ef·fect
Pas·teur treat·ment
Pas·teur·el·la
    pl pas·teur·el·las
    or pas·teur·el·lae
pas·teur·el·lo·sis
    pl pas·teur·el·lo·ses
pas·teur·i·za·tion
pas·teur·ize
pas·teur·iz·er
Pas·ti·a sign
pas·til
    or pas·tille
pas·tille
    or pas·til
pa·ta·gi·al
pa·ta·gi·ate
pa·ta·gi·um
    pl pa·ta·gi·a
Pa·tau syn·drome
patch
pate
pa·tel·la
    pl pa·tel·las
    or pa·tel·lae
pa·tel·la·pex·y
pa·tel·lar
pat·el·lec·to·my
    pl pat·el·lec·to·mies
pa·tel·li·form
pa·tel·lo·ad·duc·tor
pat·en·cy
    pl pat·en·cies
pat·ent
pa·tent·ly
pa·ter·nal
pa·ter·ni·ty
    pl pa·ter·ni·ties
Pat·er·son bod·ies

Pat·er·son-Brown-
    Kel·ly syn·
    drome
Pat·er·son-Kel·ly
    syn·drome
path
pa·the·ma
path·er·ga·si·a
path·er·gy
pa·thet·ic
pa·thet·i·cus
    pl pa·thet·i·ci
path·e·tism
path·e·tist
path·o·clis·is
path·o·don·ti·a
path·o·gen
    or path·o·gene
path·o·gene
    or path·o·gen
path·o·gen·e·sis
    pl path·o·gen·e·ses
path·o·ge·net·ic
path·o·gen·ic
path·o·gen·i·cal·ly
pa·tho·ge·nic·i·ty
    pl pa·tho·ge·nic·i·ties
pa·thog·e·ny
    pl pa·thog·e·nies
path·og·nom·ic
pa·thog·no·mon·ic
    or pa·thog·no·mon·i·cal
pa·thog·no·mon·i·cal
    or pa·thog·no·mon·ic
pa·thog·no·mon·i·cal·ly
pa·thog·no·my
    pl pa·thog·no·mies
path·og·nos·tic
path·o·le·si·a
path·o·log·ic
    or path·o·log·i·cal
path·o·log·i·cal
    or path·o·log·ic
path·o·log·i·cal·ly
pa·thol·o·gist
pa·thol·o·gy
    pl pa·thol·o·gies
path·o·ma·ni·a
path·o·mei·o·sis

pa·thom·e·ter
pa·thom·e·try
path·o·mi·me·sis
path·o·mim·ic·ry
path·o·mor·pho·log·ic
    or path·o·mor·pho·log·i·cal
path·o·mor·pho·log·i·cal
    or path·o·mor·pho·log·ic
path·o·mor·phol·o·gy
    pl path·o·mor·phol·o·gies
path·o·neu·ro·sis
    pl path·o·neu·ro·ses
path·o·phil·i·a
path·o·pho·bi·a
path·o·pho·ric
pa·thoph·o·rous
path·o·phys·i·o·log·ic
    or path·o·phys·i·o·log·i·cal
path·o·phy·s·i·o·log·i·cal
    or path·o·phys·i·o·log·ic
path·o·phys·i·ol·o·gy
    pl path·o·phys·i·ol·o·gies
path·o·plei·o·sis
path·o·psy·chol·o·gy
    pl path·o·psy·chol·o·gies
pa·tho·sis
    pl pa·tho·ses
path·way
pa·tient
pat·ri·cide
Pat·rick ar·e·as
pat·ri·lin·e·al
pat·ten
pat·tern
pat·tern·ing
pat·u·lin
pat·u·lous
pat·u·lous·ly
Paul op·er·a·tion
Paul-Bun·nell test
Paul·lin·i·a
Paul-Mik·u·licz op·er·
    a·tion
pau·lo·car·di·a
paunch
pause
pau·si·me·ni·a
Pau·trier mi·cro·ab·scess

pa·vaex
   var of pa·vex
pave·ment·ing
pa·vex
Pav·lov pouch
Pav·lov·i·an
Pav·lov·i·an·ism
pa·vor
Pa·vy dis·ease
Paw·lik folds
paw·paw
pearl
pec·cant
pec·tase
pec·ten
   pl pec·tens
   or pec·ti·nes
pec·te·no·sis
pec·tic
pec·tin
pec·tin·ase
pec·ti·nate
pec·tin·e·al
pec·tin·es·ter·ase
pec·tin·e·us
   pl pec·tin·e·i
pec·tin·i·form
pec·tin·ose
pec·ti·za·tion
pec·tize
pec·to·ral
pec·to·ra·lis
   pl pec·to·ra·les
pec·to·ril·o·quy
   pl pec·to·ril·o·quies
pec·tose
pec·tous
pec·tus
   pl pec·to·ra
ped·al
ped·a·tro·phi·a
pe·dat·ro·phy
ped·er·ast
ped·er·as·tic
ped·er·as·ti·cal·ly
ped·er·as·ty
   pl ped·er·as·ties
pe·de·sis
   pl pe·de·ses

ped·i·al·gi·a
pe·di·at·ric
pe·di·a·tri·cian
   or pe·di·at·rist
pe·di·at·rics
pe·di·at·rist
   or pe·di·a·tri·cian
pe·di·a·try
ped·i·cel
ped·i·cel·late
   or ped·i·cel·lat·ed
ped·i·cel·lat·ed
   or ped·i·cel·late
ped·i·cle
ped·i·cled
pe·dic·ter·us
pe·dic·u·lar
pe·dic·u·late
pe·dic·u·la·tion
pe·dic·u·li·ci·dal
pe·dic·u·li·cide
Pe·dic·u·loi·des
pe·dic·u·lo·pho·bi·a
pe·dic·u·lo·sis
   pl pe·dic·u·lo·ses
pe·dic·u·lous
pe·dic·u·lus
   pl pe·dic·u·li
   or pe·dic·u·lus
ped·i·cure
ped·i·palp
pe·di·tis
pe·do·don·ti·a
pe·do·don·tic
pe·do·don·tics
pe·do·don·tist
pe·do·don·tol·o·gy
ped·o·dy·na·mom·e·ter
pe·do·gen·e·sis
pe·do·log·ic
   or pe·do·log·i·cal
pe·do·log·i·cal
   or pe·do·log·ic
pe·dol·o·gist
pe·dol·o·gy
   pl pe·dol·o·gies
ped·om·e·ter
pe·dom·e·try
pe·do·no·sol·o·gy

pe·dop·a·thy
pe·do·phile
pe·do·phil·i·a
pe·do·phil·i·ac
   or pe·do·phil·ic
pe·do·phil·ic
   or pe·do·phil·i·ac
pe·do·pho·bi·a
pe·do·psy·chi·a·trist
pe·dun·cle
pe·dun·cu·lar
pe·dun·cu·late
   or pe·dun·cu·lat·ed
pe·dun·cu·lat·ed
   or pe·dun·cu·late
pe·dun·cu·la·tion
pe·dun·cu·lus
   pl pe·dun·cu·li
peel·ing
Peet op·er·a·tion
peg
peg·a·nine
pei·no·ther·a·py
Pel·cri·ses
Pel Eb·stein dis·ease
pe·la·da
pe·lade
pel·age
pel·a·gism
pel·ar·gon·ic
Pel·ger a·no·ma·ly
pel·i·com·e·ter
pel·i·di·si
pel·i·o·sis
pel·i·ot·ic
Pel·i·zae·us-Merz·bach·
   er dis·ease
pel·la·gra
pel·lag·ra·gen·ic
pel·la·gric
pel·la·grin
Pel·le·gri·ni-Stie·da
   dis·ease
pel·lag·roid
pel·lag·rous
pel·let
pel·le·tie·rine
pel·li·cle
pel·lic·u·la

pel·lic·u·lar
pel·lic·u·late
pel·lic·u·lous
pel·li·to·ry
Pel·li·zi syn·drome
pel·lo·tine
pel·lu·cid
pel·mat·o·gram
pel·oid
pe·lol·o·gy
pe·lop·si·a
pel·o·sine
pel·o·ther·a·py
  pl pel·o·ther·a·pies
Pels-Macht test
pel·ta·tin
pel·vi·ab·dom·in·al
pel·vic
pel·vi·en·ceph·a·lom·e·try
pel·vi·fem·o·ral
pel·vi·graph
pel·vim·e·ter
pel·vim·e·try
  pl pel·vim·e·tries
pel·vi·o·li·thot·o·my
pel·vi·o·ne·o·cys·tos·to·my
pel·vi·o·ra·di·og·ra·phy
pel·vi·ot·o·my
pel·vi·rec·tal
pel·vis
  pl pel·vis·es
  or pel·ves
pel·vi·sa·cral
pel·vi·scope
pel·vi·sec·tion
pel·vi·ver·te·bral
pel·vo·cal·i·ec·ta·sis
pel·vo·cal·y·ce·al
pel·vo·cal·y·cec·ta·sis
pem·o·line
pem·phi·goid
pem·phi·gus
  pl pem·phi·gus·es
  or pem·phi·gi
pem·pi·dine
pen·al·ge·si·a
pen·del·luft
Pen·dred syn·drome
pen·du·lar

pen·du·lous
pe·nec·to·my
pen·e·trance
pen·e·trat·ing
pen·e·tra·tion
pen·e·trom·e·ter
Pen·field op·er·a·tion
pe·ni·al
pen·i·ci·din
pen·i·cil·la·mine
pen·i·cil·lar
pen·i·cil·lase
pen·i·cil·late
pen·i·cil·li li·e·nis
pen·i·cil·lic
pen·i·cil·li·form
pen·i·cil·lin
pen·i·cil·li·nase
pen·i·cil·lin·ic
pen·i·cil·li·o·sis
  pl pen·i·cil·li·o·ses
Pen·i·cil·li·um
  pl Pen·i·cil·li·a
pen·i·cil·lo·ic
pen·i·cil·lus
  pl pen·i·cil·li
pe·nile
pe·nil·lic
pe·nis
  pl pe·nis·es
  or pe·nes
pen·nate
  or pen·nat·ed
pen·nat·ed
  or pen·nate
pen·ni·form
pen·ny·roy·al
pen·ny·weight
pen·ny·wort
pe·no·log·i·cal
pe·nol·o·gist
pe·nol·o·gy
pe·no·scro·tal
Pen·rose drain
pen·ta·bam·ate
pen·ta·ba·sic
pen·ta·chlo·ro·phe·nol
pen·tad

pen·ta·dac·tyl
  or pen·ta·dac·ty·late
pen·ta·dac·ty·late
  or pen·ta·dac·tyl
pen·ta·dac·tyl·ism
pen·ta·dec·yl·cat·e·chol
pen·ta·e·ryth·ri·tol tet·
  ra·ni·trate
pen·ta·e·ryth·ri·tyl tet·
  ra·ni·trate
pen·ta·gas·trin
pen·ta·gen·ic
pen·tal·o·gy
  pl pen·tal·o·gies
pen·ta·me·tho·ni·um
pen·ta·meth·yl·ene·tet·
  ra·zol
pen·ta·meth·yl·ro·san·i·line
pen·tam·i·dine
pen·tane
pen·tane·di·o·ic
pen·ta·pep·tide
pen·ta·pip·er·ide
pen·ta·quine
pen·ta·sac·cha·ride
Pen·tas·to·ma
pen·ta·stome
Pen·ta·stom·i·da
pen·ta·tom·ic
Pen·ta·trich·o·mo·nas
pen·ta·va·lent
pen·taz·o·cine
pent·dy·o·pent
pen·tene
pen·te·no·lac·tone
pen·tet·ra·zol
pen·thi·e·nate
pen·to·bar·bi·tal
pen·to·bar·bi·tone
pen·to·lin·i·um
pen·to·san
pen·to·sa·zone
pen·tose
pen·to·side
pen·to·su·ri·a
pen·to·thal
pent·ox·ide
pen·tyl
pen·ty·lene·tet·ra·zol

292

Pen·zoldt test
pe·o·til·lo·ma·ni·a
pe·po
pep·per
Pep·per syn·drome
pep·si·gogue
pep·sin
pep·sin·if·er·ous
pep·sin·o·gen
pep·si·no·ther·a·py
pep·tic
pep·ti·dase
pep·tide
pep·ti·do·gly·can
pep·ti·do·lyt·ic
pep·ti·za·tion
pep·tize
pep·to·gen·ic
pep·tog·e·nous
pep·tol·y·sis
pep·to·nae·mi·a
   var of pep·to·ne·mi·a
pep·tone
pep·to·ne·mi·a
pep·ton·ic
pep·to·ni·za·tion
pep·to·nize
pep·to·noid
pep·to·nol·y·sis
pep·to·nu·ri·a
per a·num
per os
per pri·mam
per rec·tum
per·a·ceph·a·lus
per·a·ce·tic
per·ac·id
per·a·cid·i·ty
per·a·cute
per·a·to·dyn·i·a
per·bo·rate
per·bo·ric
per·cent
per·cent·age
per·cen·tile
per·cept
per·cep·tion
per·cep·tive
per·cep·tiv·i·ty

per·cep·to·ri·um
   pl per·cep·to·ri·ums
   or per·cep·to·ri·a
per·cep·tu·al
per·chlo·rate
per·chlor·hy·dri·a
per·chlo·ric
per·chlo·ro·eth·yl·ene
per·clu·sion
per·co·late
per·co·la·tion
per·co·la·tor
per·co·morph
per·cuss
per·cus·si·ble
per·cus·sion
per·cus·sor
per·cu·ta·ne·ous
per·cu·ta·ne·ous·ly
per·fec·tion·ism
per·fla·tion
per·fo·rans
per·fo·rate
per·fo·ra·tion
per·fo·ra·tor
per·fo·ra·to·ri·um
   pl per·fo·ra·to·ri·a
per·form·ance
per·for·mic
per·fri·ca·tion
per·fus·ate
per·fuse
per·fu·sion
per·hex·i·line
per·i·ac·i·nal
   or per·i·ac·i·nous
per·i·ac·i·nar
per·i·ac·i·nous
   or per·i·ac·i·nal
per·i·ad·e·ni·tis
per·i·ad·ven·ti·tial
per·i·a·li·e·ni·tis
per·i·a·nal
per·i·an·gi·i·tis
   pl per·i·an·gi·i·ti·des
per·i·an·gi·o·cho·li·tis
per·i·a·or·tal
   or per·i·a·or·tic

per·i·a·or·tic
   or per·i·a·or·tal
per·i·a·or·ti·tis
per·i·ap·i·cal
per·i·ap·i·cal·ly
per·i·ap·pen·di·ci·tis
per·i·ap·pen·dic·u·lar
per·i·apt
per·i·aq·ue·duc·tal
per·i·a·re·o·lar
per·i·ar·te·ri·al
per·i·ar·te·ri·o·lar
per·i·ar·ter·i·tis
per·i·ar·thri·tis
   pl per·i·ar·thri·ti·des
per·i·ar·tic·u·lar
per·i·a·tri·al
per·i·au·ric·u·lar
per·i·ax·i·al
per·i·blep·si·a
per·i·blep·sis
per·i·bron·chi·al
per·i·bron·chi·o·lar
per·i·bron·chi·o·li·tis
per·i·bron·chi·tis
   pl per·i·bron·chi·ti·des
per·i·bro·sis
per·i·bur·sal
per·i·cae·cal
   var of per·i·ce·cal
per·i·cae·ci·tis
   var of per·i·ce·ci·tis
per·i·cal·y·ce·al
per·i·can·a·lic·u·lar
per·i·cap·il·lar·y
per·i·car·di·ac
per·i·car·di·a·co·phren·ic
per·i·car·di·al
per·i·car·di·ec·to·my
   pl per·i·car·di·ec·to·mies
per·i·car·di·o·cen·te·sis
per·i·car·di·ol·y·sis
per·i·car·di·o·me·di·as·ti·
   ni·tis
per·i·car·di·o·phren·ic
per·i·car·di·o·pleu·ral
per·i·car·di·or·rha·phy
per·i·car·di·os·to·my

293

per·i·car·di·ot·o·my
pl per·i·car·di·ot·o·mies
per·i·car·dit·ic
per·i·car·di·tis
pl per·i·car·di·ti·des
per·i·car·di·um
pl per·i·car·di·a
per·i·carp
per·i·car·y·on
pl par·i·car·y·a
var of per·i·kar·y·on
per·i·ca·val
per·i·ce·cal
per·i·ce·ci·tis
per·i·cel·lu·lar
per·i·ce·ment·al
per·i·ce·men·ti·tis
per·i·ce·men·to·cla·si·a
per·i·ce·men·tum
per·i·cen·tric
per·i·cen·tri·o·lar
per·i·cha·rei·a
per·i·cho·lan·gi·o·lit·ic
per·i·chol·an·git·ic
per·i·chol·an·gi·tis
pl per·i·chol·an·gi·ti·des
per·i·chol·e·cys·tic
per·i·chol·e·cys·ti·tis
per·i·chon·dral
or per·i·chon·dri·al
per·i·chon·dri·al
or per·i·chon·dral
per·i·chon·drit·ic
per·i·chon·dri·tis
per·i·chon·dri·um
pl per·i·chon·dri·a
per·i·chon·dro·ma
pl per·i·con·dro·mas
or per·i·con·dro·ma·ta
per·i·chord
per·i·chor·dal
per·i·cho·roid
per·i·cho·roi·dal
per·i·co·lic
per·i·co·li·tis
per·i·co·lon·ic
per·i·co·lon·i·tis
per·i·col·pi·tis
per·i·con·chal

per·i·con·chi·tis
per·i·cor·ne·al
per·i·cor·o·nal
per·i·cor·o·ni·tis
pl per·i·cor·o·ni·ti·des
per·i·cos·tal
per·i·cra·ni·al
per·i·cra·ni·um
pl per·i·cra·ni·a
per·i·cys·tic
per·i·cys·ti·tis
pl per·i·cys·ti·ti·des
per·i·cys·ti·um
pl per·i·cys·ti·a
per·i·cyte
per·i·cy·ti·al
per·i·cy·to·ma
pl per·i·cy·to·mas
or per·i·cy·to·ma·ta
per·i·dec·to·my
per·i·den·drit·ic
per·i·den·tal
per·i·derm
per·i·der·mal
or per·i·der·mic
per·i·der·mic
or per·i·der·mal
per·i·der·mi·um
per·i·di·as·to·le
per·i·did·y·mis
pl per·i·did·y·mi·des
per·i·di·ver·tic·u·li·tis
per·i·duc·tal
per·i·du·o·de·ni·tis
per·i·du·ral
per·i·en·ceph·a·li·tis
pl per·i·en·ceph·a·li·ti·des
per·i·en·ceph·a·lo·men·in·
gi·tis
per·i·en·ter·ic
per·i·en·ter·i·tis
pl per·i·en·ter·i·ti·ses
or per·i·en·ter·i·ti·des
per·i·en·ter·on
per·i·e·pen·dy·mal
per·i·ep·i·did·y·mi·tis
per·i·ep·i·glot·tic
per·i·e·soph·a·ge·al
per·i·e·soph·a·gi·tis

per·i·fis·tu·lar
per·i·fo·cal
per·i·fol·lic·u·lar
per·i·fol·lic·u·li·tis
per·i·for·ni·cal
per·i·fu·nic·u·lar
per·i·gan·gli·i·tis
per·i·gan·gli·on·ic
per·i·gas·tric
per·i·gas·tri·tis
per·i·gem·mal
per·i·gen·i·tal
per·i·glan·du·lar
per·i·glot·tic
per·i·glot·tis
pl per·i·glot·tis·es
or per·i·glot·ti·des
per·i·gnath·ic
per·i·he·pat·ic
per·i·hep·a·ti·tis
pl per·i·hep·a·ti·ti·des
per·i·her·ni·al
per·i·hi·lar
per·i·hy·poph·y·se·al
per·i·hy·po·phys·i·al
per·i·hys·ter·ic
per·i·in·farc·tion
per·i·je·ju·ni·tis
per·i·kar·y·al
per·i·kar·y·on
pl per·i·kar·y·a
per·i·ke·rat·ic
per·i·ky·ma
pl per·i·ky·ma·ta
per·i·lab·y·rin·thi·tis
per·i·la·ryn·ge·al
per·i·lar·yn·gi·tis
per·i·len·tic·u·lar
per·i·lymph
per·i·lym·pha
per·i·lym·phan·ge·al
or per·i·lym·phan·gi·al
per·i·lym·phan·gi·al
or per·i·lym·phan·ge·al
per·i·lym·phan·gi·tis
per·i·lym·phat·ic
per·i·mac·u·lar
per·i·mas·ti·tis
pl per·i·mas·ti·ti·des

per·i·men·in·gi·tis
pe·rim·e·ter
per·i·met·ric
pe·rim·e·trist
per·i·me·trit·ic
per·i·me·tri·tis
per·i·me·tri·um
  pl per·i·me·tri·a
per·i·me·tro·sal·pin·gi·tis
pe·rim·e·try
  pl pe·rim·e·tries
per·i·my·e·li·tis
  pl per·i·my·e·li·ti·des
per·i·my·o·si·tis
per·i·mys·i·al
per·i·my·si·um
  pl per·i·my·si·a
per·i·na·tal
per·i·ne·al
per·i·ne·o·cele
per·i·ne·om·e·ter
per·i·ne·o·plas·ty
  pl per·i·ne·o·plas·ties
per·i·ne·o·rec·tal
per·i·ne·or·rha·phy
  pl per·i·ne·or·rha·phies
per·i·ne·o·scro·tal
per·i·ne·ot·o·my
  pl per·i·ne·ot·o·mies
per·i·ne·o·vag·i·nal
per·i·ne·o·vag·i·no·rec·tal
per·i·neph·ri·al
per·i·neph·ric
per·i·ne·phrit·ic
per·i·ne·phri·tis
  pl per·i·ne·phri·ti·des
per·i·neph·ri·um
  pl per·i·neph·ri·a
per·i·neph·ros
per·i·ne·um
  pl per·i·ne·a
per·i·neu·ral
per·i·neu·ri·al
per·i·neu·ri·tis
  pl per·i·neu·ri·ti·ses
  or per·i·neu·ri·ti·des
per·i·neu·ri·um
  pl per·i·neu·ri·a
per·i·neu·ro·nal

per·i·ne·void
per·i·nu·cle·ar
per·i·oc·u·lar
pe·ri·od
per·i·o·date
pe·ri·od·ic
pe·ri·o·dic·i·ty
per·i·o·don·tal
per·i·o·don·ti·a
per·i·o·don·tic
per·i·o·don·tics
per·i·o·don·tist
per·i·o·don·ti·tis
per·i·o·don·ti·um
  pl per·i·o·don·ti·a
per·i·o·don·to·cla·si·a
per·i·o·don·tol·o·gy
  pl per·i·o·don·tol·o·gies
per·i·o·don·to·sis
  pl per·i·o·don·to·ses
pe·ri·od·o·scope
per·i·o·dyn·i·a
per·i·oe·soph·a·ge·al
  var of per·i·e·soph·a·ge·al
per·i·oe·soph·a·gi·tis
  var of per·i·e·soph·a·gi·tis
per·i·om·phal·ic
per·i·o·nych·i·a
per·i·o·nych·i·um
  pl per·i·o·nych·i·a
per·i·on·yx
per·i·o·oph·o·ri·tis
per·i·o·oph·o·ro·sal·pin·gi·tis
per·i·o·o·the·ci·tis
per·i·o·o·the·co·sal·pin·gi·tis
per·i·o·ple
per·i·op·lic
per·i·op·tom·e·try
  pl per·i·op·tom·e·tries
per·i·o·ral
per·i·or·bit
per·i·or·bi·ta
per·i·or·bit·al
per·i·or·bi·ti·tis
per·i·or·chi·tis
per·i·ost
per·i·os·te·al

per·i·os·te·i·tis
per·i·os·te·o·ma
  pl per·i·os·te·o·mas
  or per·i·os·te·o·ma·ta
per·i·os·te·o·phyte
per·i·os·te·o·ra·di·al
per·i·os·te·ot·o·my
  pl per·i·os·te·ot·o·mies
per·i·os·te·um
  pl per·i·os·te·a
per·i·os·tit·ic
per·i·os·ti·tis
per·i·os·to·ma
  pl per·i·os·to·mas
  or per·i·os·to·ma·ta
per·i·os·to·sis
  pl per·i·os·to·sis·es
  or per·i·os·to·ses
per·i·o·tic
per·i·o·va·ri·tis
per·i·o·vu·lar
per·i·pach·y·men·in·gi·tis
  pl per·i·pach·y·men·in·gi·ti·des
per·i·pan·cre·a·ti·tis
  pl per·i·pan·cre·a·ti·ti·des
per·i·pap·il·lar·y
per·i·pe·dun·cu·lar
per·i·phak·us
per·i·pha·ci·tis
per·i·pha·ryn·ge·al
pe·riph·er·ad
pe·riph·er·al
pe·riph·er·al·ly
pe·riph·er·a·phose
pe·riph·er·y
  pl pe·riph·er·ies
per·i·phle·bit·ic
per·i·phle·bi·tis
  pl per·i·phle·bi·ti·des
per·i·phlo·em
pe·riph·ra·sis
  pl pe·riph·ra·ses
per·i·phras·tic
Per·i·pla·ne·ta
per·i·pleu·ri·tis
Pe·rip·lo·ca
pe·rip·lo·cin
pe·rip·lo·cy·ma·rin

295

per·i·po·ri·tis
per·i·por·tal
per·i·proc·tal
  or per·i·proc·tic
  or per·i·proc·tous
per·i·proc·tic
  or per·i·proc·tal
  or per·i·proc·tous
per·i·proc·ti·tis
per·i·proc·tous
  or per·i·proc·tic
  or per·i·proc·tal
per·i·pros·tat·ic
per·i·pros·ta·ti·tis
per·i·py·e·li·tis
per·i·py·e·ma
per·i·py·le·phle·bi·tis
  pl per·i·py·le·phle·bi·ti·des
per·i·py·lo·ric
per·i·rec·tal
per·i·rec·ti·tis
per·i·re·nal
per·i·rhi·nal
per·i·sal·pin·gi·an
per·i·sal·pin·gi·tis
per·i·sal·pin·go·o·va·ri·tis
per·i·sal·pinx
  pl per·i·sal·pin·ges
per·i·scop·ic
per·i·sig·moid·i·tis
per·i·sin·u·ous
per·i·si·nus·i·tis
per·i·si·nu·soi·dal
per·i·sper·ma·ti·tis
per·i·sple·nic
per·i·sple·ni·tis
per·i·spon·dyl·ic
per·i·spon·dy·li·tis
per·i·stal·sis
  pl per·i·stal·ses
per·i·stal·tic
per·i·stal·ti·cal·ly
per·i·staph·y·line
per·i·staph·y·li·tis
per·i·sta·sis
per·i·stat·ic
pe·ris·to·le
per·i·stol·ic

pe·ris·to·ma
  pl pe·ris·to·mas
  or pe·ris·to·ma·ta
per·i·stome
per·i·stri·ate
per·i·sy·no·vi·al
per·i·tec·to·my
  pl per·i·tec·to·mies
per·i·ten·din·e·um
  pl per·i·ten·din·e·a
per·i·ten·di·ni·tis
per·i·ten·on
per·i·ten·o·ni·tis
per·i·the·li·al
per·i·the·li·o·ma
  pl per·i·the·li·o·mas
  or per·i·the·li·o·ma·ta
per·i·the·li·um
  pl per·i·the·li·a
per·i·thy·roid·i·tis
pe·rit·o·my
  pl pe·rit·o·mies
per·i·to·nae·al
  var of per·i·to·ne·al
per·i·to·nae·um
  pl per·i·to·nae·ums
  or per·i·to·nae·a
  var of pe·ri·to·e·um
per·i·to·ne·al
per·i·to·ne·a·li·za·tion
per·i·to·ne·a·lize
per·i·to·ne·al·ly
per·i·to·ne·a·tome
  var of per·i·to·ne·o·tome
per·i·to·ne·o·cen·te·sis
  pl per·i·to·ne·o·cen·te·ses
per·i·to·ne·op·a·thy
  pl per·i·to·ne·op·a·thies
per·i·to·ne·o·per·i·car·di·al
per·i·to·ne·o·pex·y
  pl per·i·to·ne·o·pex·ies
per·i·to·ne·o·scope
per·i·to·ne·o·scop·ic
per·i·to·ne·os·co·pist
per·i·to·ne·os·co·py
  pl per·i·to·ne·os·co·pies
per·i·to·ne·o·sub·a·rach·
  noid
per·i·to·ne·o·the·cal

per·i·to·ne·o·tome
per·i·to·ne·ot·o·my
  pl per·i·to·ne·ot·o·mies
per·i·to·ne·um
  pl per·i·to·ne·ums
  or per·i·to·ne·a
per·i·to·nit·ic
per·i·to·ni·tis
per·i·to·nize
per·i·ton·sil·lar
per·i·ton·sil·li·tis
per·i·tor·cu·lar
per·i·tra·che·al
per·i·tra·che·i·tis
pe·rit·ri·chal
per·i·trich·i·al
pe·rit·ri·chous
per·i·trun·cal
per·i·tu·bal
per·i·typh·lic
per·i·typh·lit·ic
per·i·typh·li·tis
per·i·um·bil·i·cal
per·i·un·gual
per·i·u·re·ter·al
per·i·u·re·ter·ic
per·i·u·re·ter·i·tis
per·i·u·re·thral
per·i·u·re·thri·tis
  pl per·i·u·re·thri·ti·des
per·i·u·ter·ine
per·i·u·vu·lar
per·i·vag·i·nal
per·i·vag·i·ni·tis
per·i·vas·cu·lar
per·i·vas·cu·li·tis
per·i·ve·nous
per·i·ven·tric·u·lar
per·i·ver·te·bral
per·i·ves·i·cal
per·i·ve·sic·u·lar
per·i·ve·sic·u·li·tis
per·i·vis·cer·al
per·i·vis·cer·i·tis
per·i·vi·tel·line
per·i·vul·var
per·i·xe·ni·tis
perle
per·leche

Per·li·a nu·cle·us
per·lin·gual
per·lin·gual·ly
Perls re·ac·tion
perl·sucht
per·ma·nent
per·man·ga·nate
per·man·gan·ic
per·me·a·bil·i·ty
per·me·a·ble
per·me·ase
per·me·ate
per·me·a·tion
Per·mu·tit meth·od
per·ni·cious
per·ni·o
pl per·ni·o·nes
per·ni·o·sis
per·noc·ta·tion
per·o·bra·chi·us
per·o·ceph·a·lus
per·o·chei·rus
var of per·o·chi·rus
per·o·chi·rus
per·o·cor·mus
per·o·dac·tyl·i·a
per·o·dac·ty·lus
pl per·o·dac·ty·li
per·o·me·li·a
pe·rom·e·lus
pl pe·rom·e·li
pe·rom·e·ly
per·o·ne·al
per·o·ne·o·cal·ca·ne·us
per·o·ne·o·cu·boi·de·us
per·o·ne·o·tib·i·a·lis
per·o·ne·us
pe·ro·ni·a
pe·ro·pla·si·a
pe·ro·pus
per·o·ral
per·o·ral·ly
pe·ro·sis
pl pe·ro·ses
pe·ro·so·mus
pl pe·ro·so·mus·es
or pe·ro·so·mi
pe·ro·splanch·ni·a
per·os·se·ous

pe·rot·ic
per·ox·i·dase
per·ox·ide
per·ox·i·dize
per·ox·i·som·al
per·ox·i·some
per·ox·y·a·ce·tic
per·pen·dic·u·lar
per·phen·a·zine
per·rec·tal
per·rec·tal·ly
Per·rin law
Per·rin-Fer·ra·ton dis·ease
per·salt
per·sev·er·a·tion
per·sic
per·son
per·so·na
pl per·so·nas
or per·so·nae
per·son·al
per·son·al·i·ty
pl per·son·al·i·ties
per·son·i·fi·ca·tion
per·sorp·tion
per·spi·ra·tion
per·spi·ra·to·ry
per·spire
per·sua·sion
per·sul·fate
per·su·fide
Per·thes dis·ease
Per·tik di·ver·tic·u·lum
per·tur·ba·tion
per·tus·sal
per·tus·sis
per·tus·soid
per·ver·sion
per·vert
per·vi·gil·i·um
per·vi·ous
pes
pl pe·des
pes·sa·ry
pl pes·sa·ries
pes·su·lum
pl pes·su·la
pes·sum
pl pes·sa

pest
pes·ti·ci·dal
pes·ti·cide
pes·tif·er·ous
pes·tif·er·ous·ly
pes·ti·lence
pes·ti·lent
pes·ti·len·tial
pes·ti·len·tial·ly
pes·tis
pl pes·tes
pes·tle
pe·te·chi·a
pl pe·te·chi·ae
pe·te·chi·al
pe·te·chi·ate
pe·te·chi·a·tion
pe·te·chi·om·e·ter
Pe·ters em·bry·o
Pe·ter·sen bag
peth·i·dine
pet·i·o·late
or pet·i·o·lat·ed
pet·i·o·lat·ed
or pet·i·o·late
pet·i·ole
pe·ti·o·lus
pl pe·ti·o·li
pe·tit mal
Pe·tit tri·an·gle
Pe·tri dish
pet·ri·fac·tion
pet·ri·fac·tive
pet·ri·fi·ca·tion
pet·ri·fy
pé·tris·sage
pet·ro·bas·i·lar
pet·ro·chem·i·cal
pet·ro·la·tum
pe·tro·le·um
pet·ro·mas·toid
pet·ro·oc·cip·i·tal
pet·ro·pha·ryn·ge·us
pl pet·ro·pha·ryn·ge·i
pe·tro·sa
pl pe·tro·sae
pe·tro·sal
pet·ro·si·tis
pet·ro·sphe·noid

pet·ro·squa·mous
pet·ro·tym·pan·ic
pet·rous
pe·trox·o·lin
Pet·te-Dö·ring dis·ease
Pet·ten·kof·er test
Pet·ze·ta·ki dis·ease
Petz·val the·o·ry
Peutz-Je·ghers syn·drome
pex·is
Pey·er gland, patch
pey·e·ri·an gland
pe·yo·te
 or pe·yo·tl
pe·yo·tl
 or pe·yo·te
Pey·ro·nie dis·ease
Pey·rot tho·rax
Pfan·nen·stiel in·ci·sion
Pfaund·ler-Hur·ler syn·drome
Pfeif·fer ba·cil·lus, in·flu·en·za
Pfeif·fer·el·la
Pflü·ger laws
pha·cen·to·cele
pha·ci·tis
phac·o·an·a·phy·lac·tic
phac·o·an·a·phy·lax·is
phac·o·cele
phac·o·cyst
phac·o·cys·tec·to·my
phac·o·er·i·sis
 var of phac·o·er·y·sis
phac·o·er·y·sis
phac·oid
pha·col·y·sis
 pl pha·col·y·ses
phac·o·lyt·ic
pha·co·ma
 pl pha·co·mas
 or pha·co·ma·ta
 var of pha·ko·ma
pha·co·ma·to·sis
 pl pha·co·ma·to·ses
 var of pha·ko·ma·to·sis
phac·o·met·a·cho·re·sis
phac·o·met·e·ce·sis
pha·com·e·ter

phac·o·pla·ne·sis
phac·o·scle·ro·sis
 pl phac·o·scle·ro·ses
phac·o·scope
pha·cos·co·py
phac·o·sco·tas·mus
phac·o·tox·ic
phae·na·kis·to·scope
 var of phen·a·kis·to·scope
phae·o·chrome
 var of phe·o·chrome
phae·o·chro·ma·blast
 var of phe·o·chro·mo·blast
phae·o·chro·mo·blas·to·ma
 pl phae·o·chro·mo·blas·to·mas
 or phae·o·chro·mo·blas·to·ma·ta
 var of phe·o·chro·mo·blas·to·ma
phae·o·chro·mo·cyte
 var of phe·o·chro·mo·cyte
Phae·o·phy·ce·ae
phage
 pl phag·es
 or phage
phag·e·dae·na
 var of phag·e·de·na
phag·e·daen·ic
 var of phag·e·den·ic
phag·e·de·na
phag·e·den·ic
phag·o·car·y·o·sis
 var of phag·o·kar·y·o·sis
phag·o·cyt·a·ble
phag·o·cy·tal
phag·o·cyte
phag·o·cyt·ic
phag·o·cy·tize
phag·o·cy·to·blast
phag·o·cy·to·lit·ic
phag·o·cy·tol·y·sis
phag·o·cy·tose
phag·o·cy·to·sis
 pl phag·o·cy·to·ses
phag·o·cy·tot·ic
phag·o·dy·na·mom·e·ter
phag·o·kar·y·o·sis

pha·gol·y·sis
 pl pha·gol·y·ses
phag·o·lyt·ic
phag·o·ma·ni·a
phag·o·some
phag·o·ther·a·py
pha·ko·ma
 pl pha·ko·mas
 or pha·ko·ma·ta
pha·ko·ma·to·sis
 pl pha·ko·ma·to·ses
phal·a·cro·sis
 pl phal·a·cro·ses
pha·lange
pha·lan·ge·al
phal·an·gec·to·my
 pl phal·an·gec·to·mies
pha·lan·ges
phal·an·gette
phal·an·gi·tis
pha·lan·gi·za·tion
pha·lan·go·pha·lan·ge·al
pha·lanx
 pl pha·lanx·es
 or pha·lan·ges
phal·lic
phal·li·cal·ly
phal·li·cism
phal·li·form
phal·lin
phal·lism
phal·loid
phal·loi·din
 or phal·loi·dine
phal·loi·dine
 or phal·loi·din
phal·lo·plas·ty
phal·lus
 pl phal·lus·es
 or phal·li
phan·er·o·gam
Phan·er·o·gam·i·a
phan·er·o·gam·ic
phan·er·o·ge·net·ic
 or phan·er·o·gen·ic
phan·er·o·gen·ic
 or phan·er·o·ge·net·ic
phan·er·o·ma·ni·a

298

phan·er·o·sis
pl phan·er·o·ses
phan·er·o·zo·ic
phan·er·o·zo·ite
phan·er·o·zo·it·ic
phan·quone
phan·tasm
phan·tas·ma·go·ri·a
or phan·tas·ma·go·ry
phan·tas·ma·go·ric
or phan·tas·ma·go·ri·cal
phan·tas·ma·go·ri·cal
or phan·tas·ma·go·ric
phan·tas·ma·go·ry
pl phan·tas·ma·go·ries
or phan·tas·ma·go·ri·a
phan·tas·ma·to·mo·ri·a
phan·tas·mo·sco·pi·a
phan·tast
phan·ta·sy
or fan·tasy
phan·to·geu·si·a
phan·tom
phan·tos·mi·a
phar·a·on·ic
phar·ci·dous
phar·ma·cal
phar·ma·ceu·tic
or phar·ma·ceu·ti·cal
phar·ma·ceu·ti·cal
or phar·ma·ceu·tic
phar·ma·ceu·ti·cal·ly
phar·ma·ceu·tics
phar·ma·ceu·tist
phar·ma·cist
phar·ma·co·dy·nam·ic
phar·ma·co·dy·nam·i·cal·ly
phar·ma·co·dy·nam·ics
phar·ma·co·ge·net·ic
phar·ma·co·ge·net·ics
phar·ma·cog·no·sist
phar·ma·cog·nos·tic
or phar·ma·cog·nos·ti·cal
phar·ma·cog·nos·ti·cal
or phar·ma·cog·nos·tic
phar·ma·cog·no·sy
pl phar·ma·cog·no·sies
phar·ma·co·ki·net·ics

phar·ma·co·log·ic
or phar·ma·co·log·i·cal
phar·ma·co·log·i·cal
or phar·ma·co·log·ic
phar·ma·co·log·i·cal·ly
phar·ma·col·o·gist
phar·ma·col·o·gy
pl phar·ma·col·o·gies
phar·ma·co·ma·ni·a
phar·ma·co·pae·dics
var of phar·ma·co·pe·dics
phar·ma·co·pe·di·a
phar·ma·co·pe·dic
phar·ma·co·pe·dics
phar·ma·co·pe·ia
phar·ma·co·pe·ial
phar·ma·co·pho·bi·a
phar·ma·co·phore
phar·ma·co·poe·i·a
var of phar·ma·co·pe·i·a
phar·ma·co·poe·ial
var of phar·ma·co·pe·ial
phar·ma·co·psy·cho·sis
phar·ma·co·ther·a·peu·tic
or phar·ma·co·ther·a·peu·
ti·cal
phar·ma·co·ther·a·peu·ti·
cal
or phar·ma·co·ther·a·
peu·tic
phar·ma·co·ther·a·peu·tics
phar·ma·co·ther·a·py
pl phar·ma·co·ther·a·pies
phar·ma·cy
pl phar·ma·cies
pha·ryn·gal
phar·yn·gal·gi·a
pha·ryn·ge·al
phar·yn·gec·to·my
pl phar·yn·gec·to·mies
phar·yn·gem·phrax·is
pha·ryn·ge·us
phar·yn·gism
phar·yn·gis·mus
pl phar·yn·gis·mi
phar·yn·git·ic
phar·yn·gi·tis
pl phar·yn·gi·ti·des
pha·ryn·go·bran·chi·al

pha·ryn·go·cele
pha·ryn·go·con·junc·ti·val
pha·ryn·go·dyn·i·a
pha·ryn·go·ep·i·glot·tic
pha·ryn·go·ep·i·glot·ti·cus
pl pha·ryn·go·ep·i·glot·ti·ci
pha·ryn·go·e·soph·a·ge·al
pha·ryn·go·e·soph·a·gus
pl pha·ryn·go·e·soph·a·gi
pha·ryn·go·glos·sal
pha·ryn·go·glos·sus
pl pha·ryn·go·glos·si
pha·ryn·go·ker·a·to·sis
pha·ryn·go·la·ryn·ge·al
phar·yn·go·lar·yn·gi·tis
pl pha·ryn·go·lar·yn·gi·
ti·des
pha·ryn·go·lith
pha·ryn·go·log·i·cal
phar·yn·gol·o·gy
pl phar·yn·gol·o·gies
phar·yn·gol·y·sis
pha·ryn·go·max·il·lar·y
pha·ryn·go·my·co·sis
pha·ryn·go·na·sal
pha·ryn·go·oe·soph·a·ge·al
var of pha·ryn·go·e·soph·
a·ge·al
pha·ryn·go·oe·soph·a·gus
pl pha·ryn·go·oe·soph·a·gi
var of pha·ryn·go·e·soph·
a·gus
pha·ryn·go·pal·a·tine
pha·ryn·go·pal·a·ti·nus
pl pha·ryn·go·pal·a·ti·ni
pha·ryn·go·pa·ral·y·sis
phar·yn·gop·a·thy
pha·ryn·go·pe·ris·to·le
pha·ryn·go·plas·ty
pha·ryn·go·ple·gi·a
pha·ryn·go·rhi·ni·tis
pl pha·ryn·go·rhi·ni·ti·des
pha·ryn·go·rhi·nos·co·py
pha·ryn·gor·rha·gi·a
pha·ryn·gor·rhe·a
pha·ryn·gor·rhoe·a
var of pha·ryn·gor·rhe·a
pha·ryn·go·scope
phar·yn·gos·co·py

pha·ryn·go·spasm
pha·ryn·go·spas·mod·ic
pha·ryn·go·ste·ni·a
phar·yn·gos·te·nous
pha·ryn·go·ther·a·py
phar·yn·got·o·my
   pl phar·yn·got·o·mies
pha·ryn·go·ton·sil·li·tis
pha·ryn·go·tra·che·al
pha·ryn·go·tym·pan·ic
pha·ryn·go·xe·ro·sis
phar·ynx
   pl phar·ynx·es
   or pha·ryn·ges
phase-con·trast
pha·se·o·lin
pha·sic
pha·sin
phas·mid
Phas·mid·i·a
phas·mid·i·an
phas·mo·pho·bi·a
phel·lan·drene
phem·i·tone
phen·a·caine
   or phen·o·cain
phe·nac·e·mide
phe·nac·e·tin
phe·nac·e·tu·ric
phen·a·dox·one
phen·a·gly·co·dol
phen·a·kis·to·scope
phe·nan·threne
phe·nate
phen·az·o·cine
phen·a·zone
phen·az·o·pyr·i·dine
phen·ben·i·cil·lin
phen·car·ba·mide
phen·cy·cli·dine
phen·di·met·ra·zine
phene
phen·el·zine
phen·eth·i·cil·lin
phen·eth·yl
phe·net·i·din
phe·net·i·dine
phe·net·i·di·nu·ri·a
phen·for·min

phen·go·pho·bi·a
phe·nic
phe·nin·da·mine
phen·in·di·one
phen·ir·a·mine
phen·met·ra·zine
phe·no·bar·bi·tal
phe·no·bar·bi·tone
phen·o·cain
   or phen·a·caine
phe·no·coll
phe·no·cop·y
   pl phe·no·cop·ies
phe·no·din
phe·nol
phe·no·lase
phe·no·late
phe·no·lic
phe·no·log·ic
   or phe·no·log·i·cal
phe·no·log·i·cal
   or phe·no·log·ic
phe·no·log·i·cal·ly
phe·nol·o·gist
phe·nol·o·gy
   pl phe·nol·o·gies
phe·nol·phthal·ein
phe·nol·phthal·in
phe·nol·sul·fo·nate
phe·nol·sul·fon·ic
phe·nol·sul·fon·phthal·ein
phe·nol·tet·ra·chlo·ro·
   phthal·ein
phe·nol·u·ri·a
phe·nom·e·nol·o·gy
phe·nom·e·non
   pl phe·nom·e·na
phe·no·pho·bi·a
phe·no·pro·pa·zine
phe·no·thi·a·zine
phe·no·type
phe·no·typ·ic
   or phe·no·typ·i·cal
phe·no·typ·i·cal
   or phe·no·typ·ic
phe·no·typ·i·cal·ly
phe·nox·y
phe·nox·y·a·ce·tic
phe·nox·y·ben·za·mine

phen·ox·y·meth·yl·pen·i·
   cil·lin
phe·noz·y·gous
phen·pro·cou·mon
phen·pro·pi·o·nate
phen·sux·i·mide
phen·ter·mine
phen·tol·a·mine
phe·nyl
phen·yl·a·ce·tic
phen·yl·a·ce·tyl·glu·ta·
   mine
phen·yl·a·ce·tyl·u·re·a
phen·yl·al·a·ni·nae·mi·a
   var of phen·yl·al·a·ni·ne·
   mi·a
phen·yl·al·a·nine
phen·yl·a·nine
phen·yl·al·a·ni·ne·mi·a
phen·yl·am·ine
phen·yl·bu·ta·zone
phen·yl·car·bi·nol
phen·yl·cin·cho·nin·ic
phen·yl·ene
phen·yl·en·e·di·a·mine
phen·yl·eph·rine
phen·yl·eth·yl
phen·yl·eth·yl·bar·bi·tu·ric
phen·yl·eth·yl·mal·o·nyl·
   u·re·a
phen·yl·glu·co·sa·zone
phen·yl·hy·dra·zine
phen·yl·hy·dra·zone
phe·nyl·ic
phen·yl·in·dane-1,3-di·one
phen·yl·ke·to·nu·ri·a
phen·yl·ke·to·nu·ric
phen·yl·mer·cu·ric
phen·yl·phe·nol
phen·yl·pro·pa·nol·a·mine
phe·nyl·py·ru·vic
phen·yl·thi·o·car·ba·mide
phen·yl·thi·o·u·re·a
phe·ny·to·in
phe·o·chrome
phe·o·chro·mo·blast
phe·o·chro·mo·blas·to·ma
   pl phe·o·chro·mo·blas·to·
   mas

or phe·o·chro·mo·blas·to·ma·ta
phe·o·chro·mo·cyte
phe·o·chro·mo·cy·to·ma
   pl phe·o·chro·mo·cy·to·mas
   or phe·o·chro·mo·cy·to·ma·ta
phe·ren·ta·sin
phi·al
Phi·a·loph·o·ra
phi·lo·pro·gen·i·tive
phil·ter
phil·trum
   pl phil·tra
phi·mo·sis
   pl phi·mo·ses
phi·mot·ic
phleb·an·gi·o·ma
   pl phleb·an·gi·o·mas
   or phleb·an·gi·o·ma·ta
phleb·ar·te·ri·ec·ta·si·a
phleb·ar·te·ri·o·di·al·y·sis
phleb·ec·ta·si·a
phle·bec·ta·sis
phleb·ec·tat·ic
ple·bec·to·my
   pl phle·bec·to·mies
phleb·ec·to·pi·a
phleb·em·phrax·is
phleb·ep·a·ti·tis
phleb·eu·rys·ma
phleb·ex·er·e·sis
phleb·hep·a·ti·tis
phle·bis·mus
phle·bit·ic
phle·bi·tis
   pl phle·bi·ti·des
phleb·o·car·ci·no·ma
phle·boc·ly·sis
   pl phle·boc·ly·ses
phleb·o·gram
phleb·o·graph
phleb·o·graph·ic
phle·bog·ra·phy
   pl phle·bog·ra·phies
phleb·oid
   or phle·boi·dal
phle·boi·dal
   or phleb·oid

phleb·o·lith
phleb·o·li·thi·a·sis
   pl phleb·o·li·thi·a·ses
phleb·o·lith·ic
phle·bol·o·gy
   pl phle·bol·o·gies
phleb·o·ma·nom·e·ter
phleb·o·phle·bos·to·my
phleb·o·phlo·go·sis
phleb·o·plas·ty
phleb·o·ple·ro·sis
phleb·or·rha·gi·a
phle·bor·rha·phy
phleb·or·rhex·is
phle·bo·scle·ro·sis
   pl phle·bo·scle·ro·ses
phle·bo·scle·rot·ic
phle·bos·ta·sis
phleb·o·ste·no·sis
phleb·o·strep·sis
phleb·o·throm·bo·sis
   pl phleb·o·throm·bo·ses
phleb·o·tome
phleb·o·tom·ic
   or phleb·o·tom·i·cal
phleb·o·tom·i·cal
   or phleb·o·tom·ic
phleb·o·tom·i·cal·ly
phle·bot·o·mist
phle·bot·o·mize
Phle·bot·o·mus
   pl phle·bot·o·mus·es
   or phle·bot·o·mi
phle·bot·o·my
   pl phle·bot·o·mies
phlegm
phleg·ma·si·a
   pl phleg·ma·si·ae
phleg·ma·si·a al·ba do·lens
phleg·mat·ic
   or phleg·mat·i·cal
phleg·mat·i·cal
   or phelg·mat·ic
phleg·mat·i·cal·ly
phelg·mon
phleg·mon·ic
phleg·mon·ous
phleg·mon·ous·ly

phlegm·y
phlo·gis·tic
phlo·gis·ton
phlog·o·ge·net·ic
phlog·o·gen·ic
   or phlo·gog·e·nous
phlo·gog·e·nous
   or phlog·o·gen·ic
phlo·go·sis
phlog·o·zel·o·tism
phlor·e·tin
phlo·rhi·zin
phlo·rid·zin
phlo·ro·glu·cin
phlo·ro·glu·cine
phlo·ro·glu·cin·ol
phlox·ine
phlox·in·o·phil·ic
phlyc·te·na
   pl phlyc·te·nae
phlyc·te·nar
phlyc·te·noid
phlyc·te·nu·la
   pl phlyc·te·nu·lae
phlyc·ten·u·lar
phlyc·te·nule
phlyc·ten·u·lo·sis
pho·bi·a
pho·bi·ac
pho·bic
pho·bism
pho·bo·dip·si·a
pho·bo·pho·bi·a
Pho·cas dis·ease
pho·co·me·li·a
pho·co·me·lic
pho·com·e·lus
   pl pho·com·e·li
pho·com·e·ly
phol·co·dine
Pho·ma
pho·nal
pho·nas·the·ni·a
pho·nate
pho·na·tion
pho·na·to·ry
pho·nau·to·gram
pho·nau·to·graph
pho·nau·to·graph·ic

pho·nau·to·graph·i·cal·ly
phone
pho·neme
pho·nen·do·scope
pho·net·ic
pho·net·ics
pho·ni·at·rics
pho·ni·a·try
phon·ic
pho·ni·ca
phon·ics
pho·nism
pho·no·car·di·o·gram
pho·no·car·di·o·graph
pho·no·car·di·o·graph·ic
pho·no·car·di·og·ra·phy
   pl pho·no·car·di·og·ra·phies
pho·no·chor·da
   pl pho·no·chor·dae
pho·no·cin·e·flu·o·ro·car·
   di·og·ra·phy
pho·no·gram
pho·no·gram·ic
   or pho·no·gram·mic
pho·no·gram·i·cal·ly
   or pho·no·gram·mi·cal·ly
pho·no·gram·mic
   or pho·no·gram·ic
pho·no·gram·mi·cal·ly
   or pho·no·gram·i·cal·ly
pho·no·graph
pho·no·log·ic
   or pho·no·log·i·cal
pho·no·log·i·cal
   or pho·no·log·ic
pho·no·log·i·cal·ly
pho·nol·o·gist
pho·nol·o·gy
   pl pho·nol·o·gies
pho·no·ma·ni·a
pho·no·mas·sage
pho·nom·e·ter
pho·no·met·ric
pho·nom·e·try
   pl pho·nom·e·tries
pho·no·my·oc·lo·nus
pho·no·my·og·ra·phy
pho·nop·a·thy
   pl pho·nop·a·thies

pho·no·pho·bi·a
pho·no·phore
pho·no·pho·to·gram
pho·no·pho·to·graph
pho·no·pho·tog·ra·phy
   pl pho·no·pho·tog·ra·phies
pho·nop·si·a
pho·no·re·cep·tion
pho·no·re·cep·tor
pho·no·scope
phor·bin
pho·ri·a
Phor·i·dae
Phor·mi·a
phor·a·blast
phor·o·cyte
pho·rol·o·gy
pho·rom·e·ter
pho·ro·met·ric
pho·rom·e·try
   pl pho·rom·e·tries
pho·ro·op·tom·e·ter
Phor·op·ter
phor·o·scope
phor·o·tone
phose
phos·gene
phos·gen·ic
phos·pha·gen
phos·pha·tae·mi·a
   var of phos·pha·te·mi·a
phos·pha·tase
phos·phate
phos·pha·te·mi·a
phos·pha·tide
phos·pha·tid·ic
phos·pha·tu·ri·a
phos·phene
phos·phide
phos·phine
phos·phite
phos·pho·a·mi·no·lip·id
phos·pho·ar·gi·nine
phos·pho·cre·a·tine
phos·pho·di·es·ter·ase
phos·pho·e·nol·py·ru·vic
phos·pho·fruc·to·ki·nase
phos·pho·fruc·to·mu·tase
phos·pho·ga·lac·tose

phos·pho·glu·co·mu·tase
phos·pho·glu·con·ic
phos·pho·glu·cose
phos·pho·glyc·er·al·de·
   hyde
phos·pho·gly·cer·ic
phos·pho·glyc·er·o·mu·
   tase
phos·pho·hex·o·i·som·er·
   ase
phos·pho·hex·o·ki·nase
phos·pho·i·no·si·tide
phos·pho·li·pase
phos·pho·lip·id
phos·pho·lip·in
phos·pho·mo·lyb·date
phos·pho·mo·lyb·dic
phos·pho·mon·o·es·ter·ase
phos·pho·ne·cro·sis
phos·pho·ni·um
phos·pho·pro·te·in
phos·pho·py·ru·vic
phos·phor
phos·pho·resce
phos·pho·res·cence
phos·pho·res·cent
phos·phor·hi·dro·sis
phos·pho·ri·bo·mu·tase
phos·pho·ric
phos·phor·i·dro·sis
phos·pho·rism
phos·phor·ne·cro·sis
phos·phor·ol·y·sis
phos·pho·rous
phos·pho·ryl
phos·pho·ryl·ase
phos·pho·ryl·ate
phos·pho·ryl·a·tion
phos·pho·ryl·a·tive
phos·pho·trans·a·cet·y·lase
phos·pho·tri·ose
phos·pho·tung·state
phos·pho·tung·stic
phos·vi·tin
phot
pho·taes·the·si·a
   var of pho·tes·the·si·a
pho·tal·gi·a
pho·tau·gi·o·pho·bi·a

302

pho·tes·the·si·a
pho·tic
pho·tism
pho·to·ac·tin·ic
pho·to·al·ler·gy
  pl pho·to·al·ler·gies
pho·to·bac·te·ri·um
  pl pho·to·bac·te·ri·a
pho·to·bi·o·log·ic
  or pho·to·bi·o·log·i·cal
pho·to·bi·o·log·i·cal
  or pho·to·bi·o·log·ic
pho·to·bi·ol·o·gist
pho·to·bi·ol·o·gy
  pl pho·to·bi·ol·o·gies
pho·to·bi·ot·ic
pho·to·ca·tal·y·sis
  pl pho·to·ca·tal·y·ses
pho·to·cat·a·lyst
pho·to·cat·a·lyt·ic
pho·to·chem·ical
pho·to·chem·i·cal·ly
pho·to·chem·ist
pho·to·chem·is·try
  pl pho·to·chem·is·tries
pho·to·chro·mat·ic
pho·to·chro·mo·gen
pho·to·chro·mo·gen·ic
pho·to·co·ag·u·la·tion
pho·to·co·ag·u·la·tive
pho·to·co·ag·u·la·tor
pho·to·col·or·im·e·ter
pho·to·con·duc·tive
pho·to·con·duc·tiv·i·ty
pho·to·con·junc·ti·vi·tis
pho·to·de·com·po·si·tion
pho·to·der·ma·ti·tis
pho·to·der·ma·to·sis
pho·to·dis·in·te·gra·tion
pho·tod·ro·my
pho·to·dy·nam·ic
pho·to·dy·nam·i·cal·ly
pho·to·dyn·i·a
pho·to·dys·pho·ri·a
pho·to·e·lec·tric
pho·to·e·lec·tric·i·ty
  pl pho·to·e·lec·tric·i·ties
pho·to·e·lec·tron
pho·to·e·mis·sion

pho·to·e·mis·sive
pho·to·flu·o·ro·graph·ic
pho·to·flu·o·rog·ra·phy
  pl pho·to·flu·o·rog·ra·phies
pho·to·flu·o·ros·co·py
  pl pho·to·flu·o·ros·co·pies
pho·to·gen
pho·to·gene
pho·to·gen·e·sis
  pl pho·to·gen·e·ses
pho·to·gen·ic
pho·to·gram
pho·to·graph
pho·to·graph·ic
pho·tog·ra·phy
pho·to·in·duced
pho·to·in·duc·tion
pho·to·in·duc·tive
pho·to·ki·ne·sis
  pl pho·to·ki·ne·ses
pho·to·ki·net·ic
pho·to·ky·mo·graph
pho·to·ky·mo·graph·ic
pho·to·lu·mi·nes·cence
pho·to·lu·mi·nes·cent
pho·tol·y·sis
  pl pho·tol·y·ses
pho·to·lyte
pho·to·lyt·ic
pho·to·lyt·i·cal·ly
pho·to·lyze
pho·to·mac·ro·graph
pho·to·mac·ro·graph·ic
pho·to·ma·crog·ra·phy
  pl pho·to·ma·crog·ra·phies
pho·to·mag·net·ism
pho·to·ma·ni·a
pho·to·mes·on
pho·tom·e·ter
pho·to·met·ric
  or pho·to·met·ri·cal
pho·to·met·ri·cal
  or pho·to·met·ric
pho·to·met·ri·cal·ly
pho·tom·e·try
  pl pho·tom·e·tries
pho·to·mi·cro·gram
pho·to·mi·cro·graph
pho·to·mi·crog·ra·pher

pho·to·mi·cro·graph·ic
  or pho·to·mi·cro·graph·
    i·cal
pho·to·mi·cro·graph·i·cal
  or pho·to·mi·cro·graph·ic
pho·to·mi·cro·graph·i·
    cal·ly
pho·to·mi·crog·ra·phy
  pl pho·to·mi·crog·ra·phies
pho·to·mo·tor
pho·to·mul·ti·pli·er
pho·ton
pho·to·neg·a·tive
pho·to·neu·ro·en·do·crine
pho·to·neu·tron
pho·ton·o·sus
  pl pho·ton·o·si
pho·to·nu·cle·ar
pho·to·par·aes·the·si·a
  var of pho·to·par·es·the·si·a
pho·to·par·es·the·si·a
pho·to·path·ic
pho·to·path·o·log·ic
pho·top·a·thy
  pl pho·top·a·thies
pho·to·per·cep·tive
pho·to·pe·ri·od
pho·to·pe·ri·od·ic
  or pho·to·pe·ri·od·i·cal
pho·to·pe·ri·od·i·cal
  or pho·to·pe·ri·od·ic
pho·to·pe·ri·od·i·cal·ly
pho·to·pe·ri·od·ism
pho·to·phile
  or pho·to·phil·ic
  or pho·toph·i·lous
pho·to·phil·ic
  or pho·toph·i·lous
  or pho·to·phile
pho·toph·i·lous
  or pho·to·phil·ic
  or pho·to·phile
pho·to·pho·bi·a
pho·to·pho·bic
pho·to·phone
pho·to·phore
pho·to·phos·phor·y·la·tion
pho·toph·thal·mi·a
pho·to·pi·a

pho·to·pic
pho·to·po·lym·er·i·za·tion
pho·to·pos·i·tive
pho·to·pro·ton
pho·top·si·a
pho·top·sin
pho·top·tom·e·ter
pho·top·tom·e·try
pho·to·re·ac·tion
pho·to·re·ac·ti·vat·ing
pho·to·re·ac·ti·va·tion
pho·to·re·cep·tion
pho·to·re·cep·tive
pho·to·re·cep·tor
pho·to·re·duc·tion
pho·to·ret·i·ni·tis
pho·to·scan
pho·to·scope
pho·tos·co·py
pho·to·sen·si·tive
pho·to·sen·si·tiv·i·ty
  pl pho·to·sen·si·tiv·i·ties
pho·to·sen·si·ti·za·tion
pho·to·sen·si·tize
pho·to·sen·si·tiz·er
pho·to·shock
pho·to·sta·bil·i·ty
  pl pho·to·sta·bil·i·ties
pho·to·sta·ble
pho·to·syn·the·sis
  pl pho·to·syn·the·ses
pho·to·syn·the·size
pho·to·syn·thet·ic
pho·to·syn·thet·i·cal·ly
pho·to·tac·tic
pho·to·tac·ti·cal·ly
pho·to·tax·is
  pl pho·to·tax·es
  or pho·to·tax·y
  pl pho·to·ax·ies
pho·to·tax·y
  pl pho·to·tax·ies
  or pho·to·tax·is
  pl pho·to·tax·es
pho·to·ther·a·py
  pl pho·to·ther·a·pies
pho·to·ther·mal
  or pho·to·ther·mic

pho·to·ther·mic
  or pho·to·ther·mal
pho·to·tim·er
pho·to·ton·ic
pho·to·tot·o·nus
pho·to·top·i·a
pho·to·troph
pho·to·troph·ic
pho·to·tro·pic
pho·to·tro·pi·cal·ly
pho·tot·ro·pism
pho·to·tube
pho·to·vol·ta·ic
pho·tu·ri·a
phrag·mo·plast
phren
  pl phre·nes
phre·nal·gi·a
phren·as·the·ni·a
phren·as·then·ic
phren·a·tro·phi·a
phren·em·phrax·is
  pl phren·em·phrax·es
phre·ne·si·a
phre·ne·si·ac
phre·ne·sis
phre·net·ic
  or phre·net·i·cal
  or fre·net·ic
phre·net·i·cal
  or phre·net·ic
  or fre·net·ic
phren·ic
phren·i·cec·to·my
  pl phren·i·cec·to·mies
phren·i·cla·si·a
  or phren·i·cla·sis
phren·i·cla·sis
  pl phren·i·cla·ses
  or phren·i·cla·si·a
phren·i·co·col·ic
phren·i·co·cos·tal
phren·i·co·e·soph·a·ge·al
phren·i·co·ex·er·e·sis
phren·i·co·gas·tric
phren·i·co·splen·ic
phren·i·cot·o·my
  pl phren·i·cot·o·mies
phren·i·co·trip·sy

phre·ni·tis
phren·o·bla·bi·a
phren·o·car·di·a
phren·o·car·di·ac
phren·o·col·ic
phren·o·e·soph·a·ge·al
phren·o·gas·tric
phren·o·glot·tic
phren·o·he·pat·ic
phren·o·lep·sic
phren·o·log·ic
  or phren·o·log·i·cal
phren·o·log·i·cal
  or phren·o·log·ic
phren·o·log·i·cal·ly
phre·nol·o·gist
phre·nol·o·gy
  pl phre·nol·o·gies
phren·o·pa·ral·y·sis
phren·o·path
phre·nop·a·thy
phren·o·ple·gi·a
phren·o·sin
phren·o·sin·ic
phren·o·spasm
phren·o·splen·ic
phren·sy
  var of fren·zy
phric·to·path·ic
phron·e·mo·pho·bi·a
phro·ne·sis
phryg·i·an
phry·nin
phryn·o·der·ma
phry·nol·y·sin
phthal·ate
phthal·e·in
phthal·ic
phthal·in
phthal·o·fyne
phthal·yl·sul·fa·cet·a·mide
phthal·yl·sul·fa·thi·a·zole
phthei·ri·a·sis
  pl phthei·ri·a·ses
  var of phthi·ri·a·sis
phthin·oid
phthi·o·col
phthi·o·ic

hthi·ri·a·sis
pl phthi·ri·a·ses
phthir·i·us
phthis·ic
or phthis·i·cal
hthis·i·cal
or phthis·ic
hthis·i·ol·o·gist
hthis·i·ol·o·gy
pl phthis·i·ol·o·gies
hthis·i·o·pho·bi·a
hthis·i·o·ther·a·py
hthi·sis
pl phthi·ses
hthi·sis bul·bi
hy·co·bil·in
hy·co·chrom
or phy·co·chrome
hy·co·chrome
or phy·co·chrom
hy·co·col·loid
hy·co·cy·an
or phy·co·cy·a·nin
hy·co·cy·a·nin
or phy·co·cy·an
hy·co·er·y·thrin
hy·co·my·cete
Phy·co·my·ce·tes
hy·co·my·ce·tous
hy·co·my·co·sis
phy·co·ga·lac·tic
phy·lax·is
hy·let·ic
hyl·lo·er·y·thrin
hyl·loid
hyl·lo·por·phy·rin
hyl·lo·pyr·role
hyl·lo·qui·none
hy·lo·gen·e·sis
hy·lo·ge·net·ic
hy·log·e·ny
hy·lum
pl phy·la
hy·ma
pl phy·mas
or phy·ma·ta
hy·ma·tic
hy·ma·toid
hy·ma·tor·rhy·sin

phy·ma·to·sis
pl phy·ma·to·ses
phys·a·lif·er·ous
phy·sal·i·form
phy·sal·i·phore
phy·sa·liph·o·rous
phy·sa·lis
Phy·sa·lop·ter·a
phys·co·ni·a
phys·i·an·thro·py
pl phys·i·an·thro·pies
phys·i·at·rics
phys·i·at·rist
phys·ic
pl phys·ics
or phys·icks
phys·i·cal
phy·si·cian
phys·i·cist
Phy·sick op·er·a·tion
phys·i·co·chem·i·cal
phys·i·co·chem·i·cal·ly
phys·i·co·py·rex·i·a
phys·ics
phys·i·no·sis
phys·i·o·chem·i·cal
phys·i·o·gen·ic
phys·i·og·nom·ic
or phys·i·og·nom·i·cal
phys·i·og·nom·i·cal
or phys·i·og·nom·ic
phys·i·og·nom·i·cal·ly
phys·i·og·no·mist
phys·i·og·no·my
pl phys·i·og·no·mies
phys·i·og·no·sis
phys·i·o·log·ic
or phys·i·o·log·i·cal
phys·i·o·log·i·cal
or phys·i·o·log·ic
phys·i·o·log·i·cal·ly
phys·i·o·log·i·co·an·a·
tom·ic
phys·i·ol·o·gist
phys·i·ol·o·gy
pl phys·i·ol·o·gies
phys·i·o·med·i·cal·ism
phys·i·o·path·o·log·ic
or phys·i·o·path·o·log·i·cal

phys·i·o·path·o·log·i·cal
or phys·i·o·path·o·log·ic
phys·i·o·pa·thol·o·gy
pl phys·i·o·pa·thol·o·gies
phys·i·o·psy·chic
phys·i·o·ther·a·peu·tic
phys·i·o·ther·a·peu·tics
phys·i·o·ther·a·pist
phys·i·o·ther·a·py
pl phys·i·o·ther·a·pies
phy·sique
Phy·so·ceph·a·lus
phy·so·haem·a·to·me·tra
var of phy·so·hem·a·to·
me·tra
phy·so·hem·a·to·me·tra
phy·so·hy·dro·me·tra
phy·so·me·tra
phy·so·py·o·sal·pinx
phy·so·stig·ma
phy·so·stig·mine
phy·tal·bu·mose
phy·tan·ic
phy·tase
phy·tic
phy·to·be·zo·ar
phy·to·chem·i·cal
phy·to·chem·i·cal·ly
phy·to·chem·ist
phy·to·chem·is·try
pl phy·to·chem·is·tries
phy·to·chrome
phy·to·flu·ene
phy·to·gen·e·sis
pl phy·to·gen·e·ses
phy·to·ge·net·ic
phy·to·gen·ic
phy·tog·e·nous
phy·tog·e·ny
phy·to·haem·ag·glu·ti·nin
var of phy·to·hem·ag·glu·
tin·in
phy·to·hem·ag·glu·ti·nin
phy·to·hor·mone
phy·toid
phy·tol
Phy·to·mas·ti·gi·na
phy·to·na·di·one
phy·to·par·a·site

phy·to·path·o·gen
phy·to·path·o·gen·ic
phy·to·path·o·gen·ic·i·ty
  pl phy·to·path·o·gen·ic·
  i·ties
phy·to·path·o·log·ic
  or phy·to·path·o·log·i·cal
phy·to·path·o·log·i·cal
  or phy·to·path·o·log·ic
phy·to·pa·thol·o·gist
phy·to·pa·thol·o·gy
  pl phy·to·pa·thol·o·gies
phy·toph·a·gous
phy·toph·a·gy
  pl phy·toph·a·gies
phy·to·phar·ma·co·log·i·cal
phy·to·phar·ma·col·o·gy
  pl phy·to·phar·ma·col·
  o·gies
phy·to·pho·to·der·ma·ti·tis
phy·to·pho·to·der·ma·to·sis
phy·to·pneu·mo·co·ni·o·sis
  pl phy·to·pneu·mo·co·ni·
  o·ses
phy·to·pre·cip·i·tin
phy·to·sis
  pl phy·to·ses
phy·to·ste·a·rin
phy·tos·ter·in
phy·tos·ter·ol
phy·tos·ter·o·lin
phy·to·throm·bo·ki·nase
phy·to·tox·ic
phy·to·tox·ic·i·ty
  pl phy·to·tox·ic·i·ties
phy·to·tox·in
phy·to·tron
phy·to·vi·tel·lin
phy·tyl
phy·tyl·men·a·di·one
pi·a ma·ter
pi·a-a·rach·noid
  or pi·a·rach·noid
pi·a-a·rach·noi·dal
pi·al
pi·a·ma·tral
pi·an
pi·a·rach·noid
  or pi·a-a·rach·noid

pi·as·tre·nae·mi·a
  var of pi·as·tre·ne·mi·a
pi·as·tre·ne·mi·a
pi·block·to
  or pi·blok·to
pi·blok·to
  or pi·block·to
pi·ca
Pic·co·lo·mi·ni bands
pic·e·ous
pi·chi
Pick dis·ease
Pick·wick·i·an syn·drome
Pick·worth meth·od
pic·nom·e·ter
  var of pyk·nom·e·ter
pi·e·cu·rie
pi·co·gram
pic·o·lin·ic
pi·co·pi·co·gram
pi·cor·na·vi·rus
pi·co·sec·ond
pic·ram·ic
Pic·ras·ma
pic·rate
pic·ric
pic·ro·car·mine
pic·ro·lon·ic
pic·ro·ni·gro·sin
pic·ro·pod·o·phyl·lin
Pic·ro·rhi·za
pic·ro·tin
pic·ro·tox·in
pic·ro·tox·in·in
pic·ryl
pic·to·graph
pie·bald
pie·bald·ism
pi·e·dra
Pi·erre Ro·bin syn·drome
pi·es·aes·the·si·a
  var of pi·es·es·the·si·a
pi·es·es·the·si·a
pi·e·som·e·ter
pi·e·zo·chem·is·try
  pl pi·e·zo·chem·is·tries
pi·e·zo·e·lec·tric·i·ty
pi·e·zom·e·ter
pi·e·zo·met·ric

Pif·fard paste
pig·bel
pi·geon-toed
pig·ment
pig·men·tar·y
pig·men·ta·tion
pig·ment·ed
pig·men·to·gen·e·sis
pig·men·to·phage
  or chro·mo·phage
pig·men·tum ni·grum
pig·my
  var of pyg·my
Pign·et in·dex
pig·weed
pi·i·tis
pi·lar
pi·la·ry
pi·las·ter
Pilcz re·flex
pile
pi·le·ous
pi·le·us
  pl pi·le·i
pi·li
pi·li·a·tion
pi·li·be·zoar
pi·li·form
pi·li·gan
pi·li·mic·tion
pill
pil·lar
pil·let
pil·le·um
pil·le·us
pil·lion
pil·lu·lar
  or pil·u·lar
pil·lute
  or pil·ule
pi·lo·car·pi·dine
pi·lo·car·pine
pi·lo·car·pus
  pl pi·lo·car·pi
pi·lo·cys·tic
pi·lo·e·rec·tion
pi·lo·ma·trix·o·ma
  pl pi·lo·ma·trix·o·mas
  or pi·lo·ma·trix·o·ma·ta

pi·lo·mo·tor
pi·lo·ni·dal
pi·lose
pi·lo·se·ba·ceous
pi·lo·sis
pi·los·i·ty
   pl pi·los·i·ties
pi·lous
pil·u·la
   pl pil·u·lae
pil·u·lar
   or pil·lu·lar
pil·ule
   or pil·lute
pi·lus
   pl pi·li
pi·mel·ic
pim·e·li·tis
pim·e·lo·pte·ryg·i·um
pim·e·lor·rhe·a
pim·e·lor·rhoe·a
   var of pim·e·lor·rhe·a
pim·e·lor·thop·ne·a
pim·e·lor·thop·noe·a
   var of pim·e·lor·thop·ne·a
pim·e·lu·ri·a
pi·men·ta
pi·min·o·dine
pim·o·zide
pim·pi·nel·la
pim·ple
pim·ply
pin
pin·a·coid
pi·nac·o·lone
pin·a·cy·a·nol
Pi·nard ma·neu·ver
pin·bone
pince·ment
pin·cers
Pin·cus re·a·gent
pine
pin·e·al
pin·e·al·blas·to·ma
   pl pin·e·al·blas·to·mas
   or pin·e·al·blas·to·ma·ta
pin·e·al·cy·to·ma
   pl pin·e·al·cy·to·mas
   or pin·e·al·cy·to·ma·ta

pin·e·a·lec·to·my
pin·e·al·ism
pin·e·a·lo·ma
   pl pin·e·a·lo·mas
   or pin·e·a·lo·ma·ta
Pi·nel sys·tem
pi·nene
pin·e·o·blas·to·ma
   pl pin·e·o·blas·to·mas
   or pin·e·o·blas·to·ma·ta
pin·guec·u·la
   pl pin·guec·u·lae
pin·guic·u·la
   pl pin·guic·u·lae
   var of pin·guec·u·la
pin·guid
pi·ni·form
pink·eye
pink·root
pin·na
   pl pin·nas
   or pin·nae
pin·nal
pin·o·cyte
pin·o·cy·to·sis
   pl pin·o·cy·to·ses
pin·o·cy·tot·ic
pin·o·cy·tot·i·cal·ly
pin·o·some
pin·ox·e·pin
Pins sign
pint
pin·ta
pin·tid
pin·til·lo
pin·to
Pi·nus
pin·worm
pi·o·nae·mi·a
   var of pi·o·ne·mi·a
pi·o·ne·mi·a
Pi·oph·i·la
pi·or·thop·ne·a
pi·or·thop·noe·a
   var of pi·or·thop·ne·a
Pi·o·trow·ski sign
pi·pam·a·zine
pi·pam·per·one
pi·paz·e·thate

pi·pen·zo·late
Pi·per
pip·er·a·cet·a·zine
pip·er·a·mide
pi·per·a·zine
pi·per·i·dine
pip·er·i·do·late
pip·er·ine
pip·er·o·caine
pip·er·o·nal
pip·er·ox·an
pi·pet
   or pi·pette
pi·pette
   or pi·pet
pip·o·bro·man
pip·o·sul·fan
pip·ra·drol
pip·ro·zol·in
pip·sis·se·wa
pip·syl
pip·to·nych·i·a
pi·quite
piq·ui·zil
pir·i·form
   or pyr·i·form
pir·i·for·mis
   or pyr·i·for·mis
Pi·ro·goff am·pu·ta·tion
Pir·o·nel·la
Pi·ro·plas·ma
   pl Pi·ro·plas·mas
   or Pi·ro·plas·ma·ta
pi·ro·plas·mic
pi·ro·plas·mo·sis
   pl pi·ro·plas·mo·ses
pi·ro·plas·mot·ic
Pir·quet test
pis·ci·ci·dal
pis·ci·cide
pis·cid·i·a
pi·si·an·nu·lar·is
pi·si·form
pi·si·met·a·car·pus
pi·si·un·ci·na·tus
pi·so·ha·mate
pi·so·met·a·car·pal
pi·so·tri·que·tral
pit

pitch
pitch·blende
pith·e·coid
pith·i·a·tism
pith·i·at·ic
pith·i·at·ric
pi·tom·e·ter
Pi·tot tube
Pi·tres sec·tions
pi·tu·i·cyte
pi·tu·i·cy·to·ma
  pl pi·tu·i·cy·to·mas
  or pi·tu·i·cy·to·ma·ta
pi·tu·i·ta
  pl pi·tu·i·tae
pi·tu·i·tar·y
  pl pi·tu·i·tar·ies
pit·y·ri·as·ic
pit·y·ri·a·sis
  pl pit·y·ri·a·ses
pit·y·roid
Pit·y·ro·spo·rum
pi·val·ate
pi·val·ic
piv·ot
pla·ce·bo
pla·cen·ta
  pl pla·cen·tas
  or pla·cen·tae
pla·cen·ta pre·vi·a
  pl pla·cen·tae pre·vi·ae
pla·cen·tal
plac·en·ta·tion
pla·cen·tin
plac·en·ti·tis
  pl plac·en·ti·ti·des
plac·en·tog·ra·phy
  pl plac·en·tog·ra·phies
pla·cen·toid
plac·en·tol·y·sin
plac·en·to·ma
  pl plac·en·to·mas
  or plac·en·to·ma·ta
plac·en·to·sis
pla·cen·to·ther·a·py
Pla·ci·do disk
pla·co·dal
pla·code

placque
  var of plaque
plad·a·ro·ma
  pl plad·a·ro·mas
  or plad·a·ro·ma·ta
plad·a·ro·sis
  pl plad·a·ro·ses
pla·gio·ce·phal·ic
pla·gio·ceph·a·lism
pla·gio·ceph·a·lous
pla·gio·ceph·a·ly
  pl pla·gio·o·ceph·a·lies
plague
plak·al·bu·min
plan·chet
Planck con·stant
pla·nar
plane
pla·ni·ceps
pla·ni·gram
pla·ni·graph
pla·nig·ra·phy
  pl pla·nig·ra·phies
pla·nim·e·ter
pla·ni·met·ric
plan·ing
plank·ton
pla·no·cel·lu·lar
pla·no·con·cave
pla·no·con·ic
pla·no·con·vex
plan·o·cyte
plan·o·ma·ni·a
Pla·nor·bis
pla·no·val·gus
plan·ta
  pl plan·tae
Plan·ta·go
plan·tar
plan·tar·is
  pl plan·tar·es
plan·ta·tion
plan·ti·grade
plan·u·la
  pl plan·u·lae
pla·num
  pl pla·na
plaque

plasm
plas·ma
plas·ma·blast
plas·ma·cu·les
plas·ma·cyte
plas·ma·cyt·ic
plas·ma·cy·toid
plas·ma·cy·to·ma
  pl plas·ma·cy·to·mas
  or plas·ma·cy·to·ma·ta
plas·ma·cy·to·sis
  pl plas·ma·cy·to·sis·es
  or plas·ma·cy·to·ses
plas·ma·gel
plas·ma·gene
plas·mal
plas·ma·lem·ma
plas·mal·o·gen
plas·ma·phaer·e·sis
  pl plas·ma·phaer·e·ses
  var of plas·ma·pher·e·sis
plas·ma·pher·e·sis
  pl plas·ma·pher·e·ses
plas·ma·sol
plas·ma·some
  or plas·mo·some
  or plas·mo·so·ma
plas·ma·ther·a·py
plas·mat·ic
plas·ma·tog·a·my
plas·ma·tor·rhex·is
  pl plas·ma·tor·rhex·es
plas·ma·to·sis
plas·mic
plas·mi·cal·ly
plas·mid
plas·min
plas·min·o·gen
plas·min·o·gen·o·pe·ni·a
plas·mo·crin
plas·mo·cyte
plas·mo·cyt·ic
plas·mo·cy·to·ma
  pl plas·mo·cy·to·mas
  or plas·mo·cy·to·ma·ta
  var of plas·ma·cy·to·ma
plas·mo·desm
  pl plas·mo·des·ma·ta*

308

plas·mo·di·al
  or plas·mod·ic
  or plas·mo·di·ate
plas·mo·di·a·sis
  pl plas·mo·di·a·ses
  or plas·mo·di·o·sis
  pl plas·mo·di·o·ses
plas·mo·di·ate
  or plas·mod·ic
  or plas·mo·di·al
plas·mo·di·blast
plas·mod·ic
  or plas·mo·di·al
  or plas·mo·di·ate
plas·mo·di·cide
Plas·mo·di·i·dae
plas·mo·di·o·sis
  pl plas·mo·di·o·ses
  or plas·mo·di·a·sis
  pl plas·mo·di·a·ses
plas·mo·di·tro·pho·blast
Plas·mo·di·um
  pl plas·mo·di·a
plas·mog·a·my
  pl plas·mog·a·mies
plas·mo·gen
plas·mol·y·sis
  pl plas·mol·y·ses
plas·mo·lyt·ic
plas·mo·lyt·i·cal·ly
plas·mo·lyz·a·bil·i·ty
  pl plas·mo·lyz·a·bil·i·ties
plas·mo·lyze
plas·mo·ma
  pl plas·mo·mas
  or plas·mo·ma·ta
plas·mon
  or plas·mone
plas·mone
  or plas·mon
plas·mo·nu·cle·ic
plas·moph·a·gous
plas·mop·ty·sis
  pl plas·mop·ty·ses
plas·mor·rhex·is
plas·mos·chi·sis
plas·mo·so·ma
  or plas·mo·some
  or plas·ma·some

plas·mo·some
  or plas·mo·so·ma
  or plas·ma·some
plas·mo·ther·a·py
plas·mot·o·my
  pl plas·mot·o·mies
plas·mo·trop·ic
plas·mot·ro·pism
plas·mo·zyme
plas·te·in
plas·ter of Par·is
plas·tic
plas·tic·i·ty
  pl plas·tic·i·ties
plas·ti·ciz·er
plas·tics
plas·tid
plas·tid·i·al
plas·ti·dule
plas·tin
plas·to·dy·nam·i·a
plas·tog·a·my
  pl plas·tog·a·mies
plas·to·gene
plas·to·qui·none
plas·to·some
plate
pla·teau
  pl pla·teaus
  or pla·teaux
plate·let
plate·let·phe·re·sis
pla·tin·ic
plat·i·nous
plat·i·num
plat·ode
plat·oid
plat·o·nych·i·a
plat·y·ba·si·a
plat·y·ce·li·an
  or plat·y·ce·lous
plat·y·ce·lous
  or plat·y·ce·li·an
plat·y·ce·phal·ic
  or plat·y·ceph·a·lous
plat·y·ceph·a·lism
  or plat·y·ceph·a·ly
plat·y·ceph·a·lous
  or plat·y·ce·phal·ic

plat·y·ceph·a·ly
  pl plat·y·ceph·a·lies
  or plat·y·ceph·a·lism
plat·y·cne·mi·a
plat·y·cne·mic
plat·y·cne·mism
plat·y·cne·my
  pl plat·y·cne·mies
plat·y·coe·li·an
  var of plat·y·ce·li·an
plat·y·coe·lous
  var of plat·y·ce·lous
plat·y·co·ri·a
plat·y·co·ri·a·sis
plat·y·cra·ni·a
plat·y·hel·minth
Plat·y·hel·min·thes
plat·y·hel·min·thic
plat·y·hi·er·ic
plat·y·mer·ic
plat·y·mor·phi·a
plat·y·o·pi·a
plat·y·op·ic
plat·y·pel·lic
plat·y·pel·loid
plat·y·pel·ly
  pl plat·y·pel·lies
plat·y·po·di·a
plat·yr·rhine
plat·yr·rhin·ic
plat·yr·rhi·ny
  pl plat·yr·rhi·nies
pla·tys·ma
  pl pla·tys·mas·ta
  or pla·tys·ma·ta
plat·ys·ten·ce·pha·li·a
plat·ys·ten·ce·phal·ic
plat·ys·ten·ceph·a·ly
  pl plat·ys·ten·ceph·a·lies
plec·to·ne·mic
plec·trid·i·um
  pl plec·trid·i·a
pled·get
plei·o·trop·ic
plei·ot·ro·pism
plei·ot·ro·py
  pl plei·ot·ro·pies
ple·o·chro·ic
ple·och·ro·ism

309

ple·o·chro·it·ic
ple·o·chro·mat·ic
ple·o·chrome
ple·och·ro·ous
ple·o·co·ni·al
ple·o·cy·to·sis
   pl ple·o·cy·to·ses
ple·o·mas·ti·a
ple·o·mas·tic
ple·o·ma·zi·a
ple·o·mor·phic
ple·o·mor·phism
ple·o·mor·phous
ple·o·nasm
ple·o·nas·tic
ple·o·nec·tic
ple·o·nex·i·a
ple·o·nex·y
ple·on·os·te·o·sis
ple·o·no·tus
ple·oph·a·gous
ple·ro·cer·coid
ple·ro·sis
ple·si·o·gnath·us
ple·si·o·mor·phism
ple·si·o·pi·a
ples·saes·the·si·a
   var of ples·ses·the·si·a
ples·ses·the·si·a
ples·sim·e·ter
ples·sor
ples·sus
pleth·o·ra
pleth·o·ric
ple·thys·mo·gram
ple·thys·mo·graph
ple·thys·mo·graph·ic
ple·thys·mo·graph·i·cal·ly
pleth·ys·mog·ra·phy
   pl pleth·ys·mog·ra·phies
pleu·ra
   pl pleu·ras
   or pleu·rae
pleu·ra·cen·te·sis
pleu·ra·cot·o·my
pleu·ral
pleu·ral·gi·a
pleu·ral·gic

pleur·am·ni·on
pleur·ap·o·phys·i·al
pleur·a·poph·y·sis
   pl pleur·a·poph·y·ses
pleu·ra·tome
pleu·rec·to·my
pleu·ri·sy
   pl pleu·ri·sies
pleu·rit·ic
pleu·ri·tis
   pl pleu·ri·ti·des
pleu·ro·cen·te·sis
pleu·ro·cen·tral
pleu·ro·cen·trum
   pl pleu·ro·cen·trums
   or pleu·ro·cen·ta
pleu·ro·chol·e·cys·ti·tis
pleu·ro·cu·ta·ne·ous
pleu·ro·dont
pleu·ro·dyn·i·a
pleu·ro·gen·ic
   or pleu·rog·e·nous
pleu·rog·e·nous
   or pleu·ro·gen·ic
pleu·ro·hep·a·ti·tis
pleu·ro·lith
pleu·rol·y·sis
   pl pleu·rol·y·ses
pleu·ro·ma
   pl pleu·ro·mas
   or pleu·ro·ma·ta
pleu·ro·me·lus
pleu·ro·per·i·car·di·al
pleu·ro·per·i·car·di·tis
   pl pleu·ro·per·i·car·di·ti·des
pleu·ro·per·i·to·ne·al
pleu·ro·per·i·to·ne·um
   pl pleu·ro·per·i·to·ne·ums
   or pleu·ro·per·i·to·ne·a
pleu·ro·pneu·mo·ni·a
pleu·ro·pneu·mo·nia-
   like or·gan·ism
pleu·ro·pros·o·pos·chi·sis
pleu·ro·pul·mo·nar·y
pleu·ros·co·py
pleu·ro·so·ma
pleu·ro·so·ma·tos·chi·sis
pleu·ro·so·mus

pleu·ro·spasm
pleu·ro·thot·o·nos
   or pleu·ro·thot·o·nus
pleu·ro·thot·o·nus
   or pleu·mo·thot·o·nos
pleu·rot·o·my
pleu·ro·ty·phoid
plue·ro·vis·cer·al
plex·al
plex·ec·to·my
plex·i·form
plex·im·e·ter
plex·i·met·ric
plex·im·e·try
   pl plex·im·e·tries
plex·or
plex·us
   pl plex·us·es
   or plex·us
pli·ca
   pl pli·cae
pli·ca a·lar·is
   pl pli·cae a·lar·es
pli·ca cir·cu·lar·is
   pl pli·cae cir·cu·lar·es
pli·ca po·lon·i·ca
   pl pli·cae po·lon·i·cae
pli·cal
pli·cate
pli·cate·ly
pli·cate·ness
pli·ca·tion
pli·cot·o·my
ploi·dy
   pl ploi·dies
plomb
   or plumb
plom·bage
plo·ra·tion
plug
plug·ger
plumb
   or plomb
plum·ba·gin
plum·ba·go
plum·bic
plum·bism
plum·bite

plum·bum
Plum·mer-Vin·son
  syn·drome
plu·mose
plump·er
plu·ri·de·fi·cien·cy
plu·ri·de·fi·cient
plu·ri·fo·cal
plu·ri·glan·du·lar
plu·ri·grav·i·da
plu·ri·loc·u·lar
plu·ri·or·i·fi·cial
plu·rip·a·ra
  pl plu·rip·a·rae
plu·ri·par·i·ty
plu·rip·o·tent
plu·ri·po·ten·ti·al·i·ty
  pl plu·ri·po·ten·ti·al·i·ties
plu·to·ma·ni·a
plu·to·nism
plu·to·ni·um
pne·o·car·di·ac
pne·o·dy·nam·ics
pne·o·graph
pne·om·e·ter
pne·o·pne·ic
pneu·ma
pneu·mar·thro·sis
pneu·mat·ic
pneu·mat·i·cal·ly
pneu·ma·tic·i·ty
  pl pneu·ma·tic·i·ties
pneu·mat·ics
pneu·ma·tism
pneu·ma·ti·za·tion
pneu·ma·tize
pneu·ma·to·car·di·a
pneu·ma·to·cele
pneu·ma·to·dysp·ne·a
pneu·ma·to·dysp·noe·a
  var of pneu·ma·to·dysp·
  ne·a
pneu·ma·to·gram
pneu·ma·to·graph
pneu·ma·tol·o·gy
pneu·ma·tom·e·ter
pneu·ma·tom·e·try
  pl pneu·ma·tom·e·tries

pneu·ma·tor·ra·chis
pneu·ma·to·sis
  pl pneu·ma·to·ses
pneu·ma·tu·ri·a
pneu·ma·type
pneu·mec·to·my
  pl pneu·mec·to·mies
pneu·mo·an·gi·og·ra·phy
pneu·mo·ar·thro·gram
pneu·mo·ar·throg·ra·phy
pneu·mo·ba·cil·lus
  pl pneu·mo·ba·cil·li
pneu·mo·bul·bar
pneu·mo·cele
pneu·mo·cen·te·sis
  pl pneu·mo·cen·te·ses
pneu·mo·ceph·a·lus
pneu·mo·cho·le·cys·ti·tis
pneu·mo·coc·cal
  or pneu·mo·coc·cic
pneu·mo·coc·ce·mi·a
pneu·mo·coc·cic
  or pneu·mo·coc·cal
pneu·mo·coc·ci·dal
pneu·mo·coc·co·su·ri·a
pneu·mo·coc·cus
  pl pneu·mo·coc·ci
pneu·mo·co·lon
pneu·mo·co·ni·o·sis
  pl pneu·mo·co·ni·o·ses
pneu·mo·cra·ni·um
Pneu·mo·cys·tis
pneu·mo·cys·to·gram
pneu·mo·cys·tog·ra·phy
pneu·mo·der·ma
pneu·mo·dy·nam·ics
pneu·mo·en·ceph·a·li·tis
  pl pneu·mo·en·ceph·a·li·
  ti·des
pneu·mo·en·ceph·a·lo·cele
pneu·mo·en·ceph·a·lo·
  gram
pneu·mo·en·ceph·a·lo·
  graph
pneu·mo·en·ceph·a·lo·
  graph·ic
pneu·mo·en·ceph·a·lo·
  graph·i·cal·ly

pneu·mo·en·ceph·a·log·
  ra·phy
  pl pneu·mo·en·ceph·a·log·
  ra·phies
pneu·mo·en·ter·ic
pneu·mo·en·ter·i·tis
  pl pneu·mo·en·ter·i·tis·es
  or pneu·mo·en·ter·i·ti·des
pneu·mo·gas·tric
pneu·mo·gram
pneu·mo·graph
pneu·mo·graph·ic
pneu·mo·graph·i·cal·ly
pneu·mog·ra·phy
  pl pneu·mog·ra·phies
pneu·mo·hae·mo·per·i·car·
  di·um
  var of pneu·mo·he·mo·per·
  i·car·di·um
pneu·mo·hae·mo·tho·rax
  pl pneu·mo·hae·mo·tho·
  rax·es
  or pneu·mo·hae·mo·tho·
  ra·ces
pneu·mo·he·mo·per·i·car·
  di·um
pneu·mo·he·mo·tho·rax
  pl pneu·mo·he·mo·tho·
  rax·es
  or pneu·mo·he·mo·tho·
  ra·ces
pneu·mo·hy·dro·per·i·car·
  di·um
pneu·mo·hy·dro·tho·rax
  pl pneu·mo·hy·dro·tho·
  rax·es
  or pneu·mo·hy·dro·tho·
  ra·ces
pneu·mo·hy·po·der·ma
pneu·mo·ko·ni·o·sis
  var of pneu·mo·co·ni·o·sis
pneu·mo·lip·i·do·sis
pneu·mo·lith
pneu·mo·li·thi·a·sis
pneu·mol·o·gy
  pl pneu·mol·o·gies
pneu·mol·y·sis
  pl pneu·mol·y·ses

311

pneu·mo·me·di·as·ti·num
  pl pneu·mo·me·di·as·ti·na
pneu·mom·e·try
pneu·mo·my·co·sis
  pl pneu·mo·my·co·ses
pneu·mo·nec·to·my
  pl pneu·mo·nec·to·mies
pneu·mo·ni·a
pneu·mon·ic
pneu·mo·ni·tis
  pl pneu·mo·ni·ti·des
pneu·mo·no·cele
pneu·mo·no·cen·te·sis
pneu·mo·no·co·ni·o·sis
  var of pneu·mo·co·ni·o·sis
pneu·mo·no·ko·ni·o·sis
  var of pneu·mo·co·ni·o·sis
pneu·mo·nol·y·sis
  pl pneu·mo·nol·y·ses
pneu·mo·no·my·co·sis
pneu·mo·nop·a·thy
pneu·mo·no·pex·y
pneu·mo·nor·rha·phy
pneu·mo·no·sis
  pl pneu·mo·no·ses
pneu·mo·not·o·my
pneu·mo·no·ul·tra·mi·
  crop·scop·ic·
  sil·i·co·vol·ca·no·co·
  ni·o·sis
  pl pneu·mo·no·ul·tra·mi·
    cro·scop·ic·
    sil·i·co·vol·ca·no·co·ni·
    o·ses
Pneu·mo·nys·sus
pneu·mop·a·thy
pneu·mo·per·i·car·di·tis
pneu·mo·per·i·car·di·um
  pl pneu·mo·per·i·car·di·a
pneu·mo·per·i·to·ne·um
  pl pneu·mo·per·i·to·ne·ums
  or pneu·mo·per·i·to·ne·a
pneu·mo·per·i·to·ni·tis
pneu·mo·pex·y
pneu·mo·py·e·lo·gram
pneu·mo·py·o·per·i·car·
  di·um
pneu·mo·ra·chis
  or pneu·mor·rha·chis

pneu·mo·ra·di·og·ra·phy
pneu·mor·rha·chis
  or pneu·mo·ra·chis
pneu·mor·rha·gi·a
pneu·mor·rha·phy
pneu·mo·scle·ro·sis
pneu·mo·sid·er·o·sis
pneu·mo·tach·o·gram
pneu·mo·tach·o·graph
pneu·mo·tax·ic
pneu·mo·tax·is
pneu·mo·tho·rax
  pl pneu·mo·tho·rax·es
  or pneu·mo·tho·ra·ces
pneu·mot·o·my
pneu·mo·tox·ic
pneu·mo·tox·in
pneu·mo·trop·ic
pneu·mo·ty·phoid
pneu·mo·ty·phus
pneu·mo·ven·tri·cle
pneu·mo·ven·tric·u·log·
  ra·phy
pneu·sis
pnig·ma
pni·go·pho·bi·a
pock
pocked
pock·et
pock·mark
pock·marked
po·dag·ra
po·dag·ral
po·dag·ric
po·dag·rous
po·dal·gi·a
po·dal·ic
pod·ar·thri·tis
po·dar·thrum
  pl po·dar·thra
pod·e·de·ma
pod·el·co·ma
  or pod·el·ko·ma
pod·el·ko·ma
  or pod·el·co·ma
pod·en·ceph·a·lus
po·di·at·ric
po·di·a·trist
po·di·a·try

pod·o·brom·hi·dro·sis
pod·o·cyte
pod·o·cyt·ic
pod·o·derm
pod·o·der·ma·ti·tis
  pl pod·o·der·ma·ti·tis·es
  or pod·o·der·ma·ti·ti·des
pod·o·dyn·i·a
pod·oe·de·ma
  var of pod·e·de·ma
po·dol·o·gy
  pl po·dol·o·gies
po·dom·e·ter
pod·o·phyl·lin
pod·o·phyl·lo·tox·in
pod·o·phyl·lum
  pl pod·o·phyl·lums
  or pod·o·phyl·li
po·go·ni·on
Pohl test
poi·ki·lo·blast
poi·ki·lo·blas·tic
poi·ki·lo·cyte
poi·ki·lo·cy·thae·mi·a
  var of poi·ki·lo·cy·the·mi·a
poi·ki·lo·cy·the·mi·a
poi·ki·lo·cy·to·sis
  pl poi·ki·lo·cy·to·ses
poi·ki·lo·der·ma
  pl poi·ki·lo·der·mas
  or poi·ki·lo·der·ma·ta
poi·ki·lo·der·ma·to·my·o·
  si·tis
poi·ki·lo·therm
poi·ki·lo·ther·mal
  or poi·ki·lo·ther·mic
  or poi·ki·lo·ther·mous
poi·ki·lo·ther·mic
  or poi·ki·lo·ther·mal
  or poi·ki·lo·ther·mous
poi·ki·lo·ther·mism
poi·ki·lo·ther·mous
  or poi·ki·lo·ther·mic
  or poi·ki·lo·ther·mal
poi·ki·lo·throm·bo·cyte
poi·ki·lo·zo·o·sper·mi·a
point
poin·til·lage
points dou·lou·reux

poise
Poi·seuille law
poi·son
poi·son·ous
Pois·son dis·tri·bu·tion
po·lar
po·la·rim·e·ter
po·la·ri·met·ric
po·la·rim·e·try
  pl po·la·rim·e·tries
po·lar·i·scope
po·lar·i·scop·ic
po·lar·i·scop·i·cal·ly
po·lar·i·stro·bom·e·ter
po·lar·i·ty
  pl po·lar·i·ties
po·lar·i·za·tion
po·lar·ize
po·lar·iz·er
po·lar·o·gram
po·lar·o·graph
po·lar·o·graph·ic
po·lar·o·graph·i·cal·ly
po·la·rog·ra·phy
  pl po·la·rog·ra·phies
pole
Po·len·ske val·ue
pol·i·clin·ic
po·li·o
po·li·o·dys·pla·si·a cer·e·bri
po·li·o·dys·tro·phi·a
po·li·o·dys·tro·phy
po·li·o·en·ceph·a·li·tis
  pl po·li·o·en·ceph·a·li·ti·des
po·li·o·en·ceph·a·lo·me·nin·go·my·e·li·tis
po·li·o·en·ceph·a·lo·my·e·li·tis
  pl po·li·o·en·ceph·a·lo·my·e·li·ti·des
po·li·o·en·ceph·a·lop·a·thy
po·li·o·my·el·en·ceph·a·li·tis
po·li·o·my·e·li·tis
po·li·o·my·e·lop·a·thy
po·li·o·plasm

po·li·o·sis
  pl po·li·o·ses
pol·i·o·thrix
po·li·o·vi·rus
Pol·it·z·er bar
Pol·it·zer test
po·lit·zer·i·za·tion
Pol·lack meth·od
Pol·lak test
pol·la·ki·u·ri·a
pol·len
pol·len·o·sis
  pl pol·len·o·ses
  var of pol·li·no·sis
pol·li·cal
pol·li·ci·za·tion
pol·li·cize
pol·li·co·men·tal
pol·li·no·sis
  pl pol·li·no·ses
Pol·lis·ter meth·od
pol·lu·tion
po·lo·cyte
po·lo·ni·um
pol·ox·a·lene
pol·ox·al·kol
pol·toph·a·gy
po·lus
  pl po·li
pol·y
Pol·ya op·er·a·tion
pol·y·ac·id
pol·y·a·cryl·a·mide
pol·y·ae·mia
  var of pol·y·e·mi·a
pol·y·aes·the·si·a
  var of pol·y·es·the·si·a
pol·y·al·co·hol
pol·y·a·mide
pol·y·am·ine
pol·y·a·mi·no
pol·y·an·dry
  pl pol·y·an·dries
pol·y·an·gi·i·tis
pol·y·ar·te·ri·tis
pol·y·ar·thric
pol·y·ar·thri·tis
  pl pol·y·ar·thri·ti·des
pol·y·ar·throp·a·thy

pol·y·ar·tic·u·lar
pol·y·a·tom·ic
pol·y·ax·on
  or pol·y·ax·one
pol·y·ax·one
  or pol·y·ox·on
pol·y·ba·sic
pol·y·blast
pol·y·blas·tic
pol·y·ble·phar·i·a
pol·y·bleph·a·ron
pol·y·bleph·a·ry
pol·y·car·bo·phil
pol·y·cel·lu·lar
pol·y·cen·tric
pol·y·chei·ri·a
pol·y·cho·li·a
pol·y·chon·dri·tis
pol·y·chro·ism
pol·y·chro·ma·si·a
pol·y·chro·ma·ti·a
pol·y·chro·mat·ic
pol·y·chro·mat·o·cyte
pol·y·chro·ma·to·phil
pol·y·chro·ma·to·phile
pol·y·chro·ma·to·phil·i·a
pol·y·chro·ma·to·phil·ic
pol·y·chrome
pol·y·chro·mi·a
pol·y·chro·mo·cy·to·sis
pol·y·chy·li·a
pol·y·chy·lic
pol·y·clin·ic
pol·y·clo·nal
pol·y·clo·ni·a
pol·y·co·ri·a
pol·y·crot·ic
pol·y·cy·clic
pol·y·cy·e·sis
  pl pol·y·cy·e·ses
pol·y·cys·tic
pol·y·cy·thae·mi·a
  var of pol·y·cy·the·mi·a
pol·y·cy·the·mi·a
pol·y·cy·the·mi·a ve·ra
pol·y·cy·the·mic
pol·y·dac·tyl
pol·y·dac·tyl·i·a
pol·y·dac·ty·lism

313

pol·y·dac·ty·lous
pol·y·dac·ty·ly
    pl pol·y·dac·ty·lies
pol·y·de·fi·cien·cy
pol·y·de·fi·cient
pol·y·dip·si·a
pol·y·dip·sic
pol·y·don·ti·a
pol·y·dyp·si·a
    var of pol·y·dyp·si·a
pol·y·dys·troph·ic
pol·y·dys·tro·phy
pol·y·e·lec·tro·lyte
pol·y·em·bry·o·ny
    pl pol·y·em·bry·o·nies
pol·y·e·mi·a
pol·y·ene
pol·y·en·ic
pol·y·es·the·si·a
pol·y·es·trous
pol·y·es·trus
pol·y·eth·a·dene
pol·y·eth·yl·ene
Po·lyg·a·la
pol·y·ga·lac·ti·a
pol·y·ga·lac·tu·ro·nase
po·lyg·a·mic
po·lyg·a·mist
po·lyg·a·mous
po·lyg·a·my
    pl po·lyg·a·mies
pol·y·gas·tri·a
pol·y·gas·tric
pol·y·gene
pol·y·gen·ic
pol·y·glan·du·lar
pol·y·glob·u·lia
pol·y·glob·u·lism
pol·y·gly·col·ic
pol·y·gnath·us
po·lyg·o·nal
Po·lyg·o·num
pol·y·gram
pol·y·graph
pol·y·graph·ic
pol·y·graph·i·cal·ly
po·lyg·y·nist
po·lyg·y·nous

po·lyg·y·ny
    pl po·lyg·y·nies
pol·y·gy·ria
pol·y·hae·mi·a
    var of pol·y·he·mi·a
pol·y·he·dral
pol·y·he·mi·a
pol·y·hi·dro·sis
    pl pol·y·hi·dro·ses
pol·y·hy·brid
pol·y·hy·dram·ni·os
pol·y·hy·dric
pol·y·hy·drox·y
pol·y·hy·dru·ri·a
pol·y·i·dro·sis
    pl pol·y·i·dro·ses
    var of pol·y·hi·dro·sis
pol·y·in·fec·tion
pol·y·lec·i·thal
pol·y·lep·tic
pol·y·lob·u·lar
pol·y·mas·ti·a
    or pol·y·mas·ty
pol·y·mas·ti·gate
Pol·y·mas·tig·i·da
Pol·y·mas·ti·gi·na
pol·y·mas·ti·gote
pol·y·mas·ti·gous
pol·y·mas·ty
    pl pol·y·mas·ties
    or pol·y·mas·ti·a
pol·y·ma·zi·a
pol·y·me·li·a
    or pol·y·me·ly
    pl pol·y·me·lies
pol·y·me·lus
pol·y·me·ly
    pl pol·y·me·lies
    or pol·y·me·li·a
pol·y·me·ni·a
pol·y·men·or·rhe·a
pol·y·men·or·rhoe·a
    var of pol·y·men·or·rhe·a
pol·y·mer
pol·ym·er·ase
pol·y·me·ri·a
pol·y·mer·ic
pol·y·mer·i·cal·ly
po·lym·er·ide

po·lym·er·ism
po·lym·er·i·za·tion
po·lym·er·ize
pol·y·met·a·car·pal·ism
pol·y·mi·cro·bi·al
    or pol·y·mi·cro·bic
pol·y·mi·cro·bic
    or pol·y·mi·cro·bi·al
pol·y·mi·cro·gy·ri·a
pol·y·morph
pol·y·mor·phic
pol·y·mor·phi·cal·ly
pol·y·mor·phism
pol·y·mor·pho·cel·lu·lar
pol·y·mor·pho·cyte
pol·y·mor·pho·nu·cle·ar
pol·y·mor·phous
pol·y·mor·phous·ly
pol·y·my·al·gi·a
pol·y·my·oc·lo·nus
pol·y·my·op·a·thy
pol·y·my·o·si·tis
pol·y·myx·in
pol·y·ne·sic
pol·y·neu·ral
pol·y·neu·ral·gi·a
pol·y·neu·ric
poly·neu·rit·ic
pol·y·neu·ri·tis
    pl pol·y·neu·ri·tis·es
    or pol·y·neu·ri·ti·des
pol·y·neu·ro·my·o·si·tis
pol·y·neu·rop·a·thy
    pl pol·y·neu·rop·a·thies
pol·y·neu·ro·ra·dic·u·li·tis
pol·y·nu·cle·ar
pol·y·nu·cle·ate
pol·y·nu·cle·o·sis
    pl pol·y·nu·cle·o·ses
pol·y·nu·cle·o·ti·dase
pol·y·nu·cle·o·tide
pol·y·o·don·ti·a
pol·y·oes·trus
    var of pol·y·es·trus
pol·y·o·ma
pol·y·o·nych·i·a
pol·y·o·pi·a
pol·y·op·ic
pol·y·or·chi·dism

pol·y·or·chis
pol·y·o·rex·i·a
pol·y·or·ga·no·sil·ox·ane
pol·y·or·rho·men·in·gi·tis
pol·y·or·rhy·me·ni·tis
pol·y·os·tot·ic
pol·y·o·ti·a
pol·y·ov·u·lar
pol·y·ov·u·la·tion
pol·y·ox·yl
pol·yp
pol·y·pap·il·lo·ma
pol·y·pa·re·sis
pol·y·path·i·a
pol·y·pec·to·my
　pl pol·y·pec·to·mies
pol·y·pep·ti·dae·mi·a
　var of pol·y·pep·ti·de·mi·a
pol·y·pep·ti·dase
pol·y·pep·tide
pol·y·pep·ti·de·mi·a
pol·y·pep·ti·dor·rha·chi·a
pol·y·pha·gi·a
po·lyph·a·gous
pol·y·pha·lan·gism
pol·y·phar·ma·cy
　pl pol·y·phar·ma·cies
pol·y·phe·nol
pol·y·pho·bi·a
pol·y·phy·let·ic
pol·y·phy·let·i·cal·ly
pol·y·phy·le·tism
pol·y·phy·le·tist
pol·y·phy·o·dont
pol·y·pif·er·ous
pol·y·plast
pol·y·plas·tic
pol·y·ploid
pol·y·ploi·dy
　pl pol·y·ploi·dies
pol·yp·ne·a
pol·yp·ne·ic
pol·yp·noe·a
　var of pol·yp·ne·a
pol·y·pod
pol·y·po·di·a
pol·y·poid
　or poly·poi·dal

pol·y·poi·dal
　or pol·y·poid
po·lyp·o·rous
Po·lyp·o·rus
pol·y·po·sis
　pl pol·y·po·ses
pol·y·pous
pol·y·pro·pyl·ene
pol·y·pty·chi·al
pol·y·pus
　pl pol·y·pus·es
　or pol·y·pi
pol·y·py·ram·i·dal
pol·y·ra·dic·u·li·tis
pol·y·ra·dic·u·lo·neu·ri·tis
pol·y·ra·dic·u·lo·neu·rop·
　a·thy
pol·y·ri·bo·nu·cle·o·tide
pol·y·ri·bo·som·al
pol·y·ri·bo·some
pol·y·sac·cha·ride
pol·y·sce·li·a
po·lys·ce·lus
pol·y·scle·ro·sis
pol·y·scope
pol·y·sco·pic
pol·y·se·ro·si·tis
pol·y·si·nus·i·tis
pol·y·so·ma·tous
pol·y·some
pol·y·so·mic
pol·y·so·mus
pol·y·so·my
　pl pol·y·so·mies
pol·y·sor·bate
pol·y·sper·mi·a
pol·y·sper·mic
pol·y·sper·mism
pol·y·sper·my
　pl pol·y·sper·mies
pol·y·sphyg·mo·graph
pol·y·sphyg·mo·graph·ic
pol·y·stich·i·a
pol·y·sto·ma·tous
pol·y·sty·rene
pol·y·sus·pen·soid
pol·y·symp·to·mat·ic
pol·y·syn·ap·tic
pol·y·syn·ap·ti·cal·ly

pol·y·syn·dac·ty·lism
pol·y·tene
pol·y·ter·pene
pol·y·the·li·a
pol·y·the·lism
pol·y·thi·a·zide
po·lyt·o·cous
pol·y·trich·i·a
pol·y·tri·cho·sis
pol·y·tro·phi·a
pol·y·troph·ic
po·lyt·ro·phy
pol·y·trop·ic
pol·y·typ·ic
pol·y·un·sat·u·rat·ed
pol·y·u·ri·a
pol·y·u·ric
pol·y·va·lence
　or pol·y·va·len·cy
pol·y·va·len·cy
　pl pol·y·va·len·cies
　or pol·y·va·lence
pol·y·va·lent
pol·y·vi·nyl
pol·y·vi·nyl·pyr·rol·i·done
po·made
po·man·der
po·ma·tum
Pom·pe dis·ease
pom·pho·ly·hae·mi·a
　var of pom·pho·ly·he·mi·a
pom·pho·ly·he·mi·a
pom·pho·lyx
pom·phus
po·mum A·da·mi
pon·ceau
Pon·cet dis·ease
pon·der·a·ble
Pon·der-Kin·youn stain
Pon·fick sha·dow
Pon·gi·dae
Pon·go
po·no·graph
po·no·pal·mo·sis
pons
　pl pon·tes
pons Va·ro·li·i
　pl pon·tes Va·ro·li·i
pon·tic

pon·tic·u·lus
    pl pon·tic·u·li
pon·tile
pon·tine
pon·to·bul·bar
pon·to·cer·e·bel·lar
Pool-Schles·in·ger sign
pop·les
pop·lit·e·al
pop·lit·e·us
    pl pop·lit·e·i
por·ad·e·no·lym·phi·tis
por·ce·lain
por·cine
pore
por·en·ce·pha·li·a
por·en·ce·phal·ic
por·en·ceph·a·li·tis
por·en·ceph·a·lus
por·en·ceph·a·ly
por·fi·ro·my·cin
Por·ges-Pol·lat·schek
    re·ac·tion
po·ri·o·ma·ni·a
po·ri·on
    pl po·ri·ons
    or po·ri·a
por·no·graph·ic
por·no·graph·i·cal·ly
por·nog·ra·phy
    pl por·nog·ra·phies
po·ro·ceph·a·li·a·sis
    pl po·ro·ceph·a·li·a·ses
Po·ro·ce·phal·i·dae
Po·ro·ceph·a·lus
po·ro·ker·a·to·sis
po·ro·ma
    pl po·ro·ma·ta
po·ro·plas·tic
po·ro·sis
    pl po·ro·sis·es
    or po·ro·ses
po·ros·i·ty
    pl po·ros·i·ties
po·rot·ic
po·rous
por·phin
    or por·phine

por·phine
    or por·phin
por·pho·bi·lin
por·pho·bi·lin·o·gen
por·phyr·i·a
por·phy·rin
por·phy·ri·nu·ri·a
por·phy·ri·za·tion
por·phy·rop·sin
por·phy·ry
por·rig·i·nous
por·ri·go
Por·ro op·er·a·tion
port
porta
    pl por·tae
por·ta·ca·val
    or por·to·ca·val
por·tal
por·ta·re·nal
porte·pol·ish·er
Por·ter sign
Por·ter-Sil·ber re·ac·tion
Por·tes op·er·a·tion
por·ti·o
    pl por·ti·o·nes
por·to·ca·val
    or por·ta·ca·val
por·to·gram
por·tog·ra·phy
por·to·sys·tem·ic
por·to·ve·no·gram
por·to·ve·nog·ra·phy
po·rus
    pl po·rus·es
    or po·ri
po·si·o·ma·ni·a
po·si·tion
po·si·tion·al
po·si·tive
pos·i·tron
pos·i·tro·ni·um
po·so·log·ic
    or po·so·log·i·cal
po·so·log·i·cal
    or po·so·log·ic
po·sol·o·gy
    pl po·sol·o·gies
post·a·bor·tal

post·an·aes·thet·ic
    var of post·an·es·thet·ic
post·a·nal
post·an·es·thet·ic
post·an·ox·ic
post·ap·o·plec·tic
post·ar·te·ri·o·lar
post·au·di·to·ry
post·ax·i·al
post·ax·i·al·ly
post·bra·chi·al
post·cap·il·lar·y
post·car·di·ac
post·car·di·nal
post·car·di·ot·o·my
post·ca·va
post·ca·va·val
post·cen·tral
post·chrom·ing
post·ci·bal
post·cla·vic·u·lar
post·co·i·tal
post·com·mis·sure
post·com·mis·sur·ot·o·my
post·con·cep·tu·al
post·con·cus·sion
post·con·dy·lar
post·con·i·za·tion
post·con·nu·bi·al
post·con·vul·sive
post·cor·di·al
post·cor·nu
post·cos·tal
post·cri·coid
post·dam
post·di·crot·ic
post·di·ges·tive
post·diph·the·rit·ic
post·dor·mi·tal
post·em·bry·o·nal
    or post·em·bry·on·ic
post·em·bry·on·ic
    or post·em·bry·o·nal
post·en·ceph·a·lit·ic
post·ep·i·lep·tic
pos·te·ri·ad
pos·te·ri·or
pos·te·ri·or·ly
pos·ter·o·an·te·ri·or

pos·ter·o·ex·ter·nad
pos·ter·o·ex·ter·nal
pos·ter·o·in·ter·nad
pos·ter·o·in·ter·nal
pos·ter·o·lat·er·ad
pos·ter·o·lat·er·al
pos·ter·o·mar·gi·nal
pos·ter·o·me·di·ad
pos·ter·o·me·di·al
pos·ter·o·me·di·an
pos·ter·o·su·pe·ri·or
pos·ter·o·tem·po·ral
pos·ter·o·trans·verse
post·e·rup·tive
post·e·soph·a·ge·al
post·e·vac·u·a·tion
post·ex·an·them·a·tous
post·fas·ci·al
post·fe·brile
post·gan·gli·on·ic
post·gas·trec·to·my
post·gle·noid
  or post·gle·noi·dal
post·gle·noi·dal
  or post·gle·noid
post·grav·id
post·hem·i·ple·gic
post·hem·or·rhag·ic
post·he·pat·ic
post·hep·a·tit·ic
post·her·pet·ic
pos·thet·o·my
pos·thi·tis
  pl pos·thi·ti·des
pos·tho·lith
post·hu·mous
post·hu·mous·ly
post·hyp·not·ic
post·hyp·not·i·cal·ly
post·hy·poph·y·sis
  pl post·hy·poph·y·ses
post·ic·tal
post·ic·ter·ic
pos·ti·cus
post·in·farc·tion
post·in·fec·tious
post·in·fec·tive
post·in·flu·en·zal

Post·Lau·der·milk
  meth·od
post·ir·ra·di·a·tion
post·ma·lar·i·al
post·mam·ma·ry
post·mas·tec·to·my
post·ma·ture
post·ma·tu·ri·ty
  pl post·ma·tu·ri·ties
post·me·di·al
  or post·me·di·an
post·me·di·an
  or post·me·di·al
post·men·ar·che
post·men·o·pau·sal
post·men·stru·al
post·mor·tal
post·mor·tem
post·mu·coid
post·na·ris
  pl post·na·res
post·na·sal
post·na·tal
post·na·tal·ly
post·ne·crot·ic
post·neu·rit·ic
post·nod·u·lar
post·oc·u·lar
post·oe·soph·a·ge·al
  var of post·e·soph·a·ge·al
post·ol·i·var·y
post·op·er·a·tive
post·o·ral
post·or·bit·al
post·pal·a·tine
post·pa·lu·dal
post·par·a·lyt·ic
post·par·tal
  or post·par·tum
post·par·tum
  or post·par·tal
post·per·fu·sion
post·pha·ryn·ge·al
post·phle·bit·ic
post·pi·tu·i·tar·y
post·pran·di·al
post·pran·di·al·ly
post·pros·tat·ic
post·pu·ber·al

post·pu·ber·tal
post·pu·bes·cent
post·pyc·not·ic
post·py·ram·i·dal
post·ra·di·a·tion
post·re·duc·tion
post·re·nal
post·rhi·nal
post·ro·lan·dic
post·ro·ta·to·ry
post·scap·u·la
  pl post·scap·u·las
  or post·scap·u·lae
post·scap·u·lar
post·scar·la·ti·nal
post·sphyg·mic
post·sple·nec·to·my
post·ste·not·ic
post·syn·ap·tic
post·syn·ap·ti·cal·ly
post·syph·i·lit·ic
post·trau·mat·ic
post·tre·mat·ic
post·treat·ment
post·tus·sive
pos·tu·late
pos·tur·al
pos·ture
post·vac·ci·nal
post·val·vu·lot·o·my
post·ves·i·cal
po·ta·ble
Po·tain dis·ease
Pot·a·mon
pot·a·mo·pho·bi·a
pot·ash
pot·as·sae·mi·a
  var of pot·as·se·mi·a
pot·as·se·mi·a
po·tas·sic
po·tas·si·um
po·ten·cy
  pl po·ten·cies
po·tent
po·ten·ti·a
po·ten·tial
po·ten·ti·ate
po·ten·ti·a·tion
po·ten·ti·a·tor

po·ten·ti·om·e·ter
po·ten·ti·o·met·ric
po·ten·ti·o·met·ri·cal·ly
po·tion
po·to·ma·ni·a
Pott dis·ease
pouch
pou·drage
Pou·let dis·ease
poul·tice
pound
Pou·part lig·a·ment
pov·er·ty
pl pov·er·ties
po·vi·done
po·vi·done-i·o·dine
Pow·as·san vi·rus
pow·der
pow·er
Pow·er test
pox
pl pox·es
or pox
pox·vi·rus
pl pox·vi·rus·es
Poz·zi syn·drome
prac·tice
prac·tise
var of prac·tice
prac·ti·tion·er
Pra·der-Wil·li syn·drome
prae·cox
var of pre·cox
prae·cu·ne·us
var of pre·cu·ne·us
prae·pu·ti·um
pl prae·pu·ti·a
var of pre·pu·ti·um
prae·vi·a
var of pre·vi·a
prag·mat·ag·no·si·a
prag·mat·am·ne·si·a
Prague ma·neu·ver
pral·i·dox·ime
pra·mox·ine
pran·di·al
pran·di·al·i·ty
pra·se·o·dym·i·um
pra·tique

Praus·nitz-Küst·ner
re·ac·tion
prax·e·o·log·i·cal
prax·e·ol·o·gy
pl prax·e·ol·o·gies
var of prax·i·ol·o·gy
prax·in·o·scope
prax·i·ol·o·gy
pl prax·i·ol·o·gies
prax·is
pl prax·es
pra·ze·pam
pra·zo·sin
pre·ad·o·les·cence
pre·ad·o·les·cent
pre·ag·o·nal
pre·al·bu·mi·nu·ric
pre·am·pul·lar·y
pre·an·aes·thet·ic
var of pre·an·es·thet·ic
pre·a·nal
pre·an·es·thet·ic
pre·an·ti·sep·tic
pre·a·or·tic
pre·a·sep·tic
pre·a·tax·ic
pre·au·ric·u·lar
pre·ax·i·al
pre·be·ta·lip·o·pro·te·in
pre·be·ta·lip·o·pro·te·in·
ae·mi·a
var of pre·be·ta·lip·o·pro·
te·in·e·mi·a
pre·be·ta·lip·o·pro·te·in·
e·mi·a
pre·can·cer·ous
pre·cap·il·lar·y
pre·car·di·ac
pre·car·di·nal
pre·car·ti·lage
pre·car·ti·lag·i·nous
pre·ca·va
pl pre·ca·vae
pre·ca·val
pre·cen·tral
pre·cer·vi·cal
pre·chor·dal
pre·cip·i·ta·bil·i·ty
pl pre·cip·i·ta·bil·i·ties

pre·cip·i·ta·ble
pre·cip·i·tant
pre·cip·i·tate
pre·cip·i·ta·tion
pre·cip·i·ta·tor
pre·cip·i·tin
pre·cip·i·tin·o·gen
pre·cip·i·tin·o·gen·ic
pre·cip·i·tin·oid
pre·clin·i·cal
pre·coc·cyg·e·al
pre·co·cious
pre·coc·i·ty
pre·cog·ni·tion
pre·co·i·tal
pre·col·lag·e·nous
pre·com·a·tose
pre·com·mis·sur·al
pre·com·mis·sure
pre·con·scious
pre·con·scious·ly
pre·con·vul·sant
pre·con·vul·sive
pre·cop·u·la·to·ry
pre·cor·di·al
pre·cor·di·um
pl pre·cor·di·a
pre·cor·nu
pl pre·cor·nu·a
pre·cos·tal
pre·cox
pre·cri·coid
pre·crit·i·cal
pre·cu·ne·us
pl pre·cu·ne·i
pre·cur·sor
pre·den·tin
pre·di·a·be·tes
pre·di·a·bet·ic
pre·di·a·stol·ic
pre·di·crot·ic
pre·di·gest
pre·di·ges·ted
pre·di·ges·tion
pre·dis·pose
pre·dis·po·si·tion
pred·nis·o·lone
pred·ni·sone
pred·ni·val

pre·dor·mi·tal
pre·dor·mi·tion
pre·e·clamp·si·a
pre·e·clamp·tic
pre·ep·i·glot·tic
pre·e·rup·tive
pre·ex·ci·ta·tion
pre·fi·brot·ic
pre·for·ma·tion
pre·fron·tal
pre·gan·gli·ar
    or pre·gan·gli·on·ic
pre·gan·gli·on·ic
    or pre·gan·gli·ar
pre·gen·i·tal
pre·gle·noid
preg·nan·cy
    pl preg·nan·cies
preg·nane
preg·nane·di·ol
preg·nant
preg·nene
preg·nen·in·o·lone
preg·nen·o·lone
preg·no·pho·bi·a
pre·hal·lux
    pl pre·hal·lu·ces
pre·hem·i·ple·gic
pre·hen·sile
pre·hen·sil·i·ty
    pl pre·hen·sil·i·ties
pre·hen·sion
pre·he·pat·ic
pre·hy·poph·y·sis
    pl pre·hy·poph·y·ses
pre·ic·ter·ic
pre·in·cu·ba·tion
pre·in·duc·tion
pre·in·farc·tion
pre·in·su·la
    pl pre·in·su·lae
pre·in·va·sive
Prei·ser dis·ease
pre·lac·ri·mal
pre·lar·val
pre·leu·kae·mi·a
    var of pre·leu·ke·mi·a
pre·leu·ke·mi·a
pre·leu·ke·mic

pre·lo·co·mo·tion
pre·lum
pre·ma·lig·nant
pre·mam·mil·lar·y
pre·ma·ni·a·cal
pre·mar·i·tal
pre·ma·ture
pre·ma·ture·ly
pre·ma·tur·i·ty
    pl pre·ma·tur·i·ties
pre·max·il·la
    pl pre·max·il·lae
pre·max·il·lar·y
pre·me·di·an
pre·med·i·cal
pre·med·i·cant
pre·med·i·cate
pre·med·i·ca·tion
pre·mel·a·no·some
pre·men·o·paus·al
pre·men·o·pause
pre·men·stru·al
pre·men·stru·al·ly
pre·men·stru·um
    pl pre·men·stru·ums
    or pre·men·stru·a
pre·mo·lar
pre·mon·i·ta·ry
    or pre·mon·i·to·ry
pre·mon·i·to·ry
    or pre·mon·i·ta·ry
pre·mon·o·cyte
pre·mor·bid
pre·mor·tal
pre·mo·tor
pre·mune
pre·mu·ni·tion
    or pre·mu·ni·ty
pre·mu·ni·ty
    pl pre·mu·ni·ties
    or pre·mu·ni·tion
pre·mu·nize
pre·mus·cle
pre·my·e·lo·blast
pre·my·e·lo·cyte
pre·nar·co·sis
pre·na·ris
    pl pre·na·res
pre·na·tal

pre·na·tal·ly
pre·ne·o·plas·tic
pre·nid·a·to·ry
pre·nod·u·lar
pre·nyl·a·mine
pre·oc·cip·i·tal
pre·ol·i·var·y
pre·op·er·a·tive
pre·op·er·a·tive·ly
pre·op·tic
pre·op·ti·cus
pre·o·ral
pre·o·ral·ly
pre·ov·u·la·to·ry
prep
pre·pal·a·tal
pre·par·a·lyt·ic
prep·a·ra·tion
prep·ar·a·tor
pre·pa·ret·ic
pre·par·tal
    or pre·par·tum
pre·par·tum
    or pre·par·tal
pre·pa·tel·lar
pre·pat·ent
pre·pel·vic
pre·per·cep·tion
pre·per·cep·tive
pre·per·i·to·ne·al
pre·phe·nic ac·id
pre·pla·cen·tal
pre·pol·lex
pre·pon·der·ance
pre·pon·tine
pre·po·ten·cy
    pl pre·po·ten·cies
pre·po·tent
pre·po·tent·ly
pre·psy·chot·ic
pre·pu·ber·al
    or pre·pu·ber·tal
pre·bu·ber·tal
    or pre·pu·ber·al
pre·pu·ber·ty
    pl pre·pu·ber·ties
pre·pu·bes·cence
pre·pu·bes·cent

319

pre·pu·bi·an
or pre·pu·bic
pre·pu·bic
or pre·pu·bi·an
pre·puce
pre·pu·cial
or pre·pu·tial
pre·pu·cot·o·my
pre·pu·tial
or pre·pu·cial
pre·pu·ti·um
pl pre·pu·ti·a
pre·py·lo·ric
pre·py·ram·i·dal
pre·rec·tal
pre·re·nal
pre·re·pro·duc·tive
pre·ret·i·nal
pre·sa·cral
pres·by·a·cou·si·a
or pres·by·a·cu·si·a
or pres·by·cu·sis
pres·by·a·cu·si·a
or pres·by·a·cou·si·a
or pres·by·cu·sis
pres·by·at·rics
pres·by·car·di·a
pres·by·cu·sis
pl pres·by·cu·ses
or pres·by·a·cu·si·a
or pres·by·a·cou·si·a
pres·by·der·ma
pres·by·ope
pres·by·o·phre·ni·a
pres·by·o·phren·ic
pres·by·o·pi·a
pres·by·op·ic
pres·by·o·sphac·e·lus
pres·by·ti·a
pres·by·ti·at·rics
pres·byt·ic
Pres·by·tis
pres·by·tism
pre·sca·lene
pre·schiz·o·phren·ic
pre·scle·ro·sis
pre·scle·rot·ic
pre·scribe
pre·scrip·tion

pre·se·nile
pre·se·nil·i·ty
pl pre·se·nil·i·ties
pres·en·ta·tion
pre·ser·va·tive
pre·so·mite
pre·spas·tic
pre·sphe·noid
pre·sphyg·mic
pres·sor
pres·so·re·cep·tor
pres·so·sen·si·tive
pres·sure
pre·ster·nal
pre·ster·num
pl pre·ster·nums
or pre·ster·na
pre·su·bic·u·lum
pl pre·su·bic·u·la
pre·sump·tive
pre·sup·pu·ra·tive
pre·syl·vi·an
pre·symp·to·mat·ic
pre·syn·ap·tic
pre·syn·ap·ti·cal·ly
pre·sys·to·le
pre·sys·tol·ic
pre·tec·tal
pre·tem·po·ral
pre·ter·mi·nal
pre·ter·nat·u·ral
pre·thy·roi·de·an
pre·tib·i·al
pre·tra·gal
pre·trans·fer·ence
pre·treat·ment
pre·tre·mat·ic
pre·tu·ber·cu·lous
pre·u·re·thri·tis
pre·va·lence
pre·ven·ta·tive
pre·ven·tive
pre·ven·to·ri·um
pl pre·ven·to·ri·ums
or pre·ven·to·ri·a
pre·ver·te·bral
pre·ver·tig·i·nous
pre·ves·i·cal
pre·vi·a

pre·vil·lous
pre·vi·ral
Prey·er re·flex
pre·zone
pre·zon·u·lar
pre·zyg·a·poph·y·sis
pri·a·pism
pri·a·pis·mic
pri·a·pus
pl pri·a·pus·es
or pri·a·pi
Price-Jones curve
pril·o·caine
pri·mal
pri·ma·quine
pri·mar·y
pri·mate
Pri·ma·tes
pri·mi·done
pri·mi·grav·i·da
pl pri·mi·grav·i·das
or pri·mi·grav·i·dae
pri·mip·a·ra
pl pri·mip·a·ras
or pri·mip·a·rae
pri·mi·par·i·ty
pl pri·mi·par·i·ties
pri·mip·a·rous
pri·mite
pri·mi·ti·ae
prim·i·tive
pri·mor·di·al
pri·mor·di·al·ly
pri·mor·di·um
pl pri·mor·di·a
prin·ceps
prin·ci·pal
prin·ci·ple
Prin·gle ad·e·no·ma se·ba·ce·um
Pri·o·nu·rus
pri·sil·i·dene
prism
pris·ma
pl pris·ma·ta
pris·ma·ta ad·a·man·ti·na
pris·mat·ic
pris·moid
pris·mop·tom·e·ter

pris·mo·sphere
pro·ac·cel·er·in
pro·ac·ro·so·mal
pro·ac·ti·va·tor
pro·ac·tive
pro·ag·glu·ti·noid
pro·al
pro·am·ni·on
  pl pro·am·ni·ons
  or pro·am·ni·a
pro·am·ni·ot·ic
pro·at·las
pro·bac·te·ri·o·phage
pro·band
pro·bang
pro·bar·bi·tal
probe
pro·ben·e·cid
pro·bit
pro·bos·cis
  pl pro·bos·cis·es
  or pro·bos·ci·des
pro·cain·a·mide
pro·caine
pro·cal·lus
pro·car·ba·zine
pro·car·y·ote
  var of pro·kar·y·ote
pro·car·y·ot·ic
  var of pro·kar·y·ot·ic
pro·ca·tarc·tic
pro·ce·lous
pro·cen·tri·ole
pro·ce·phal·ic
pro·cer·coid
pro·ce·rus
  pl pro·ce·rus·es
  or pro·ce·ri
proc·ess
proc·ces·so·ma·ni·a
proc·ces·sus
  pl pro·ces·sus
pro·chei·li·a
pro·chei·lon
pro·chlor·per·a·zine
pro·chon·dral
pro·chord·al
pro·cho·re·sis
Pro·chow·nick meth·od

pro·ci·den·ti·a
pro·clo·nol
pro·co·ag·u·lant
pro·con·dy·lism
pro·con·ver·tin
pro·cre·ate
pro·cre·a·tion
pro·cre·a·tive
proc·tag·ra
proc·tal·gi·a
proc·ta·tre·si·a
proc·tec·ta·si·a
proc·tec·to·my
  pl proc·tec·to·mies
proc·ten·cli·sis
proc·teu·ryn·ter
proc·ti·tis
proc·to·cele
proc·toc·ly·sis
  pl proc·toc·ly·ses
proc·to·co·li·tis
proc·to·co·lon·os·co·py
proc·to·col·po·plas·ty
proc·to·cys·to·plas·ty
proc·to·dae·um
  pl proc·to·dae·ums
  or proc·to·dae·a
  var of proc·to·de·um
proc·to·de·um
  pl proc·to·de·ums
  or proc·to·de·a
proc·to·dyn·ia
proc·to·log·ic
  or proc·to·log·i·cal
proc·to·log·i·cal
  or proc·to·log·ic
proc·tol·o·gist
proc·tol·o·gy
  pl proc·tol·o·gies
proc·to·pa·ral·y·sis
proc·to·pex·y
proc·to·phil·i·a
proc·to·pho·bi·a
proc·to·plas·ty
proc·to·ple·gi·a
proc·top·to·si·a
proc·top·to·sis
proc·tor·rha·phy
proc·tor·rhe·a

proc·tor·rhoe·a
  var of proc·tor·rhe·a
proc·to·scope
proc·to·scop·ic
proc·to·scop·i·cal·ly
proc·tos·co·py
  pl proc·tos·co·pies
proc·to·sig·moid·ec·to·my
  pl proc·to·sig·moid·ec·to·
  mies
proc·to·sig·moi·di·tis
proc·to·sig·moi·do·scope
proc·to·sig·moi·do·scop·ic
proc·to·sig·moi·dos·co·py
  pl proc·to·sig·moi·dos·co·
  pies
proc·to·spasm
proc·tos·ta·sis
proc·to·ste·no·sis
proc·tos·to·my
  pl proc·tos·to·mies
proc·tot·o·my
pro·cum·ben·cy
pro·cum·bent
pro·cur·sive
pro·cur·va·tion
pro·cy·cli·dine
pro·dig·i·o·sin
pro·dil·i·dine
pro·dro·ma
  pl pro·dro·mas
  or pro·dro·ma·ta
pro·dro·mal
  or pro·drom·ic
pro·drome
  pl pro·drom·es
  or pro·dro·ma·ta
pro·drom·ic
  or pro·dro·mal
prod·ro·mous
pro·duct
pro·duc·tive
pro·e·mi·al
pro·en·ceph·a·lus
pro·en·ceph·a·ly
pro·en·zyme
pro·e·ryth·ro·blast
pro·e·ryth·ro·cyte
pro·es·tro·gen

pro·es·trum
   or pro·es·trus
pro·es·trus
   pl pro·es·trus·es
   or pro·es·trum
Proetz treat·ment
pro·fen·a·mine
pro·fer·ment
pro·fes·sion·al
pro·fi·bri·no·ly·sin
Pro·fi·chet syn·drome
pro·file
pro·fla·vine
pro·flu·vi·um
   pl pro·flu·vi·ums
   or pro·flu·vi·a
pro·fun·da
   pl pro·fun·dae
pro·fun·dus
pro·gas·ter
pro·gen·er·ate
pro·gen·e·sis
pro·gen·i·tor
prog·e·ny
pro·ge·ri·a
pro·ges·ta·tion·al
pro·ges·ter·one
pro·ges·ter·on·ic
pro·ges·tin
pro·ges·to·gen
pro·glot·tid
pro·glot·tid·e·an
pro·glot·tis
   pl pro·glot·ti·des
prog·nath·ic
prog·na·thism
   or prog·na·thy
prog·na·thous
prog·na·thy
   pl prog·na·thies
   or prog·na·thism
prog·nose
prog·no·sis
   pl prog·no·ses
prog·nos·tic
prog·nos·ti·cate
prog·nos·ti·cian
pro·go·nal

pro·go·no·ma
   pl pro·go·no·mas
   or pro·go·no·ma·ta
pro·gran·u·lo·cyte
pro·grav·id
pro·gress
pro·gres·sion
pro·gres·sive
pro·gua·nil
pro·in·su·lin
pro·i·o·sys·to·le
pro·i·o·ti·a
pro·jec·tile
pro·jec·tion
pro·jec·tive
pro·kar·y·o·cyte
pro·kar·y·ote
pro·kar·y·ot·ic
pro·ki·nase
pro·la·bi·um
   pl pro·la·bi·a
pro·lac·tin
pro·la·min
   or pro·la·mine
pro·la·mine
   or pro·la·min
pro·lan
pro·lapse
pro·lap·sus
pro·late
pro·lep·sis
   pl pro·lep·ses
pro·lep·tic
   or pro·lep·ti·cal
pro·lep·ti·cal
   or pro·lep·tic
pro·leu·co·cyte
   var of pro·leu·ko·cyte
pro·leu·ko·cyte
pro·lif·er·ate
pro·lif·er·a·tion
pro·lif·er·a·tive
pro·lif·er·ous
pro·lif·ic
pro·lig·er·ous
pro·li·nae·mi·a
   var of pro·li·ne·mi·a
pro·lin·ase
pro·line

pro·li·ne·mi·a
pro·lin·tane
pro·li·nu·ri·a
pro·li·pase
pro·lon·gev·i·ty
pro·lo·ther·a·py
   pl pro·lo·ther·a·pies
pro·lyl
pro·lym·pho·cyte
pro·ma·zine
pro·meg·a·kar·y·o·cyte
pro·meg·a·lo·blast
pro·meg·a·lo·kar·y·o·cyte
pro·mes·o·bil·i·fus·cin
pro·met·a·phase
pro·meth·a·zine
pro·meth·es·trol
pro·me·thi·um
pro·meth·oes·trol
   var of pro·meth·es·trol
prom·i·nence
prom·i·nen·ti·a
   pl prom·i·nen·ti·ae
prom·ne·si·a
pro·mon·o·cyte
prom·on·to·ri·um
   pl prom·on·to·ri·a
prom·on·to·ry
   pl prom·on·to·ries
pro·mot·er
pro·mo·tor
pro·my·e·lo·cyte
pro·nase
pro·nate
pro·na·tion
pro·na·tor
pro·na·tor qua·dra·tus
pro·na·tor te·res
prone
pro·neph·ric
pro·neph·ron
   pl pro·neph·ra
   or pro·neph·ros
   pl pro·neph·roi
pro·neph·ros
   pl pro·neph·roi
   or pro·neph·ron
   pl pro·neph·ra
pro·neth·al·ol

pro·no·grade
pro·nor·mo·blast
pro·nor·mo·cyte
pro·nounced
pro·nu·cle·us
  pl pro·nu·cle·us·es
  or pro·nu·cle·i
pro·oes·trus
  var of pro·es·trus
pro·o·tic
pro·o·var·i·um
pro·pa·di·ene
pro·pae·deu·tic
  var of pro·pe·deu·tic
pro·pae·deu·tics
  var of pro·pe·deu·tics
prop·a·gate
prop·a·ga·tion
prop·a·ga·tive
pro·pal·i·nal
pro·pam·i·dine
pro·pane
pro·pan·i·did
pro·pa·no·ic
pro·pa·nol
pro·pa·none
pro·pan·the·line
pro·par·a·caine
pro·pa·tyl
pro·pe·deu·tic
pro·pe·deu·tics
pro·pene
pro·pe·no·ic
pro·pen·dy·o·pent
pro·pe·nyl
pro·pen·zo·late
pro·pep·sin
pro·pep·tone
pro·pep·to·nu·ri·a
pro·per·din
pro·per·i·to·ne·al
pro·phage
pro·phase
pro·phen·py·rid·a·mine
pro·phy·lac·tic
pro·phy·lac·ti·cal·ly
pro·phy·lax·is
  pl pro·phy·lax·es
pro·pi·cil·lin

pro·pi·o·lac·tone
pro·pi·o·ma·zine
pro·pi·o·nate
Pro·pi·on·i·bac·te·ri·um
  pl Pro·pi·on·i·bac·te·ri·a
pro·pi·on·ic
pro·pi·ram
pro·pit·o·caine
pro·plas·ma·cyte
pro·pos·i·tus
  pl pro·pos·i·ti
pro·pox·y·caine
pro·pox·y·phene
pro·pran·o·lol
pro·pri·e·tar·y
  pl pro·pri·e·tar·ies
pro·pri·o·cep·tion
pro·pri·o·cep·tive
pro·pri·o·cep·tor
pro·pri·o·spi·nal
pro·pri·us
prop·tom·e·ter
prop·to·sis
  pl prop·to·ses
prop·tot·ic
pro·pul·sion
pro·pul·sive
pro·pyl
pro·pyl·a·ce·tic
pro·pyl·ene
pro·pyl·hex·e·drine
pro·pyl·i·o·done
pro·pyl·par·a·ben
pro·pyl·thi·o·u·ra·cil
pro·pyne
pro·ren·nin
pro·ru·bri·cyte
pro·sce·ni·o·pho·bi·a
pro·scil·lar·i·din
pro·sco·lex
  pl pro·sco·li·ces
pro·se·cre·tin
pro·sect
pro·sec·tion
pro·sec·tor
pros·en·ce·phal·ic
pros·en·ceph·a·lon
  pl pros·en·ceph·a·la
pro·se·ro·zyme

pro·sim·i·an
Pro·sim·i·i
pros·o·cele
  var of pros·o·coele
pros·o·coel
  var of pros·o·coele
pros·o·coele
pros·o·dem·ic
pros·op·ag·no·si·a
pro·sop·a·gus
pros·o·pal·gi·a
pros·o·pal·gic
pros·op·ic
pro·sop·i·cal·ly
pro·so·pla·si·a
pros·o·plas·tic
pros·o·po·a·nos·chi·sis
  pl pros·o·po·a·nos·chi·ses
pros·o·po·di·ple·gi·a
pros·o·po·dyn·i·a
pros·o·po·neu·ral·gi·a
pros·o·pop·a·gus
pros·o·po·ple·gi·a
pros·o·po·ple·gic
pros·o·pos·chi·sis
  pl pros·o·pos·chi·sis·es
  or pros·o·pos·chi·ses
pros·o·po·spasm
pros·o·po·ster·no·did·y·
  mus
pros·o·po·ster·no·dyn·i·a
pros·o·po·tho·ra·cop·a·gus
pros·o·po·to·ci·a
pros·o·pus var·us
pros·ta·glan·din
pros·ta·ta
pros·tate
pros·ta·tec·to·my
  pl pros·ta·tec·to·mies
pros·tat·ic
pros·tat·i·co·ves·i·cal
pros·ta·tism
pros·ta·tit·ic
pros·ta·ti·tis
pros·ta·to·cys·ti·tis
  pl pros·ta·to·cys·ti·ti·des
pros·tat·o·gram
pros·ta·tog·ra·phy
  pl pros·ta·tog·ra·phies

pros·tat·o·lith
pros·ta·to·li·thot·o·my
pros·ta·tor·rhe·a
pros·ta·tor·rhoe·a
var of pros·ta·tor·rhe·a
pros·ta·tot·o·my
pros·ta·to·ve·sic·u·li·tis
pro·ster·na·tion
pro·ster·num
pl pro·ster·nums
or pro·ster·na
pros·the·sis
pl pros·the·ses
pros·thet·ic
pros·thet·i·cal·ly
pros·thet·ics
pros·the·tist
pros·thi·on
pros·tho·don·ti·a
pros·tho·don·tics
pros·tho·don·tist
Pros·tho·gon·i·mus
pros·tig·mine
pros·ti·tu·tion
pros·trate
pros·tra·tion
pro·tac·tin·i·um
or pro·to·ac·tin·i·um
pro·ta·gon
pro·tag·o·nist
pro·tal
pro·tal·bu·mose
pro·ta·mine
pro·ta·nom·a·ly
pl pro·tan·om·a·lies
pro·ta·nope
pro·ta·no·pi·a
pro·ta·nop·ic
pro·te·an
pro·te·ase
pro·tec·tive
pro·te·ic
pro·te·id
or pro·te·ide
pro·te·ide
or pro·te·id
pro·te·i·form
pro·te·in
pro·te·i·na·ceous

pro·te·i·nae·mi·a
var of pro·te·i·ne·mi·a
pro·te·i·nase
pro·te·i·nate
pro·te·i·ne·mi·a
pro·te·in·ic
pro·te·in·o·chro·mo·gen
pro·te·in·oid
pro·te·in·o·sis
pro·te·in·o·ther·a·py
pro·te·i·nu·ri·a
pro·te·o·clas·tic
pro·te·o·lip·id
pro·te·ol·y·sis
pro·te·o·lyt·ic
pro·te·o·met·a·bol·ic
pro·te·o·me·tab·o·lism
pro·te·o·pep·tic
pro·te·ose
pro·te·o·su·ri·a
Pro·ter·o·glyph·a
pro·te·u·ri·a
Pro·te·us
pl Pro·te·i
pro·the·sis
pl pro·the·ses
pro·throm·base
pro·throm·bin
pro·throm·bi·nae·mi·a
var of pro·throm·bi·ne·mi·a
pro·throm·bi·ne·mi·a
pro·throm·bi·no·gen·ic
pro·throm·bi·no·pe·ni·a
pro·throm·bo·gen·ic
pro·throm·bo·ki·nase
pro·thy·mi·a
pro·tide
pro·ti·des
pro·tist
Pro·tis·ta
pro·tis·tan
pro·tis·tol·o·gist
pro·tis·tol·o·gy
pl pro·tis·tol·o·gies
pro·ti·um
pro·to·ac·tin·i·um
or pro·tac·tin·i·um
pro·to·al·bu·mose

Pro·to·bi·os bac·te·ri·oph·a·gus
pro·to·blast
pro·to·blas·tic
pro·to·car·di·ac
pro·to·cat·e·chu·ic
pro·to·chlo·ride
pro·to·col
pro·to·cone
pro·to·co·nid
pro·to·cop·ro·por·phyr·i·a he·red·i·tar·i·a
pro·to·derm
pro·to·der·mal
pro·to·di·a·stol·ic
pro·to·e·las·tose
pro·to·fi·bril
pro·to·fil·a·ment
pro·tog·a·la
pro·to·gas·ter
pro·to·gen
pro·to·glob·u·lose
pro·to·heme
pro·to·i·o·dide
pro·tok·y·lol
pro·to·leu·ko·cyte
pro·tol·y·sis
pl pro·tol·y·ses
pro·to·me·rite
pro·tom·e·ter
pro·to·me·tro·cyte
Pro·to·mon·a·di·na
pro·to·my·o·sin·ose
pro·ton
pro·to·neu·ron
pro·ton-syn·chro·tron
pro·to·path·ic
pro·to·pec·tin
pro·to·pep·si·a
pro·to·phile
Pro·toph·y·ta
pro·to·phyte
pro·to·pla·sis
pro·to·plasm
pro·to·plas·mal
or pro·to·plas·mat·ic
pro·to·plas·mat·ic
or pro·to·plas·mal
pro·to·plas·mic

pro·to·plast
pro·to·por·phyr·i·a
pro·to·por·phy·rin
pro·to·por·phy·ri·nu·ri·a
pro·to·pro·te·ose
pro·to·sid·er·in
pro·to·spasm
Pro·to·stron·gy·lus
pro·to·sul·fate
pro·to·troph
pro·to·troph·ic
pro·tot·ro·py
    pl pro·tot·ro·pies
pro·to·ver·a·trine
pro·to·ver·ine
pro·to·ver·te·bra
    pl pro·to·ver·te·bras
    or pro·to·ver·te·brae
pro·to·ver·te·bral
pro·tox·ide
pro·tox·in
Pro·to·zo·a
pro·to·zo·a·cide
pro·to·zo·al
pro·to·zo·an
pro·to·zo·i·a·sis
    pl pro·to·zo·i·a·ses
pro·to·zo·ol·o·gist
pro·to·zo·ol·o·gy
    pl pro·to·zo·ol·o·gies
pro·to·zo·on
    pl pro·to·zo·a
pro·to·zo·o·phage
pro·tract
pro·trac·tion
pro·trac·tor
pro·trip·ty·line
pro·trude
pro·tru·si·o ac·e·tab·u·li
pro·tru·sion
pro·tru·sive
pro·tryp·sin
pro·tu·ber·ance
pro·tu·ber·ant
pro·tu·be·ran·ti·a
pro·ty·ros·in·ase
Proust-Licht·heim ma·
    neu·ver
pro·ven·tri·cule

pro·ven·tric·u·lus
    pl pro·ven·tric·u·li
pro·vi·ral
pro·vi·rus
pro·vi·ta·min
prov·o·ca·tion
pro·voc·a·tive
pro·voke
Pro·wa·zek-Hal·ber·
    staed·ter bod·
    ies
Prow·er fac·tor
prox·a·zole
prox·i·mad
prox·i·mal
prox·i·mal·ly
prox·i·mate
prox·i·mate·ly
prox·i·mo·a·tax·i·a
prox·i·mo·buc·cal
prox·i·mo·la·bi·al
prox·i·mo·lin·gual
pro·zone
pro·zy·go·sis
pro·zy·mo·gen
pru·i·nate
Pru·nus
pru·rig·i·nous
pru·ri·go
pru·rit·ic
pru·ri·tus
Prus·sak fi·bers
Prus·sian blue
prus·si·ate
prus·sic
Pryce slide-cul·ture
    meth·od
psal·te·ri·al
psal·te·ri·um
    pl psal·te·ri·a
psam·mism
psam·mo·na
    pl psam·mo·mas
    or psam·mo·ma·ta
psam·mom·a·tous
psam·mo·sar·co·ma
    pl psam·mo·sar·co·mas
    or psam·mo·sar·co·ma·ta
psam·mous

psel·a·phe·si·a
psel·a·phe·sis
psel·lism
psel·lis·mus mer·cu·ri·a·lis
pseu·da·cous·ma
pseu·dac·ro·meg·a·ly
pseu·da·cu·sis
pseu·daes·the·si·a
    var of pseu·des·the·si·a
pseu·da·graph·i·a
psue·dal·bu·mi·nu·ri·a
pseu·dam·ne·si·a
pseu·dan·gi·na
pseu·dan·ky·lo·sis
pseu·da·phe
pseu·daph·i·a
pseu·dar·thri·tis
pseud·ar·thro·sis
    pl pseud·ar·thros·es
Pseu·dech·is
Pseu·de·laps
pseu·del·minth
pseu·den·ceph·aly
pseu·des·the·si·a
pseu·do·a·con·i·tine
pseu·do·ab·scess
pseu·do·ac·an·tho·sis nig·
    ri·cans
pseu·do·a·ceph·a·lus
pseu·do·ac·ro·meg·a·ly
pseu·do·aes·the·si·a
    var of pseu·do·es·the·si·a
pseu·do·ag·glu·ti·na·tion
pseu·do·a·gram·ma·tism
pseu·do·a·graph·i·a
pseu·do·al·bu·mi·nu·ri·a
pseu·do·al·lele
pseu·do·al·lel·ism
pseu·do·al·ve·o·lar
pseu·do·a·nae·mi·a
    var of pseu·do·a·ne·mi·a
pseu·do·a·ne·mi·a
pseu·do·an·eu·rysm
pseu·do·an·gi·na
pseu·do·an·gi·o·ma
pseu·do·an·o·rex·i·a
pseu·do·a·pha·ki·a
pseu·do·ap·o·plex·y
pseu·do·ap·pen·di·ci·tis

pseu·do·ar·thri·tis
pseu·do·ar·thro·sis
   pl pseu·do·ar·thro·ses
   var of pseud·ar·thro·sis
pseu·do·a·ste·re·og·no·sis
pseu·do·a·tax·i·a
pseu·do·ath·er·o·ma
pseu·do·ath·e·to·sis
pseu·do·at·ro·pho·der·ma
   col·li
pseu·do·blep·si·a
pseu·do·blep·sis
pseu·do·bul·bar
pseu·do·car·ti·lage
pseu·do·casts
pseu·do·cele
   or pseu·do·coele
pseu·do·chan·cre
pseu·do·chol·e·stane
pseu·do·cho·les·te·a·to·ma
pseu·do·cho·lin·es·ter·ase
pseu·do·cho·re·a
pseu·do·chro·maes·the·si·a
   var of pseu·do·chro·mes·
   the·si·a
pseu·do·chrom·es·the·si·a
pseu·do·chro·mi·a
pseu·do·chro·mo·some
pseu·do·chy·lous
pseu·do·cir·rho·sis
   pl pseu·do·cir·rho·ses
pseu·do·co·arc·ta·tion
pseu·do·coele
   or pseu·do·cele
pseu·do·col·loid
pseu·do·col·o·bo·ma
pseu·do·cop·u·la·tion
pseu·do·cox·al·gi·a
pseu·do·cri·sis
pseu·do·croup
pseu·do·cryp·to·chism
pseu·do·cy·e·sis
   pl pseu·do·cy·e·ses
pseu·do·cyl·in·droid
pseu·do·cyst
pseu·do·de·cid·u·a
pseu·do·de·men·ti·a
pseu·do·diph·the·ri·a
pseu·do·di·ver·tic·u·lum

pseu·do·e·de·ma
pseu·do·en·do·me·tri·tis
pseu·do·e·o·sin·o·phil
pseu·do·e·phed·rine
pseu·do·ep·i·lep·sy
pseu·do·ep·i·the·li·om·a·
   tous
pseu·do·e·rec·tile
pseu·do·es·the·si·a
pseu·do·ex·fo·li·a·tion
pseu·do·far·cy
   pl pseu·do·far·cies
pseu·do·fluc·tu·a·tion
pseu·do·fol·lic·u·lar
pseu·do·frac·ture
pseu·do·gan·gli·on
pseu·do·geu·saes·the·si·a
   var of pseu·do·geu·ses·
   the·si·a
pseu·do·geu·ses·the·si·a
pseu·do·geu·si·a
pseu·do·glan·ders
pseu·do·gli·o·ma
pseu·do·glob·u·lin
pseu·do·gon·or·rhe·a
pseu·do·gon·or·rhoe·a
   var of pseu·do·gon·or·rhe·a
pseu·do·gout
pseu·do-Grae·fe phe·nom·
   e·non
pseu·do·gyn·ae·co·mas·ti·a
   var of pseu·do·gyn·e·co·
   mas·ti·a
pseu·do·gyn·e·co·mas·ti·a
pseu·do·hae·mo·phil·i·a
   var of pseu·do·he·mo·phil·
   i·a
Pseu·do·ha·je
pseu·do·hal·lu·ci·na·tion
pseu·do·hem·i·a·car·di·us
pseu·do·he·mo·phil·i·a
pseu·do·her·maph·ro·dite
pseu·do·her·maph·ro·dit·ic
pseu·do·her·maph·ro·dit·
   ism
pseu·do·her·maph·ro·di·
   tis·mus
pseu·do·hy·dro·ceph·a·ly
pseu·do·hy·dro·ne·phro·sis

pseu·do·hy·dro·pho·bi·a
pseu·do·hy·o·scy·a·mine
pseu·do·hy·per·troph·ic
pseu·do·hy·per·tro·phy
   pl pseu·do·hy·per·tro·phies
pseu·do·hy·po·na·trae·mi·a
   var of pseu·do·hy·po·na·
   tre·mi·a
pseu·do·hy·po·na·tre·mi·a
pseu·do·hy·po·par·a·thy·
   roid·ism
pseu·do·il·e·us
pseu·do·i·so·chro·mat·ic
pseu·do·jaun·dice
pseu·do·ke·loid
pseu·do·ker·a·tin
pseu·do·ker·a·to·sis
pseu·do·lep·ra
pseu·do·leu·kae·mi·a
   var of pseu·do·leu·ke·mi·a
pseu·do·leu·ke·mi·a
pseu·do·li·thi·a·sis
pseu·do·lo·gi·a fan·tas·ti·
   ca
pseu·do·lys·sa
pseu·do·mal·a·dy
pseu·do·ma·lar·i·a
pseu·do·mam·ma
pseu·do·ma·ni·a
pseu·do·mel·a·no·sis
   pl pseu·do·mel·a·no·ses
pseu·do·mem·brane
pseu·do·mem·bra·nous
pseu·do·men·in·gi·tis
pseu·do·me·ninx
pseu·do·men·stru·a·tion
pseu·do·me·tam·er·ism
pseu·do·met·hae·mo·glo·
   bin
   var of pseu·do·met·he·
   mo·glo·bin
pseu·do·met·he·mo·glo·bin
pseu·do·mi·cro·ceph·a·ly
pseu·dom·ne·si·a
pseu·do·mo·nad
Pseu·dom·o·na·da·ce·ae
Pseu·dom·o·nas
   pl pseu·dom·o·na·des
pseu·do·mon·gol·ism

pseu·do·mon·gol·oid
pseu·do·mu·cin
pseu·do·mu·cin·ous
pseu·do·my·as·then·ic
pseu·do·myx·o·ma
  pl pseu·do·myx·o·mas
  or pseu·do·myx·o·ma·ta
pseu·do·myx·om·a·tous
pseu·do·nar·co·tism
pseu·do·ne·o·plasm
pseu·do·ne·o·plas·tic
pseu·do·neu·ri·tis
pseu·do·neu·ro·ma
  pl pseu·do·neu·ro·mas
  or pseu·do·neu·ro·ma·ta
pseu·do·neu·rot·ic
pseu·do·nu·cle·in
pseu·do·nu·cle·o·lus
  pl pseu·do·nu·cle·o·li
pseu·do·nys·tag·mus
pseu·do·oe·de·ma
  var of pseu·do·e·de·ma
pseu·do·oph·thal·mo·ple·
  gi·a
pseu·do·os·te·o·ma·la·ci·a
pseu·do·pap·il·le·de·ma
pseu·do·pap·il·loe·de·ma
  var of pseu·do·pap·il·le·
  de·ma
pseu·do·pa·ral·y·sis
  pl pseu·do·pa·ral·y·ses
pseu·do·par·a·ple·gi·a
pseu·do·par·a·site
pseu·do·pa·re·sis
pseu·do·pe·lade
pseu·do·pep·tone
pseu·do·pho·tes·the·si·a
Pseu·do·phyl·lid·e·a
pseu·do·ple·gi·a
pseu·do·pock·et
pseu·do·pod
pseu·do·po·di·o·spore
pseu·do·po·di·um
  pl pseu·do·po·di·a
pseu·do·pol·y·co·ri·a
pseu·do·pol·y·po·sis
pseu·do·po·en·ceph·a·ly
pseu·do·preg·nan·cy
  pl pseu·do·preg·nan·cies

pseu·do·preg·nant
pseu·do·pseu·do·hy·po·
  par·a·thy·roid·ism
pseu·dop·si·a
pseu·do·psy·cho·path·ic
pseu·do·pte·ryg·i·um
  pl pseu·do·pte·ryg·i·ums
  or pseu·do·pte·ryg·i·a
pseu·do·pto·sis
  pl pseu·do·pto·ses
pseu·do·pus
pseu·do·ra·bies
  pl pseu·do·ra·bies
pseu·do·re·ac·tion
pseu·do·re·tar·da·tion
pseu·do·rhon·cus
  pl pseu·do·rhon·ci
pseu·do·rick·ets
pseu·do·ro·sette
pseu·do·ru·bel·la
pseu·do·sar·co·ma
  pl pseu·do·sar·co·mas
  or pseu·do·sar·co·ma·ta
pseu·do·scar·la·ti·na
pseu·do·sci·ence
pseu·do·scle·re·ma
pseu·do·scle·ro·sis
  pl pseu·do·scle·ro·ses
pseu·do·se·rous
pseu·do·sil·i·cot·i·cum
pseu·do·small·pox
pseu·dos·mi·a
pseu·do·spi·der
pseu·do·spon·ta·ne·ous
pseu·do·sto·ma
  pl pseu·do·sto·mas
  or pseu·do·sto·ma·ta
pseu·do·stra·bis·mus
pseu·do·strat·i·fied
pseu·do·ta·bes
pseu·do·ta·bet·ic
pseu·do·tet·a·nus
Pseu·do·thel·phu·sa
pseu·do·tho·rax
pseu·do·tin·ni·tus
pseu·do·trich·i·no·sis
pseu·do·tri·loc·u·lar
pseu·do·tro·pine

pseu·do·trun·cus ar·te·ri·
  o·sus
pseu·do·tu·ber·cle
pseu·do·tu·ber·cu·lo·sis
  pl pseu·do·tu·ber·cu·lo·ses
pseu·do·tu·ber·cu·lous
pseu·do·tu·mor
pseu·do·tym·pa·ni·tes
pseu·do·tym·pa·ny
pseu·do·ty·phoid
pseu·do·vac·u·oles
pseu·do·vag·i·nal
pseu·do·ven·tri·cle
pseu·do·vom·it·ing
pseu·do·xan·tho·ma e·las·
  ti·cum
pseu·dy·drops
psi
psi·co·fu·ra·nine
psi·lo·cin
psi·lo·cy·bin
psi·lo·sis
  pl psi·lo·ses
psit·ta·co·sis
  pl psit·ta·co·ses
pso·as
  pl pso·ai
  or pso·ae
psod·y·mus
pso·i·tis
pso·mo·pha·gi·a
pso·mo·phag·ic
pso·moph·a·gy
pso·ra
pso·ra·len
Psor·er·gates
pso·ri·a·si·form
pso·ri·a·sis
  pl pso·ri·a·ses
pso·ri·at·ic
psor·oph·thal·mi·a
Pso·rop·tes
pso·ro·sperm
pso·ro·sper·mi·a
  pl pso·ro·sper·mi·ae
pso·ro·sper·mi·al
pso·ro·sper·mic
pso·ro·sper·mo·sis
psy·cha·go·gi·a

psy·cha·gog·ic
psy·cha·go·gy
   pl psy·cha·go·gies
psy·chal·gi·a
psy·cha·li·a
psych·as·the·ni·a
psych·as·then·ic
psych·a·tax·i·a
psych·au·di·to·ry
psy·che
psy·che·del·ic
psy·che·ism
psy·chen·to·ni·a
psy·chi·a·ter
psy·chi·at·ric
   or psy·chi·at·ri·cal
psy·chi·at·ri·cal
   or psy·chi·at·ric
psy·chi·at·ri·cal·ly
psy·chi·at·rics
psy·chi·a·trist
psy·chi·a·try
   pl psy·chi·a·tries
psy·chic
psy·chi·cal
psy·chi·no·sis
psy·chlamp·si·a
psy·cho·a·cous·tic
psy·cho·a·cous·tics
psy·cho·ac·ti·va·tor
psy·cho·ac·tive
psy·cho·an·al·ge·si·a
psy·cho·a·nal·y·sis
   pl psy·cho·a·nal·y·ses
psy·cho·an·a·lyst
psy·cho·an·a·lyt·ic
   or psy·cho·an·a·lyt·i·cal
psy·cho·an·a·lyt·i·cal
   or psy·cho·an·a·lyt·ic
psy·cho·an·a·lyze
psy·cho·au·di·to·ry
psy·cho·bi·o·log·ic
   or psy·cho·bi·o·log·i·cal
psy·cho·bi·o·log·i·cal
   or psy·cho·bi·o·log·ic
psy·cho·bi·ol·o·gist
psy·cho·bi·ol·o·gy
   pl psy·cho·bi·ol·o·gies
psy·cho·car·di·ac

psy·cho·ca·thar·sis
   pl psy·cho·ca·thar·ses
psy·cho·chem·i·cal
psy·cho·ci·ne·si·a
psy·cho·co·ma
psy·cho·cor·ti·cal
psy·cho·del·ic
psy·cho·di·ag·no·sis
   pl psy·cho·di·ag·no·ses
psy·cho·di·ag·nos·tic
psy·cho·di·ag·nos·tics
Psy·chod·i·dae
psy·cho·dom·e·ter
psy·cho·dom·e·try
psy·cho·dra·ma
psy·cho·dy·nam·ic
psy·cho·dy·nam·i·cal·ly
psy·cho·dy·nam·ics
psy·cho·ep·i·lep·sy
psy·cho·gal·van·ic
psy·cho·gal·va·nom·e·ter
psy·cho·gen·e·sis
   pl psy·cho·gen·e·ses
psy·cho·ge·net·ic
psy·cho·gen·ic
psy·cho·gen·i·cal·ly
psy·chog·e·ny
   pl psy·chog·e·nies
psy·cho·geu·sic
psy·chog·no·sis
   pl psy·chog·no·ses
psy·chog·nos·tic
psy·cho·gram
psy·cho·graph·ic
psy·cho·graph·i·cal·ly
psy·chog·ra·phy
   pl psy·chog·ra·phies
psy·cho·ki·ne·si·a
psy·cho·ki·ne·sis
   pl psy·cho·ki·ne·ses
psy·cho·lag·ny
psy·cho·lep·sy
   pl psy·cho·lep·sies
psy·cho·lep·tic
psy·cho·log·ic
   or psy·cho·log·i·cal
psy·cho·log·i·cal
   or psy·cho·log·ic
psy·cho·log·i·cal·ly

psy·chol·o·gist
psy·chol·o·gize
psy·chol·o·gy
   pl psy·chol·o·gies
psy·cho·math·e·mat·ics
psy·cho·met·ric
psy·cho·met·ri·cal·ly
psy·cho·me·tri·cian
psy·cho·met·rics
psy·chom·e·try
   pl psy·chom·e·tries
psy·cho·mo·tor
psy·cho·neu·ro·log·ic
   or psy·cho·neu·ro·log·i·cal
psy·cho·neu·ro·log·i·cal
   or psy·cho·neu·ro·log·ic
psy·cho·neu·ro·sis
   pl psy·cho·neu·ro·ses
psy·cho·neu·rot·ic
psy·cho·nom·ic
psy·cho·nom·ics
psy·chon·o·my
   pl psy·chon·o·mies
psy·cho·no·se·ma
psy·cho·pa·re·sis
psy·cho·path
psy·cho·path·i·a
psy·cho·path·ic
psy·cho·path·i·cal·ly
psy·chop·a·thist
psy·cho·path·o·log·ic
   or psy·cho·path·o·log·i·cal
psy·cho·path·o·log·i·cal
   or psy·cho·path·o·log·ic
psy·cho·pa·thol·o·gist
psy·cho·pa·thol·o·gy
   pl psy·cho·pa·thol·o·gies
psy·chop·a·thy
   pl psy·chop·a·thies
psy·cho·phar·ma·ceu·ti·cal
psy·cho·phar·ma·co·log·ic
   or psy·cho·phar·ma·co·log·i·cal
psy·cho·phar·ma·co·log·i·cal
   or psy·cho·phar·ma·co·log·ic
psy·cho·phar·ma·col·o·gist

psy·cho·phar·ma·col·o·gy
  pl psy·cho·phar·ma·col·
  o·gies
psy·cho·pho·nas·the·ni·a
psy·cho·phys·i·cal
psy·cho·phys·i·cal·ly
psy·cho·phys·i·cist
psy·cho·phys·ics
psy·cho·phys·i·o·log·i·cal
  or psy·cho·phys·i·o·log·ic
psy·cho·phys·i·o·log·i·cal
  or psy·cho·phys·i·o·log·ic
psy·cho·phys·i·ol·o·gy
  pl psy·cho·phys·i·ol·o·gies
psy·cho·ple·gi·a
psy·cho·ple·gic
psy·cho·rhyth·mi·a
psy·chor·rha·gi·a
psy·cho·sen·so·ri·al
psy·cho·sen·so·ry
psy·cho·sex·u·al
psy·cho·sex·u·al·i·ty
  pl psy·cho·sex·u·al·i·ties
psy·cho·sex·u·al·ly
psy·cho·sine
psy·cho·sis
  pl psy·cho·ses
psy·cho·so·cial
psy·cho·so·cial·ly
psy·cho·so·mat·ic
psy·cho·so·mat·i·cal·ly
psy·cho·so·mat·ics
psy·cho·sur·geon
psy·cho·sur·ger·y
  pl psy·cho·sur·ger·ies
psy·cho·sur·gi·cal
psy·cho·syn·the·sis
  pl psy·cho·syn·the·ses
psy·cho·tech·ni·cian
psy·cho·tech·nics
psy·cho·ther·a·peu·tic
psy·cho·ther·a·peu·ti·cal·ly
psy·cho·ther·a·peu·tics
psy·cho·ther·a·pist
psy·cho·ther·a·py
  pl psy·cho·ther·a·pies
psy·chot·ic
psy·chot·i·cal·ly
psy·chot·o·gen

psy·chot·o·gen·ic
psy·chot·o·mi·met·ic
psy·chot·o·mi·met·i·cal·ly
psy·cho·tox·ic
psy·cho·trop·ic
psy·cho·vi·su·al
psy·chral·gi·a
psy·chro·aes·the·si·a
  var of psy·chro·es·the·si·a
psy·chro·es·the·si·a
psy·chro·lu·si·a
psy·chrom·e·ter
psy·chrom·e·try
  pl psy·chrom·e·tries
psy·chro·phil·ic
psy·chro·pho·bi·a
psy·chro·phore
psy·chro·ther·a·py
  pl psy·chro·ther·a·pies
psyl·li·um
ptar·mic
ptar·mus
ptel·e·or·rhine
pter·i·dine
pter·i·do·phyte
pter·in
pter·i·on
pte·ro·ic
pter·o·yl·glu·tam·ic
pte·ryg·i·al
pte·ryg·i·um
  pl pte·ryg·i·ums
  or pte·ryg·i·a
pter·y·go·a·lar
pter·y·goid
  or pter·y·goi·dal
pter·y·goi·dal
  or pter·y·goid
pter·y·go·man·di·bu·lar
pter·y·go·max·il·lar·y
pter·y·go·pal·a·tine
pter·y·go·pha·ryn·ge·us
pter·y·go·spi·nous
pti·lo·sis
  pl pti·lo·ses
pto·maine
pto·mat·i·nu·ri·a
ptosed
  or ptot·ic

pto·sis
  pl pto·ses
ptot·ic
  or ptosed
pty·al·a·gogue
pty·a·lase
pty·a·lec·ta·sis
pty·a·lin
pty·a·lin·o·gen
pty·a·lism
pty·a·lith
pty·a·lo·cele
pty·a·lo·gen·ic
pty·al·o·gog·ue
pty·a·log·ra·phy
  pl pty·a·log·ra·phies
pty·a·lo·lith
pty·a·lo·li·thi·a·sis
pty·a·lor·rhe·a
pty·a·lor·rhoe·a
  var of pty·a·lor·rhe·a
pty·a·lose
pty·a·lo·sis
pty·o·crine
pty·oc·ri·nous
ptys·ma
ptys·ma·gogue
pu·ber
pu·ber·al
  or pu·ber·tal
pu·ber·tal
  or pu·ber·al
pu·ber·tas
pu·ber·ty
  pl pu·ber·ties
pu·ber·u·lic
pu·ber·u·lon·ic
pu·bes
  pl pu·bes
pu·bes·cence
pu·bes·cent
pu·be·trot·o·my
pu·bic
pu·bi·ot·o·my
  pl pu·bi·ot·o·mies
pu·bis
  pl pu·bes
pu·bo·ad·duc·tor
pu·bo·cap·su·lar

pu·bo·cav·er·no·sus
pu·bo·coc·cyg·e·al
pu·bo·coc·cyg·e·us
pu·bo·fem·o·ral
pu·bo·per·i·to·ne·a·lis
pu·bo·pros·tat·ic
pu·bo·rec·ta·lis
pu·bo·scro·tal
pu·bo·trans·ver·sa·lis
pu·bo·tu·ber·ous
pu·bo·ves·i·cal
pu·bo·ves·i·ca·lis
pu·den·dag·ra
pu·den·dal
pu·den·dum
   pl pu·den·da
pu·dic
Pu·en·te dis·ease
pu·er·i·cul·ture
pu·er·ile
pu·er·il·ism
pu·er·i·ti·a
pu·er·per·a
   pl pu·er·per·ae
pu·er·per·al
pu·er·per·al·ism
pu·er·per·ant
pu·er·pe·ri·um
   pl pu·er·pe·ri·a
Pugh test
pu·le·gone
Pu·lex
pu·li·car·is
pu·li·ca·ti·o
Pu·lic·i·dae
pu·li·ci·dal
pu·li·cide
pul·lo·rum dis·ease
Pul·lu·lar·i·a
pul·lu·late
pul·lu·la·tion
pul·mo
   pl pul·mo·nes
pul·mo·car·di·ac
pul·mo·gas·tric
pul·mo·he·pat·ic
pul·mom·e·ter
pul·mom·e·try
   pl pul·mom·e·tries

pul·mo·nar·y
pul·mo·nate
pul·mo·nec·to·my
   pl pul·mo·nec·to·mies
pul·mon·ic
pul·mo·ni·tis
pul·mo·tor
pul·mo·vas·cu·lar
pulp
pul·pa
pulp·al
   or pulp·ar
pulp·al·ly
pulp·ar
   or pulp·al
pul·pa·tion
pul·pec·to·my
   pl pul·pec·to·mies
pul·pi·tis
pul·pot·o·my
   pl pul·pot·o·mies
pulp·stone
pulp·y
pul·que
pul·sate
pul·sa·tile
pul·sa·til·la
pul·sa·tion
pul·sa·tor
pul·sa·to·ry
pulse
pulse·less
pul·sim·e·ter
pul·sion
pul·sion di·ver·tic·u·lum
pul·sus
   pl pul·sus
pul·ta·ceous
pul·ver·i·za·tion
pul·ver·ize
pul·ver·u·lent
pul·vi·nar
pul·vi·nate
   or pul·vi·nat·ed
pul·vi·nat·ed
   or pul·vi·nate
pul·vis
pu·mex
pum·ice

pump
pu·na
punch
punc·ta
punc·tate
punc·tat·ed
punc·tic·u·lum
punc·ti·form
punc·to·graph
punc·tum
   pl punc·ta
punc·ture
pun·gent
pu·ni·cine
punk·tal
pu·nu·dos
pu·pa
   pl pu·pas
   or pu·pae
pu·pal
pu·pil
pu·pil·la
   pl pu·pil·lae
pu·pil·lar·y
pu·pil·lo·con·stric·tor
pu·pil·lo·di·la·tor
pu·pil·lom·e·ter
pu·pil·lom·e·try
   pl pu·pil·lom·e·tries
pu·pil·lo·mo·tor
pu·pil·lo·sta·tom·e·ter
pu·pil·lo·to·ni·a
pu·pil·lo·ton·ic
pure
pur·ga·tion
pur·ga·tive
purge
pu·ri·form
pu·ri·fy
pu·rine
pu·ri·ty
Pur·kin·je af·ter·im·age
Pur·kin·je cell
Pur·kin·je fi·ber
Pur·kin·je fig·ure
Pur·kin·je net·work
Pur·kin·je phe·nom·e·non
Pur·kin·je-San·son
   im·a·ges

pu·ro·mu·cous
pu·ro·my·cin
pur·po·sive
pur·pu·ra
pur·pu·ra hem·or·rhag·i·ca
pur·pu·ric
pur·pu·rin
pur·pu·ri·nur·i·a
purr
pu·ru·lence
 or pu·ru·len·cy
pu·ru·len·cy
 pl pu·ru·len·cies
 or pu·ru·lence
pu·ru·lent
pu·ru·loid
pu·ru·pu·ru
pus
pus·tu·lant
pus·tu·lar
pus·tu·late
pus·tu·la·tion
pus·tule
pus·tu·li·form
pus·tu·lo·der·ma
pus·tu·lo·sis
 pl pus·tu·lo·sis·es
 or pus·tu·lo·ses
pu·ta·men
 pl pu·ta·mi·na
Put·nam-Da·na syn·drome
Put·nam scle·ro·sis
pu·tre·fac·tion
pu·tre·fac·tive
pu·tre·fy
pu·tres·cence
pu·tres·cent
pu·tres·cine
pu·trid
pu·tro·maine
Pu·us·sepp op·er·a·tion
py·ae·mi·a
 var of py·e·mi·a
py·ae·mic
 var of py·e·mic
py·ar·thro·sis
 pl py·ar·thro·ses
pyc·nic
 var of pyk·nic

pyc·no·dys·os·to·sis
 var of pyk·no·dys·os·to·sis
pyc·no·ep·i·lep·sy
 var of pyk·no·ep·i·lep·sy
pyc·no·lep·sy
 var of pyk·no·lep·sy
pyc·nom·e·ter
 var of pyk·nom·e·ter
pyc·no·mor·phic
 var of pyk·no·mor·phous
pyc·no·mor·phous
 var of pyk·no·mor·phous
pcy·no·phra·si·a
 var of pyk·no·phra·si·a
pyc·no·sis
 var of pyk·no·sis
pyc·not·ic
 var of pyk·not·ic
py·ec·chy·sis
py·e·lec·ta·si·a
py·e·lec·ta·sis
 pl py·e·lec·ta·ses
py·el·ic
py·e·lit·ic
py·e·li·tis
py·e·lo·cys·ti·tis
 pl py·e·lo·cys·ti·ti·des
py·e·lo·gen·ic
py·e·lo·gram
 or py·e·lo·graph
py·e·lo·graph
 or py·e·lo·gram
py·e·lo·graph·ic
py·e·log·ra·phy
 pl py·e·log·ra·phies
py·e·lo·li·thot·o·my
py·e·lo·ne·phrit·ic
py·e·lo·ne·phri·tis
 pl py·e·lo·ne·phri·ti·des
py·e·lo·ne·phro·sis
 pl py·e·lo·ne·phro·ses
py·e·lo·plas·ty
py·e·lo·pli·ca·tion
py·e·los·to·my
 pl py·e·los·to·mies
py·e·lot·o·my
py·e·lo·tu·bu·lar
py·e·lo·u·re·ter·al
py·e·lo·u·re·ter·ic

py·e·lo·u·re·ter·o·gram
py·e·lo·u·re·ter·og·ra·phy
py·e·lo·ve·nous
py·em·e·sis
py·e·mi·a
py·e·mic
py·en·ceph·a·lus
py·e·sis
py·gal
py·gal·gi·a
pyg·ma·li·on·ism
pyg·my
py·go·a·mor·phus
py·go·did·y·mus
py·gom·e·lus
py·gop·a·gus
 pl py·gop·a·gi
py·go·par·a·si·tus
py·go·ter·a·toi·des
py·ic
py·in
pyk·nic
pyk·no·dys·os·to·sis
pyk·no·ep·i·lep·sy
 pl pyk·no·ep·i·lep·sies
pyk·no·lep·sy
 pl pyk·no·lep·sies
pyk·nom·e·ter
pyk·no·mor·phous
pyk·no·phra·si·a
pyk·no·sis
pyk·not·ic
py·la
 pl py·las
 or py·lae
py·lar
py·lem·phrax·is
py·le·phleb·ec·ta·si·a
py·le·phle·bec·ta·sis
 pl py·le·phle·bec·ta·ses
py·le·phle·bi·tis
 pl py·le·phle·bi·ti·des
py·le·throm·bo·phle·bi·tis
py·le·throm·bo·sis
 pl py·le·throm·bo·ses
py·lic
py·lon
py·lo·ral·gi·a
py·lo·rec·to·my

py·lor·ic
py·lo·ri·ste·no·sis
py·lo·ri·tis
py·lo·ro·col·ic
py·lo·ro·di·la·tor
py·lo·ro·di·o·sis
py·lo·ro·du·o·de·nal
py·lo·ro·gas·trec·to·my
  pl py·lo·ro·gas·trec·to·mies
py·lo·ro·my·ot·o·my
  pl py·lo·ro·my·ot·o·mies
py·lo·ro·plas·ty
  pl py·lo·ro·plas·ties
py·lor·op·to·si·a
py·lor·op·to·sis
py·lo·ro·sche·sis
py·lo·ros·co·py
py·lo·ro·spasm
py·lo·ro·ste·no·sis
py·lo·ros·to·my
py·lo·rot·o·my
  pl py·lo·rot·o·mies
py·lo·rus
  pl py·lo·rus·es
  or py·lo·ri
py·o·ar·thro·sis
py·o·cele
py·o·ceph·a·lus
py·o·che·zi·a
py·o·coc·cus
  pl py·o·coc·ci
py·o·col·po·cele
py·o·col·pos
py·o·cy·a·nase
py·o·cy·an·ic
py·o·cy·a·nin
  or py·o·cy·a·nine
py·o·cy·a·nine
  or py·o·cy·a·nin
py·o·cy·a·nol·y·sin
py·o·cyst
py·o·cys·tis
py·o·der·ma
  or py·o·der·mi·a
py·o·der·ma·ti·tis
py·o·der·ma·to·sis
py·o·der·ma·tous
py·o·der·mi·a
  or py·o·der·ma

py·o·gen
py·og·e·nes
py·o·gen·e·sis
py·o·ge·net·ic
py·o·gen·ic
py·og·e·nous
py·o·he·mo·tho·rax
  pl py·o·he·mo·tho·rax·es
  or py·o·he·mo·tho·ra·ces
py·oid
py·o·lab·y·rin·thi·tis
py·o·me·tra
py·o·me·tri·um
py·o·my·o·si·tis
py·o·ne·phri·tis
  pl py·o·ne·phri·ti·des
py·o·neph·ro·li·thi·a·sis
py·o·ne·phro·sis
  pl py·o·ne·phro·ses
py·o·ne·phrot·ic
py·o·o·var·i·um
py·o·per·i·car·di·tis
py·o·per·i·car·di·um
py·o·per·i·to·ne·um
py·o·per·i·to·ni·tis
py·o·pha·gi·a
py·oph·thal·mi·a
py·o·phy·lac·tic
py·o·phy·so·me·tra
py·o·pneu·mo·per·i·car·
  di·tis
py·o·pneu·mo·per·i·car·
  di·um
py·o·pneu·mo·per·i·to·
  ne·um
py·o·pneu·mo·per·i·to·
  ni·tis
py·o·pneu·mo·tho·rax
  pl py·o·pneu·mo·tho·rax·es
  or py·o·pneu·mo·tho·ra·ces
py·o·poi·e·sis
  pl py·o·poi·e·ses
py·o·poi·et·ic
py·op·ty·sis
py·or·rhe·a
py·or·rhea·al·ve·o·lar·is
py·or·rhoe·a
  var of py·or·rhe·a
py·o·sal·pin·gi·tis

py·o·sal·pin·go·o·o·pho·
  ri·tis
py·o·sal·pinx
  pl py·o·sal·pin·ges
py·o·sep·ti·ce·mi·a
py·o·sis
py·o·sper·mi·a
py·o·stat·ic
py·o·ther·a·py
py·o·tho·rax
  pl py·o·tho·rax·es
  or py·o·tho·ra·ces
py·o·u·ra·chus
py·o·u·re·ter
py·o·xan·thin
py·o·xan·those
py·ra·hex·yl
pyr·a·mid
py·ram·i·dal
py·ram·i·dale
py·ram·i·da·lis
  pl py·ram·i·da·lis·es
  or py·ram·i·da·les
py·ram·i·des re·na·les
pyr·a·mi·dot·o·my
  pl pyr·a·mi·dot·o·mies
pyr·a·min
pyr·a·mis
  pl py·ra·mi·des
py·ran
py·ra·nis·a·mine
py·ra·nose
py·ran·tel
pyr·a·zin·a·mide
pyr·a·zine
pyr·a·zole
py·raz·o·lone
py·rec·tic
py·rene
py·re·nin
py·re·thrum
py·ret·ic
py·ret·o·gen
pyr·e·to·ge·ne·si·a
pyr·e·to·gen·e·sis
pyr·e·to·ge·net·ic
pyr·e·to·gen·ic
  or pyr·e·tog·e·nous

pyr·e·tog·e·nous
or pyr·e·to·gen·ic
pyr·e·tol·o·gist
pyr·e·tol·o·gy
pyr·e·tol·y·sis
pyr·e·to·ther·a·py
pl pyr·e·to·ther·a·pies
pyr·e·to·ty·pho·sis
py·rex·i·a
py·rex·i·al
py·rex·ic
py·rex·in
py·rex·i·o·pho·bi·a
pyr·go·ce·phal·ic
pyr·go·ceph·a·lous
pyr·go·ceph·a·ly
pyr·he·li·om·e·ter
py·rid·a·zine
pyr·i·dine
pyr·i·do·stig·mine
pyr·i·dox·al
pyr·i·dox·a·mine
pyr·i·dox·ic
pyr·i·dox·in
or pyr·i·dox·ine
pyr·i·dox·ine
or pyr·i·dox·in
pyr·i·dyl
pyr·i·form
or pir·i·form
pyr·i·form·is
or pi·ri·form·is

pyr·il·a·mine
pyr·i·meth·a·mine
py·rim·i·dine
pyr·in·o·line
pyr·i·thi·a·mine
py·ro·cat·e·chase
py·ro·cat·e·chin
py·ro·cat·e·chi·nu·ri·a
py·ro·cat·e·chol
py·ro·gal·lic
py·ro·gal·lol
py·ro·gen
py·ro·gen·ic
py·ro·glo·bu·lin
py·ro·glob·u·li·nae·mi·a
var of py·ro·glob·u·li·
ne·mi·a
py·ro·glob·u·li·ne·mi·a
py·ro·glos·si·a
py·ro·lag·ni·a
py·ro·lig·ne·ous
py·rol·y·sis
pl py·rol·y·ses
py·ro·lyt·ic
py·ro·ma·ni·a
py·ro·ma·ni·ac
py·ro·ma·ni·a·cal
py·rom·e·ter
py·ro·mu·cic
py·rone
py·ro·nine

py·ro·nin·o·phil·ic
py·ro·pho·bi·a
py·ro·phos·pha·tase
py·ro·phos·phate
py·ro·phos·pho·ric
py·rop·to·thy·mi·a
py·ro·punc·ture
py·ro·ra·ce·mic
py·ro·scope
py·ro·sis
py·ro·sul·fite
py·rot·ic
py·ro·tox·in
py·ro·va·ler·one
py·rox·a·mine
py·rox·y·lin
pyr·rhol
pyr·ro·bu·ta·mine
pyr·ro·caine
pyr·role
pyr·rol·i·done
pyr·rol·i·phene
pyr·rol·ni·trin
pyr·ro·lo·por·phyr·i·a
py·ru·vate
py·ru·vic
pyr·vin·i·um pam·o·ate
py·tho·gen·ic
py·u·ri·a
py·u·ric

Q

quack
quack·er·y
pl quack·er·ies
quack·sal·ver
qua·dran·gu·lar

quad·rant
quad·ran·ta·no·pi·a
quad·ran·ta·nop·si·a
quad·ran·tic
quad·rate

qua·dra·tus
pl qua·dra·ti
quad·ri·ceps, ex·ten·sor,
fem·o·ris
quad·ri·cip·i·tal

333

quad·ri·cus·pid
quad·ri·gem·i·na
quad·ri·gem·i·nal
quad·ri·gem·i·nate
quad·ri·lat·er·al
qua·drip·a·ra
quad·ri·pa·re·sis
quad·ri·par·i·ty
qua·drip·a·rous
quad·ri·ple·gi·a
quad·ri·ple·gic
quad·ri·sect
quad·ri·tu·ber·cu·lar
quad·ri·u·rate
quad·ri·va·lence
quad·ri·va·lent
quad·roon
quad·ru·ped
qua·dru·pe·dal
quad·ru·ple
quad·ru·plet
Quain fat·ty de·gen·er·a·tion
qua·lim·e·ter
qual·i·ta·tive
qual·i·ty
quan·tal
quan·ta·some
quan·tim·e·ter
quan·ti·ta·tive
quan·ti·ty
quan·tum
    pl quan·ta
quar·an·tine
quark
quart
quar·tan
quar·ter
quar·tip·a·ra
quar·tip·a·rous
quartz

quas·si·a
quat
    or khat
    or kat
qua·ter in di·e
qua·ter·nar·y
quat·tu·or
qua·zo·dine
que·bra·bun·da
que·bra·chine
que·bra·cho
Queck·en·stedt ma·neu·ver
quel·lung
Qué·nu op·er·a·tion
que·nu·tho·ra·co·plas·ty
quer·ce·tin
    or quer·ci·tin
quer·ci·tan·ic
quer·ci·tan·nin
quer·ci·tin
    or quer·ce·tin
Quer·cus
quer·u·lent
Quer·vain dis·ease
Qué·venne i·ron
Quey·rat e·ryth·ro·pla·si·a
quick
Quick test
quick·en
quick·lime
quick·sil·ver
qui·es·cence
qui·es·cent
quil·la·ja
qui·na
quin·a·crine
quin·al·bar·bi·tone
quin·al·dine
quin·az·o·sin
quin·bo·lone

Quin·cke dis·ease
quin·dec·a·mine
quin·do·ni·um
quin·es·trol
quin·eth·a·zone
quin·ges·ta·nol
quin·ges·trone
quin·i·cine
quin·i·dine
qui·nine
qui·nin·ism
quin·i·no·der·ma
qui·none
quin·ism
quin·o·chrome
quin·oid
quin·o·line
qui·nol·o·gist
qui·nol·o·gy
    pl qui·nol·o·gies
qui·no·lone
qui·none
quin·o·tan·nic
qui·no·va·tine
quin·o·vin
qui·no·vose
Quin·quaud dis·ease
quin·que·tu·ber·cu·lar
quin·qui·na
quin·sy
    pl quin·sies
quin·tan
quin·tip·a·ra
quin·tip·a·rous
quin·tu·plet
qui·nu·cli·dine
quip·a·zine
qui·tiq·ua
quit·tor
quo·tid·i·an
quo·tient

R

rab·bet·ing
ra·bic
rab·id
ra·bies
 pl ra·bies
ra·bi·form
race
Race-Coombs test
ra·ce·mase
ra·ce·mate
ra·ceme
ra·ce·mic
ra·ce·mi·za·tion
rac·e·mose
rac·e·phed·rine
ra·ce·phen·i·col
ra·chi·al
 or ra·chid·i·al
ra·chi·al·gi·a
ra·chi·an·aes·the·si·a
 var of ra·chi·an·es·the·si·a
ra·chi·an·es·the·si·a
ra·chi·as·mus
ra·chi·cele
ra·chi·cen·te·sis
 pl ra·chi·cen·te·ses
ra·chid·i·al
 or ra·chi·al
ra·chid·i·an
ra·chi·graph
ra·chil·y·sis
 pl ra·chil·y·ses
ra·chi·o·camp·sis
ra·chi·o·cen·te·sis
ra·chi·o·dyn·i·a
ra·chi·om·e·ter
ra·chi·op·a·thy
ra·chi·o·ple·gi·a
ra·chi·o·sco·li·o·sis
ra·chi·o·tome
ra·chi·ot·o·my
ra·chip·a·gus
ra·chi·re·sis·tance

ra·chis
 pl ra·chis·es
 or rach·i·des
ra·chis·chi·sis
 pl ra·chis·chi·ses
ra·chit·a·min
ra·chi·ter·a·ta
ra·chit·ic
ra·chi·tis
 pl ra·chi·ti·des
 or rah·chi·tis
 pl rha·chi·ti·des
ra·chi·tism
rach·i·to·gen·ic
ra·cial
ra·clage
ra·cle·ment
rad
ra·dar·ky·mo·gram
ra·dar·ky·mog·ra·phy
ra·dec·to·my
 pl ra·dec·to·mies
ra·di·a·bil·i·ty
 pl ra·di·a·bil·i·ties
ra·di·ad
ra·di·al
ra·di·a·le
 pl ra·di·a·li·a
ra·di·a·lis
ra·di·al·ly
ra·di·an
ra·di·ant
Ra·di·a·ta
ra·di·ate
ra·di·a·ti·o
 pl ra·di·a·ti·o·nes
ra·di·a·tion
rad·i·cal
rad·i·cle
rad·i·cot·o·my
ra·dic·u·lal·gi·a
ra·dic·u·lar
ra·dic·u·lec·to·my
 pl ra·dic·u·lec·to·mies
ra·dic·u·li·tis

ra·dic·u·lo·gang·li·o·ni·tis
ra·dic·u·lo·me·nin·go·my·e·
 li·tis
ra·dic·u·lo·my·e·lop·a·thy
ra·dic·u·lo·neu·ri·tis
ra·dic·u·lo·neu·rop·a·thy
ra·dic·u·lop·a·thy
ra·dif·er·ous
ra·di·o·ab·la·tion
ra·di·o·ac·tin·i·um
ra·di·o·ac·tive
ra·di·o·ac·tive·ly
ra·di·o·ac·tiv·i·ty
 pl ra·di·o·ac·tiv·i·ties
ra·di·o·ar·te·ri·o·gram
ra·di·o·au·to·gram
ra·di·o·au·to·graph
ra·di·o·au·to·graph·ic
ra·di·o·au·tog·ra·phy
 pl ra·di·o·au·tog·ra·phies
ra·di·obe
ra·di·o·bi·cip·i·tal
ra·di·o·bi·o·log·ic
 or ra·di·o·bi·o·log·i·cal
ra·di·o·bi·o·log·i·cal
 or ra·di·o·bi·o·log·ic
ra·di·o·bi·o·log·i·cal·ly
ra·di·o·bi·ol·o·gist
ra·di·o·bi·ol·o·gy
 pl ra·di·o·bi·ol·o·gies
ra·di·o·cal·ci·um
ra·di·o·car·bon
ra·di·o·car·di·o·gram
ra·di·o·car·di·og·ra·phy
ra·di·o·car·pal
ra·di·o·car·pe·us
ra·di·o·chem·i·cal
ra·di·o·chem·i·cal·ly
ra·di·o·chem·ist
ra·di·o·chem·is·try
 pl ra·di·o·chem·is·tries
ra·di·o·chro·ma·to·graph·ic
ra·di·o·chro·ma·tog·ra·phy
 pl ra·di·o·cro·ma·tog·ra·
 phies

ra·di·o·cin·e·mat·o·graph
ra·di·o·co·balt
ra·di·o·col·loid
ra·di·o·cur·a·bil·i·ty
ra·di·o·cur·a·ble
ra·di·o·cys·ti·tis
ra·di·ode
ra·di·o·dense
ra·di·o·der·ma·ti·tis
   pl ra·di·o·der·ma·ti·ti·ses
   or ra·di·o·der·ma·ti·ti·des
ra·di·o·don·ti·a
ra·di·o·don·tic
ra·di·o·don·tics
ra·di·o·don·tist
ra·di·o·e·col·o·gist
ra·di·o·e·col·o·gy
   pl ra·di·o·e·col·o·gies
ra·di·o·el·e·ment
ra·di·o·gen·i
ra·di·o·gold
ra·di·o·gram
ra·di·o·graph
ra·di·og·ra·pher
ra·di·o·graph·ic
ra·di·o·graph·i·cal·ly
ra·di·og·ra·phy
   pl ra·di·og·ra·phies
ra·di·o·hu·mer·al
ra·di·o·im·mu·ni·ty
ra·di·o·im·mu·no·as·say
ra·di·o·im·mu·no·dif·fu·
   sion
ra·di·o·i·o·dine
ra·di·o·i·ron
ra·di·o·i·so·tope
ra·di·o·i·so·top·ic
ra·di·o·i·so·to·pi·cal·ly
ra·di·o·ky·mog·ra·phy
ra·di·o·lead
ra·di·o·log·ic
   or ra·di·o·log·i·cal
ra·di·o·log·i·cal
   or ra·di·o·log·ic
ra·di·o·log·i·cal·ly
ra·di·ol·o·gist
ra·di·ol·o·gy
   pl ra·di·ol·o·gies

ra·di·o·lu·cen·cy
   pl ra·di·o·lu·cen·cies
ra·di·o·lu·cent
ra·di·o·lu·mi·nes·cence
ra·di·ol·y·sis
   pl ra·di·ol·y·ses
ra·di·om·e·ter
ra·di·o·met·ric
ra·di·o·met·ri·cal·ly
ra·di·om·e·try
   pl ra·di·om·e·tries
ra·di·o·mi·crom·e·ter
ra·di·o·mi·met·ic
ra·di·on
ra·di·o·ne·cro·sis
   pl ra·di·o·ne·cro·ses
ra·di·o·ne·crot·ic
ra·di·o·neu·ri·tis
ra·di·o·ni·tro·gen
ra·di·o·nu·clide
ra·di·o·o·paque
ra·di·o·pac·i·ty
   pl ra·di·o·pac·i·ties
ra·di·o·paque
ra·di·o·pa·thol·o·gy
ra·di·o·pel·vim·e·try
ra·di·o·phar·ma·ceu·ti·cal
ra·di·o·phos·pho·rus
ra·di·o·po·ten·ti·a·tion
ra·di·o·prax·is
ra·di·o·pro·tec·tion
ra·di·o·pro·tec·tive
ra·di·o·pro·tec·tor
ra·di·o·re·cep·tor
ra·di·o·re·sis·tance
ra·di·o·re·sis·tant
ra·di·o·re·spon·sive
ra·di·o·scope
ra·di·o·scop·ic
   or ra·di·o·scop·i·cal
ra·di·o·scop·i·cal
   or ra·di·o·scop·ic
ra·di·os·co·py
   pl ra·di·os·co·pies
ra·di·o·sen·si·tive
ra·di·o·sen·si·tiv·i·ty
   pl ra·di·o·sen·si·tiv·i·ties
ra·di·o·so·di·um
ra·di·o·ster·e·os·co·py

ra·di·o·ster·il·i·za·tion
ra·di·o·ster·il·i·zed
ra·di·o·stron·ti·um
ra·di·o·sur·ger·y
   pl ra·di·o·sur·ger·ies
ra·di·o·tel·e·met·ric
ra·di·o·te·lem·e·try
   pl ra·di·o·te·lem·e·tries
ra·di·o·ther·a·peu·tic
ra·di·o·ther·a·peu·tics
ra·di·o·ther·a·pist
ra·di·o·ther·a·py
   pl ra·di·o·ther·a·pies
ra·di·o·ther·my
   pl ra·di·o·ther·mies
ra·di·o·tho·ri·um
ra·di·o·thy·roid·ec·to·mize
ra·di·o·tox·e·mi·a
ra·di·o·trans·par·ent
ra·di·o·tro·pic
ra·di·o·tro·pism
ra·di·o·ul·nar
ra·di·um
ra·di·us
   pl ra·di·us·es
   or ra·di·i
ra·dix
   pl ra·dix·es
   or ra·dix·ces
ra·don
Ra·do·vi·ci re·flex
Rae·der syn·drome
raf·fi·nase
raf·fi·nose
rag·weed
Rail·li·eti·na
Rai·mist sign
Rain·ey cor·pus·cle
rale
Ralph meth·od
ra·mal
Ram·an ef·fect
ram·i·fi·ca·tion
ram·i·fy
ram·i·sec·tion
ram·i·sec·to·my
ra·mose
Ram·say Hunt syn·drome
Rams·den eye·piece

Rams·den oc·u·lar
Ram·stedt op·er·a·tion
ram·u·lus
  pl ram·u·li
ra·mus
  pl ra·mi
ra·mus com·mu·ni·cans
  pl ra·mi com·mu·ni·can·tes
Ra·na
ran·cid
ran·cid·i·fi·ca·tion
ran·cid·i·fy
ran·cid·i·ty
  pl ran·cid·i·ties
Ran·di·a
ra·ni·my·cin
ra·nine
Ran·ke hy·poth·e·sis
Ran·kin op·er·a·tion
Ran·kine scale
Ran·so·hoff op·er·a·tion
Ran·son pyr·i·dine sil·ver
  stain
ran·u·la
Ra·nun·cu·lus
ra·nun·cu·la·ceous
Ran·vier node
Ra·oult law
rape
ra·pha·ni·a
raph·a·nin
ra·phe
  or rha·phe
ra·pid eye move·ment
Rap·kine meth·od
rap·port
rap·tus
  pl rap·ti
rar·e·fac·tion
rar·e·fy
  or rar·i·fy
rar·i·fy
  or rar·e·fy
rar·i·tas
Rasch sign
rash
ra·sion
Ras·mus·sen an·eu·rysm

Ra·so·ri·an·ism
ra·sor·ite
ras·pa·to·ry
  pl ras·pa·to·ries
rasp·ber·ry
rat-bite fe·ver
rate
Rath·ke pouch
ra·ti·o
ra·tion
ra·tion·al
ra·tion·al·i·ty
  pl ra·tion·al·i·ties
ra·tion·al·i·za·tion
ra·tion·al·ize
rats·bane
rat·tle
rat·tle·snake
Rat·tus
Rau·ber cell
Rau·wol·fi·a
rau·wol·fine
Ra·va·ton am·pu·ta·tion
ray
Ray ma·ni·a
Ray·gat test
Ray·leigh e·qua·tion
Ray·mond syn·drome
Ray·mond-
  Ces·tan syn·drome
Ray·naud dis·ease
rays of Sa·gnac
re·ab·sorb
re·ab·sorp·tion
re·ac·quired
re·act
re·ac·tance
re·ac·tant
re·ac·tion
re·ac·ti·vate
re·ac·ti·va·tion
re·ac·tive
re·ac·tiv·i·ty
  pl re·ac·tiv·i·ties
re·ac·tor
re·a·gent
re·ag·gre·ga·tion
re·a·gin
re·a·gin·ic

re·al·gar
re·al·i·ty
  pl re·al·i·ties
ream·er
re·am·i·na·tion
re·am·pu·ta·tion
re·an·i·mate
re·at·tach·ment
Ré·au·mur scale ther·
  mom·e·ter
re·bel·lion
re·bound
re·branch
re·breath·ing
re·cal·ci·fi·ca·tion
re·cal·ci·fy
re·cal·ci·trant
re·call
Ré·ca·mier op·er·a·tion
re·ca·nal·i·za·tion
re·ca·pit·u·la·tion
re·cep·tac·u·lum
  pl re·cep·tac·u·la
re·cep·tive
re·cep·to·ma
  pl re·cep·to·mas
  or re·cep·to·ma·ta
re·cep·tor
re·cess
re·ces·sion
re·ces·sive
re·ces·sus
  pl re·ces·sus
re·cid·i·va·tion
re·cid·i·vism
re·cid·i·vist
re·cid·i·vis·tic
rec·i·div·i·ty
rec·i·pe
re·cip·i·ent
re·cip·ro·cal
re·cip·ro·ca·tion
rec·i·proc·i·ty
Reck·ling·hau·sen dis·ease
rec·li·na·ti·o
rec·li·na·tion
Re·clus dis·ease
re·coil
re·com·bi·nant

re·com·bi·na·tion
re·com·po·si·tion
re·com·pres·sion
re·con
re·con·di·tion
re·con·stit·u·ent
re·con·sti·tute
re·con·sti·tu·tion
re·son·struct
re·con·struc·tion
re·con·struc·tive
re·cov·er
re·cov·er·y
 pl re·cov·er·ies
rec·re·ment
rec·re·men·tal
rec·re·men·ti·tial
rec·re·men·ti·tious
re·cru·des·cence
re·cru·des·cent
re·cruit·ment
rec·tal
rec·tal·gi·a
rec·tal·ly
rec·tec·to·my
rec·ti·fi·ca·tion
rec·ti·fy
rec·ti·lin·e·ar
rec·ti·tis
rec·to·ab·dom·i·nal
rec·to·a·nal
rec·to·cele
rec·toc·ly·sis
 pl rec·toc·ly·ses
rec·to·coc·cyg·e·al
rec·to·coc·cyg·e·us
 pl rec·to·coc·cyg·e·i
rec·to·co·li·tis
rec·to·co·lon·ic
rec·to·cu·ta·ne·ous
rec·to·fis·tu·la
rec·to·gen·i·tal
rec·to·la·bi·al
rec·to·per·i·ne·al
rec·to·pex·y
rec·to·pho·bi·a
rec·to·plas·ty
rec·to·rec·tos·to·my
rec·to·ro·man·o·scope

rec·to·scope
rec·tos·co·py
rec·to·sig·moid
rec·to·sig·moi·dec·to·my
rec·to·sig·moi·do·scope
rec·to·sig·moi·do·scop·ic
rec·to·sig·moi·dos·co·py
 pl rec·to·sig·moi·dos·co·pies
rec·to·ste·no·sis
rec·tos·to·my
rec·tot·o·my
rec·to·u·re·thral
rec·to·u·re·thra·lis
rec·to·u·ter·ine
rec·to·vag·i·nal
rec·to·vag·i·no·ab·dom·i·nal
rec·to·ves·i·cal
rec·to·ves·i·ca·lis
rec·tum
 pl rec·tums
 or rec·ta
rec·tus
 pl rec·ti
re·cum·ben·cy
 pl re·cum·ben·cies
re·cum·bent
re·cu·per·ate
re·cu·per·a·tion
re·cu·per·a·tive
re·cur
re·cur·rence
re·cur·rent
re·cur·va·tion
Red Cross
red-green blind·ness
re·di·a
 pl re·di·as
 or re·di·ae
re·di·al
re·dif·fer·en·ti·a·tion
re·din·te·gra·tion
re·din·te·gra·tive
red·out
re·dox
re·dresse·ment
re·duce
re·duc·er

re·duc·i·bil·i·ty
 pl re·duc·i·bil·i·ties
re·duc·i·ble
re·duc·tant
re·duc·tase
re·duc·tic
re·duc·tion
re·duc·tone
re·dun·dan·cy
re·dun·dant
re·du·pli·cate
re·du·pli·ca·tion
re·du·vi·id
Red·u·vi·i·dae
Re·du·vi·us
Reed-Frost the·o·ry
Reed-Stern·berg cell
re·ed·u·ca·tion
reef·ing
Reen·stier·na test
re·en·try
 pl re·en·tries
re·ep·i·the·li·al·i·za·tion
re·ep·i·the·li·al·ize
Rees and Eck·er di·lu·ting
 flu·id
re·ev·o·lu·tion
re·ex·cise
re·ex·ci·ta·tion
re·ex·pand
re·fec·tion
re·fer
re·fer·ral
re·fill
re·fine
re·flect
re·flec·tance
re·flect·ed
re·flec·tion
re·flec·tor
re·flex
re·flex·i·o
re·flex·o·gen·ic
 or re·flex·og·e·nous
re·flex·og·e·nous
 or re·flex·o·gen·ic
re·flex·o·graph
re·flex·o·log·ic
re·flex·o·log·i·cal·ly

re·flex·ol·o·gist
re·flex·ol·o·gy
   pl re·flex·ol·o·gies
re·flex·om·e·ter
re·flex·o·ther·a·py
re·flux
re·fract
re·frac·ta do·si
re·frac·tile
re·frac·tion
re·frac·tion·ist
re·frac·tive
re·frac·tive·ness
re·frac·tiv·i·ty
   pl re·frac·tiv·i·ties
re·frac·tom·e·ter
re·frac·to·met·ric
re·frac·tom·e·try
   pl re·frac·tom·e·tries
re·frac·to·ri·ness
re·frac·to·ry
re·frac·ture
re·fran·gi·bil·i·ty
   pl re·fran·gi·bil·i·ties
re·fran·gi·ble
re·fresh
re·frig·er·ant
re·frig·er·ate
re·frig·er·a·tion
re·frin·gence
   or re·frin·gen·cy
re·frin·gen·cy
   pl re·frin·gen·cies
   or re·frin·gence
re·frin·gent
Ref·sum dis·ease
re·fu·sion
Re·gaud stain
re·gen·er·a·ble
re·gen·er·ate
re·gen·er·a·tion
re·gen·er·a·tive
reg·i·men
re·gi·o
   pl re·gi·o·nes
re·gion·al
reg·is·ter
reg·is·trant
reg·is·trar

reg·is·tra·tion
reg·is·try
   pl reg·is·tries
reg·li·men·ta·tion
reg·nan·cy
   pl reg·nan·cies
re·gress
re·gres·sion
re·gres·sive
re·grow
   re·grew
   re·grown
reg·u·lar
reg·u·lar·i·ty
   pl reg·u·lar·i·ties
reg·u·late
reg·u·la·tion
reg·u·la·tive
reg·u·la·tor
re·gur·gi·tant
re·gur·gi·tate
re·gur·gi·ta·tion
re·gur·gi·ta·tive
re·ha·bil·i·tant
re·ha·bil·i·tate
re·ha·bil·i·ta·tion
re·ha·bil·i·ta·tive
re·ha·bil·i·ta·tor
re·ha·bil·i·tee
re·ha·la·tion
Reh·berg test
Reh·fuss tube
Rehn-De·lorme
   op·er·a·tion
re·hy·drate
re·hy·dra·tion
Rei·chel duct
Rei·chert mem·brane
Rei·chert-Meissl
   num·ber, val·ue
Reich·mann dis·ease
Reich·stein sub·stance
Reil·ly bod·ies
re·im·plan·ta·tion
Rein ther·mo·stro·muhr
Rein·ke crys·tals, salt
re·in·fec·tion
re·in·force
re·in·force·ment

re·in·forc·er
re·in·fu·sion
Rein·hold meth·od
re·in·ner·va·tion
re·in·oc·u·late
re·in·oc·u·la·tion
Reinsch test
re·in·te·grate
re·in·te·gra·tion
re·in·te·gra·tive
re·in·ver·sion
Rei·sin·ger meth·od
Reiss·ner fi·ber
Rei·ter dis·ease, syn·
   drome
re·ject
re·jec·tion
re·ju·ve·nate
re·ju·ve·na·tion
re·ju·ve·nes·cence
re·ju·ve·nes·cent
re·lapse
re·late
re·la·tion
re·la·tion·al
re·la·tion·ship
rel·a·tive
re·lax
re·lax·ant
re·lax·a·tion
re·lax·in
re·lease
re·leas·er
re·lief
re·lieve
re·line
re·lo·my·cin
REM sleep
Re·mak fi·ber
re·me·di·a·ble
re·me·di·al
re·me·di·al·ly
rem·e·dy
   pl rem·e·dies
Re·mij·i·a
re·min·er·al·i·za·tion
re·mis·sion
re·mit
re·mit·tence

re·mit·tent
re·mit·tent·ly
rem·nant
re·mote
re·move
ren
   pl re·nes
re·nal
re·na·tur·a·tion
re·na·ture
Ren·du tre·mor
Ren·du-Os·ler-
   Web·er dis·ease
re·ni·fleur
ren·i·form
re·nin
ren·i·pel·vic
ren·i·por·tal
re·ni·punc·ture
ren·net
ren·nin
ren·nin·o·gen
re·no·gas·tric
re·no·gram
re·no·graph·ic
re·nog·ra·phy
   pl re·nog·ra·phies
Rén·on-
   De·lille syn·drome
re·nop·a·thy
re·no·pri·val
re·no·re·nal
re·no·tro·phic
re·no·tro·pic
re·no·vas·cu·lar
Ren·shaw cell
re·or·gan·i·za·tion
re·o·vi·rus
   pl re·o·vi·rus·es
rep
re·pair
re·par·a·tive
re·pel·lant
   or re·pel·lent
re·pel·lent
   or re·pel·lant
re·pel·ler
re·per·co·la·tion
re·per·cus·sion

re·per·cus·sive
rep·e·ti·tion com·pul·sion
re·place·ment
re·plan·ta·tion
re·plete
re·ple·tion
re·pli·ca·ble
rep·li·case
rep·li·cate
rep·li·ca·tion
rep·li·ca·tive
re·po·lar·i·za·tion
re·port
re·po·si·tion
re·pos·i·tor
re·pos·i·to·ry
   pl re·pos·i·to·ries
re·press
re·press·i·bil·i·ty
   pl re·press·i·bil·i·ties
re·press·i·ble
re·pres·sion
re·pres·sor
re·pro·duce
re·pro·duc·tion
re·pro·duc·tive
re·pro·duc·tive·ly
Rep·til·i·a
rep·til·i·an
re·pul·lu·la·tion
re·pul·sion
res·az·u·rin
res·cin·na·mine
re·search
re·sect
re·sect·a·bil·i·ty
   pl re·sect·a·bil·i·ties
re·sect·a·ble
re·sec·tion
re·sec·to·scope
re·ser·pine
re·ser·pin·i·za·tion
re·ser·pin·iz·ed
re·serve
res·er·voir
res·i·den·cy
   pl res·i·den·cies
res·i·dent
re·sid·u·al

res·i·due
re·sid·u·um
   pl re·sid·u·a
re·sil·ience
re·sil·ient
res·in
re·si·na
res·in·oid
res·in·ous
re·sis·tance
re·sis·tant
re·sis·to·my·cin
res·o·lu·tion
re·solve
re·sol·vent
res·o·nance
res·o·nant
res·o·na·tor
re·sorb
re·sorb·ent
re·sor·cin
re·sor·cin·fuch·sin
re·sor·cin·ism
re·sor·cin·ol
re·sor·cin·ol·phthal·ein
re·sorp·tion
re·sorp·tive
res·pi·ra·bil·i·ty
res·pi·ra·ble
res·pi·rat·ing
res·pi·ra·tion
res·pi·ra·tor
res·pi·ra·to·ry
re·spire
res·pi·rom·e·ter
res·pi·ro·met·ric
res·pi·rom·e·try
   pl res·pi·rom·e·tries
re·spon·dent
re·sponse
re·spon·si·bil·i·ty
rest
re·ste·no·sis
res·ti·bra·chi·um
res·ti·form
res·tis
   pl res·tes
res·ti·tu·ti·o ad in·te·grum
res·ti·tu·tion

res·to·ra·tion
re·stor·a·tive
re·store
re·strain
re·straint
re·strin·gent
re·sul·tant
re·su·pi·nate
or re·su·pi·nat·ed
re·su·pi·nat·ed
or re·su·pi·nate
re·su·pi·na·tion
res·ur·rec·tion·ism
res·ur·rec·tion·ist
re·sus·ci·tate
re·sus·ci·ta·tion
re·sus·ci·ta·tive
re·sus·ci·ta·tor
re·su·ture
re·tain·er
re·tar·date
re·tar·da·tion
re·tard·ed
re·tard·er
retch
re·te
pl re·ti·a
re·te mi·ra·bi·le
pl re·ti·a mi·ra·bi·li·a
re·ten·tion
re·ti·al
re·tic·u·lar
re·tic·u·late
or re·tic·u·lat·ed
re·tic·u·lat·ed
or re·tic·u·late
re·tic·u·la·tion
re·tic·u·lin
re·tic·u·li·tis
re·tic·u·lo·bul·bar
re·tic·u·lo·cyte
re·tic·u·lo·cyt·ic
re·tic·u·lo·cy·to·pe·ni·a
re·tic·u·lo·cy·to·sis
pl re·tic·u·lo·cy·to·ses
re·tic·u·lo·en·do·the·li·al
re·tic·u·lo·en·do·the·li·o·ma
pl re·tic·u·lo·en·do·the·li·o·
mas

or re·tic·u·lo·en·do·the·li·o·
ma·ta
re·tic·u·lo·en·do·the·li·o·sis
pl re·tic·u·lo·en·do·the·li·o·
ses
re·tic·u·lo·en·do·the·li·um
pl re·tic·u·lo·en·do·the·li·a
re·tic·u·lo·his·ti·o·cy·to·ma
re·tic·u·lo·ol·i·var·y
re·tic·u·lo·pe·ni·a
re·tic·u·lo·po·di·um
pl re·tic·u·lo·po·di·a
re·tic·u·lo·re·tic·u·lar
re·tic·u·lo·sar·co·ma
pl re·tic·u·lo·sar·co·mas
or re·tic·u·lo·sar·co·ma·ta
re·tic·u·lose
re·tic·u·lo·sis
pl re·tic·u·lo·ses
re·tic·u·lo·spi·nal
re·tic·u·lo·the·li·o·ma
pl re·tic·u·lo·the·li·o·mas
or re·tic·u·lo·the·li·o·ma·ta
re·tic·u·lo·the·li·um
re·tic·u·lum
pl re·tic·u·la
re·tif·ism
ret·i·form
ret·i·na
pl ret·i·nas
or ret·i·nae
ret·i·nac·u·lum
pl ret·i·nac·u·la
ret·i·nal
ret·ine
ret·i·nene
ret·i·ni·tis
pl ret·i·ni·ti·des
ret·i·no·blas·to·ma
pl ret·i·no·blas·to·mas
or ret·i·no·blas·to·ma·ta
ret·i·no·cho·roid·i·tis
ret·i·no·cy·to·ma
pl ret·i·no·cy·to·mas
or ret·i·no·cy·to·ma·ta
ret·i·no·di·al·y·sis
ret·i·no·ic
ret·i·noid
ret·i·nol

ret·i·no·ma·la·ci·a
ret·i·no·pap·il·li·tis
ret·i·nop·a·thy
pl ret·i·nop·a·thies
ret·i·no·pex·y
ret·i·nos·chi·sis
pl ret·i·nos·chi·ses
ret·i·no·scope
ret·i·no·scop·ic
ret·i·nos·co·py
pl ret·i·nos·co·pies
ret·i·no·sis
ret·i·no·ski·as·co·py
re·tort
ret·o·the·li·al
re·to·the·li·o·ma
pl re·to·the·li·o·mas
or re·to·the·li·o·ma·ta
re·to·the·li·o·sar·co·ma
pl re·to·the·li·o·sar·co·mas
or re·to·the·li·o·sar·co·ma·
ta
ret·o·the·li·um
re·tract
re·trac·tile
re·trac·til·i·ty
re·trac·tion
re·trac·tor
re·trad
ret·ra·hens au·rem
re·tra·hent
re·trench·ment
ret·ro·ac·tion
ret·ro·an·ter·o·am·ne·si·a
ret·ro·an·ter·o·grade
ret·ro·au·ric·u·lar
ret·ro·bul·bar
ret·ro·cae·cal
var of ret·ro·ce·cal
ret·ro·cal·ca·ne·al
ret·ro·cal·ca·ne·o·bur·si·tis
ret·ro·car·di·ac
ret·ro·ca·val
ret·ro·ce·cal
ret·ro·cede
ret·ro·cele
ret·ro·cer·vi·cal
ret·ro·ces·sion
ret·ro·chei·li·a

ret·ro·co·lic
ret·ro·col·lic
ret·ro·col·lis
ret·ro·con·dy·lism
ret·ro·cop·u·la·tion
ret·ro·cur·sive
ret·ro·de·vi·a·tion
ret·ro·dis·place·ment
re·tro·du·o·de·nal
ret·ro·e·soph·a·ge·al
ret·ro·flec·tion
   or ret·ro·flex·ion
ret·ro·flex
   or ret·ro·flexed
ret·ro·flexed
   or ret·ro·flex
ret·ro·flex·ion
   or ret·ro·flec·tion
ret·ro·gas·se·ri·an
ret·ro·gnath·i·a
ret·ro·gnath·ism
ret·ro·grade
ret·ro·grade·ly
re·trog·ra·phy
ret·ro·gres·sion
ret·ro·gres·sive
re·tro·in·gui·nal
re·tro·in·su·lar
ret·ro·ject
ret·ro·jec·tion
ret·ro·jec·tor
ret·ro·len·tal
ret·ro·len·tic·u·lar
ret·ro·lin·gual
ret·ro·ma·lar
ret·ro·mam·ma·ry
ret·ro·man·dib·u·lar
ret·ro·mas·toid
ret·ro·max·il·lar·y
ret·ro·mo·lar
ret·ro·mor·pho·sis
ret·ro·na·sal
ret·ro·oc·u·lar
ret·ro·oe·soph·a·ge·al
   var of ret·ro·e·soph·a·ge·al
ret·ro·or·bi·tal
ret·ro·pa·rot·id
ret·ro·per·i·to·ne·al
ret·ro·per·i·to·ne·al·ly

ret·ro·per·i·to·ne·um
ret·ro·per·i·to·ni·tis
ret·ro·pha·ryn·ge·al
ret·ro·phar·yn·gi·tis
ret·ro·phar·ynx
ret·ro·pla·cen·tal
ret·ro·pla·si·a
ret·ro·posed
ret·ro·po·si·tion
ret·ro·pros·tat·ic
ret·ro·pu·bic
ret·ro·pul·sion
ret·ro·py·ram·i·dal
ret·ro·spec·tion
ret·ro·spec·tive
ret·ro·stal·sis
   pl ret·ro·stal·ses
ret·ro·tar·sal
ret·ro·ten·di·nous
ret·ro·ten·do·a·chil·lis
ret·ro·thy·roid
ret·ro·ton·sil·lar
ret·ro·tra·che·al
ret·ro·u·ter·ine
ret·ro·vac·ci·na·tion
ret·ro·ver·si·o·flex·ion
ret·ro·ver·sion
ret·ro·vert·ed
ret·ro·ves·i·cal
re·trude
re·tru·sion
re·tru·sive
Ret·ter·er stain
Ret·zi·us vein
re·un·ion
re·vac·ci·nate
re·vac·ci·na·tion
re·vas·cu·lar·i·za·tion
re·vel·lent
re·ver·ber·ate
re·ver·ber·a·tion
Re·ver·din graft
rev·er·ie
   pl rev·er·ies
   or rev·er·y
re·ver·sal
re·verse
re·verse tran·scrip·tase
re·vers·i·ble

re·ver·sion
re·vert
re·ver·tant
rev·er·y
   or rev·er·ie
Re·vil·liod sign
re·vi·tal·i·za·tion
re·vive
re·viv·i·fi·ca·tion
re·viv·i·fy
rev·o·lute
re·vul·sant
re·vul·sion
re·vul·sive
Reye syn·drome
Rhab·di·tis
Rhab·di·toi·de·a
rhab·do·cyte
rhab·doid
rhab·dom
   or rhab·dome
rhab·dome
   or rhab·dom
rhab·do·mere
rhab·do·my·o·blast·ic
rhab·do·my·o·blas·to·ma
   pl rhab·do·my·o·blas·to·
     mas
   or rhab·do·my·o·blas·to·
     ma·ta
rhab·do·my·ol·y·sis
rhab·do·my·o·ma
   pl rhab·do·my·o·mas
   or rhab·do·my·o·ma·ta
rhab·do·my·o·sar·co·ma
   pl rhab·do·my·o·sar·co·mas
   or rhab·do·my·o·sar·co·ma·
     ta
rhab·do·pho·bi·a
rhab·do·sar·co·ma
rhab·do·vi·rus
rha·cous
rhae·bo·sce·li·a
   var of rhe·bo·sce·li·a
rhae·bo·sce·lic
   var of rhe·bo·sce·lic
rhag·a·des
rhag·di·a
rha·gad·i·form

342

rhag·i·o·crin
  or rhag·i·o·crine
rhag·i·o·crine
  or rhag·i·o·crin
rhag·oid
rham·ni·nose
rham·no·glu·co·side
rham·nose
rham·no·side
rham·no·xan·thin
Rham·nus
rha·phe
  or ra·phe
rha·pon·tic
rhat·a·ny
  pl rhat·a·nies
rha·thy·mi·a
rhe
rhe·a·dine
rhe·bo·sce·li·a
rhe·bo·sce·lic
rheg·ma
rheg·ma·tog·e·nous
rhe·in
rhem·bas·mus
rhe·ni·um
rhe·o·base
rhe·o·ba·sic
rhe·o·car·di·og·ra·phy
rhe·o·en·ceph·a·log·ra·phy
rhe·o·log·ic
rhe·ol·o·gist
rhe·ol·o·gy
  pl rhe·ol·o·gies
rhe·om·e·ter
rhe·om·e·try
  pl rhe·om·e·tries
rhe·o·nome
rhe·o·pex·y
rhe·o·stat
rhe·os·to·sis
rhe·o·ta·chyg·ra·phy
rhe·o·tax·is
  pl rhe·o·tax·es
rhe·o·trope
rhe·ot·ro·pism
rhes·to·cy·the·mi·a
rhe·sus mon·key
  or rhe·sus ma·ca·que

Rhe·um
rheu·mar·thri·tis
rheu·ma·tal·gi·a
rheu·mat·ic
rheu·mat·i·cal·ly
rheu·ma·tid
rheu·ma·tism
rheu·ma·toid
rheu·ma·to·log·ic
rheu·ma·tol·o·gist
rheu·ma·tol·o·gy
  pl rheu·ma·tol·o·gies
rheu·mo·cri·nol·o·gy
rhex·is
  pl rhex·es
rhi·chi·tis
  pl rhi·chi·ti·des
  or ra·chi·tis
  pl ra·chi·ti·des
rhi·go·sis
rhi·nal
rhi·nal·gi·a
rhi·nan·tral·gi·a
rhi·nel·cos
rhin·en·ce·phal·ic
  or rhin·en·ceph·a·lous
rhin·en·ceph·a·lon
  pl rhin·en·ceph·a·la
rhin·en·ceph·a·lous
  or rhin·en·ce·phal·ic
rhi·nen·chy·sis
rhi·nes·the·si·a
rhi·neu·ryn·ter
rhin·hae·ma·to·ma
  var of rhin·he·ma·to·ma
rhin·he·ma·to·ma
rhi·ni·a·try
rhin·i·on
rhi·nism
rhi·ni·tis
  pl rhi·ni·ti·des
rhi·no·an·tri·tis
rhi·no·by·on
rhi·no·can·thec·to·my
rhi·no·cele
  var of rhi·no·coele
rhi·no·ce·pha·li·a
rhi·no·ceph·a·lus
rhi·no·ceph·a·ly

rhi·no·chei·lo·plas·ty
rhi·no·clei·sis
rhi·no·cnes·mus
rhi·no·coele
rhi·no·dac·ry·o·lith
rhi·no·der·ma
rhi·no·dym·i·a
rhi·nod·y·mus
rhi·no·dyn·i·a
Rhi·noes·trus
rhi·no·gen·ic
  or rhi·nog·e·nous
rhi·nog·e·nous
  or rhi·no·gen·ic
rhi·no·ky·pho·sis
rhi·no·la·li·a
rhi·no·lar·yn·gi·tis
rhi·no·lar·yn·gol·o·gy
  pl rhi·no·lar·yn·gol·o·gies
rhi·no·lar·yn·go·scope
rhi·no·lite
rhi·no·lith
rhi·no·li·thi·a·sis
rhi·no·lith·ic
rhi·no·log·ic
  or rhi·no·log·i·cal
rhi·no·log·i·cal
  or rhi·no·log·ic
rhi·nol·o·gist
rhi·nol·o·gy
  pl rhi·nol·o·gies
rhi·no·ma·nom·e·ter
rhi·nom·e·ter
rhi·no·mi·o·sis
rhi·nom·mec·to·my
rhi·no·my·co·sis
rhi·no·ne·cro·sis
rhi·nop·a·thy
rhi·no·pha·ryn·ge·al
rhi·no·phar·yn·gi·tis
  pl rhi·no·phar·yn·gi·ti·des
rhi·no·pha·ryn·go·lith
rhi·no·phar·ynx
  pl rhi·no·phar·ynx·es
  or rhi·no·pha·ryn·ges
rhi·no·pho·ni·a
rhi·no·phore
rhi·no·phy·co·my·co·sis

rhi·no·phy·ma
   pl rhi·no·phy·mas
   or rhi·no·phy·ma·ta
rhi·no·plas·tic
rhi·no·plas·ty
   pl rhi·no·plas·ties
rhi·no·pol·yp
rhi·no·pol·y·pus
rhi·nop·si·a
rhi·nor·rha·gi·a
rhi·nor·rha·phy
rhi·nor·rhe·a
rhi·nor·rhoe·a
   var of rhi·nor·rhe·a
rhi·no·sal·pin·gi·tis
rhi·nos·chi·sis
rhi·no·scle·ro·ma
   pl rhi·no·scle·ro·ma·ta
rhi·no·scope
rhi·no·scop·ic
rhi·nos·co·py
   pl rhi·nos·co·pies
rhi·no·si·nu·si·tis
rhi·no·si·nus·o·path·i·a
rhi·no·spo·rid·i·o·sis
   pl rhi·no·spo·rid·i·o·ses
Rhi·no·spo·rid·i·um
   pl Rhi·no·spo·rid·i·a
rhi·no·ste·no·sis
rhi·no·thrix
rhi·not·o·my
rhi·no·vi·rus
Rhi·pi·ceph·a·lus
rhip·tas·mus
rhi·ti·do·sis
   var of rhyt·i·do·sis
Rhi·zo·bi·um
   pl Rhi·zo·bi·a
Rhi·zog·ly·phus
rhi·zoid
rhi·zome
rhi·zo·mel·ic
rhi·zo·me·nin·go·my·e·li·
   tis
rhi·zo·mor·phoid
rhi·zo·neure
rhi·zo·nych·i·a
rhi·zo·nych·i·um
rhi·zo·pod

Rhi·zop·o·da
rhi·zop·ter·in
Rhi·zo·pus
rhi·zot·o·my
   pl rhi·zot·o·mies
Rh-neg·a·tive
rho·da·mine
rho·da·nate
rho·da·nese
rho·dan·ic
Rho·din fix·a·tive
rho·di·um
Rhod·ni·us
rho·do·gen·e·sis
rho·do·phy·lac·tic
rho·do·phy·lax·is
rho·dop·sin
rhoe·a·dine
   var of rhe·a·dine
rhoeb·de·sis
rhom·ben·ce·phal·ic
rhom·ben·ceph·a·lon
   pl rhom·ben·ceph·a·la
rhom·bic
rhom·bo·coele
rhom·boid
rhom·boi·dal
rhom·boi·de·su
   pl rhom·boi·de·i
rhom·bo·mere
rhon·chal
rhon·chi·al
rhon·chus
   pl rhon·chi
rho·phe·o·cy·to·sis
rho·ta·cism
   or rho·ta·cis·mus
   or ro·ta·cism
rho·ta·cis·mus
   or rho·ta·cism
   or ro·ta·cism
Rh-pos·i·tive
rhu·barb
rhus
   pl Rhus·es
   or rhus
Rhus gla·bra
rhy·poph·a·gy
rhy·po·pho·bi·a

rhy·se·ma
rhythm
rhyth·mic
   or rhyth·mi·cal
rhyth·mi·cal
   or rhyth·mic
rhyth·mi·cal·ly
rhyth·mic·i·ty
   pl rhyth·mic·i·ties
rhyt·i·dec·tom·y
rhyt·i·do·plas·ty
   pl rhyt·i·do·plas·ties
rhyt·i·do·sis
rib
ri·bam·in·ol
rib·bon
ri·bi·tol
ri·bo·des·ose
ri·bo·fla·vin
ri·bo·nu·cle·ase
ri·bo·nu·cle·ic
ri·bo·nu·cle·o·pro·te·in
ri·bo·nu·cle·o·side
ri·bo·nu·cle·o·tide
ri·bo·prine
ri·bose
ri·bo·side
ri·bo·som·al
ri·bo·some
ri·bo·syl
ri·bu·lose
Ric·co law
rice
Rich·ter her·ni·a
ri·cin
ric·i·nine
ric·in·ism
ric·in·o·le·ate
ric·in·o·le·ic
ric·in·o·le·in
Ric·i·nus
rick·ets
Rick·etts or·gan·ism
rick·ett·si·a
   pl rick·ett·si·as
   or rick·ett·si·ae
Rick·ett·si·a·ce·ae
rick·ett·si·al
rick·ett·si·al·pox

rick·ett·si·ci·dal
rick·ett·si·o·sis
    pl rick·ett·si·o·ses
rick·ett·si·o·stat·ic
rick·e·ty
Ri·cord meth·od
ric·tal
ric·tus
    pl ric·tus·es
    or ric·tus
Rid·doch syn·drome
Rid·e·al-Walk·er meth·od
ri·deau
ridge
ridge·ling
    or ridg·ling
ridg·ling
    or ridge·ling
Rie·del dis·ease
Rie·gel test
Rie·ger a·nom·a·ly
Riehl mel·a·no·sis
Ries-Clark op·er·a·tion
Ries·man sign
Rieux her·ni·a
rif·a·mide
ri·fam·pi·cin
rif·am·pin
ri·fa·my·cin
R̶ ̶a dis·ease
Ri·ga-F de dis·ease
Riggs and Sta·die meth·
    od
right-eyed
right-foot·ed
right-hand
right-hand·ed
rig·id
ri·gid·i·tas
ri·gid·i·ty
    pl ri·gid·i·ties
rig·or
rig·or mor·tis
Ri·ley-Day syn·drome
ri·ma
    pl ri·mae
ri·ma glot·ti·dis
ri·man·ta·dine

ri·mose
    or ri·mous
ri·mous
    or ri·mose
rim·u·la
    pl rim·u·lae
rin·der·pest
Rine·hart and A·bul-
    Haj stain
ring
ring·bin·den
ring·bone
ring·boned
Ring·er so·lu·tion
ring·hals
ring·schwie·le
ring·worm
Rin·ne test
ri·no·lite
Ri·o·lan arc
ri·par·i·an
Ris·ley prism
ri·so·ri·us
    pl ri·so·ri·i
ris·to·ce·tin
ri·sus
ri·sus sar·don·i·cus
Rit·gen ma·neu·ver
Rit·ter dis·ease
Rit·ter-Val·li law
rit·u·al
ri·val·ry
Ri·val·ta test
Ri·vi·nus ducts
ri·vus
    pl ri·vi
riz·i·form
RNA·ase
    or RNase
RNase
    or RNA·ase
roar·ing
Rob·ert pel·vis
Rob·erts test
Rob·in·son dis·ease
Rob·in·son-Kep·ler-
    Pow·er test
rob·o·rant
Ro·chelle salt

Rock·ley sign
Rocky Moun·tain spot·ted
    fe·ver
rod
Ro·den·ti·a
ro·den·ti·cide
Rod·man in·ci·sion
rod·mon·o·chro·mat
ro·do·nal·gi·a
rods of Gor·ti
Roe·der·er o·bliq·ui·ty
Roe-Kahn meth·od
Roen·ne na·sal step
roent·gen
roent·gen·i·za·tion
roent·gen·ize
roent·gen·ky·mo·gram
roent·gen·ky·mo·graph
roent·gen·ky·mo·graph·ic
roent·gen·ky·mog·ra·phy
    pl roent·gen·ky·mog·ra·
    phies
roent·gen·o·der·ma
roent·gen·o·gram
roent·gen·o·graph
roent·gen·o·graph·ic
roent·gen·o·graph·i·cal·ly
roent·gen·og·ra·phy
    pl roent·gen·og·ra·phies
roent·gen·o·ky·mo·gram
roent·gen·o·ky·mog·ra·phy
roent·gen·o·log·ic
    or roent·gen·o·log·i·cal
roent·gen·o·log·i·cal
    or roent·gen·o·log·i·cal
roent·gen·o·log·i·cal·ly
roent·gen·ol·o·gist
roent·gen·ol·o·gy
    pl roent·gen·ol·o·gies
roent·gen·o·lu·cent
roent·gen·om·e·ter
roent·gen·om·e·try
    pl roent·gen·om·e·tries
roent·gen·o·scope
roent·gen·o·scop·ic
roent·gen·o·scop·i·cal·ly
roent·ge·nos·co·py
    pl roent·ge·nos·co·pies

roent·gen·o·ther·a·py
  pl roent·gen·o·ther·a·pies
roent·gen·ther·a·py
  pl roent·gen·ther·a·pies
roe·then
ro·flu·rane
Ro·ger dis·ease
Ro·gers re·flex
Rohr stri·a
Ro·ki·tan·sky-
  Asch·off si·nus·es
Ro·ki·tan·sky dis·ease
ro·lan·dic
Ro·lan·do ar·e·a
ro·let·a·mide
ro·li·cy·prine
ro·li·tet·ra·cy·cline
roll·er
Rol·ler nu·cle·us
Roll·e·ston rule
Rol·let cell
Rol·lett dis·ease
Rol·lier meth·od
ro·lo·dine
Ro·ma·na sign
ro·man·o·scope
Ro·ma·nov·sky stains
Rom·berg sign
rom·berg·ism
Ro·mieu re·ac·tion
ron·geur
ro·ni·da·zole
Roñ·ne na·sal step
ron·nel
root
Ror·schach test
ro·sa·ce·a
ro·sa·ce·i·form
ro·sa·li·a
ro·san·i·line
ro·sa·ry
rose ben·gal
Rose op·er·a·tion
ro·se·in
ro·sel·la
Ro·sen·bach dis·ease
Ro·sen·muel·ler fos·sa
Ro·sen·thal ca·nal
ro·se·o·la

ro·se·o·la in·fan·tum
ro·se·o·lous
Ro·ser sign
Ro·ser-Braun sign
ro·sette
ros·in
ro·so·lic
Ross bod·ies
Ross-Jones test
Ross·bach dis·ease
Ross·man flu·id
Ros·so·li·mo re·flex
Ros·tan asth·ma
ros·tel·lar
ros·tel·late
ros·tel·lum
ros·trad
ros·tral
ros·tral·most
ros·trate
ros·trum
  pl ros·trums
  or ros·tra
rot
ro·ta·cism
  or rho·ta·cism
  or rho·ta·cis·mus
ro·tam·e·ter
ro·ta·ry
ro·tate
ro·ta·tion
ro·ta·tor
  pl ro·ta·tors
  or ro·ta·to·res
ro·ta·to·ri·a
ro·ta·to·ry
Rotch sign
ro·te·none
Roth dis·ease
Roth-Bern·hardt dis·ease
Roth·er·a test
Roth-Kva·le test
Roth·mund syn·drome
Roth·mund-
  Thom·son syn·drome
Ro·tor syn·drome
ro·tox·a·mine
Rot·ter test
rott·ler·a

rot·u·lar
Rou·get cell
rough·age
Rough·ton-
  Scho·lan·der meth·od
Roug·non-
  Heb·er·den dis·ease
rou·leau
  pl rou·leaus
  or rou·leaux
round-shoul·der·ed
round·worm
roup
Rous sar·co·ma
Rous·sy-
  De·je·rine syn·drome
Rous·sy-Le·vy dis·ease
Roux en Y by·pass
Roux op·er·a·tion
Roux-Y by·pass
Rov·sing sign
Rowe di·ets
Rown·tree-Ger·agh·ty test
Ru·barth dis·ease
rub·ber-dam
ru·be·an·ic
ru·be·do
ru·be·fa·cient
ru·be·fac·tion
ru·bel·la
ru·bel·li·form
ru·be·o·la
ru·be·o·lar
ru·be·o·sis
ru·ber
ru·bes·cence
ru·bes·cent
ru·bid·i·um
ru·big·i·nous
ru·bi·jer·vine
Ru·bin·stein-
  Tay·bi syn·drome
Ru·bin test
Rub·ner test
ru·bor
ru·bres·er·ine
ru·bri·blast
ru·bric
ru·bri·cyte

ru·bri·u·ri·a
ru·bro·bul·bar
ru·bro·ol·i·var·y
ru·bro·re·tic·u·lar
ru·bro·spi·nal
ru·bro·sta·sis
ru·bro·tha·lam·ic
ru·brum scar·la·ti·num
Ru·bus
ruc·ta·tion
ruc·tus
Rud syn·drome
ru·di·ment
ru·di·men·ta·ry
ru·di·men·tum
   pl ru·di·men·ta
rue
Ruf·fi·ni cell
ru·fous
ru·ga
   pl ru·gae
ru·gal
ru·gi·tus
ru·gose

ru·gose·ly
ru·gos·i·ty
   pl ru·gos·i·ties
ru·gous
Ruhm·korff coil
rule
rum·ba·tron
ru·men
   pl ru·mens,
   or ru·mi·na
ru·men·i·tis
ru·me·not·o·my
   pl ru·me·not·o·mies
Ru·mex
ru·mi·nant
ru·mi·nate
ru·mi·na·tion
ru·mi·na·tive
Rum·mo dis·ease
rump
Rum·pel-Leede
   phe·nom·e·non
run

Ru·otte op·er·a·tion
ru·pi·a
ru·pi·al
ru·po·pho·bi·a
rup·ti·o
rup·ture
Rus·sel meth·od, vi·per
rust
Rust dis·ease
rut
Ru·ta·ce·ae
ru·ta·my·cin
Rut·gers 612
Ruth meth·od
ru·the·ni·um
ruth·er·ford
Ruth·er·ford-
   Bohr a·tom mod·el
ru·tin
ru·tin·ose
Ry·a·ni·a
ry·an·o·dine
Ryd·y·gier op·er·a·tion

S

sab·a·dil·la
sa·bad·i·nine
sa·bal
Sab·a·ne·ev-
   Frank op·er·a·tion
Sa·be·thes
Sab·e·thi·ni
Sa·bin vac·cine
Sa·bin-Feld·man dye test
Sa·bou·raud a·gar
sab·u·line
   or sab·u·lous
   or sab·u·lose

sab·u·lose
   or sab·u·lous
   or sab·u·line
sab·u·lous
   or sab·u·lose
   or sab·u·line
sa·bur·ra
sa·bur·ral
sac
sac·cade
sac·cad·ic
sac·cate
sac·cha·rase

sac·cha·rate
sac·cha·rat·ed
sac·char·eph·i·dro·sis
sac·char·ic
sac·cha·ride
sac·cha·rif·er·ous
sac·char·i·fi·ca·tion
sac·char·i·fy
sac·cha·rim·e·ter
sac·cha·ri·met·ric
   or sac·cha·ri·met·ri·cal
sac·cha·ri·met·ri·cal
   or sac·cha·ri·met·ric

sac·cha·rim·e·try
sac·cha·rin
sac·cha·rine
sac·cha·rin·i·ty
   pl sac·cha·rin·i·ties
sac·cha·ro·bi·ose
sac·cha·ro·ga·lac·tor·rhe·a
sac·cha·ro·ga·lac·tor·rhoe·a
   var of sac·cha·ro·ga·lac·tor·
    rhe·a
sac·cha·ro·lyt·ic
sac·cha·ro·met·a·bol·ic
sac·cha·ro·me·tab·o·lism
sac·cha·rom·e·ter
sac·cha·ro·met·ric
sac·cha·rom·e·try
   pl sac·cha·rom·e·tries
Sac·cha·ro·my·ces
Sac·cha·ro·my·ce·ta·ce·ae
sac·cha·ro·my·ce·ta·ceous
sac·cha·ro·my·ce·ta·les
sac·cha·ro·my·cete
sac·cha·ro·my·ce·tic
sac·cha·ro·my·co·sis
sac·char·o·pine
sac·cha·ro·pi·nu·ri·a
sac·cha·ror·rhe·a
sac·cha·ror·rhoe·a
   var of sac·cha·ror·rhe·a
sac·cha·rose
sac·cha·ro·su·ri·a
sac·cha·rum
sac·ci·form
sac·cu·lar
sac·cu·late
sac·cu·lat·ed
sac·cu·la·tion
sac·cule
sac·cu·li
sac·cu·lo·coch·le·ar
sac·cu·lus
   pl sac·cu·li
sac·cus
   pl sac·ci
Sachs dis·ease
Sachs-Geor·gi test
sa·crad
sa·cral
sa·cral·gi·a

sa·cral·i·za·tion
sa·cral·ize
sa·crec·to·my
   pl sac·crec·to·mies
sa·cro·an·te·ri·or
sa·cro·coc·cyg·e·al
sa·cro·coc·cyg·e·us
sa·cro·cox·al·gi·a
sa·cro·cox·i·tis
sa·cro·dyn·i·a
sa·cro·gen·i·tal
sa·cro·il·i·ac
sa·cro·lum·ba·lis
sa·cro·lum·bar
sa·cro·per·i·ne·al
sa·cro·pos·te·ri·or
sa·cro·pu·bic
sa·cro·sci·at·ic
sa·cro·spi·na·lis
sa·cro·spi·nous
sa·cro·tu·ber·ous
sa·cro·u·ter·ine
sa·cro·ver·te·bral
sa·crum
   pl sa·cra
sac·to·sal·pinx
sad·dle
sad·dle·back
sad·dle·nose
sa·dism
sa·dist
sa·dis·tic
sa·dis·ti·cal·ly
sa·do·mas·o·chism
sa·do·mas·o·chist
sa·do·mas·o·chis·tic
Saen·ger op·er·a·tion
saf·fron
saf·ra·nine
saf·ra·no·phil
saf·role
sa·fu
sage
sage·brush
sa·git·ta
sag·it·tal
sag·it·tal·ly
Sa·gnac rays
sa·go

sag·u·lum
Sah·li meth·od
Sah·yun meth·od
Sai·mir·i
Saint Ag·a·tha di·sease
Saint Ag·nan dis·ease
Saint Am·an dis·ease
Saint An·tho·ny dance,
   fire
Saint A·ver·tin dis·ease
Saint Blaize dis·ease
St. Clair meth·od
Saint E·ras·mus dis·ease
Saint Fi·a·cre dis·ease
Saint Ger·va·si·us dis·ease
Saint Giles dis·ease
Saint Goth·ard dis·ease
Saint Guy dance
Saint Ig·na·ti·us itch
Saint Lou·is en·ceph·a·li·
   tis
Saint Main e·vil
Saint Mar·tin dis·ease
Saint Roch dis·ease
Saint Sa·bas·ti·an dis·ease
Saint Val·en·tine dis·ease
Saint Vi·tus dance
Saint Zach·a·ry dis·ease
Sak·el meth·od
sal
sal vol·a·tile
sa·laam
sa·la·cious
sa·lac·i·ty
sal·ep
sal·eth·a·mide
sal·i·cin
sal·i·cyl
sal·i·cyl·al·de·hyde
sal·i·cyl·am·ide
sal·i·cyl·an·i·lide
sa·lic·y·late
sa·lic·y·lat·ed
sal·i·cyl·a·zo·sul·fa·pyr·i·
   dine
sal·i·cyl·ic
sal·i·cyl·ism
sal·i·cyl·i·za·tion
sal·i·cyl·ize

sal·i·cyl·u·ric ac·id
sa·lic·y·lyl
sa·li·ent
sal·i·fi·a·ble
sal·i·fi·ca·tion
sal·i·fy
sal·i·gen·in
sal·i·jen·in
sa·lim·e·ter
sa·line
sa·li·nom·e·ter
sa·li·va
sal·i·vant
sal·i·var·y
sal·i·vate
sal·i·va·tion
sal·i·va·tor
sal·i·va·to·ry
sal·i·vo·li·thi·a·sis
sa·li·vous
Salk vac·cine
sal·mine
sal·mone
Sal·mo·nel·la
    pl sal·mo·nel·las
    or sal·mo·nel·lae
    or sal·mo·nel·la
Sal·mo·nel·le·ae
sal·mo·nel·lo·sis
    pl sal·mo·nel·lo·ses
sal·ol
sal·pin·ge·al
sal·pin·gec·to·my
sal·pin·gem·phrax·is
sal·pin·gi·an
sal·pin·git·ic
sal·pin·gi·tis
sal·pin·go·cath·e·ter·ism
sal·pin·go·cele
sal·pin·go·cy·e·sis
    pl sal·pin·go·cy·e·ses
sal·pin·go·gram
sal·pin·gog·ra·phy
sal·pin·gol·y·sis
sal·pin·go·o·o·pho·rec·
    to·my
sal·pin·go·o·o·pho·ri·tis
sal·pin·go·o·oph·o·ro·cele

sal·pin·go·o·o·the·
    cec·to·my
sal·pin·go·o·o·the·ci·tis
sal·pin·go·o·o·the·co·cele
sal·pin·go·o·var·i·ec·to·my
sal·pin·go·o·var·i·ot·o·my
sal·pin·go·o·va·ri·tis
sal·pin·go·pal·a·tine
sal·pin·go·per·i·to·ni·tis
sal·pin·go·pex·y
    pl sal·pin·go·pex·ies
sal·pin·go·pha·ryn·ge·al
sal·pin·go·pha·ryn·ge·us
sal·pin·go·plas·ty
    pl sal·pin·go·plas·ties
sal·pin·gor·rha·phy
sal·pin·go·sal·pin·gos·to·
    my
sal·pin·go·scope
sal·pin·go·sten·o·cho·ri·a
sal·pin·go·sto·mat·o·my
sal·pin·gos·to·my
    pl sal·pin·gos·to·mies
sal·pin·go·the·cal
sal·pin·got·o·my
sal·pin·gys·ter·o·cy·e·sis
    pl sal·pin·gys·ter·o·cy·e·ses
sal·pinx
    pl sal·pin·ges
salt
sal·ta·tion
sal·ta·to·ric
sal·ta·to·ry
Sal·ter lines
salt·pe·ter
salt·pe·tre
    var of salt·pe·ter
salt-sen·si·tive
sa·lu·bri·ous
sa·lu·bri·ous·ly
sa·lu·bri·ty
    pl sa·lu·bri·ties
sal·u·ret·ic
sal·u·ret·i·cal·ly
sal·u·tar·i·ly
sal·u·tar·y
sal·vage
salve
sal·vi·a

Salz·mann no·du·lar cor·
    ne·al dys·tro·phy
sa·mar·i·um
sam·bu·cus
sam·ple
Samp·son cysts
San Joa·quin Val·ley fe·ver
San·a·rel·li vi·rus
san·a·tar·i·um
    pl san·a·tar·i·ums
    or san·a·tar·i·a
san·a·tive
san·a·to·ri·um
    pl san·a·to·ri·ums
    or san·a·to·ri·a
san·a·to·ry
sand crack
san·da·rac
sand-blind
sand·fly fe·ver
San·der dis·ease
San·ders sign
San·ders-Ho·gan dis·ease
Sand·hoff dis·ease
sane
San·fi·lip·po syn·drome
san·guic·o·lous
san·guif·er·ous
san·gui·fi·ca·tion
san·gui·nar·i·a
san·guin·a·rine
san·gui·nar·y
san·guine
san·guine·ly
san·guin·e·ous
san·guin·o·lent
san·gui·no·pu·ru·lent
san·gui·no·se·rous
san·gui·nous
san·guis
san·gui·suc·tion
san·gui·su·ga
san·guiv·o·rous
san·i·cle
sa·ni·es
    pl sa·ni·es
sa·ni·ous
san·i·tar·i·an

349

san·i·tar·i·ly
san·i·ta·ri·um
   pl san·i·ta·ri·ums
   or san·i·ta·ri·a
san·i·tar·y
san·i·tate
san·i·ta·tion
san·i·ta·tion·ist
san·i·ti·za·tion
san·i·tize
san·i·to·ri·um
   pl san·i·to·ri·ums
   or san·i·to·ri·a
san·i·ty
   pl san·i·ties
San·som sign
san·ton·i·ca
san·to·nin
san·to·nism
San·to·ri·ni car·ti·lag·es
sap
sa·phe·na
sa·phe·no·fem·o·ral
sa·phe·nous
sap·id
sa·po
sap·o·gen·in
sap·o·na·ceous
Sap·o·nar·i·a
sap·o·nat·ed
sa·pon·i·fi·a·ble
sa·pon·i·fi·ca·tion
sa·pon·i·fi·er
sa·pon·i·form
sa·pon·i·fy
sap·o·nin
sa·po·ta
sap·o·tox·in
sap·pan·wood
Sap·pey mus·cle
sap·phic
sap·phism
sa·prae·mi·a
   var of sa·pre·mi·a
sa·pre·mi·a
sa·pre·mic
sap·rine
sap·ro·gen
sap·ro·gen·ic

sap·ro·ge·nic·i·ty
   pl sap·ro·ge·nic·i·ties
sa·prog·e·nous
sa·proph·a·gous
sap·ro·phile
   or sa·proph·i·lous
sa·proph·i·lous
   or sap·ro·phile
sap·ro·phyte
sap·ro·phyt·ic
sap·ro·phyt·i·cal·ly
sap·ro·zo·ic
sar·a·pus
Sar·ci·na
   pl Sar·ci·nas
   or Sar·ci·nae
sar·ci·tis
sar·co·ad·e·no·ma
   pl sar·co·ad·e·no·mas
   or sar·co·ad·e·no·ma·ta
sar·co·bi·ont
sar·co·blast
sar·co·car·ci·no·ma
   pl sar·co·car·ci·no·mas
   or sar·co·car·ci·no·ma·ta
sar·co·cele
Sar·co·cys·tis
   pl Sar·co·cys·tis
   or Sar·co·cys·tis·es
sar·code
Sar·co·di·na
sar·co·din·i·an
sar·co·en·do·the·li·o·ma
   pl sar·co·en·do·the·li·o·mas
   or sar·co·en·do·the·li·o·
     ma·ta
sar·co·fe·tal
sar·co·gen·ic
sar·cog·li·a
sar·co·hy·dro·cele
sar·co·hys·ter·ic
sar·coid
sar·coid·o·sis
   pl sar·coid·o·ses
sar·co·lac·tic
sar·co·lem·ma
sar·co·lem·mal
sar·co·lem·mic
sar·co·lem·mous

sar·co·leu·kae·mi·a
   var of sar·co·leu·ke·mi·a
sar·co·leu·ke·mi·a
sar·co·ly·sin
sar·col·y·sis
   pl sar·col·y·ses
sar·co·ma
   pl sar·co·mas
   or sar·co·ma·ta
sar·co·ma·gen·ic
sar·co·ma·toid
sar·co·ma·to·sis
   pl sar·co·ma·to·ses
sar·co·ma·tous
sar·co·mere
sar·co·mer·ic
sar·co·mes·o·the·li·o·ma
   pl sar·co·mes·o·the·li·o·mas
   or sar·co·mes·o·the·li·o·
     ma·ta
sar·co·my·ces
Sar·co·phag·i·dae
sar·co·plasm
sar·co·plas·ma
   pl sar·co·plas·ma·ta
sar·co·plas·mat·ic
sar·co·plas·mic
sar·co·plast
sar·co·poi·e·sis
sar·co·poi·et·ic
Sar·cop·tes
sar·cop·tic
Sar·cop·ti·dae
sar·cop·toid
Sar·cop·toi·de·a
sar·co·sine
sar·co·si·ne·mi·a
sar·co·sis
sar·co·som·al
sar·co·some
Sar·co·spo·rid·i·a
sar·co·spo·rid·i·o·sis
   pl sar·co·spo·rid·i·o·ses
sar·co·style
sar·co·thal·sis
sar·co·tu·bule
sar·cous
sar·don·ic
sa·rin

sar·men·to·cy·ma·rin
sar·men·tog·e·nin
sar·men·tose
sar·sap·a·ril·la
sar·sa·sap·o·gen·in
sar·sa·sap·o·nin
sar·to·ri·us
   pl sar·to·ri·i
sas·sa·fras
sa·tan·o·pho·bia
sat·el·lite
sat·el·li·to·sis
   pl sat·el·li·to·ses
sa·ti·ate
sa·ti·a·tion
sa·ti·e·ty
   pl sa·ti·e·ties
Sat·ter·thwaite meth·od
sat·u·rate
sat·u·ra·tion
sat·ur·nine
sat·urn·ism
sat·y·ri·a·sis
   pl sat·y·ri·a·ses
sat·y·ro·ma·ni·a
sau·cer·i·za·tion
sau·cer·ize
sau·na
Saun·ders dis·ease
sau·ri·a·sis
sau·ri·o·sis
sau·rop·sid
Sau·rop·si·da
sau·rop·si·dan
sau·rox·ine
sau·ru·rine
sau·sa·rism
Sau·vi·neau oph·thal·mo·
   ple·gi·a
sav·in
Sa·vi·no test
saw
Sa·wah itch
sax·i·tox·in
scab
scab·by
sac·bet·ic
   or sca·bi·et·ic
scab·i·ci·dal

sca·bi·cide
   or sca·bi·et·i·cide
sca·bies
   pl sca·bies
sca·bi·et·ic
   or sca·bet·ic
sca·bi·et·i·cide
   or sca·bi·cide
sca·bi·o·pho·bia
sca·bi·ous
sca·bri·ti·es
sca·la
   pl sca·lae
sca·la me·di·a
   pl sca·lae me·di·ae
sca·la tym·pa·ni
   pl sca·lae tym·pa·no·rum
sca·la ves·tib·u·li
   pl sca·lae ves·tib·u·lo·rum
scald
scale
sca·lene
sca·le·nec·to·my
   pl sca·le·nec·to·mies
sca·le·not·o·my
   pl sca·le·not·o·mies
sca·le·nus
   pl sca·le·ni
scal·er
scal·ing
sca·lo·gram
scal·pel
scal·pri·form
scal·prum
   pl scal·pra
scal·y
scam·mo·ny
   pl scam·mo·nies
scan
scan·di·um
scan·ning e·lec·tron mi·
   cro·scope
scan·so·ri·us
Scan·zo·ni ma·neu·ver
sca·pha
scaph·o·ce·phal·ic
scaph·o·ceph·a·lism

scaph·o·ceph·a·lous
scaph·o·ceph·a·ly
   pl scaph·o·ceph·a·lies
scaph·oid
scaph·oid·i·tis
scap·u·la
   pl scap·u·las
   or scap·u·lae
scap·u·lal·gi·a
scap·u·lar
scap·u·lar·y
   pl scap·u·lar·ies
scap·u·lec·to·my
scap·u·lo·cla·vic·u·lar·is
scap·u·lo·cos·tal
scap·u·lo·hu·mer·al
scap·u·lo·per·i·os·te·al
scap·u·lo·pex·y
sca·pus
   pl sca·pi
scar
scar·a·bi·a·sis
scarf·skin
scar·i·fi·ca·tion
scar·i·fi·ca·tor
scar·i·fi·er
scar·i·fy
scar·la·ti·na
scar·la·ti·nal
scar·la·ti·nel·la
scar·la·ti·ni·form
scar·la·ti·no·gen·ic
scar·la·ti·noid
scar·la·ti·nous
scar·let
Scar·pa fas·ci·a
scat·a·cra·ti·a
sca·te·mi·a
scat·ol
scat·ole
   var of skat·ole
scat·o·lo·gi·a
scat·o·log·ic
   or scat·o·log·i·cal
scat·o·log·i·cal
   or scat·o·log·ic
sca·tol·o·gy
   pl sca·tol·o·gies

sca·to·ma
  pl sca·to·mas
  or sca·to·ma·ta
sca·toph·a·gous
sca·toph·a·gy
  pl sca·toph·a·gies
scat·o·pho·bi·a
sca·tos·co·py
scat·ter
scat·u·la
  pl scat·u·lae
scav·eng·er
scav·eng·ing
Scha·fer meth·od
Schä·fer syn·drome
Schä·fer re·flex
Schales and Schales
  meth·od
Scham·berg dis·ease
Schanz syn·drome
Schar·lach R stain
Schat·ski ring
Schau·dinn fix·ing flu·id
Schau·mann bod·ies
Schau·ta-Wert·heim
  op·er·a·tion
Sche·de meth·od
sched·ule
Scheib·ler re·a·gent
Scheie syn·drome
Schell·ong-
  Stri·sow·er phe·nom·e·
  non
sche·ma
  pl sche·ma·ta
sche·mat·ic
sche·mat·o·gram
sche·mat·o·graph
sche·mo·graph
Schenck dis·ease
Scher·er test
sche·ro·ma
Scheu·er·mann dis·ease
Schick test
Schiff re·a·gent
Schiff-
  Sher·ring·ton phe·nom·
  e·non

Schil·der-Ad·di·son
  com·plex
Schil·ler test
Schil·ling test
Schim·mel·busch dis·ease
schin·dy·le·sis
  pl schin·dy·le·ses
Schir·mer test
schir·rhus
  pl schir·rhus·es
  var of scir·rhus
schis·ten·ceph·al·y
schis·to·ce·li·a
schis·to·ce·phal·ic
schis·to·ceph·a·lus
schis·to·cor·mus
schis·to·cyte
schis·to·cys·tis
schis·to·cyte
schis·to·cy·to·sis
  pl schis·to·cy·to·sis·es
  or schis·to·cy·to·ses
schis·to·glos·si·a
schis·tom·e·lus
  pl schis·tom·e·li
schis·tom·e·ter
schis·to·pro·so·pi·a
schis·to·pros·o·pus
schis·to·pros·o·py
schis·tor·ra·chis
  or schis·tor·rha·chis
schis·tor·rha·chis
  or schis·tor·ra·chis
schis·to·sis
  pl schis·to·ses
Schis·to·so·ma
schis·to·so·mal
schis·to·some
schis·to·so·mi·a·sis
  pl schis·to·so·mi·a·ses
schis·to·so·mi·a·sis ja·pon·
  i·ca
shis·to·so·mi·a·sis man·so·
  ni
Schis·to·so·moph·o·ra
schis·to·so·mus
schis·to·ster·ni·a
schis·to·tho·rax
schis·to·tra·che·lus

schiz·am·ni·on
schiz·ax·on
schiz·en·ceph·a·ly
schiz·o·af·fec·tive
schiz·o·ble·phar·i·a
schiz·o·cyte
schiz·o·cy·to·sis
schiz·o·gen·e·sis
schiz·o·ge·net·ic
  or schiz·o·gen·ic
schiz·o·ge·net·i·cal·ly
schiz·o·gen·ic
  or schiz·o·ge·net·ic
schi·zog·e·nous
schi·zog·e·nous·ly
schi·z·o·gnath·ism
schiz·o·gnath·ous
schiz·o·gon·ic
  or schi·zog·o·nous
schi·zog·o·nous
  or schiz·o·gon·ic
schi·zog·o·ny
  pl schi·zog·o·nies
schiz·o·gy·ri·a
schiz·oid
schiz·oid·man·ic
  or schiz·o·man·ic
schiz·o·ma·ni·a
schiz·o·man·ic
  or schiz·oid·man·ic
schiz·o·my·cete
Schiz·o·my·ce·tes
schiz·o·my·cet·ic
schiz·o·my·ce·tous
schiz·ont
schi·zon·ti·ci·dal
schi·zon·ti·cide
schiz·o·nych·i·a
schiz·o·pha·si·a
schiz·o·phre·ni·a
schiz·o·phre·nic
schiz·o·phre·nic·al·ly
schiz·o·so·ma si·re·noi·des
schiz·o·the·mi·a
schiz·o·tho·rax
schiz·o·thy·mi·a
schiz·o·thy·mic
  or schiz·o·thy·mous

352

schiz·o·thy·mous
    or schiz·o·thy·mic
schiz·o·try·pan·o·so·mi·a·
    sis
Schiz·o·tryp·a·num
schiz·o·type
Schla·er test
Schlange sign
Schlat·ter dis·ease
Schlemm ca·nal
Schle·sin·ger sign
Schlof·fer op·er·a·tion
Schlös·ser treat·ment
Schmidt test
Schmin·cke tu·mor
Schmitz ba·cil·lus
Schmorl grooves
Schmutz py·or·rhe·a
Schna·bel at·ro·phy
Schnei·der meth·od
Schnei·de·ri·an mem·
    brane
Schoen·bein test
Schoen·hei·mer and Sper·
    ry meth·od
Scholz dis·ease
Scholz-Biel·schow·sky-
    Hen·ne·berg dis·ease
Schön·lein dis·ease
Schott·mül·er dis·ease
Schre·ger-Hun·ter bands
Schrid·de can·cer hairs
Schroe·der meth·od
Schüff·ner dots
Schul·ler-Chris·tian
    syn·drome
Schultz syn·drome
Schultz-
    Charl·ton blanch·ing
    test
Schultz-Dale test
Schult·ze meth·od
Schwa·bach test
Schwal·be nu·cle·us
Schwann cell, sheath
Schwann·i·an
schwan·no·gli·o·ma
    pl schwan·no·gli·o·mas
    or schwan·no·gli·o·ma·ta

schwan·no·ma
    pl schwan·no·mas
    or schwan·no·ma·ta
schwan·no·sar·co·ma
    pl schwan·no·sar·co·mas
    or schwan·no·sar·co·ma·ta
Schwartz-
    Bart·ter syn·drome
Schwartz-
    Jam·pel syn·drome
Schweig·ger-
    Sei·del sheath
Schwein·furth green
Schwei·zer-Fo·ley Y-
    plas·ty
Schwen·in·ger meth·od
sci·age
sci·ap·o·dy
sci·a·sco·pi·a
sci·as·co·py
sci·at·ic
sci·at·i·ca
sci·ence
sci·en·tif·ic
sci·en·tist
sci·e·ro·pi·a
scil·la
scil·lism
scil·lo·ceph·a·lus
scil·lo·ceph·a·ly
scin·ti·gram
scin·ti·graph·ic
scin·tig·ra·phy
    pl scin·tig·ra·phies
scin·til·late
scin·til·la·tion
scin·til·la·tor
scin·til·lom·e·ter
scin·ti·pho·tog·ra·phy
scin·ti·scan
scin·ti·scan·ner
scin·ti·scan·ning
sci·on
scir·rhoid
scir·rhous
scir·rhus
    pl scir·rhus·es
    or scir·rhi
scis·sile

scis·sion
scis·si·par·i·ty
    pl scis·si·par·i·ties
scis·sor·ing
scis·sors
scis·su·ra
    pl scis·su·rae
scis·sure
scle·ra
    pl scle·ras
    or scle·rae
scler·ac·ne
scle·ral
scle·ra·ti·tis
scle·ra·tog·e·nous
scler·ec·ta·si·a
scle·rec·to·ir·i·dec·to·my
    pl scle·rec·to·ir·i·dec·to·
    mies
scle·rec·to·my
    pl scle·rec·to·mies
scler·e·de·ma
    pl scler·e·de·mas
    or scler·e·de·ma·ta
scle·re·ma
scle·re·ma ad·i·po·sum
scle·re·ma ne·o·na·to·rum
scle·re·mi·a
scle·re·mus
scle·ren·ce·pha·li·a
scle·ren·ceph·a·ly
scle·ren·chy·ma
    pl scle·ren·chy·mas
    or scle·ren·chy·ma·ta
scle·ren·chym·a·tous
scle·ri·a·sis
scle·rit·ic
scle·ri·tis
    pl scle·ri·tis·es
scle·ro·a·troph·ic
scle·ro·blas·tem
    var of scle·ro·blas·te·ma
scle·ro·blas·te·ma
    or scle·ro·blas·te·ma·ta
    pl scle·ro·blas·to·mas
scle·ro·blas·tem·ic
scle·ro·con·junc·ti·val
scle·ro·con·junc·ti·vi·tis
scle·ro·cor·ne·a

scle·ro·cor·ne·al
scle·ro·dac·tyl·i·a
  or scle·ro·dac·ty·ly
scle·ro·dac·ty·ly
  pl scle·ro·dac·ty·lies
  or scle·ro·dac·tyl·i·a
scle·ro·der·ma
  pl scle·ro·der·mas
  or scle·ro·der·ma·ta
scle·ro·der·ma·ti·tis
  pl scle·ro·der·ma·ti·tis·es
  or scle·ro·der·ma·ti·ti·des
scle·ro·der·ma·tous
scle·ro·gen·ic
  or scle·rog·e·nous
scle·rog·e·nous
  or scle·ro·gen·ic
scle·ro·gy·ri·a
scle·roid
scle·ro·ker·a·ti·tis
  pl scle·ro·ker·a·ti·ti·des
scle·ro·ma
  pl scle·ro·mas
  or scle·ro·ma·ta
scle·ro·ma·la·ci·a
scle·ro·me·ninx
  pl scle·ro·me·nin·ges
scle·ro·mere
scle·rom·e·ter
scle·ro·myx·e·de·ma
scle·ro·nych·i·a
scle·ro·nyx·is
scle·ro·o·o·pho·ri·tis
scle·ro·plas·ty
  pl scle·ro·plas·ties
scle·ro·pro·te·in
scle·ro·sant
scle·rose
scle·ro·sis
  pl scle·ro·ses
scle·ro·ste·no·sis
  pl scle·ro·ste·no·ses
scle·ros·to·my
  pl scle·ros·to·mies
scle·ro·ther·a·py
  pl scle·ro·ther·a·pies
scle·ro·thrix
scle·rot·ic

scle·rot·i·ca
scle·rot·i·cec·to·my
scle·rot·i·co·nyx·is
scle·rot·i·co·punc·ture
scle·rot·i·cot·o·my
scle·rot·i·dec·to·my
scle·ro·ti·tis
  pl scle·ro·ti·tis·es
scle·ro·ti·um
  pl scle·ro·ti·a
scle·ro·tome
scle·ro·tom·ic
scle·rot·o·my
  pl scle·rot·o·mies
scle·rous
scob·i·nate
sco·lec·i·form
scol·e·coid
sco·lex
  pl sco·lex·es
  or scol·i·ces
  or sco·le·ces
sco·li·o·lor·do·sis
sco·li·o·si·om·e·try
sco·li·o·sis
  pl sco·li·o·ses
sco·li·o·som·e·ter
sco·li·o·som·e·try
sco·li·ot·ic
sco·li·o·tone
Scol·o·pen·dra
scom·brine
scom·brone
scoop
sco·pa·rin
sco·par·i·us
sco·pine
sco·po·la
  or sco·po·li·a
sco·pol·a·mine
sco·po·li·a
  or sco·po·la
sco·po·phil·i·a
sco·po·phil·i·ac
sco·po·phil·ic
sco·po·pho·bi·a
Scop·u·lar·i·op·sis
scor·a·cra·ti·a

scor·bu·tic
scor·bu·ti·cal·ly
scor·bu·ti·gen·ic
scor·bu·tus
scor·di·ne·ma
score
scor·e·te·mi·a
Scor·pi·o
scor·pi·on
Scor·pi·on·i·da
scot·o·chro·mo·gen
scot·o·din·i·a
scot·o·gram
scot·o·graph
sco·to·ma
  pl sco·to·mas
  or sco·to·ma·ta
sco·to·ma·graph
sco·to·ma·tous
sco·tom·e·ter
scot·o·phil·i·a
scot·o·pho·bi·a
sco·to·pi·a
sco·top·ic
sco·top·sin
sco·tos·co·py
sco·to·sis
scrap·er
screen
screw·worm
scro·bic·u·late
scro·bic·u·lus
  pl scro·bic·u·li
scrof·u·la
scrof·u·lo·der·ma
scrof·u·lo·der·mi·a
scrof·u·lo·der·mic
scrof·u·lo·sis
  pl scof·u·lo·ses
scrof·u·lous
scrot·al
scro·tec·to·my
  pl scro·tec·to·mies
scro·to·cele
scro·to·plas·ty
scro·tum
  pl scro·tums
  or scro·ta

354

scrub ty·phus
scru·ple
scru·pu·los·i·ty
  pl scru·pu·los·i·ties
scurf
scur·vy
  pl scur·vies
scu·tate
scute
scu·tel·lum
  pl scu·tel·la
scu·ti·form
Scu·tig·e·ra
scu·tu·late
scu·tu·lum
  pl scu·tu·la
scu·tum
  pl scu·ta
scyb·a·lous
scyb·a·lum
  pl scyb·a·la
scy·phi·form
scy·ti·tis
Sea·bright-
  Ban·tam syn·drome
seal
seam
sea·sick·ness
seat·worm
se·ba·ce·o·fol·lic·u·lar
se·ba·ceous
se·bac·ic
se·bas·to·ma·ni·a
se·bif·er·ous
se·bip·a·rous
se·bo·cys·to·ma·to·sis
seb·o·lith
seb·or·rha·gi·a
seb·or·rhe·a
seb·or·rhe·al
seb·or·rhe·ic
seb·or·rhoe·a
  var of seb·or·rhe·a
seb·or·rhoe·al
  var of seb·or·rhe·al
seb·or·rhoe·ic
  var of seb·or·rhe·ic
se·bum

se·cern·ment
Seck·el syn·drome
se·clu·sion
sec·o·bar·bi·tal
sec·o·dont
sec·on·dar·y
sec·ond-de·gree burn
sec·on·dines
  or sec·und·ines
sec·ond-set
se·cre·ta
se·cre·ta·gogue
  or sec·re·to·gogue
Se·cré·tan dis·ease
se·crete
se·cre·tin
se·cre·tin·ase
se·cre·tion
se·cre·to·gogue
  or se·cre·ta·gogue
se·cre·to·in·hib·i·tor
sec·re·to·mo·tor
se·cre·tor
se·cre·to·ry
sec·tar·i·an
sec·tile
sec·ti·o
  pl sec·ti·o·nes
sec·tion
sec·tion·al
sec·to·ri·al
se·cun·di·grav·i·da
  pl se·cun·di·grav·i·das
  or se·cun·di·grav·i·dae
se·cun·di·nae
sec·un·dines
  or sec·on·dines
sec·un·dip·a·ra
  pl sec·un·dip·a·ras
  or sec·un·dip·a·rae
sec·un·di·par·i·ty
sec·un·dip·a·rous
se·cun·dum ar·tem
se·cure
se·cu·ri·ty
  pl se·cu·ri·ties
se·date
se·da·tion

sed·a·tive
sed·en·tar·y
sed·i·ment
sed·i·men·ta·ry
sed·i·men·ta·tion
sed·i·men·tom·e·ter
se·do·hep·tu·lose
seed
See·lig·muel·ler sign
seg·ment
seg·men·ta
seg·men·tal
seg·men·tar·y
seg·men·ta·tion
seg·men·tec·to·my
  pl seg·men·tec·to·mies
seg·men·ter
Seg·men·ti·na
seg·men·tum
  pl seg·men·ta
seg·re·gant
seg·re·gate
seg·re·ga·tion
seg·re·ga·tion·al
seg·re·ga·tor
Sé·guin sign
sei·aes·the·si·a
  var of sei·es·the·si·a
Seid·litz pow·ders
sei·es·the·si·a
Sei·gnette salt
seis·mo·ther·a·py
Seitz fil·ter
sei·zure
se·junc·tion
sel·a·chyl
se·la·pho·bi·a
Sel·din·ger tech·nique
se·lec·tion
se·lec·tor
se·le·ne
  pl se·le·nai
se·le·nic
sel·e·nif·er·ous
se·le·ni·ous
sel·e·nite
se·le·ni·um
se·len·o·dont

se·le·no·gam·i·a
se·le·no·sis
self-ab·sorp·tion
self-a·buse
self-ac·cu·sa·tion
self-al·li·en·a·tion
self-a·nal·y·sis
    pl self-a·nal·y·ses
self-an·a·lyt·ic
    or self-an·a·lyt·i·cal
self-an·a·lyt·i·cal
    or self-an·a·lyt·ic
self-a·ware
self-a·ware·ness
self-con·cept
self-con·cep·tion
self-dif·fer·en·ti·a·tion
self-di·ges·tion
self-fer·men·ta·tion
self-fer·til·i·za·tion
self-hyp·no·sis
    pl self-hyp·no·ses
self-i·den·ti·fi·ca·tion
self-im·age
self-in·duc·tance
self-in·fec·tion
self-in·flict·ed
self-in·oc·u·la·tion
self-lim·it·ed
    or self-lim·it·ing
self-lim·it·ing
    or self-lim·it·ed
self-mu·ti·la·tion
self-per·cep·tion
self-pol·lu·tion
self-rep·li·cat·ing
self-re·pres·sion
self-re·pro·duc·ing
self-stim·u·la·tion
self-sug·gest·i·bil·i·ty
self-sug·ges·tion
self-sus·pen·sion
self-treat·ment
Sel·i·wa·noff test
sel·la
    pl sel·las
    or sel·lae
sel·la tur·ci·ca
    pl sel·lae tur·ci·cae

sel·lar
Sel·ter dis·ease
Sel·ye syn·drome
se·man·tic
se·man·tics
Semb op·er·a·tion
se·mei·og·ra·phy
    pl se·mei·og·ra·phies
se·mei·o·log·ic
se·mei·ol·o·gy
    pl se·mei·ol·o·gies
se·mei·ot·ic
    or se·mei·ot·i·cal
se·mei·ot·i·cal
    or se·mei·ot·ic
se·mei·ot·ics
se·men
    pl se·mens
    or sem·i·na
Sem·e·noff meth·od
se·me·nu·ri·a
    var of se·mi·nu·ri·a
sem·i·a·ceph·a·lus
sem·i·ca·nal
sem·i·ca·na·lis
    pl sem·i·ca·na·les
sem·i·car·ba·zide
sem·i·car·ba·zone
sem·i·car·ti·lag·i·nous
sem·i·cir·cu·lar
sem·i·co·ma
sem·i·com·a·tose
sem·i·con·scious
sem·i·con·scious·ly
sem·i·con·scious·ness
sem·i·dom·i·nant
sem·i·flex·ion
sem·i·le·thal
sem·i·lu·nar
sem·i·lux·a·tion
sem·i·mem·bra·no·sus
    pl sem·i·mem·bra·no·si
sem·i·mem·bra·nous
sem·i·nal
sem·i·nal·ly
sem·i·nate
sem·i·na·tion
sem·i·nif·er·al
    or sem·i·nif·er·ous

sem·i·nif·er·ous
    or sem·i·nif·er·al
sem·i·no·ma
    pl sem·i·no·mas
    or sem·i·no·ma·ta
sem·i·nor·mal
se·mi·nu·ri·a
se·mi·og·ra·phy
    pl se·mi·og·ra·phies
    var of se·mei·og·ra·phy
se·mi·o·log·ic
    var of se·mei·o·log·ic
se·mi·o·log·i·cal
    var of se·mei·o·log·i·cal
se·mi·ol·o·gy
    pl se·mi·ol·o·gies
    var of se·mei·o·lo·gy
se·mi·ot·ics
    var of se·mei·ot·ics
sem·i·pen·ni·form
sem·i·per·me·a·ble
sem·i·pla·cen·ta
sem·i·ple·gi·a
sem·i·pri·vate
semi·pro·na·tion
sem·i·prone
sem·i·pto·sis
sem·i·quin·one
Se·mir·a·mid·i·an op·er·a·tion
se·mis
sem·i·sid·e·ra·ti·o
sem·i·som·nus
sem·i·so·por
sem·i·spi·na·lis
    pl sem·i·spi·na·les
sem·i·su·pi·na·tion
sem·i·syn·thet·ic
sem·i·ten·di·no·sus
    pl sem·i·ten·di·no·si
sem·i·ten·di·nous
Se·mon law
Se·mon-Ro·sen·bach law
Sen meth·od
Sen·e·ar-
    Ush·er syn·drome
Se·ne·ci·o
se·ne·ci·o·sis
    pl se·ne·ci·o·ses

se·nec·ti·tude
sen·e·ga
sen·e·gin
Sen·ek·jie me·di·um
se·nes·cence
se·nes·cent
se·nile
se·nile·ly
se·nil·ism
se·nil·i·ty
pl se·nil·i·ties
se·ni·um
sen·na
sen·no·side
se·no·pi·a
sen·sa·tion
sen·sa·tion·al
sense
sen·sib·a·mine
sen·si·bil·i·a
sen·si·bil·i·ty
pl sen·si·bil·i·ties
sen·si·bil·iz·er
sen·sib·i·lus pro·pri·us nu·cle·us
sen·si·ble
sen·si·tive
sen·si·tiv·i·ty
pl sen·si·tiv·i·ties
sen·si·ti·za·tion
sen·si·tize
sen·si·tiz·er
sen·so·mo·tor
sen·so·pa·ral·y·sis
sen·sor
sen·so·ri·al
sen·so·ri·al·ly
sen·so·ri·mo·tor
sen·so·ri·neu·ral
sen·so·ri·um
pl sen·so·ri·ums
or sen·so·ri·a
sen·so·ry
pl sen·so·ries
sen·su·al
sen·su·al·ism
sen·su·al·i·ty
pl sen·su·al·i·ties
sen·su·al·ly

sen·sum
pl sen·sa
sen·sus
sen·ti·ent
sen·ti·ment
sep·a·ra·tor
sep·sis
pl sep·ses
sep·tae·mi·a
var of sep·te·mi·a
sep·tal
sep·tate
sep·ta·tion
sep·tec·to·my
sep·te·mi·a
sep·tic
sep·ti·cae·mi·a
var of sep·ti·ce·mi·a
sep·ti·cae·mic
var of sep·ti·ce·mic
sep·ti·ce·mi·a
sep·ti·ce·mic
sep·ti·co·phle·bi·tis
sep·ti·co·py·e·mi·a
sep·ti·co·py·e·mic
sep·ti·grav·i·da
sep·tile
sep·ti·me·tri·tis
sep·tip·a·ra
sep·to·mar·gi·nal
sep·tom·e·ter
sep·to·na·sal
sep·to·plas·ty
sep·to·tome
sep·tot·o·my
sep·tu·la tes·tis
sep·tu·lum
pl sep·tu·la
sep·tum
pl sep·tums
or sep·ta
sep·tum pel·lu·ci·dum
pl sep·ta pel·lu·ci·da
sep·tum trans·ver·sum
pl sep·ta trans·ver·sa
sep·tup·let
sep·tu·plex
sep·ul·ture

se·quel·a
pl se·quel·ae
se·quence
se·quen·tial
se·ques·ter
se·ques·tra·tion
se·ques·trec·to·my
pl se·ques·trec·to·mies
se·ques·trot·o·my
se·ques·trum
pl se·ques·trums
or se·ques·tra
se·quoi·o·sis
ser·al·bu·min
se·rem·pi·on
ser·e·no·a
Ser·gent sign
se·ri·al
se·ri·al·o·graph
ser·i·ceps
ser·i·cin
se·ries
pl se·ries
ser·i·flux
ser·ine
se·ro·al·bu·min·ous
se·ro·che
se·ro·chrome
se·ro·co·li·tis
se·ro·cul·ture
se·ro·cys·tic
se·ro·der·ma·ti·tis
se·ro·der·ma·to·sis
se·ro·der·mi·tis
se·ro·di·ag·no·sis
pl se·ro·di·ag·no·ses
se·ro·di·ag·nos·tic
se·ro·en·ter·i·tis
se·ro·fi·brin·ous
se·ro·lem·ma
se·ro·li·pase
se·ro·log·ic
or se·ro·log·i·cal
se·ro·log·i·cal
or se·ro·log·ic
se·ro·log·i·cal·ly
se·rol·o·gist
se·rol·o·gy
pl se·rol·o·gies

se·rol·y·sin
se·ro·ma
se·ro·mem·bra·nous
se·ro·mu·ci·nous
se·ro·mu·cous
se·ro·mus·cu·lar
se·ro·neg·a·tive
se·ro·neg·a·tiv·i·ty
  pl se·ro·neg·a·tiv·i·ties
se·ro·per·i·to·ne·um
se·ro·pos·i·tive
se·ro·pos·i·tiv·i·ty
  pl se·ro·pos·i·tiv·i·ties
se·ro·prog·no·sis
se·ro·pu·ru·lent
se·ro·pus
se·ro·re·ac·tion
se·ro·re·sis·tance
se·ro·re·sis·tant
se·ro·sa
  pl se·ro·sas
  or se·ro·sae
se·ro·sal
se·ro·sa·mu·cin
se·ro·san·guin·e·ous
se·ro·se·rous
se·ro·si·tis
  pl se·ro·si·tis·es
se·ros·i·ty
  pl se·ros·i·ties
se·ro·syn·o·vi·tis
se·ro·ther·a·py
  pl se·ro·ther·a·pies
se·ro·to·nin
se·ro·tox·in
se·ro·type
se·rous
se·ro·zy·mo·gen·ic
ser·pens
ser·pent
ser·pen·tar·i·a
ser·pig·i·nous
ser·pig·i·nous·ly
ser·ra
ser·rate
Ser·ra·ti·a
ser·ra·tion
ser·ra·tus
  pl ser·ra·ti

serre·fine
Ser·res an·gle
ser·ru·late
ser·ru·la·tion
Ser·ti·li cells
se·rum
  pl se·rums
  or se·ra
se·rum·al
ser·vo·mech·a·nism
ser·yl
ses·a·me
ses·a·moid
ses·a·moi·di·tis
  pl ses·a·moi·dit·is·es
Se·sar·ma
ses·qui·chlo·ride
ses·qui·ho·ra
ses·qui·ox·ide
ses·qui·salt
ses·qui·sul·fide
ses·qui·sul·phide
  var of ses·qui·sul·fide
ses·qui·ter·pene
ses·sile
set
se·ta
  pl se·tae
se·ta·ceous
se·ta·ceous·ly
se·tal
Se·tar·i·a
set·fast
  var of sit·fast
se·tig·er·ous
se·ton
set·up
Se·ver dis·ease
Se·vip·a·rous
se·vum
sex
sex·i·dig·i·tal
  or sex·i·dig·i·tate
sex·i·dig·i·tate
  or sex·i·dig·i·tal
sex·in·ter·grade
sex·lim·it·ed
sex·link·age
sex·linked

sex·o·aes·thet·ic
  var of sex·o·es·the·tic
sex·o·es·thet·ic
sex·o·log·ic
sex·o·log·i·cal
sex·ol·o·gist
sex·ol·o·gy
  pl sex·ol·o·gies
sex·ti·grav·i·da
sex·tip·a·ra
  pl sex·tip·a·ras
  or sex·tip·a·rae
sex·tup·let
sex·u·al
sex·u·al·i·ty
  pl sex·u·al·i·ties
sex·u·al·i·za·tion
sex·u·al·ize
sex·u·al·ly
Sé·za·ry cell
shad·ow·cast·ing
Shaf·fer meth·od
shaft
sha·green
shank
shark-liv·er oil
Shar·pey fi·bers
Sha·ver dis·ease
sheath
sheathe
shed
Shee·han syn·drome
shelf
shell
shel·lac
shell·shock
Shen·stone op·er·a·tion
Shep·herd frac·ture
Sher·man-Mun·sell u·nit
Sher·ren tri·an·gle
Sher·ring·ton law
Shev·sky test
Shib·ley sign
shield
shift
Shi·ga ba·cil·lus
Shi·gel·la
  pl shi·gel·las
  or shi·gel·lae

shig·el·lo·sis
  pl shig·el·lo·ses
shi·kim·ic
shi·ma·mu·shi
  or shi·mu·mu·shi
shi·mu·mu·shi
  or shi·ma·mu·shi
shin
shin·bone
shin·gles
shin·splints
shiv·er
shock
Shock and Has·tings
  meth·od
shod·dy
Shohl and King meth·od
Shope pa·pil·lo·ma
Shorr tri·chrome stain
short·sight·ed
short·sight·ed·ly
short·sight·ed·ness
short·wind·ed
shot·ty
shoul·der
shoul·der·blade
Shrap·nell mem·brane
shreds
shriv·el
shud·der
Shumm test
Shunk stain
shunt
Shwartz·man phe·nom·e·non
Shy-Dra·ger syn·drome
si·a·go·nag·ra
si·al·a·den
si·al·ad·e·ni·tis
si·al·ad·e·nog·ra·phy
si·al·ad·en·on·cus
si·al·a·gog
si·al·a·gog·ic
si·al·a·gogue
  var of si·al·a·gog
si·al·an·gi·og·ra·phy
si·al·a·po·ri·a
si·al·ec·ta·si·a
si·al·ic

si·al·ine
si·a·li·thot·o·my
si·a·li·tis
si·a·lo·ad·e·nec·to·my
si·a·lo·ad·e·ni·tis
si·a·lo·ad·e·not·o·my
si·a·lo·aer·oph·a·gy
si·a·lo·an·gi·ec·ta·sis
si·a·lo·an·gi·ec·ta·sis
si·a·lo·an·gi·og·ra·phy
si·a·lo·an·gi·tis
si·a·lo·do·chi·tis
si·a·lo·do·chi·um
  pl si·a·lo·do·chi·a
si·a·lo·do·cho·li·thi·a·sis
si·a·lo·do·cho·plas·ty
si·a·lo·gas·trone
si·a·log·e·nous
si·a·lo·gogue
  var of si·a·la·gog
si·a·lo·gram
si·a·log·ra·phy
  pl si·a·log·ra·phies
si·a·loid
si·al·o·lith
si·a·lo·li·thi·a·sis
  pl si·a·lo·li·thi·a·ses
si·a·lo·li·thot·o·my
si·a·lo·mu·cin
si·a·lon
si·a·lor·rhe·a
si·a·lor·rhoe·a
  var of si·a·lor·rhe·a
si·a·los·che·sis
si·a·lo·se·mei·ol·o·gy
si·a·lo·sis
si·a·lo·ste·no·sis
si·a·lo·syr·inx
Si·a·mese twins
Si·a wa·ter test
sib
sib·i·lant
sib·i·la·tion
sib·i·lis·mus
sib·i·lus
sib·ling
sib·ship
Sib·son fas·ci·a
Si·card syn·drome

sic·ca
sic·cant
sic·ca·tive
sic·cha·si·a
sic·cus
sick
Sick·a meth·od
sick·en
sick·lae·mi·a
  var of sick·le·mi·a
sick·le
sick·le-cell a·ne·mi·a
sick·le·form
sick·le-hammed
sick·le-hocked
sick·le·mi·a
sick·le·mic
sick·ness
sick·room
Sid·bur·y syn·drome
Sid·dall test
side
sid·er·a·tion
sid·er·ism
sid·er·ite
sid·er·o·cyte
sid·er·o·cy·to·sis
sid·er·o·dro·mo·pho·bi·a
sid·er·o·fi·bro·sis
  pl sid·er·o·fi·bro·ses
sid·er·o·pe·ni·a
sid·er·o·pe·nic
sid·er·o·phage
sid·er·o·phil
  or sid·er·o·phile
sid·er·o·phile
  or sid·er·o·phil
sid·er·o·phil·i·a
sid·er·oph·i·lin
sid·er·oph·i·lous
sid·er·o·phyl·lin
sid·er·o·sil·i·co·sis
sid·er·o·sis
  pl sid·er·o·sis·es
sid·er·ot·ic
Sie·gert sign
Sie·mens syn·drome
sigh
sight

sig·ma
sig·ma·tism
sig·moid
    or sig·moi·dal
sig·moi·dal
    or sig·moid
sig·moi·dal·ly
sig·moi·dec·to·my
    pl sig·moi·dec·to·mies
sig·moi·di·tis
sig·moi·do·pex·y
sig·moi·do·proc·tos·to·my
sig·moi·do·rec·tos·to·my
sig·moid·o·scope
sig·moid·o·scop·ic
sig·moi·dos·co·py
    pl sig·moi·dos·co·pies
sig·moi·do·sig·moi·dos·to·
    my
sig·moi·dos·to·my
    pl sig·moi·dos·to·mies
sig·moi·dot·o·my
sig·moi·do·ves·i·cal
sign
sig·na·ture
sig·num
    pl sig·na
sil·lan·drone
Si·las·tic
si·lent
si·lex
sil·i·ca
sil·i·cate
sil·i·ca·to·sis
si·li·ceous
    var of si·li·cious
si·lic·ic
si·li·cious
si·li·ci·um
sil·i·co·flu·o·ride
sil·i·con
sil·i·cone
sil·i·co·sid·er·o·sis
sil·i·co·sis
    pl sil·i·co·ses
sil·i·cot·ic
sil·i·co·tu·ber·cu·lo·sis
    pl sil·i·co·tu·ber·cu·lo·ses
sil·i·co·tung·stic

si·lique
sil·i·quose
    or sil·i·quous
sil·i·quous
    or sil·i·quose
sil·o·drate
sil·ver
Sil·ver syn·drome
Sil·ves·ter meth·od
Sim·a·rou·ba
    var of sim·a·ru·ba
sim·a·ru·ba
si·meth·i·cone
Sim·i·ae
sim·i·an
si·mil·i·a si·mil·i·bus cu·
    ran·tur
si·mil·i·mum
Sim·monds dis·ease
Sim·mons ci·trate a·gar
Si·mon op·er·a·tion
Si·mo·nart threads
Si·mon·sen phe·nom·e·
    non
sim·ple
Simp·son syn·drome
sim·tra·zene
si·mul
sim·u·late
sim·u·la·tion
sim·u·la·tor
Si·mu·li·um
si·mul·tag·no·si·a
si·nal
si·na·pis
sin·a·pis·co·py
sin·a·pism
sin·cip·i·tal
sin·ci·put
    pl sin·ci·puts
    or sin·cip·i·ta
Sin·ding-Lar·sen dis·ease
sin·ew
sin·gle-blind
sin·gul·ta·tion
sin·gul·tus
    pl sin·gul·ti
sin·i·grin
sin·is·ter

sin·is·trad
sin·is·tral
sin·is·tral·i·ty
    pl sin·is·tral·i·ties
si·nis·tral·ly
sin·is·tra·tion
sin·is·trau·ral
si·nis·tro·car·di·a
sin·is·tro·cer·e·bral
sin·is·troc·u·lar
sin·is·troc·u·lar·i·ty
    pl sin·is·troc·u·lar·i·ties
sin·is·tro·gy·ra·tion
sin·is·tro·gy·ric
sin·is·tro·man·u·al
sin·is·trop·e·dal
sin·is·trorse
sin·is·trorse·ly
sin·is·tro·tor·sion
sin·is·trous
si·no·a·tri·al
si·no·au·ric·u·lar
si·no·bron·chi·tis
si·no·ca·rot·id
si·no·gram
si·nog·ra·phy
si·no·vag·i·nal
sin·u·ous
sin·u·ous·ly
sinus
    pl sinus·es
    or si·nus
si·nus·al
si·nus·i·tis
sin·us·oid
si·nus·oi·dal
si·nus·oi·dal·ly
si·nus·oi·dal·i·za·tion
si·nus·ot·o·my
    pl si·nus·ot·o·mies
si·phon
si·phon·age
Si·pho·nap·ter·a
si·phon·ap·ter·ous
Si·phun·cu·la·ta
Si·phun·cu·li·na
Sip·py di·et
si·ren
si·ren·i·form

si·ren·limb
si·ren·oid
si·re·no·me·li·a
si·re·nom·e·lus
   pl si·re·nom·e·li
si·re·nom·e·ly
si·ri·a·sis
   pl si·ri·a·ses
sir·ih
sir·kar·i
sir·up
   var of sy·rup
sis·mo·ther·a·py
Sis·to sign
Sis·tru·rus
site
sit·fast
sit·i·eir·gi·a
si·tol·o·gy
   pl si·tol·o·gies
si·to·ma·ni·a
si·to·pho·bi·a
si·to·stane
si·tos·ter·ol
si·to·ther·a·py
si·tu
sit·u·a·tion
sit·u·a·tion·al
sit·us
   pl si·tus
si·tus in·ver·sus
sitz bath
Sjö·gren-
   Lars·son syn·drome
skat·ol
   or skat·ole
skat·ole
   or skat·ol
ska·tol·o·gy
   pl ska·tol·o·gies
   var of sca·to·lo·gy
skat·ox·yl
skein
ske·lal·gi·a
ske·le·tal
skel·e·tal·ly
ske·le·ti·za·tion
skel·e·tog·e·nous
skel·e·to·mus·cu·lar

skel·e·ton
Skene duct
skene·i·tis
   var of ske·ni·tis
skene·o·scope
ske·ni·tis
ske·o·cy·to·sis
skew
skew·foot
ski·a·gram
ski·a·graph
ski·ag·ra·pher
ski·ag·ra·phy
   pl ski·ag·ra·phies
ski·am·e·try
   pl ski·am·e·tries
ski·a·po·res·co·py
ski·a·scope
ski·as·co·py
   pl ski·as·co·pies
skin
Skin·ner box
Skin·ner·i·an
skin·ny
skle·ri·a·sis
Sklow·sky symp·tom
sko·da·ic
sko·li·o·lor·do·sis
   var of sco·li·o·lor·do·sis
sko·li·o·si·om·e·try
   var of sco·li·o·si·om·e·try
sko·li·o·sis
   pl sko·li·o·ses
   var of sco·li·o·sis
sko·li·o·som·e·ter
   var of sco·li·o·som·e·ter
sko·li·o·som·e·try
   var of sco·li·o·som·e·try
sko·li·ot·ic
   var of sco·li·ot·ic
skull
skull·cap
Skutsch op·er·a·tion
slake
slant
slap·ping
slav·er
sleep
sleep·less·ness

sleep·walk·er
sleep·walk·ing
slide
slime mold
sling
slip
slit
sliv·er
slob·ber
slough
slow vi·rus
Slu·der meth·od
sludge
sluice·way
slum·ber
slur
slur·ry
   pl slur·ries
small·pox
smear
smeg·ma
smeg·mat·ic
Smel·lie meth·od
smi·lax
Smith test
Smith-Die·trich meth·od
Smith-Lem·li-
   O·pitz syn·drome
Smith-Pe·ter·son nail
Smith·wick op·er·a·tion
smudg·ing
smut
snake·root
snap
snare
sneeze
Snel·len chart
snif·fle
snore
snow-blind
snow-blind·ness
snuff·box
snuf·fles
soap·stone
sob
so·cal·o·in
so·ci·a
so·cial
so·cial·i·za·tion

so·cial·ize
so·cial·ly
so·ci·o·cen·tric
so·ci·o·cen·tric·i·ty
   pl so·ci·o·cen·tric·i·ties
so·ci·o·cen·trism
so·ci·o·gen·e·sis
   pl so·ci·o·gen·e·ses
so·ci·o·ge·net·ic
so·ci·o·gen·ic
so·ci·o·gram
so·ci·o·log·ic
   or so·ci·o·log·i·cal
so·ci·o·log·i·cal
   or so·cio·log·ic
so·ci·ol·o·gist
so·ci·ol·o·gy
   pl so·ci·ol·o·gies
so·ci·o·med·i·cal
so·ci·o·met·ric
so·ci·om·e·trist
so·ci·om·e·try
   pl so·ci·om·e·tries
so·ci·o·path
so·ci·o·path·ic
so·ci·op·a·thy
   pl so·ci·op·a·thies
so·ci·o·sex·u·al
so·ci·o·sex·u·al·i·ty
   pl so·ci·o·sex·u·al·i·ties
sock·et
so·cor·di·a
so·da
so·da·mide
Sö·der·bergh pres·sure re·
   flex
so·di·um
so·do·ku
sod·o·mist
sod·o·mite
sod·o·my
   pl sod·o·mies
Soem·mer·ing bone
soil·borne
so·ja bean
sol
So·la·na·ce·ae
so·la·na·ceous

so·lan·i·dine
so·la·nin
   or so·la·nine
so·la·nine
   or so·la·nin
So·la·num
so·lap·sone
so·lar
so·lar plex·us
so·lar·i·um
   pl so·lar·i·ums
   or so·lar·i·a
so·lar·i·za·tion
so·lar·ize
sol·a·tion
sole
so·le·al
so·le·no·glyph
So·le·nog·ly·pha
so·le·no·glyph·ic
   or so·le·nog·ly·phous
so·le·nog·ly·phous
   or so·le·no·glyph·ic
sole·plate
sole·print
So·ler·a re·ac·tion
so·le·us
   pl so·le·us·es
   or so·le·i
sol·id
sol·i·da·go
so·lid·i·fi·ca·tion
so·lid·i·fy
sol·id·un·gu·late
sol·i·dus
   pl sol·i·di
sol·i·ped
sol·ip·sism
sol·i·tar·y
sol·lu·nar
Sol·o·mon rule
Sol·pu·gi·da
sol·u·bil·i·ty
   pl sol·u·bil·i·ties
sol·u·bi·li·za·tion
sol·u·bi·lize
sol·u·ble
sol·u·bly
so·lum tym·pa·ni

so·lute
so·lu·tion
sol·vate
sol·va·tion
sol·vent
sol·vol·y·sis
   pl sol·vol·y·ses
sol·vo·lyt·ic
sol·y·per·tine
so·ma
   pl so·mas
   or so·ma·ta
so·maes·the·si·a
   var of so·mes·the·si·a
so·maes·thet·ic
   var of so·mes·thet·ic
so·maes·the·to·psy·chic
   var of so·mes·the·to·psy·
   chic
so·mal
so·mas·the·ni·a
so·mat·aes·the·si·a
   var of so·mat·es·the·si·a
so·mat·aes·thet·ic
   var of so·mat·es·thet·ic
so·mat·es·the·si·a
so·mat·es·thet·ic
so·mat·ic
so·mat·i·cal·ly
so·mat·i·co·splanch·nic
so·mat·i·co·vis·cer·al
so·ma·tist
so·ma·ti·za·tion
so·ma·tize
so·mat·o·chrome
so·ma·to·did·y·mus
so·ma·to·dym·i·a
so·ma·to·ge·net·ic
   or so·ma·to·gen·ic
so·ma·to·gen·ic
   or so·ma·to·ge·net·ic
so·ma·tog·e·ny
so·ma·to·log·ic
so·ma·to·log·i·cal
so·ma·tol·o·gy
   pl so·ma·tol·o·gies
so·ma·tome
so·ma·to·meg·a·ly
so·ma·to·met·ric

so·ma·tom·e·try
   pl so·ma·tom·e·tries
so·ma·tom·ic
so·ma·top·a·gus
so·ma·to·path·ic
so·ma·to·plasm
so·ma·to·plas·tic
so·ma·to·pleu·ral
so·ma·to·pleure
so·ma·to·pleu·ric
so·ma·to·psy·chic
so·ma·to·sen·so·ry
so·ma·to·splanch·nic
so·ma·to·splanch·no·pleu·
   ric
so·ma·to·ther·a·pist
so·ma·to·ther·a·py
   pl so·ma·to·ther·a·pies
so·ma·to·to·ni·a
so·ma·to·ton·ic
so·ma·to·top·ag·no·si·a
so·ma·to·top·ic
   or so·ma·to·top·i·cal
so·ma·to·top·i·cal
   or so·ma·to·top·ic
so·ma·to·trid·y·mus
so·ma·to·tro·phic
so·ma·to·tro·phin
so·ma·to·trop·ic
so·ma·to·tro·pin
so·ma·to·type
so·ma·to·typ·ic
so·ma·to·typ·i·cal·ly
so·ma·to·ty·pol·o·gy
   pl so·ma·to·ty·pol·o·gies
so·mes·the·si·a
so·mes·thet·ic
so·mes·the·tog·no·sis
so·mes·the·to·psy·chic
so·mite
som·nam·bu·lance
som·nam·bu·lant
som·nam·bu·lar
som·nam·bu·late
som·nam·bu·la·tion
som·nam·bu·la·tor
som·nam·bu·lism
som·nam·bu·lisme pro·vo·
   qué

som·nam·bu·list
som·nam·bu·lis·tic
som·nam·bu·lis·ti·cal·ly
som·ni·al
som·ni·a·tion
som·ni·a·tive
som·nic·u·lous
som·ni·fa·cient
som·nif·er·ous
som·nif·er·ous·ly
som·nif·ic
som·nif·u·gous
som·nil·o·quence
som·nil·o·quism
som·nil·o·quist
som·nil·o·quy
   pl som·nil·o·quies
som·nip·a·thist
som·nip·a·thy
   pl som·nip·a·thies
som·no·cin·e·mat·o·graph
som·no·form
som·no·lence
   or som·no·len·cy
som·no·len·cy
   pl som·no·len·cies
   or som·no·lence
som·no·lent
som·no·lent·ly
som·no·len·ti·a
som·no·les·cent
som·no·lism
som·nop·a·thist
som·nop·a·thy
som·no·vig·il
som·nus
So·mo·gyi meth·od
sone
son·ic
son·i·cate
son·i·ca·tion
son·i·ca·tor
son·i·tus
Son·ne dys·en·ter·y
son·o·chem·i·cal
son·o·chem·is·try
son·o·en·ceph·a·lo·gram
son·o·gram

so·nog·ra·phy
so·nom·e·ter
so·no·rous
so·nus
soor
so·phis·ti·cate
so·phis·ti·ca·tion
soph·o·ma·ni·a
So·pho·ra
soph·o·rine
so·por
so·po·rate
so·po·rif·er·ous
so·po·rif·er·ous·ness
so·po·rif·ic
so·po·rose
sor·be·fa·cient
sor·bic
sor·bi·tan
sor·bite
sor·bi·tol
sor·bose
Sor·by cell
sor·des
   pl sor·des
sor·did
sore
sor·ghum
so·ro·ri·a·tion
sorp·tion
sor·rel
so·ta·lol
so·ter·e·nol
souf·fle
sound
Souques sign
so·ya
soy·bean
so·zo·i·od·o·late
so·zo·i·o·dol·ic
spa
space of Burns
spaces
spa·cial
   var of spa·tial
Spal·ding sign
Spal·lan·za·ni law
spal·la·tion

Span·ish fly
Span·ish in·flu·en·za
spar·a·drap
spare
spar·ga·no·sis
 pl spar·ga·no·ses
Spar·ga·num
 pl Spar·ga·nums
 or Spar·ga·na
spar·go·sis
 pl spar·go·sis·es
 or spar·go·ses
spar·so·my·cin
spar·te·ine
spasm
spas·mat·ic
 or spas·mat·i·cal
spas·mat·i·cal
 or spas·mat·ic
spas·mod·ic
 or spas·mod·i·cal
spas·mod·i·cal
 or spas·mod·ic
spas·mod·i·cal·ly
spas·mo·gen·ic
spas·mol·o·gy
spas·mo·lyg·mus
spas·mol·y·sis
 pl spas·mol·y·ses
spas·mo·lyt·ic
spas·mo·lyt·i·cal·ly
spas·mo·phe·mi·a
spas·mo·phile
 or spas·mo·phil·ic
spas·mo·phil·i·a
spas·mo·phil·ic
 or spas·mo·phile
spas·mus
spas·tic
spas·ti·cal·ly
spas·tic·i·ty
 or spas·tic·i·ties
spa·ti·a
spa·tial
spa·tial sum·ma·tion
spa·tial·ly
spa·ti·um
 pl spa·ti·a
spat·u·la

spat·u·late
spat·u·la·tion
spa·tule
spav·in
 or spav·ine
spav·ine
 or spav·in
spav·ined
spay
spe·cial·ism
spe·cial·ist
spe·cial·i·za·tion
spe·cial·ize
spe·cial·ty
 pl spe·ci·al·i·ties
spe·cies
 pl spe·cies
spe·cies-spe·ci·fic
spe·cies-spe·ci·fic·i·ty
 pl spe·cies-spe·ci·fic·i·ties
spe·cif·ic
spe·cif·i·cal·ly
spec·i·fic·i·ty
 pl spec·i·fic·i·ties
spec·i·men
spec·ta·cles
spec·ti·no·my·cin
spec·tral
spec·tral·ly
spec·tro·chem·i·cal
spec·tro·chem·is·try
 pl spec·tro·chem·is·tries
spec·tro·col·o·rim·e·ter
spec·tro·gram
spec·tro·graph
spec·trog·ra·pher
spec·tro·graph·ic
spec·tro·graph·i·cal·ly
spec·trog·ra·phy
 pl spec·trog·ra·phies
spec·trom·e·ter
spec·trom·e·try
 pl spec·trom·e·tries
spec·tro·mi·cro·scope
spec·tro·pho·tom·e·ter
spec·tro·pho·to·met·ric
 or spec·tro·pho·to·met·ri·
  cal

spec·tro·pho·to·met·ri·cal
 or spec·tro·pho·to·met·ric
spec·tro·pho·to·met·ri·cal·
  ly
spec·tro·pho·tom·e·try
 pl spec·tro·pho·tom·e·tries
spec·tro·po·la·rim·e·ter
spec·tro·scope
spec·tro·scop·ic
 or spec·tro·scop·i·cal
spec·tro·scop·i·cal
 or spec·tro·scop·ic
spec·tro·scop·i·cal·ly
spec·tros·co·pist
spec·tros·co·py
 pl spec·tros·co·pies
spec·trum
 pl spec·trums
 or spec·tra
spec·u·lar
spec·u·lum
 pl spec·u·lums
 or spec·u·la
Spee curve
speech
spe·le·os·to·my
spel·ter
Spen·cer-Par·ker vac·cine
Speng·ler frag·ments
Spens syn·drome
sperm
 pl sperms
 or sperm
sper·ma·ce·ti
sper·ma·cra·si·a
sper·ma·ry
 pl sper·ma·ries
sper·ma·ta·cra·si·a
sper·ma·ta·gen·ic
 or sper·ma·to·gen·ic
sper·ma·te·li·o·sis
sper·mat·ic
sper·mat·i·cal·ly
sper·ma·ti·ci·dal
sper·ma·tid
sper·ma·tin
sper·ma·to·blast
sper·ma·to·blas·tic
sper·mat·o·cele

364

sper·ma·to·ce·lec·to·my
sper·ma·to·ci·dal
 or sper·mi·cid·al
sper·ma·to·cide
 or sper·mi·cide
sper·ma·to·cyst
sper·ma·to·cys·tec·to·my
sper·ma·to·cys·tic
sper·ma·to·cys·ti·tis
sper·ma·to·cys·tot·o·my
sper·ma·to·cy·tal
sper·ma·to·cyte
sper·ma·to·cy·to·ma
 pl sper·ma·to·cy·to·mas
 or sper·ma·to·cy·to·ma·ta
sper·ma·to·gen·e·sis
 pl sper·ma·to·gen·e·ses
sper·ma·to·gen·ic
 or sper·ma·ta·gen·ic
sper·ma·tog·e·nous
sper·ma·tog·e·ny
 pl sper·ma·tog·e·nies
sper·ma·to·go·ni·al
 or sper·ma·to·gon·ic
sper·ma·to·gon·ic
 or sper·ma·to·go·ni·al
sper·ma·to·go·ni·um
 pl sper·ma·to·go·ni·a
sper·ma·toid
sper·ma·tol·y·sin
sper·ma·tol·y·sis
 pl sper·ma·tol·y·ses
sper·ma·to·lyt·ic
sper·ma·top·a·thy
 pl sper·ma·top·a·thies
sper·mat·o·phore
sper·ma·tor·rhe·a
sper·ma·tor·rhoe·a
 var of sper·ma·tor·rhe·a
sper·ma·tox·in
sper·ma·to·zo·al
sper·ma·to·zo·an
sper·ma·to·zo·i·cide
sper·ma·to·zo·id
sper·ma·to·zo·on
 pl sper·ma·to·zo·a
sper·ma·tu·ri·a
sper·mec·to·my

sper·mi·a·tion
sper·mi·cid·al
 or sper·ma·to·ci·dal
sper·mi·cide
 or sper·ma·to·cide
sper·mi·dine
sper·mine
sper·mi·o·gen·e·sis
 pl sper·mi·o·gen·e·ses
sper·mi·o·gram
sperm·ism
sperm·ist
sper·mi·um
 pl sper·mi·a
sper·mo·lith
sper·mol·y·sin
sper·mol·y·sis
 pl sper·mol·y·ses
sper·mo·tox·in
Sper·ry meth·od
spes phthis·i·ca
sphac·e·late
sphac·e·la·tion
sphac·e·lism
sphac·e·lo·der·ma
 pl sphac·e·lo·der·mas
 or sphac·e·lo·der·ma·ta
sphac·e·loid
sphac·e·lus
sphaer·oid
 var of sphe·roid
Sphae·roph·o·rus
spha·gi·as·mus
spha·gi·tis
sphen·eth·moid
sphe·ni·on
sphe·no·bas·i·lar
 or sphe·no·bas·i·lic
sphe·no·bas·i·lic
 or sphe·no·bas·i·lar
sphe·no·ce·phal·ic
 or sphe·no·ceph·a·lous
sphe·no·ceph·a·lous
 or sphe·no·ce·phal·ic
sphe·no·ceph·a·lus
sphe·no·ceph·a·ly
 pl sphe·no·ceph·a·lies
sphe·no·eth·moid
sphe·no·fron·tal

sphe·noid
 or sphe·noi·dal
sphe·noi·dal
 or sphe·noid
sphe·noid·i·tis
sphe·noid·ot·o·ny
sphe·no·ma·lar
sphe·no·man·dib·u·lar
sphe·no·max·il·lar·y
sphe·no·oc·cip·i·tal
sphe·nop·a·gus par·a·sit·i·cus
sphe·no·pal·a·tine
spheno·pa·ri·e·tal
sphe·no·pe·tro·sal
sphe·no·sal·pin·go·staph·y·li·nus
sphe·no·sis
sphe·no·squa·mo·sal
sphe·no·tem·po·ral
sphe·not·ic
sphe·no·tre·si·a
sphe·no·tribe
sphe·no·trip·sy
sphe·no·tur·bi·nal
sphe·no·zy·go·mat·ic
sphe·raes·the·si·a
 var of sphe·res·the·si·a
sphere
sphe·res·the·si·a
spher·ic
 or spher·i·cal
spher·i·cal
 or spher·ic
sphe·ro·ceph·a·lus
sphe·ro·cyl·in·der
sphe·ro·cyte
sphe·ro·cyt·ic
sphe·ro·cy·to·sis
sphe·roid
sphe·roi·dal
sphe·rom·e·ter
sphe·ro·pha·ki·a
Sphe·roph·o·rus
sphe·ro·plast
spher·ule
sphinc·ter
sphinc·ter pu·pil·lae
sphinc·ter vag·i·nae

365

sphinc·ter·al
sphinc·ter·al·gi·a
sphinc·ter·ec·to·my
    pl sphinc·ter·ec·to·mies
sphinc·ter·ic
sphinc·ter·is·mus
sphinc·ter·i·tis
sphinc·ter·ol·y·sis
    pl sphinc·ter·ol·y·ses
sphinc·ter·o·plas·ty
sphinc·ter·ot·o·my
    pl sphinc·ter·ot·o·mies
sphin·go·lip·id
    or sphin·go·lip·ide
sphin·go·lip·ide
    or sphin·go·lip·id
sphin·go·lip·i·do·sis
sphin·go·my·e·lin
sphin·go·sine
sphyg·mic
    or sphyg·mi·cal
sphyg·mi·cal
    or sphyg·mic
sphyg·mo·bo·lom·e·ter
sphyg·mo·bo·lom·e·try
sphyg·mo·chron·o·graph
sphyg·mo·chro·nog·ra·phy
sphyg·mod·ic
sphyg·mo·dy·na·mom·e·ter
sphyg·mo·gram
sphyg·mo·graph
sphyg·mo·graph·ic
sphyg·mog·ra·phy
    pl sphyg·mog·ra·phies
sphyg·moid
sphyg·mo·ma·nom·e·ter
sphyg·mo·ma·no·met·ric
sphygo·mo·ma·no·met·ri·cal·ly
sphyg·mo·ma·nom·e·try
    pl sphyg·mo·ma·nom·e·tries
sphyg·mom·e·ter
sphyg·mo·os·cil·lom·e·ter
sphyg·mo·pal·pa·tion
sphyg·mo·phone
sphyg·mo·scope
sphyg·mos·co·py
sphyg·mo·sys·to·le

sphyg·mo·tech·ny
sphyg·mo·to·no·graph
sphyg·mo·to·nom·e·ter
sphyg·mus
    pl sphyg·mi
sphynx-neck
spi·ca
    pl spi·cas
    or spi·caa
spic·u·la
    pl spic·u·lae
spic·u·lar
spic·u·late
spic·u·la·tion
spic·ule
spic·u·lum
    pl spic·u·la
spi·der
Spie·gler test
Spie·gler-Fendt sar·coid
Spiel·mey·er-Vogt
    dis·ease
Spi·ge·li·a
Spi·ge·li·an
spike
spike·nard
spi·lo·ma
    pl spi·lo·mas
    or spi·lo·ma·ta
spi·lo·pla·ni·a
spi·lus
    pl spi·li
spi·na
    pl spi·nae
spi·na bi·fi·da
spi·na·cene
spi·nae pal·a·ti·nae
spi·nal
spi·na·lis
    pl spi·na·les
spi·nal·ly
spi·nate
spin·dle
spine
spine·less
spi·no·bul·bar
spi·no·cel·lu·lar
spi·no·cer·e·bel·lar
spi·no·col·lic·u·lar

spi·no·gal·va·ni·za·tion
spi·no·ol·i·var·y
spi·no·sal
spi·nose
spi·nose·ly
spi·no·spi·nal
spi·no·sus
spi·no·tec·tal
spi·no·tha·lam·ic
spi·no·trans·ver·sar·i·us
spi·nous
spin·thar·i·con
spin·thar·i·scope
spin·ther·ism
spi·nu·lose
spi·ny
spi·ny-head·ed worm
spip·er·one
spir·a·cle
spi·rad·e·ni·tis sup·pu·ra·ti·va
spi·rad·e·no·ma
    pl spi·rad·e·no·mas
    or spi·rad·e·no·ma·ta
spi·ral
spi·ra·my·cin
spi·rem
    or spi·reme
spi·reme
    or spi·rem
Spi·ril·la·ce·ae
spi·ril·la·ce·ous
spi·ril·lar
spi·ril·lar·y
spi·ril·li·ci·dal
spi·ril·lo·sis
    pl spi·ril·lo·sis·es
    or spi·ril·lo·ses
spi·ril·um
    pl spi·ril·la
spir·it
spir·i·tu·ous
spir·i·tus
spir·i·tus fru·men·ti
spi·ro·cer·ca
Spi·ro·chae·ta
    pl Spi·ro·chae·tae
    or Spi·ro·che·ta
Spi·ro·chae·ta·ce·ae

spi·ro·chae·tae·mi·a
  var of spi·ro·che·te·mi·a
spi·ro·chae·tal
  var of spi·ro·che·tal
Spi·ro·chae·ta·les
spi·ro·chaete
  var of spi·ro·chete
spi·ro·chae·ti·cide
  var of spi·ro·che·ti·cide
spi·ro·chae·tol·y·sis
  var of spi·ro·che·tol·y·sis
spi·ro·chae·to·sis
  pl spi·ro·chae·to·ses
  var of spi·ro·che·to·sis
spi·ro·chae·tot·ic
  var of spi·ro·che·tot·ic
Spi·ro·chae·ta
  pl Spi·ro·che·tae
  or Spi·ro·chae·ta
spi·ro·che·tal
spi·ro·chete
spi·ro·che·te·mi·a
spi·ro·che·ti·ci·dal
spi·ro·che·ti·cide
spi·ro·che·tol·y·sis
spi·ro·che·to·sis
  pl spi·ro·che·to·ses
spi·ro·che·tot·ic
spi·ro·gram
spi·ro·graph
spi·ro·graph·ic
spi·ro·me·ter
spi·ro·met·ric
spi·rom·e·try
  pl spi·rom·e·tries
spi·ro·no·lac·tone
Spi·rop·ter·a
spi·rox·a·sone
spis·sat·ed
spis·si·tude
spit·al
spit·tle
splanch·naes·the·si·a
  var of splanch·nes·the·si·a
splanch·nec·to·pi·a
splanch·nem·phrax·is
splanch·nes·the·si·a
splanch·nic

splanch·ni·cec·to·my
  pl splanch·ni·cec·to·mies
splanch·ni·cot·o·my
  pl splanch·ni·cot·o·mies
splanch·no·cele
splanch·no·coel
  or splanch·no·coele
splanch·no·coele
  or splanch·no·coel
splanch·no·di·as·ta·sis
splanch·nog·ra·phy
splanch·no·lith
splanch·no·li·thi·a·sis
splanch·no·lo·gi·a
splanch·nol·o·gy
  pl splanch·nol·o·gies
splanch·no·meg·a·ly
  pl splanch·no·meg·a·lies
splanch·no·mi·cri·a
splanch·nop·a·thy
splanch·no·pleu·ral
splanch·no·pleure
splanch·no·pleu·ric
splanch·nop·to·si·a
splanch·nop·to·sis
splanch·no·scle·ro·sis
splanch·nos·co·py
  pl splanch·nos·co·pies
splanch·no·skel·e·ton
splanch·no·so·mat·ic
splanch·not·o·my
splanch·no·tribe
splay·foot
  pl splay·feet
spleen
sple·nal·gi·a
sple·nal·gic
sple·nec·to·mize
sple·nec·to·my
  pl sple·nec·to·mies
splen·ec·to·pi·a
sple·nec·to·py
sple·ne·o·lus
  pl sple·ne·o·li
sple·net·ic
sple·net·i·cal·ly
sple·ni·al
splen·ic
  or splen·i·cal

splen·i·cal
  or splen·ic
splen·i·co·pan·cre·at·ic
splen·i·fi·ca·tion
splen·i·form
sple·ni·tis
  pl sple·ni·tis·es
sple·ni·um
  pl sple·ni·a
sple·ni·us
  pl sple·ni·i
splen·i·za·tion
sple·no·cele
sple·no·clei·sis
sple·no·cyte
sple·no·dyn·i·a
sple·no·gen·ic
sple·no·gram
sple·no·gran·u·lo·ma·to·sis
  sid·er·ot·i·ca
sple·no·hep·a·to·meg·a·ly
  pl sple·no·hep·a·to·meg·a·
   lies
sple·noid
sple·nol·y·sis
sple·no·ma·la·ci·a
sple·no·me·ga·li·a
sple·no·meg·a·ly
  pl sple·no·meg·a·lies
sple·no·my·e·log·e·nous
sple·nop·a·thy
  pl sple·nop·a·thies
sple·no·pex·y
  pl sple·no·pex·ies
sple·no·pneu·mo·ni·a
sple·no·por·to·gram
sple·no·por·tog·ra·phy
sple·nop·to·sis
  pl sple·nop·to·ses
sple·nor·rha·phy
sple·not·o·my
  pl sple·not·o·mies
sple·no·tox·in
sple·no·ty·phoid
splen·u·lus
  pl splen·u·li
  or sple·nun·cu·lus
  pl sple·nun·cu·li

sple·nun·cu·lus
  pl sple·nun·cu·li
  or splen·u·lus
  pl splen·u·li
splice
splint
splint·age
splin·ter
splint·ing
split-brain
split·ters of Spen·gler
split-thick·ness graft
split·ting
spo·di·o·my·e·li·tis
spod·o·gram
spo·dog·ra·phy
spon·dy·lal·gi·a
spon·dyl·ar·thri·tis
spon·dyl·ar·throc·a·ce
spon·dyl·ex·ar·thro·sis
spon·dy·lit·ic
spon·dy·li·tis
spon·dy·li·ze·ma
spon·dy·lo·ar·thi·tis
spon·dy·lo·loc·a·ce
spon·dy·lo·di·dym·i·a
spon·dy·lod·y·mus
spon·dy·lo·dyn·i·a
spon·dy·lo·lis·the·sis
spon·dy·lo·lis·thet·ic
spon·dy·lol·y·sis
  pl spon·dy·lol·y·ses
spon·dy·lop·a·thy
  pl spon·dy·lop·a·thies
spon·dy·lo·py·o·sis
spon·dy·lo·sis
  pl spon·dy·lo·sis·es
  or spon·dy·lo·ses
spon·dy·lo·syn·de·sis
spon·dy·lot·o·my
  pl spon·dy·lot·o·mies
spon·dy·lous
spon·dy·lus
  pl spon·dy·li
spon·gi·form
spon·gin
spon·gi·o·blast

spon·gi·o·blas·to·ma
  pl spon·gi·o·blas·to·mas
  or spon·gi·o·blas·to·ma·ta
spon·gi·o·cyte
spon·gi·o·cy·to·ma
  pl spon·gi·o·cy·to·mas
  or spon·gi·o·cy·to·ma·ta
spon·gi·o·form
spon·gi·oid
spon·gi·o·neu·ro·blas·toma
  pl spon·gi·o·neu·ro·blas·to·
    mas
  or spon·gi·o·neu·ro·blas·to·
    ma·ta
spon·gi·o·plasm
spon·gi·o·plas·mic
spon·gi·o·sa
spon·gi·ose
spon·gi·o·sis
spon·gi·o·si·tis
spon·gi·ot·ic
spon·gy
spon·ta·ne·ous
spon·ta·ne·ous·ly
spoon
spoon·er·ism
spo·rad·ic
spo·ran·gi·o·phore
spo·ran·gi·o·spore
spo·ran·gi·um
  pl spo·ran·gi·a
spore
spo·ric·i·dal
spo·ri·cide
spo·rid·i·um
  pl spo·rid·i·a
spo·ro·ag·glu·ti·na·tion
spo·ro·blast
spo·ro·cyst
spo·ro·cys·tic
spo·ro·cyte
spo·ro·gen·e·sis
  pl spo·ro·gen·e·ses
spo·ro·gen·ic
spo·rog·e·nous
spo·rog·o·ny
  pl spo·rog·e·nies
spo·ro·gon·ic
  or spo·rog·o·nous

spo·rog·o·nous
  or spo·ro·gon·ic
spo·rog·o·ny
  pl spo·rog·o·nies
spo·ront
spo·ro·phose
spo·ro·phyte
spo·ro·plasm
spo·rot·ri·chin
spo·ro·tri·cho·sis
  pl spo·ro·tri·cho·ses
Spo·rot·ri·chum
  pl Spo·rot·ri·cha
Spo·ro·zo·a
spo·ro·zo·an
spo·ro·zo·ite
spo·ro·zo·on
  pl spo·ro·zo·a
spor·u·lar
spor·u·late
spor·u·la·tion
spor·u·la·tive
spor·ule
spot
sprain
spray
spread·er
Spren·gel de·for·mi·ty
sprue
spud
spur
spu·ri·ous
spu·tum
  pl spu·tums
  or spu·ta
squa·lene
squa·ma
  pl squa·mae
squa·mate
squame
squa·mo·ba·sal
squa·mo·co·lum·nar
squa·moid
squa·mo·oc·cip·i·tal
squa·mo·pa·ri·e·tal
squa·mo·sa
  pl squa·mo·sas
  or squa·mo·sae
squa·mo·sal

squa·mose
squa·mo·sphe·noid
squa·mo·tym·pan·ic
squa·mous
squar·rose
  or squar·rous
squar·rous
  or squar·rose
squill
squint
squint-eyed
stab
sta·bile
stab·i·lim·e·ter
sta·bi·lize
sta·bi·li·zer
sta·ble
stac·ca·to
  pl stac·ca·tos
  or stac·ca·ti
stach·y·drine
stach·y·ose
stac·tom·e·ter
Sta·der splint
Sta·die meth·od
sta·di·um
  pl sta·di·ums
  or sta·di·a
Staeh·li pig·ment line
staff
staff of Aes·cu·la·pi·us
stage
stag·gers
stag·nate
stag·na·tion
Stahl ear
stain
stain·a·bil·i·ty
  pl stain·a·bil·i·ties
stal·ag·mom·e·ter
stale
stalk
sta·men
  pl sta·mens
  or sta·mi·na
Stam·ey test
stam·i·na
stam·i·nate
stam·mer

stamp·er
stan·dard
stan·dard·i·za·tion
stan·dard·ize
Stan·ford-Bi·net test
stand·still
stan·nate
stan·nic
stan·nous
stan·num
stan·o·lone
stan·o·zo·lol
sta·pe·dec·to·mized
sta·pe·dec·to·my
  pl sta·pe·dec·to·mies
sta·pe·dial
sta·pe·di·o·te·not·o·my
sta·pe·di·o·ves·tib·u·lar
sta·pe·di·us
  pl sta·pe·di·i
sta·pes
  pl sta·pes
  or sta·pe·des
staph·i·sa·gri·a
staph·y·le
staph·y·lec·to·my
  pl staph·y·lec·to·mies
staph·yl·e·de·ma
  pl staph·yl·ede·mas
  or staph·yl·ede·ma·ta
staph·y·le·us
staph·yl·hae·ma·to·ma
  var of staph·yl·he·ma·to·
    ma
staph·yl·he·ma·to·ma
staph·y·line
staph·y·li·no·pha·ryn·ge·us
staph·y·li·nus
sta·phyl·i·on
staph·y·li·tis
staph·y·lo·coc·cae·mi·a
  var of staph·y·lo·coc·ce·mi·
    a
staph·y·lo·coc·cal
staph·y·lo·coc·ce·mi·a
staph·y·lo·coc·ce·mic
staph·y·lo·coc·cic
staph·y·lo·coc·cus
  pl staph·y·lo·coc·ci

Staph·y·lo·coc·cus
staph·y·lo·co·sis
staph·y·lo·der·ma
staph·y·lo·der·ma·ti·tis
  pl staph·y·lo·der·ma·ti·ti·
    ses
  or staph·y·lo·der·ma·ti·ti·
    des
staph·y·lo·di·al·y·sis
staph·yl·oe·de·ma
  var of staph·yl·e·de·ma
staph·y·lo·ki·nase
staph·y·lol·y·sin
staph·y·lo·ma
staph·y·lo·mat·ic
staph·y·lom·a·tous
staph·y·lon·cus
staph·y·lo·pha·ryn·ge·us
staph·y·lo·phar·yn·gor·rha·
  phy
staph·y·lo·plas·ty
  pl staph·y·lo·plas·ties
staph·y·lop·to·sis
staph·y·lor·rha·phy
staph·y·los·chi·sis
staph·y·lot·o·my
  pl staph·y·lot·o·mies
staph·y·lo·tox·in
staph·y·ly·gro·ma
starch
starch·i·ness
starch·y
Star·gardt dis·ease
Star·ling law
star·ter
star·tle
star·va·tion
starve
star·wort
stas·i·bas·i·pho·bi·a
stas·i·pho·bi·a
sta·sis
  pl sta·ses
state
stat·ic
stat·ics
stat·im
sta·tion
sta·tion·ar·y

sta·tis·ti·cal
sta·tis·tics
stat·o·co·ni·um
  pl stat·o·co·ni·a
stat·o·cyst
stat·o·ki·net·ic
stat·o·lith
stato·lith·ic
sta·to·lon
stat·om·e·ter
stat·ure
sta·tus
sta·tus asth·mat·i·cus
sta·tus ep·i·lep·ti·cus
sta·tus lym·phat·i·cus
sta·tus thy·mi·co·lym·phat·i·cus
sta·tu·vo·lence
sta·tu·vo·lent
Staub-Trau·gott ef·fect
stau·ri·on
staves·a·cre
stax·is
ste·ap·sin
ste·a·rate
ste·ar·ic ac·id
ste·ar·i·form
ste·a·rin
ste·a·ro·der·mi·a
ste·a·rop·ten
  or ste·a·rop·tene
ste·a·rop·tene
  or ste·a·rop·ten
ste·ar·rhe·a
ste·a·ryl
ste·a·tite
ste·a·tit·ic
ste·a·ti·tis
ste·a·to·cryp·to·sis
ste·a·to·cys·to·ma mul·ti·plex
ste·a·tog·e·nous
ste·a·tol·y·sis
  pl ste·a·tol·y·ses
ste·a·to·lyt·ic
ste·a·to·ma
  pl ste·a·to·mas
  or ste·a·to·ma·ta
ste·a·to·ma·tous

ste·a·to·pyg·a
  or ste·a·to·pyg·i·a
ste·a·to·pyg·i·a
  or ste·a·to·pyg·a
ste·a·to·pyg·a
  or ste·a·top·y·gous
ste·a·top·y·gous
  or ste·a·to·pyg·ic
ste·a·tor·rhe·a
ste·a·tor·rhoe·a
  var of ste·a·tor·rhe·a
ste·a·to·sis
  pl ste·a·to·ses
Steele-Rich·ard·son-Ol·szew·ski syn·drome
Steen·bock u·nit
stef·fi·my·cin
steg·no·sis
steg·not·ic
Steg·o·my·i·a
Stein test
Stei·nach meth·od
Steind·ler op·er·a·tion
Stei·ner tu·mor
Stei·nert dis·ease
Stein-Lev·en·thal syn·drome
Stein·mann pin
stel·la
  pl stel·lae
stel·lar
stel·late
stel·late·ly
stel·lec·to·my
  pl stel·lec·to·mies
Stell·wag op·er·a·tion
stem
ste·nag·mus
sten·bo·lone
Sten·der dish
Sten·ger test
ste·ni·on
  pl ste·ni·a
Sten·o duct
sten·o·car·di·a
sten·o·car·di·ac
sten·o·ce·phal·i·a
  or sten·o·ceph·a·ly
sten·o·ce·phal·ic

sten·o·ceph·a·lous
sten·o·ceph·a·ly
  pl sten·o·ceph·a·lies
  or sten·o·ce·phal·i·a
sten·o·chas·mus
sten·o·cho·ri·a
sten·o·co·ri·a·sis
sten·o·crot·a·phy
sten·o·dont
sten·o·mer·ic
sten·o·myc·te·ri·a
Ste·no·ni·an duct
sten·o·pae·ic
  var of sten·o·pe·ic
sten·o·pa·ic
  var of sten·o·pe·ic
sten·o·pe·ic
ste·no·sal
ste·nose
ste·no·sis
  pl ste·no·ses
sten·os·to·my
sten·o·therm
sten·o·ther·mal
  or sten·o·ther·mic
sten·o·ther·mic
  or sten·o·ther·mal
sten·o·ther·my
  pl sten·o·ther·mies
sten·o·tho·rax
  pl sten·o·tho·rax·es
  or sten·o·tho·ra·ces
ste·not·ic
Sten·sen duct
stent
sten·to·roph·o·nous
Sten·ver pro·jec·tion
ste·pha·ni·al
ste·phan·ic
ste·pha·ni·on
Steph·a·no·fi·lar·i·a
steph·a·no·fil·a·ri·a·sis
  pl steph·a·no·fil·a·ri·a·ses
steph·a·nu·ri·a·sis
Steph·a·nu·rus
step·page
ste·rad
  or ste·ra·di·an

ste·ra·di·an
or ste·rad
ster·co·bi·lin
ster·co·bi·lin·o·gen
ster·co·lith
ster·co·ra·ceous
ster·co·ral
ster·co·rar·y
ster·co·ro·ma
  pl ster·co·ro·mas
  or ster·co·ro·ma·ta
Ster·cu·li·a
ster·cus
  pl ster·co·ra
stere
ster·e·o·ag·no·sis
ster·e·o·an·aes·the·si·a
  var of ster·e·o·an·es·the·si·a
ster·e·o·an·es·the·si·a
ster·e·o·ar·throl·y·sis
ster·e·o·blas·tu·la
  pl ster·e·o·blas·tu·las
  or ster·e·o·blas·tu·lae
ster·e·o·cam·pim·e·ter
ster·e·o·chem·i·cal
ster·e·o·chem·is·try
  pl ster·e·o·chem·is·tries
ster·e·o·cil·i·um
  pl ster·e·o·cil·i·a
ster·e·o·en·ceph·a·lo·tome
ster·e·o·en·ceph·a·lot·o·my
ster·e·og·no·sis
ster·e·og·nos·tic
ster·e·o·gram
ster·e·o·graph
ster·e·og·ra·phy
ster·e·o·i·so·mer
ster·e·o·i·so·mer·ic
ster·e·o·i·som·er·ism
ster·e·om·e·ter
ster·e·o·met·ric
ster·e·om·e·try
  pl ster·e·om·e·tries
ster·e·o·pho·to·mi·cro·
  graph
ster·e·o·mon·o·scope
ster·e·o·oph·thal·mo·scope
ster·e·o·phan·to·scope
ster·e·o·pho·ro·scope

ster·e·o·plasm
ster·e·op·sis
ster·e·op·ter
ster·e·o·ra·di·o·graph
ster·e·o·ra·di·o·graph·ic
ster·e·o·ra·di·og·ra·phy
  pl ster·e·o·ra·di·og·ra·phies
ster·e·o·roent·gen·og·ra·
  phy
ster·e·o·scope
ster·e·o·scop·ic
  or ster·e·o·scop·i·cal
ster·e·o·scop·i·cal
  or ster·e·o·scop·ic
ster·e·o·scop·i·cal·ly
ster·e·os·co·py
  pl ster·e·os·co·pies
ster·e·o·spec·if·ic
ster·e·o·spe·cif·i·cal·ly
ster·e·o·spec·i·fic·i·ty
  pl ster·e·o·spec·i·fic·i·ties
ster·e·o·stro·bo·scope
ster·e·o·tac·tic
ster·e·o·tac·ti·cal·ly
ster·e·o·tax·i·a
ster·e·o·tax·ic
ster·e·o·tax·i·cal·ly
ster·e·o·tax·is
  pl ster·e·o·tax·es
ster·e·o·tax·y
ster·e·o·trop·ic
ster·e·ot·ro·pism
ster·e·o·type
ster·e·o·ty·py
  pl ster·e·o·ty·pies
ster·e·o·vec·tor·car·di·o·
  graph
ste·ric
ste·rid
  or ste·ride
ste·ride
  or ste·rid
ste·rig·ma
  pl ste·rig·mas
  or ste·rig·ma·ta
ster·ig·mat·ic
Ste·rig·ma·to·cys·tis
ster·ile
ster·ile·ly

ste·ril·i·ty
  pl ste·ril·i·ties
ster·il·i·za·tion
ster·il·ize
ster·il·iz·er
ster·nad
ster·nal
ster·nal·gi·a
ster·na·lis
  pl ster·na·les
Stern·berg cell
Stern·berg-Reed cell
Stern·heim·er-
  Mal·bin cells
ster·no·chon·dro·scap·u·
  lar·is
ster·no·cla·vic·u·lar
ster·no·cla·vic·u·lar·is
ster·no·clei·dal
ster·no·clei·do·mas·toid
ster·no·cos·tid
ster·no·cos·ta·lis
ster·no·dym·i·a
ster·nod·y·mus
ster·no·dyn·i·a
ster·no·fa·ci·a·lis
  pl ster·no·fa·ci·a·les
ster·no·hy·oid
ster·no·hy·oi·de·us az·y·
  gos
ster·no·mas·toid
ster·no·om·pha·lo·dym·i·a
ster·no·pa·gi·a
ster·nop·a·gus
ster·nop·a·gy
ster·no·per·i·car·di·al
ster·nos·chi·sis
ster·no·thy·roid
ster·not·o·my
  pl ster·not·o·mies
ster·num
  pl ster·nums
  or ster·na
ster·nu·ta·tion
ster·nu·ta·tive
  or ster·nu·ta·to·ry
ster·nu·ta·tor

ster·nu·ta·to·ry
  or ster·nu·ta·tive
ste·roid
ste·roi·dal
ste·roi·do·gen·e·sis
  pl ste·roi·do·gen·e·ses
ste·roi·do·gen·ic
ste·rol
ste·rone
ster·tor
ster·to·rous
ster·to·rous·ly
steth·ar·te·ri·tis
steth·o·gram
steth·o·graph
steth·o·graph·ic
ste·thog·ra·phy
ste·thom·e·ter
steth·o·met·ric
steth·o·phone
steth·o·pol·y·scope
steth·o·scope
steth·o·scop·ic
  or steth·o·scop·i·cal
steth·o·scop·i·cal
  or steth·o·scop·ic
steth·o·scop·i·cal·ly
ste·thos·co·py
  pl ste·thos·co·pies
Ste·vens-
  John·son syn·drome
Stew·art-Holmes
  phe·nom·e·non
Stew·art-Mo·rel-
  Mor·ga·gni syn·drome
Stew·art-Treves-
  syn·drome
sthe·ni·a
sthen·ic
stib·a·mine
stib·i·ac·ne
stib·i·al·ism
stib·ine
stib·i·um
sti·bo·ni·um
stib·o·phen
stich·o·chrome
Stick·er dis·ease

stic·tac·ne
Stie·da frac·ture
sti·fle
stig·ma
  pl stig·mas
  or stig·ma·ta
stig·mal
stig·mas·ter·ol
stig·mat·ic
stig·ma·tism
stig·ma·ti·za·tion
stig·ma·tize
stig·ma·tose
stil·bam·i·dine
stil·baz·i·um
stil·bene
stil·bes·trol
stil·boes·trol
  var of stil·bes·trol
Stiles-Craw·ford ef·fect
sti·let
  var of sty·let
sti·lette
  var of sty·let
sti·let·ted
Still dis·ease
still·birth
still·born
Stil·ler dis·ease
stil·li·cid·i·um
Stil·ling ca·nal
stil·lin·gi·a
Still·man cleft
sti·lus
  var of sty·lus
Stim·son meth·od
stim·u·lant
stim·u·late
stim·u·la·tion
stim·u·la·tive
stim·u·la·tor
stim·u·la·to·ry
stim·u·lin
stim·u·lus
  pl stim·u·li
sting
stipe
stip·ple

stip·pling
stir·rup
stitch
sto·chas·tic
stock
Stock re·ti·nal a·tro·phy
Stock·ert phe·nom·e·non
stock·i·net
  or stock·i·nette
stock·i·nette
  or stock·i·net
stock·ing
Stof·fel op·er·a·tion
stoi·chi·o·met·ric
  or stoi·chi·o·met·ri·cal
stoi·chi·o·met·ri·cal
  or stoi·chi·o·met·ric
stoi·chi·o·met·ri·cal·ly
stoi·chi·om·e·try
  pl stoi·chi·om·e·tries
Stokes law
Stokes-
  Ad·ams syn·drome
Stok·vis dis·ease
Stoll meth·od
sto·lon
Stoltz op·er·a·tion
sto·ma
  pl sto·mas
  or sto·ma·ta
sto·mac·a·ce
sto·ma·ceph·a·lus
stom·ach
stom·ach·ache
stom·ach·al
sto·mach·ic
  or sto·mach·i·cal
sto·mach·i·cal
  or sto·mach·ic
sto·mach·i·cal·ly
sto·mal
sto·ma·tal
sto·ma·tal·gi·a
sto·mat·ic
sto·ma·ti·tis
  pl sto·ma·ti·ti·es
  or sto·ma·ti·ti·des
sto·ma·toc·a·ce

372

sto·ma·to·ca·thar·sis
sto·ma·to·ceph·a·lus
sto·ma·to·dyn·i·a
sto·ma·to·dy·so·di·a
sto·ma·to·gas·tric
sto·ma·to·glos·si·tis
sto·ma·to·log·ic
  or sto·ma·to·log·i·cal
sto·ma·to·log·i·cal
  or sto·ma·to·log·ic
sto·ma·tol·o·gist
sto·ma·tol·o·gy
  pl sto·ma·tol·o·gies
sto·ma·to·ma·la·ci·a
sto·ma·to·me·ni·a
sto·ma·to·mi·a
sto·mat·o·my
  pl sto·mat·o·mies
sto·ma·to·my·co·sis
sto·ma·to·ne·cro·sis
sto·ma·to·no·ma
sto·ma·top·a·thy
sto·ma·to·plas·tic
sto·ma·to·plas·ty
sto·ma·tor·rha·gi·a
sto·ma·to·scope
sto·ma·to·sis
  pl sto·ma·to·sis·es
  or sto·ma·to·ses
sto·ma·tot·o·my
sto·men·or·rha·gi·a
sto·mo·dae·al
  var of sto·mo·de·al
sto·mo·dae·um
  pl sto·mo·dae·ums
  or sto·mo·dae·a
  var of sto·mo·de·um
sto·mo·de·um
  pl sto·mo·de·ums
  or sto·mo·de·a
sto·mos·chi·sis
Sto·mox·ys
stone
Stone op·er·a·tion
stone-blind
stone-blind·ness
stone-deaf
stone-deaf·ness

Stook·ey re·flex
stool
stop·cock
stop·page
sto·rax
sto·ri·form
storm
stra·bi·lis·mus
stra·bil·i·za·tion
  or stro·bi·la·tion
stra·bis·mal
stra·bis·mal·ly
stra·bis·mic
stra·bis·mom·e·ter
stra·bis·mom·e·try
  pl stra·bis·mom·e·tries
stra·bis·mus
stra·bom·e·ter
stra·bom·e·try
strab·o·tome
stra·bot·o·my
Stra·chan syn·drome
strag·u·lum
  pl strag·u·la
strain
strain·er
strait
strait·jack·et
stra·mo·ni·um
strand·ed
strand·ed·ness
stran·gle
stran·gles
stran·gu·late
stran·gu·la·tion
stran·gu·ry
  pl stran·gu·ries
strap
Strass·mann phe·nom·e·
  non
strat·i·fi·ca·tion
strat·i·fied
stra·ti·graph·ic
stra·tig·ra·phy
stra·to·sphere
stra·tum
  pl stra·tums
  or stra·ta

stra·tum cor·ne·um
  pl stra·ta cor·ne·a
stra·tum ger·mi·na·ti·vum
  pl stra·ta ger·mi·na·ti·va
stra·tum gran·u·lo·sum
  pl stra·ta gran·u·lo·sa
stra·tum lu·ci·dum
  pl stra·ta lu·ci·da
Strauss re·ac·tion
Strauss syn·drome
straw·ber·ry mark
streak
streph·o·sym·bo·li·a
streph·o·sym·bol·ic
strep·i·tus
  pl strep·i·ti
strep·o·gen·in
strep·ti·cae·mi·a
  var of strep·ti·ce·mi·a
strep·ti·ce·mi·a
strep·ti·dine
strep·to·an·gi·na
strep·to·bac·il·lar·y
strep·to·ba·cil·lus
  pl strep·to·ba·cil·li
strep·to·bi·o·sa·mine
strep·to·coc·cae·mi·a
  var of strep·to·coc·ce·mi·a
strep·to·coc·cal
  or strep·to·coc·cic
Strep·to·coc·ce·ae
strep·to·coc·ce·mi·a
strep·to·coc·cic
  or strep·to·coc·cal
strep·to·coc·co·sis
strep·to·coc·cus
  pl strep·to·coc·ci
strep·to·co·ly·sin
strep·to·dor·nase
strep·to·gen·in
strep·to·he·mol·y·sin
strep·to·ki·nase
strep·to·ly·sin
Strep·to·my·ces
  pl Strep·to·my·ces
  or Strep·to·my·ce·tes
Strep·to·my·ce·ta·ce·ae
strep·to·my·cin

373

strep·to·nic·o·zid
strep·to·ni·grin
strep·tose
strep·to·sep·ti·cae·mi·a
   var of strep·to·sep·ti·ce·
     mi·a
strep·to·sep·ti·ce·mi·a
strep·to·so·mus
strep·to·thri·cin
strep·to·thri·co·sis
   or strep·to·tri·co·sis
Strep·to·thrix
   pl Strep·to·thri·ces
strep·to·tri·cho·sis
   or strep·to·thri·cho·sis
stress
stres·sor
stretch·er
stri·a
   pl stri·ae
stri·a lon·gi·tu·di·na·lis
   pl stri·ae lon·gi·tu·di·na·les
stri·a·tal
stri·ate
stri·at·ed
stri·a·tion
stri·a·to·ni·gral
stri·a·to·pal·li·dal
stri·a·to·tha·lam·ic
stri·a·tum
   pl stri·a·ta
strick·en
stric·ture
stri·dent
stri·dent·ly
stri·dor
strid·u·lous
strin·gent
string·halt
string·halt·ed
stri·o·cel·lu·lar
stri·o·cer·e·bel·lar
stri·o·ni·gral
stri·o·tha·lam·ic
strip
stripe
stripes of Bail·lar·ger
strip·per

strob·ic
strob·il
   or strob·ile
stro·bi·la
   pl stro·bi·lae
stro·bi·lar
stro·bi·la·tion
   or stra·bil·i·za·tion
strob·ile
   or strob·il
strob·i·loid
strob·i·lus
   pl strob·i·li
stro·bo·scope
stro·bo·scop·ic
stro·bo·scop·i·cal·ly
stro·bo·ster·e·o·scope
Stro·ga·nov meth·od
stroke
stro·ma
   pl stro·ma·ta
stro·mal
stro·ma·tal
stro·mat·ic
stro·ma·tin
stro·ma·to·sis
stro·muhr
stron·gyl
   or stron·gyle
stron·gyle
   or stron·gyl
Stron·gy·loi·de·a
Stron·gy·loi·des
stron·gy·loi·di·a·sis
   or stron·gy·loi·do·sis
stron·gy·loi·do·sis
   or stron·gy·loi·di·a·sis
stron·gy·lo·sis
stron·gy·lus
stron·ti·a
stron·ti·um
stro·phan·thi·din
stro·phan·thin
stro·phan·thus
stroph·o·ceph·a·lus
stroph·o·ceph·a·ly
stroph·u·lus
   pl stroph·u·li

struc·tur·al
struc·ture
stru·ma
   pl stru·mas
   or stru·mae
Stru·mi·a u·ni·ver·sal stain
stru·mi·form
stru·mi·pri·val
stru·mi·pri·vic
stru·mi·pri·vous
stru·mi·tis
stru·mous
Strüm·pell sign
Strüm·pell-
    Ma·rie di·sease
Strüm·pell-
    West·phal pseu·do·scle·
    ro·sis
strych·nine
strych·nin·ism
strych·nin·i·za·tion
Strych·nos
Stu·art fac·tor
stul·ti·ti·a
stump
stunt
stu·pe·fa·cient
stu·pe·fac·tion
stu·pe·fac·tive
stu·pe·fy
stu·pe·ma·ni·a
stu·por
stu·por·ous
stur·dy
   pl stur·dies
Sturge-Web·er dis·ease
stur·in
   or stur·ine
stur·ine
   or stur·in
Sturm·dorf op·er·a·tion
stut·ter
stut·ter·er
sty
   pl sties
   var of stye
stye
sty·let

sty·li·form
sty·lo·glos·sus
   pl sty·lo·glos·si
sty·lo·hy·al
sty·lo·hy·oid
sty·lo·hy·oi·de·us
   pl sty·lo·hy·oi·de·i
sty·loid
sty·lo·man·dib·u·lar
sty·lo·mas·toid
sty·lo·pha·ryn·ge·us
   pl sty·lo·pha·ryn·ge·i
sty·lus
   pl sty·lus·es
   or sty·li
sty·ma·to·sis
styp·sis
styp·tic
sty·ra·cin
sty·ra·mate
sty·rax
sty·rene
sty·rol
sub·ab·dom·i·nal
sub·ac·e·tate
sub·a·cro·mi·al
sub·a·cute
sub·a·cute·ly
sub·al·i·men·ta·tion
sub·an·co·ne·us
sub·a·or·tic
sub·ap·i·cal
sub·api·cal·ly
sub·ap·o·neu·rot·ic
sub·a·que·ous
sub·a·rach·noid
sub·ar·cu·ate
sub·a·re·o·lar
sub·as·trag·a·lar
sub·as·trin·gent
sub·a·tom·ic
sub·au·di·tion
sub·au·ral
sub·au·ric·u·lar
sub·ax·il·lar
   or sub·ax·il·lar·y
sub·ax·il·lar·y
   or sub·ax·il·lar

sub·bas·al
sub·brach·i·al
   or sub·bra·chi·an
sub·bra·chi·an
   or sub·bra·chi·al
sub·brach·y·ce·phal·ic
sub·cal·car·e·ous
sub·cal·ca·rine
sub·cal·lo·sal
sub·cap·su·lar
sub·car·bon·ate
sub·car·di·nal
sub·car·ti·lag·i·nous
sub·cel·lu·lar
sub·cer·vi·cal
sub·chlo·ride
sub·chon·dral
sub·cho·ri·al
sub·cho·ri·on·ic
sub·cho·roi·dal
sub·chron·ic
sub·class
sub·cla·vi·an
sub·cla·vi·us
   pl sub·cla·vi·i
sub·clin·i·cal
sub·clin·i·cal·ly
sub·cli·noid
sub·col·lat·er·al
sub·co·ma
sub·con·junc·ti·val
sub·con·junc·ti·val·ly
sub·con·scious
sub·con·scious·ly
sub·con·scious·ness
sub·con·tin·u·ous
sub·cor·a·coid
sub·cor·ne·al
sub·cor·tex
   pl sub·cor·tex·es
   or sub·cor·ti·ces
sub·cor·ti·cal
sub·cor·ti·cal·ly
sub·cos·tal
sub·cos·tal·gi·a
sub·crep·i·tant
sub·crep·i·ta·tion
sub·cur·re·us

sub·cul·ture
sub·cu·ra·tive
sub·cu·ta·ne·ous
sub·cu·ta·ne·ous·ly
sub·cu·tic·u·lar
sub·cu·tis
   pl sub·cu·tis·es
   or sub·cu·tes
sub·de·lir·i·um
sub·del·toid
sub·der·mal
sub·der·mic
sub·di·a·phrag·mat·ic
sub·dol·i·cho·ce·phal·ic
   or sub·dol·i·cho·ceph·a·
    lous
sub·dol·i·cho·ceph·a·lous
   or sub·dol·i·cho·ce·phal·ic
sub·dor·sal
sub·dor·sal·ly
sub·duct
sub·duc·tion
sub·du·ral
sub·du·ral·ly
sub·du·ro·per·i·to·ne·al
sub·du·ro·pleu·ral
sub·en·ceph·a·lon
   pl sub·en·ceph·a·la
sub·en·do·car·di·al
sub·en·do·the·li·al
sub·en·er·get·ic
sub·e·pen·dy·mal
sub·e·pen·dy·mo·ma
   pl sub·e·pen·dy·mo·mas
   or sub·e·pen·dy·mo·ma·ta
sub·ep·i·der·mal
sub·ep·i·the·li·al
su·ber·in
su·be·ri·za·tion
su·be·rized
su·ber·o·sis
su·ber·yl·ar·gi·nine
sub·fam·i·ly
sub·fas·ci·al
sub·ga·le·al
sub·gal·late
sub·ger·mi·nal
sub·gin·gi·val

sub·gle·noid
sub·glos·si·tis
sub·glot·tic
sub·gron·da·tion
sub·he·pat·ic
sub·hy·a·loid
sub·hy·oid
sub·ic·ter·ic
su·bic·u·lar
su·bic·u·lum
   pl su·bic·u·la
sub·in·ci·sion
sub·in·fec·tion
sub·in·gui·nal
sub·in·teg·u·men·tal
sub·in·ti·mal
sub·in·vo·lu·tion
sub·i·o·dide
sub·ja·cent
sub·ja·cent·ly
sub·jec·tive
sub·jec·tive·ly
sub·la·tion
sub·le·thal
sub·le·thal·ly
sub·leu·kae·mic
   var of sub·leu·ke·mic
sub·leu·ke·mic
sub·li·mate
sub·li·ma·tion
sub·lime
sub·lim·i·nal
sub·lim·i·nal·ly
sub·li·mis
sub·line
sub·lin·gual
sub·lin·gui·tis
sub·lob·u·lar
sub·lob·u·lar·ly
sub·lux
sub·lux·at·ed
sub·lux·a·tion
sub·mal·le·o·lar
sub·mam·ma·ry
sub·man·dib·u·lar
sub·mar·gin·al
sub·max·il·la
   pl sub·max·il·las
   or sub·max·il·lae

sub·max·il·lar·i·tis
sub·max·il·lar·y
sub·me·di·al
sub·me·di·al·ly
sub·me·di·an
sub·men·tal
sub·mes·a·ti·ce·phal·ic
sub·met·a·cen·tric
sub·me·tal·lic
sub·mi·cron
sub·mi·cro·scop·ic
sub·mil·i·ary
sub·min·i·mal
sub·mi·to·chon·dri·al
sub·mor·phous
sub·mu·co·sa
   pl sub·mu·co·sas
   or sub·mu·co·sae
sub·mu·co·sal
sub·mu·cous
sub·nar·cot·ic
sub·na·sal
sub·na·sa·le
sub·neu·ral
sub·ni·trate
sub·nor·mal
sub·nor·mal·i·ty
sub·nor·mal·ly
sub·no·to·chord·al
sub·nu·cle·us
   pl sub·nu·cle·us·es
   or sub·nu·cle·i
sub·nu·tri·tion
sub·oc·cip·i·tal
sub·oc·cip·i·tal·ly
sub·oc·cip·i·to·breg·mat·ic
sub·o·per·cu·lum
sub·op·ti·mal
sub·op·ti·mum
sub·or·bit·al
sub·or·der
sub·or·di·na·tion
sub·ox·ide
sub·pap·il·lary
sub·pap·u·lar
sub·par·a·lyt·ic
sub·pa·ri·e·tal
sub·pec·to·ral
sub·pe·dun·cu·lar

sub·per·i·car·di·al
sub·per·i·os·te·al
sub·pha·ryn·ge·al
sub·phren·ic
sub·phy·lum
sub·pi·al
sub·pla·cen·ta
   pl sub·pla·cen·tas
   or sub·pla·cen·tae
sub·pla·cen·tal
sub·plan·ti·grade
sub·plat·y·hi·er·ic
sub·pleu·ral
sub·pleu·ral·ly
sub·po·ten·cy
   pl sub·po·ten·cies
sub·po·tent
sub·pu·bic
sub·ros·tral
sub·sar·to·ri·al
sub·scap·u·lar
sub·scap·u·lar·is
sub·scle·ral
sub·scle·rot·ic
sub·scrip·tion
sub·sen·sa·tion
sub·se·ro·sa
sub·se·rous
sub·sib·i·lant
sub·side
sub·si·dence
sub·sig·moid
sub·sist·ence
sub·spe·cies
sub·spi·nous
sub·stage
sub·stance
sub·stan·ti·a
   pl sub·stan·ti·ae
sub·stan·ti·a ni·gra
   pl sub·stan·ti·ae ni·grae
sub·stan·ti·a pro·pri·a
   pl sub·stan·ti·ae pro·pri·ae
sub·stan·tive
sub·ster·nal
sub·stit·u·ent
sub·sti·tute
sub·sti·tu·tion
sub·sti·tu·tive

sub·strate
sub·stra·tum
   pl sub·stra·ta
sub·struc·ture
sub·sul·fate
sub·sul·to·ry
sub·sul·tus
sub·syn·ap·tic
sub·ta·lar
sub·tem·po·ral
sub·ten·to·ri·al
sub·ter·mi·nal
sub·ter·tian
sub·the·tan·ic
sub·tha·lam·ic
sub·thal·a·mus
   pl sub·thal·a·mi
sub·thresh·old
sub·thy·roid·ism
sub·ti·lin
sub·til·i·sin
sub·to·tal
sub·tra·pe·zi·al
sub·trig·o·nal
sub·tro·chan·ter·ic
sub·trop·i·cal
sub·u·ber·is
   pl sub·u·ber·es
sub·um·bil·i·cal
sub·un·gual
   or sub·un·gui·al
sub·un·gui·al
   or sub·un·gual
sub·u·re·thral
sub·vag·i·nal
sub·val·vu·lar
sub·vi·ral
sub·vir·ile
sub·vi·ta·min·o·sis
sub·vo·la
sub·vo·lu·tion
sub·vo·mer·ine
sub·wak·ing
suc·ce·da·ne·ous
suc·ce·da·ne·um
   pl suc·ce·da·ne·ums
   or suc·ce·da·ne·a
suc·cen·tu·ri·ate
suc·cif·er·ous

suc·ci·nate
suc·cin·chlor·im·ide
suc·cin·ic
suc·cin·ox·i·dase
suc·ci·nyl·cho·line
suc·cor·ance
suc·cor·ant
suc·cor·rhe·a
suc·cor·rhoe·a
   var of suc·cor·rhe·a
suc·cu·bus
   pl suc·cu·bi
suc·cu·lent
suc·cur·sal
suc·cus
   pl suc·ci
suc·cus en·ter·i·cus
suc·cuss
suc·cus·sion
suck
suck·le
Suc·quet-Hoy·er ca·nal
su·crase
su·crate
su·crose
su·cro·su·ri·a
suc·tion
Suc·to·ri·a
suc·to·ri·al
su·da·men
   pl su·dam·i·na
su·dam·i·nal
Su·dan stain
su·dan·o·phil
su·dan·o·phil·i·a
su·dan·o·phil·ic
su·da·tion
su·da·to·ri·um
   pl su·da·to·ri·a
Su·deck at·ro·phy
su·do·i·ker·a·to·sis
su·do·lor·rhe·a
su·do·lor·rhoe·a
   var of su·do·lor·rhe·a
su·do·mo·tor
su·dor
su·do·re·sis
su·do·rif·er·ous

su·do·rif·ic
su·do·rip·a·rous
suf·fo·cate
suf·fo·ca·tion
suf·fuse
suf·fu·sion
sug·ar
sug·ar·ine
sug·gest·i·bil·i·ty
sug·gest·i·ble
sug·ges·tion
sug·ges·tion·ist
sug·gil·la·tion
su·i·ci·dal
su·i·ci·dal·ly
su·i·cide
su·i·ci·dol·o·gist
su·i·ci·dol·o·gy
   pl su·i·ci·dol·o·gies
su·i·gen·der·ism
su·int
Su·ker sign
sul·a·za·pam
sul·cal
   or sul·car
sul·car
   or sul·cal
sul·cate
sul·ci
sul·ci·form
sul·cu·lus
   pl sul·cu·li
sul·cus
   pl sul·ci
sul·cus lu·na·tus
   pl sul·ci lu·na·ti
sul·cus of Ro·lan·do
sul·cus ter·mi·na·lis
   pl sul·ci ter·mi·na·les
sul·fa
sul·fa·cet·a·mide
   or sul·fa·cet·i·mide
sul·fa·cet·i·mide
   or sul·fa·cet·a·mide
sul·fa·chlor·py·rid·a·zine
sulf·ac·id
sul·fa·di·a·zine
sul·fa·di·meth·ox·ine
sul·fa·di·me·tine

sul·fa·dox·ine
sul·fa·the·i·dole
sul·fa·eth·yl·thi·a·di·a·zole
sul·fa·gua·ni·dine
sul·fa·lene
sul·fa·mer·a·zine
sul·fa·met·a·zine
sul·fa·me·ter
sul·fa·meth·a·zine
sul·fa·meth·i·zole
sul·fa·meth·ox·a·zole
sul·fa·me·thox·y·di·a·zine
sul·fa·me·thox·y·py·rid·a·zine
sul·fa·mez·a·thine
sul·fa·mon·o·meth·ox·ine
sul·fa·mox·ole
sul·fa·nil·a·mide
sul·fan·i·late
sul·fa·nil·ic
sul·fa·pyr·a·zine
sul·fa·pyr·a·zole
sul·fa·pyr·i·dine
sul·fa·qui·nox·a·line
sulf·ars·phen·a·mine
sul·fa·som·i·zole
sul·fa·tase
sul·fate
sul·fa·thi·a·zole
sul·fat·ide
sul·fat·i·do·sis
sul·faz·a·met
sulf·ben·za·mine
sulf·hae·mo·glo·bin
    var of sulf·he·mo·glo·bin
sulf·hae·mo·glo·bi·nae·
    mi·a
    var of sulf·he·mo·glo·bi·ne·
    mi·a
sulf·he·mo·glo·bin
sulf·he·mo·glo·bi·ne·mi·a
sulf·hy·drate
sulf·hy·dryl
sul·fide
sul·fine
sul·fin·pyr·a·zone
sul·fi·som·i·dine
sul·fi·sox·a·zole
sul·fite

sul·fit·ic
sulf·met·hae·mo·glo·bin
    var of sulf·met·he·mo·glo·
    bin
sulf·met·he·mo·glo·bin
sul·fo·ac·id
sul·fo·bro·mo·phthal·e·in
sul·fo·car·bo·late
sul·fo·car·bol·ic
sul·fo·cy·a·nate
sul·fo·cy·an·ic
sul·fo·mu·cin
sul·fon·a·mide
sul·fo·nate
sul·fo·na·tion
sul·fone
sul·fone·phthal·e·in
sul·fon·eth·yl·meth·ane
sul·fon·ic
sul·fo·ni·um
sul·fon·meth·ane
sul·fo·nyl
sul·fo·nyl·u·re·a
sul·fo·phe·nate
sul·fo·phen·yl·ate
sul·fo·sal·i·cyl·ic
sul·fo·salt
sulf·ox·ide
sulf·ox·one
sul·fur
sul·fu·rate
sul·fu·ra·tor
sul·fu·ret
sul·fu·ric
sul·fu·rize
sul·fu·rous
sul·fu·ryl
sul·fy·drate
sul·i·so·ben·zone
Sul·ko·witch test
sul·lage
Sul·li·van test
sul·pha
    var of sul·fa
sul·pha·dim·i·dine
sul·pha·fu·ra·zole
sul·phate
    var of sul·fate

sul·phide
    var of sul·fide
sul·phite
    var of sul·fite
sul·pho·nate
    var of sul·fo·nate
sul·phur
    var of sul·fur
sul·phu·rate
    var of sul·fu·rate
sul·phu·rize
    var of sul·fu·rize
sul·phu·rous
    var of sul·fu·rous
sul·phy·drate
    var of sulf·hy·drate
sul·phy·dryl
    var of sulf·hy·dryl
sul·thi·ame
Sulz·ber·ger-Garbe
    dis·ease
su·mac
su·mach
    var of su·mac
sum·bul
sum·mate
sum·ma·tion
sum·ma·tion·al
Sum·mer·son-
    Bar·ker meth·od
Sum·ner meth·od
sump
sun·burn
sun·spots
sun·stroke
su·per·ab·duc·tion
su·per·ac·id
su·per·a·cid·i·ty
su·per·ac·tiv·i·ty
su·per·a·cute
su·per·al·bu·mi·no·sis
su·per·al·i·men·ta·tion
su·per·al·ka·lin·i·ty
su·per·bus
su·per·cen·tral
su·per·cer·e·bel·lar
su·per·cil·i·ar·y
su·per·cil·i·um
    pl su·per·cil·i·a

su·per·di·crot·ic
su·per·dis·ten·tion
su·per·duct
su·per·duc·tion
su·per·e·go
su·per·e·vac·u·a·tion
su·per·ex·ci·ta·tion
su·per·ex·ten·sion
su·per·fe·cun·da·tion
su·per·fe·cun·di·ty
su·per·fe·ta·tion
su·per·fi·cial
su·per·fi·ci·es
   pl su·per·fi·ci·es
su·per·foe·ta·tion
   var of su·per·fe·ta·tion
su·per·fu·sion
su·per·gene
su·per·im·preg·nate
su·per·im·preg·na·tion
su·per·in·duce
su·per·in·duc·tion
su·per·infect
su·per·in·fec·tion
su·per·in·vo·lu·tion
su·pe·ri·or
su·pe·ri·or·ly
su·per·lac·ta·tion
su·per·le·thal
su·per·mo·lec·u·lar
su·per·mol·e·cule
su·per·mo·ron
su·per·na·tant
su·per·nate
su·per·nor·mal
su·per·nu·mer·ar·y
   pl su·per·nu·mer·ar·ies
su·per·nu·tri·tion
su·per·o·in·fe·ri·or
su·per·o·lat·er·al
su·per·o·me·di·al
su·per·ov·u·late
su·per·ov·u·la·tion
su·per·par·a·site
su·per·par·a·sit·ic
su·per·par·a·sit·ism
su·per·phos·phate
su·per·pig·men·ta·tion

su·per·po·ten·cy
   pl su·per·po·ten·cies
su·per·po·tent
su·per·salt
su·per·sat·u·rate
su·per·sat·u·ra·tion
su·per·scrip·tion
su·per·se·cre·tion
su·per·sen·si·tive
su·per·sen·si·ti·za·tion
su·per·sep·tal
su·per·son·ic
su·per·son·i·cal·ly
su·per·struc·ture
su·per·tem·po·ral
su·per·ten·sion
su·per·ve·nos·i·ty
su·per·ven·tion
su·per·ver·sion
su·per·vi·sor
su·per·volt·age
su·pi·nate
su·pi·na·tion
su·pi·na·tor
su·pine
sup·pe·da·ne·ous
sup·pe·da·ne·um
sup·ple·ment
sup·ple·men·tal
sup·ple·men·ta·ry
sup·port
sup·port·er
sup·por·tive
sup·pos·i·to·ry
   pl sup·pos·i·to·ries
sup·press
sup·pres·sant
sup·pres·sion
sup·pres·sive
sup·pres·sor
sup·pu·rant
sup·pu·rate
sup·pu·ra·tion
sup·pu·ra·tive
su·pra·a·or·tic
su·pra·ar·tic·u·lar
su·pra·au·ric·u·lar
su·pra·cal·lo·sal
su·pra·car·di·nal

su·pra·cel·lu·lar
su·pra·cer·vi·cal
su·pra·cho·roid
   or su·pra·cho·roi·dal
su·pra·cho·roi·dal
   or su·pra·cho·roid
su·pra·cho·roi·de·a
su·pra·cil·i·ar·y
su·pra·cla·vic·u·lar
su·pra·cla·vic·u·lar·is pro·
   pri·us
su·pra·cli·noid
su·pra·clu·sion
su·pra·com·mis·sure
su·pra·con·dy·lar
su·pra·cos·ta·lis
   pl su·pra·cos·ta·les
su·pra·di·a·phrag·mat·ic
su·pra·di·a·phrag·mat·i·cal·
   ly
su·pra·ge·nic·u·late
su·pra·gin·gi·val
su·pra·gle·noid
su·pra·glot·tal
   or su·pra·glot·tic
su·pra·glot·tic
   or su·pra·glot·tal
su·pra·gran·u·lar
su·pra·he·pat·ic
su·pra·hy·oid
su·pra·in·gui·nal
su·pra·le·thal
su·pra·le·va·tor
su·pra·lim·i·nal
su·pra·lim·i·nal·ly
su·pra·mal·le·o·lar
su·pra·mam·mil·lar·y
su·pra·man·dib·u·lar
su·pra·mar·gin·al
su·pra·mas·toid
su·pra·max·il·la
   pl su·pra·max·il·las
   or su·pra·max·il·lae
su·pra·max·il·lar·y
su·pra·me·a·tal
su·pra·men·tal
su·pra·na·sal
su·pra·nu·cle·ar
su·pra·oc·cip·i·tal

su·pra·oc·clu·sion
su·pra·om·pha·lo·dym·i·a
su·pra·op·tic
su·pra·op·ti·co·hy·poph·y·se·al
su·pra·or·bit·al
su·pra·pa·tel·lar
su·pra·pel·vic
su·pra·pin·e·al
su·pra·mas·toid
su·pra·max·il·lary
su·pra·me·a·tal
su·pra·nu·cle·ar
su·pra·oc·cip·i·tal
su·pra·oc·clu·sion
su·pra·om·pha·lo·dym·ia
su·pra·op·tic
su·pra·op·ti·co·hy·poph·y·se·al
su·pra·or·bit·al
su·pra·pa·tel·lar
su·pra·pel·vic
su·pra·pin·e·al
su·pra·pleu·ral
su·pra·pu·bic
su·pra·re·nal
su·pra·re·nal·ec·to·my
   pl su·pra·re·nal·ec·to·mies
su·pra·re·na·lis ab·er·ra·ta
su·pra·re·nal·ism
su·pra·re·nal·op·a·thy
su·pra·scap·u·la
   pl su·pra·scap·u·las
   or su·pra·scap·u·lae
su·pra·scap·u·lar
su·pra·scle·ral
su·pra·sel·lar
su·pra·son·ic
su·pra·spi·nal
su·pra·spi·na·tus
su·pra·spi·nous
su·pra·sple·ni·al
su·pra·sta·pe·di·al
su·pra·ster·nal
su·pra·ste·rol
su·pra·tem·po·ral
su·pra·ten·to·ri·al
su·pra·ton·sil·lar
su·pra·tri·gem·i·nal

su·pra·troch·le·ar
su·pra·um·bil·i·cal
su·pra·vag·i·nal
su·pra·val·vu·lar
su·pra·ven·tric·u·lar
su·pra·ver·gence
su·pra·ves·i·cal
su·pra·vi·tal
su·ra
   pl su·rae
su·ral
sur·al·i·men·ta·tion
sur·a·min
sur·cin·gle
sur·di·tas
sur·di·ty
   pl sur·di·ties
sur·do·car·di·ac
sur·ex·ci·ta·tion
sur·face
sur·face-ac·tive
sur·fac·tant
sur·geon
sur·geon a·poth·e·car·y
   pl sur·geon a·poth·e·car·ies
sur·geon gen·er·al
   pl sur·geons gen·er·al
sur·ger·y
   pl sur·ger·ies
sur·gi·cal
sur·gi·cal·ly
Su·ri·nam bark
sur·ra
sur·rah
   var of sur·ra
sur·ro·gate
sur·sum·duc·tion
sur·sum·ver·gence
sur·sum·ver·gent
sur·sum·ver·sion
sur·veil·lance
sus·cep·ti·bil·i·ty
   pl sus·cep·ti·bil·i·ties
sus·cep·ti·ble
sus·cep·ti·bly
sus·ci·tate
sus·ci·ta·tion
sus·pend·ed
sus·pen·sion

sus·pen·soid
sus·pen·so·ri·um
   pl sus·pen·so·ri·a
sus·pen·so·ry
   pl sus·pen·so·ries
sus·pi·ra·tion
sus·pi·ri·um
   pl sus·pi·ri·a
sus·ten·tac·u·lar
sus·ten·tac·u·lum
   pl sus·ten·tac·u·la
su·sur·ra·tion
su·sur·rus
su·ti·lains
Sut·ter blood group
su·tu·ra
   pl su·tu·rae
su·tu·rae cra·ni·i
su·tur·al
su·ture
sux·a·me·tho·ni·um
Sved·berg flo·ta·tion u·nit
swab
swage
swal·low
swathe
sway·back
sweat
Swe·di·aur dis·ease
swee·ney
   var of swee·ny
swee·ny
   pl swee·nies
sweet·bread
swell·head
swell·ing
Swift dis·ease
swim·mer's itch
swin·ney
   var of swee·ny
sy·co·ma
   pl sy·co·mas
   or sy·co·ma·ta
sy·co·si·form
sy·co·sis
   pl sy·co·ses
Syd·en·ham cho·re·a

syl·la·bus
 pl syl·la·bus·es
 or syl·la·bi
syl·lep·si·ol·o·gy
 pl syl·lep·si·ol·o·gies
syl·lep·sis
 pl syl·lep·ses
syl·van
syl·vat·ic
syl·vi·an
Syl·vi·an aq·ue·duct
Syl·vi·an fis·sure
sym·bal·lo·phone
sym·bi·o·gen·ic
sym·bi·on
sym·bi·ont
sym·bi·o·sis
 pl sym·bi·o·ses
sym·bi·ot
 or sym·bi·ote
sym·bi·ote
 or sym·bi·ot
sym·bi·ot·ic
 or sym·bi·ot·i·cal
sym·bi·ot·i·cal
 or sym·bi·ot·ic
sym·bi·ot·i·cal·ly
sym·bleph·a·ron
sym·bleph·a·ro·sis
sym·bol
sym·bo·li·a
sym·bol·ic
sym·bol·ism
sym·bol·i·za·tion
sym·bo·lo·pho·bi·a
sym·clo·sene
sym·di·chlo·ro·eth·yl·ene
sy·me·li·a
sym·e·lus
Syme am·pu·ta·tion
sym·e·tine
sym·me·lus
 pl sym·me·li
sym·met·ric
 or sym·met·ri·cal
sym·met·ri·cal
 or sym·met·ric
sym·me·try
 pl sym·me·tries

sym·pa·ral·y·sis
sym·pa·thec·to·my
 pl sym·pa·thec·to·mies
sym·path·e·o·neu·ri·tis
sym·pa·thet·ic
sym·pa·thet·i·cal·ly
sym·pa·thet·i·co·mi·met·ic
sym·pa·thet·i·co·to·ni·a
sym·pa·thet·i·co·ton·ic
sym·pa·thet·o·blast
sym·path·i·cec·to·my
sym·path·i·co·blast
sym·path·i·co·blas·to·ma
 pl sym·path·i·co·blas·to·
   mas
 or sym·path·i·co·blas·to·
   ma·ta
sym·path·i·co·cy·to·ma
 pl sym·path·i·co·cy·to·mas
 or sym·path·i·co·cy·to·ma·
   ta
sym·path·i·co·go·ni·o·ma
 pl sym·path·i·co·go·ni·o·
   mas
 or sym·path·i·co·go·ni·o·
   ma·ta
sym·path·i·co·lyt·ic
sym·path·i·co·mi·met·ic
sym·path·i·co·neu·ri·tis
sym·path·i·cop·a·thy
sym·path·i·co·to·ni·a
sym·path·i·co·ton·ic
sym·path·i·co·trop·ic
sym·path·i·cus
sym·pa·thin
sym·pa·thism
sym·pa·thist
sym·pa·thiz·er
sym·path·o·blast
sym·pa·tho·blas·to·ma
 pl sym·pa·tho·blas·to·mas
 or sym·pa·tho·blas·to·ma·ta
sym·pa·tho·chro·maf·fin
sym·path·o·gone
sym·pa·tho·go·ni·a
sym·pa·tho·go·ni·o·ma
 pl sym·pa·tho·go·ni·o·mas
 or sym·pa·tho·go·ni·o·ma·
   ta

sym·pa·tho·lyt·ic
sym·pa·tho·ma
 pl sym·pa·tho·mas
 or sym·pa·tho·ma·ta
sym·pa·tho·mi·met·ic
sym·pa·thy
 pl sym·pa·thies
sym·pet·al·ous
sym·pex·i·on
sym·pex·is
sym·phal·an·gism
sym·phy·o·ceph·a·lus
sym·phy·se·al
 or sym·phy·si·al
sym·phy·si·al
 or sym·phy·se·al
sym·phys·ic
sym·phys·i·ec·to·my
sym·phys·i·on
sym·phys·i·or·rha·phy
sym·phys·i·o·tome
sym·phys·i·ot·o·my
 pl sym·phys·i·ot·o·mies
sym·phy·sis
 pl sym·phy·ses
sym·phy·sis pu·bis
sym·phy·so·dac·ty·li·a
sym·phy·sop·si·a
sym·phy·so·ske·li·a
sym·plasm
sym·plast
sym·po·di·a
sym·po·sium
 pl sym·po·si·ums
 or sym·po·si·a
symp·tom
symp·to·mat·ic
symp·to·mat·i·cal·ly
symp·to·mat·o·log·ic
 or symp·to·mat·o·log·i·cal
symp·to·mat·o·log·i·cal
 or symp·to·mat·o·log·ic
symp·to·mat·o·log·i·cal·ly
symp·to·ma·tol·o·gy
 pl symp·to·ma·tol·o·gies
symp·tom·less
symp·to·sis
sym·pus
sym·sep·a·lous

381

syn·ac·to·sis
syn·a·del·phus
syn·aer·e·sis
  pl syn·aer·e·ses
  var of syn·er·e·sis
syn·aes·the·si·a
  var of syn·es·the·si·a
syn·aes·the·si·al·gi·a
  var of syn·es·the·si·al·gi·a
syn·aes·thet·ic
  var of syn·as·thet·ic
syn·al·gi·a
syn·al·gic
syn·a·nas·to·mo·sis
  pl syn·a·nas·to·mo·ses
sy·nan·che
syn·an·the·ma
  pl syn·an·the·mas
  or syn·an·the·ma·ta
syn·an·throp·ic
syn·an·thro·py
  pl syn·an·thro·pies
syn·an·throse
syn·apse
  pl sy·nap·ses
syn·ap·sis
  pl syn·ap·ses
syn·ap·tase
syn·ap·tene
syn·ap·tic
  or syn·ap·ti·cal
syn·ap·ti·cal
  or syn·ap·tic
syn·ap·to·lem·ma
syn·ap·tol·o·gy
  pl syn·ap·tol·o·gies
syn·ap·to·ne·mal com·plex
syn·ap·to·som·al
syn·ap·to·some
syn·ar·thro·di·a
syn·ar·thro·di·al
syn·ar·thro·di·al·ly
syn·ar·thro·phy·sis
  pl syn·ar·thro·phy·ses
syn·ar·thro·sis
  pl syn·ar·thro·ses
syn·can·thus
syn·car·y·on
  or syn·kar·y·on

syn·ceph·a·lus
  pl syn·ceph·a·li
syn·chei·li·a
  var of syn·chi·li·a
syn·che·sis
  var of syn·chy·sis
shy·chi·li·a
syn·chon·dro·ses
syn·chon·dro·si·al
syn·chon·dro·sis
  pl syn·chon·dro·ses
syn·chon·drot·o·my
  pl syn·chon·drot·o·mies
syn·cho·pex·i·a
syn·cho·pex·y
syn·chro·cy·clo·tron
syn·chro·nism
syn·chro·nous
syn·chro·ny
  pl syn·chro·nies
syn·chro·tron
syn·chy·sis
syn·ci·ne·sis
syn·cli·nal
syn·clit·ic
syn·cli·tism
syn·clon·ic
syn·clo·nus
  pl syn·clo·ni
syn·co·pal
syn·co·pe
syn·cop·ic
syn·cy·ti·al
syn·cy·ti·o·ly·sin
syn·cy·ti·o·ma
  pl syn·cy·ti·o·mas
  or syn·cy·ti·o·ma·ta
syn·cy·ti·o·tox·in
syn·cy·ti·o·tro·pho·blast
syn·cy·ti·um
  pl syn·cy·ti·a
syn·dac·tyl
  or syn·dac·tyle
syn·dac·tyle
  or syn·dac·tyl
syn·dac·tyl·i·a
syn·dac·tyl·ic
  or syn·dac·ty·lous
syn·dac·ty·lism

syn·dac·ty·lous
  or syn·dac·tyl·ic
syn·dac·ty·lus
syn·dac·ty·ly
  pl syn·dac·ty·lies
syn·de·sis
syn·des·mec·to·pi·a
syn·des·mi·tis
syn·des·mo·cho·ri·al
syn·des·mo·di·as·ta·sis
syn·des·mo·lo·gi·a
syn·des·mol·o·gy
syn·des·mo·pex·y
syn·des·mor·rha·phy
syn·des·mo·sis
  pl syn·des·mo·ses
syn·des·mot·ic
syn·des·mot·o·my
  pl syn·des·mot·o·mies
syn·det
syn·drome
syn·drom·ic
syn·ech·i·a
  pl syn·ech·i·ae
syn·ech·i·al
syn·ech·o·tome
syn·e·chot·o·my
syn·en·ceph·a·lo·cele
syn·eph·rine
syn·er·e·sis
  pl syn·er·e·ses
syn·er·get·ic
syn·er·gi·a
syn·er·gic
  or syn·er·gi·cal
syn·er·gi·cal
  or syn·er·gic
syn·er·gi·cal·ly
syn·er·gism
syn·er·gist
syn·er·gis·tic
  or syn·er·gis·ti·cal
syn·er·gis·ti·cal
  or syn·er·gis·tic
syn·er·gis·ti·cal·ly
syn·er·gy
  pl syn·er·gies
syn·es·the·si·a
syn·es·the·si·al·gi·a

syn·es·thet·ic
syn·e·ze·sis
var of syn·i·ze·sis
Syn·ga·mus la·ryn·ge·us
syn·gam·ic
syn·ga·mous
syn·ga·my
syn·ge·ne·ic
syn·ge·ne·si·o·plas·tic
syn·ge·ne·si·o·plas·ty
syn·ge·ne·si·o·trans·plan·ta·tion
syn·ge·ne·si·ous
syn·gen·e·sis
pl syn·gen·e·ses
syn·ge·net·ic
syn·gig·no·scism
syn·hex·yl
syn·hi·dro·sis
sy·ni·a·trist
syn·i·dro·sis
syn·i·ze·sis
syn·kar·y·on
or syn·car·y·on
syn·ki·ne·si·a
syn·ki·ne·sis
pl syn·ki·ne·ses
syn·ki·net·ic
syn·ne·ma·tin
syn·o·don·ti·a
syn·oph·rys
syn·oph·thal·mi·a
syn·oph·thal·mus
syn·op·si·a
syn·op·to·phore
syn·or·chi·dism
or syn·or·chism
syn·or·chism
or syn·or·chi·dism
syn·os·che·os
syn·os·te·o·phyte
syn·os·te·o·sis
pl syn·os·te·o·ses
or syn·os·to·sis
syn·os·tose
syn·os·to·sis
pl syn·os·to·ses
syn·os·tot·ic
syn·os·tot·ic·al·ly

syn·o·ti·a
syn·o·tus
syn·o·vec·to·my
pl syn·o·vec·to·mies
syn·o·vi·a
syn·o·vi·al
syn·o·vi·al·ly
syn·o·vi·al·o·ma
pl syn·o·vi·al·o·mas
or syn·o·vi·al·o·ma·ta
syn·o·vi·o·en·do·the·li·o·ma
pl syn·o·vi·o·en·do·the·li·o·mas
or syn·o·vi·o·en·do·the·li·o·ma·ta
syn·o·vi·o·ma
pl syn·o·vi·o·mas
or syn·o·vi·o·ma·ta
syn·o·vip·a·rous
syn·o·vi·tis
syn·tac·tic
or syn·tac·ti·cal
syn·tac·ti·cal
or syn·tac·tic
syn·tac·tics
syn·tal·i·ty
pl syn·tal·i·ties
syn·ta·sis
syn·tax·is
syn·tec·tic
or syn·tec·ti·cal
syn·tec·ti·cal
or syn·tec·tic
syn·thase
syn·ther·mal
syn·the·sis
pl syn·the·ses
syn·the·size
syn·the·tase
syn·thet·ic
or syn·thet·i·cal
syn·thet·i·cal
or syn·thet·ic
syn·thet·i·cal·ly
syn·tho·rax
syn·ton·ic
syn·to·nin
syn·tro·phism

syn·tro·pho·blast
syn·tro·pho·blas·tic
syn·trop·ic
syn·tro·phus
pl syn·tro·phi
syn·tro·py
pl syn·tro·pies
Sy·pha·ci·a
syph·i·lel·cos
syph·i·lel·cus
syph·i·le·mi·a
syph·i·lid
syph·i·li·on·thus
pl syph·i·li·on·thi
syph·i·lis
syph·i·lit·ic
syph·i·li·za·tion
syph·i·lize
syph·i·lo·derm
or syph·i·lo·der·ma
syph·i·lo·der·ma
pl syph·i·lo·der·ma·ta
or syph·i·lo·derm
syph·i·lo·der·ma·tous
syph·i·lo·gen·e·sis
syph·i·log·ra·pher
syph·i·log·ra·phy
pl syph·i·log·ra·phies
syph·i·loid
syph·i·lol·o·gist
syph·i·lol·o·gy
pl syph·i·lol·o·gies
syph·i·lo·ma
pl syph·i·lo·mas
or syph·i·lo·ma·ta
syph·i·lom·a·tous
syph·i·lo·nych·i·a
syph·i·lop·a·thy
syph·i·lo·phobe
syph·i·lo·pho·bi·a
syph·i·lo·phy·ma
pl syph·i·lo·phy·mas
or syph·i·lo·phy·ma·ta
syph·i·lo·psy·cho·sis
pl syph·i·lo·psy·cho·ses
syph·i·lo·ther·a·py
pl syph·i·lo·ther·a·pies
sy·rig·mo·pho·ni·a
sy·rig·mus

syr·in·gad·e·no·ma
  pl syr·in·gad·e·no·mas
  or syr·in·gad·e·no·ma·ta
syr·in·gad·e·no·sus
sy·ringe
sy·rin·go·bul·bi·a
sy·rin·go·car·ci·no·ma
  pl sy·rin·go·car·ci·no·mas
  or sy·rin·go·car·ci·no·ma·ta
sy·rin·go·cele
  or sy·rin·go·coele
sy·rin·go·coele
  or sy·rin·go·cele
sy·rin·go·coe·li·a
sy·rin·go·cyst·ad·e·no·ma
  pl sy·rin·go·cyst·ad·e·no·mas
  or sy·rin·go·cyst·ad·e·no·ma·ta
sy·rin·go·cys·to·ma
  pl sy·rin·go·cys·to·mas
  or sy·rin·go·cys·to·ma·ta
sy·rin·goid

syr·in·go·ma
  pl syr·in·go·mas
  or syr·in·go·ma·ta
sy·rin·go·me·nin·go·cele
sy·rin·go·my·e·li·a
sy·rin·go·my·el·ic
sy·rin·go·my·e·lo·cele
syr·inx
  pl sy·rinx·es
  or sy·rin·ges
syr·o·sing·o·pine
syr·up
sys·sar·co·sis
  pl sys·sar·co·ses
sys·sar·cot·ic
sys·so·ma
sys·so·mic
sys·so·mus
sys·tal·tic
sys·ta·sis
sys·tem
sys·te·ma

sys·te·mat·ic
  or sys·te·mat·i·cal
sys·te·mat·i·cal
  or sys·te·mat·ic
sys·te·mat·i·cal·ly
sys·te·ma·ti·za·tion
sys·tem·a·tize
sys·tem·ic
sys·tem·i·cal·ly
sys·tem·oid
sys·to·le
sys·tol·ic
sys·trem·ma
  pl sys·trem·mas
  or sys·trem·ma·ta
sy·zyg·i·al
syz·y·gy
  pl syz·y·gies
Sza·bo sign
Szent-Györ·gyi test
Syz·ma·now·ski op·er·a·tion

T

T cell
T lym·pho·cyte
Taarn·hoj op·er·a·tion
tab·a·co·sis
ta·ba·cum
tab·a·gism
tab·a·nid
Ta·ban·i·dae
Ta·ba·nus
ta·bar·di·llo
ta·ba·tière a·na·to·mique
ta·bel·la
  pl ta·bel·lae

ta·bes
  pl ta·bes
ta·bes dor·sa·lis
ta·bes·cence
ta·bes·cent
ta·bet·ic
ta·bet·i·form
tab·ic
tab·id
tab·la·ture
ta·ble
ta·ble·spoon

ta·ble·spoon·ful
  pl ta·ble·spoon·fuls
  or ta·ble·spoons·ful
tab·let
ta·boo
ta·bo·pa·ral·y·sis
  pl ta·bo·pa·ral·y·ses
ta·bo·pa·re·sis
  pl ta·bo·pa·re·ses
ta·bu
  var of ta·boo
tab·u·lar
tache noire
  pl taches noires

384

tach·e·om·e·ter
taches ro·sées len·ti·cu·
  laires
ta·chet·ic
ta·chis·to·scope
ta·chis·to·scopic
ta·chis·to·scop·i·cal·ly
tach·o·gram
ta·chog·ra·phy
  pl ta·chog·ra·phies
ta·chom·e·ter
tach·y·al·i·men·ta·tion
tach·y·ar·rhyth·mi·a
tach·y·aux·e·sis
  pl tach·y·aux·e·ses
tach·y·car·di·a
tach·y·car·di·ac
tach·y·graph
ta·chyg·ra·phy
tach·y·la·li·a
tach·y·lo·gi·a
ta·chym·e·ter
tach·y·pha·gi·a
tach·y·pha·si·a
tach·y·phe·mi·a
tach·y·phra·si·a
tach·y·phre·ni·a
tach·y·phy·lax·i·a
tach·y·phy·lax·is
  pl tach·y·phy·lax·es
tach·y·pne·a
tach·y·pnoe·a
  var of tach·y·pne·a
tach·y·pne·ic
tach·y·rhyth·mi·a
ta·chys·ter·ol
tach·y·sys·to·le
tac·tile
tac·til·i·ty
  pl tac·til·i·ties
tac·tion
tac·toid
tac·tom·e·ter
tac·tu·al
tac·tu·al·ly
tac·tus
tae·di·um vi·tae
tae·ni·a
  var of te·ni·a

tae·ni·a·cide
  var of te·ni·a·cide
tae·ni·a·fuge
  var of te·ni·a·fuge
Tae·ni·a·rhyn·chus
tae·ni·a·sis
  var of te·ni·a·sis
tae·ni·form
  var of te·ni·form
tae·ni·oid
  var of te·ni·oid
tae·ni·o·la
  var of te·ni·o·la
tae·ni·o·pho·bi·a
  var of te·ni·o·pho·bi·a
tag
tag·a·tose
tag·ma
  pl tag·ma·ta
tail
tail·bone
taint
tai·pan
Ta·ka·ta-A·ra test
Ta·ka·ya·su dis·ease
ta·ko·sis
ta·lal·gi·a
ta·lar
tal·bu·tal
talc
talc·o·sis
  pl talc·o·ses
tal·cum
tal·i·on
tal·i·pes
tal·i·pom·a·nus
Tall·er·man treat·ment
tal·low
Tall·quist meth·od
Tal·ma-
  Mor·i·son op·er·a·tion
ta·lo·cal·ca·ne·al
ta·lo·cal·ca·ne·o·na·vic·u·
  lar
ta·lo·cru·ral
ta·lo·fib·u·lar
ta·lo·mal·le·o·lar
ta·lo·na·vic·u·lar
tal·o·nid

ta·lose
ta·lo·tib·i·al
ta·lus
  pl ta·li
ta·ma
tam·a·rin
tam·a·rind
tam·bour
tam·pan
tam·pon
tam·pon·ade
  or tam·pon·age
tam·pon·age
  or tam·pon·ade
tam·pon·ing
tam·pon·ment
ta·na·pox
tan·dem
tan·gent
Tan·gi·er dis·ease
tan·nase
tan·nate
tan·nic
tan·nin
tan·no·phil
Tan·ret-May·er test
Tan·ret re·a·gent
tan·ta·lum
tan·trum
tap
ta·pei·no·ceph·a·ly
ta·pe·tal
ta·pe·to·ret·i·nal
ta·pe·tum
  pl ta·pe·ta
tape·worm
taph·e·pho·bi·a
  or taph·i·pho·bi·a
taph·i·pho·bi·a
  or taph·e·pho·bi·a
Ta·pi·a syn·drome
tap·i·no·ce·phal·ic
tap·i·no·ceph·a·ly
  pl tap·i·no·ceph·a·lies
tap·i·o·ca
ta·pir
ta·pir·oid
ta·pote·ment
tap·root

tar
Tar·ak·tog·e·nos
tar·an·tism
ta·ran·tu·la
   pl ta·ran·tu·las
   or ta·ran·tu·lae
ta·ras·sis
ta·rax·a·cum
ta·rax·e·in
ta·rax·is
tar·ba·gan
Tar·dieu ec·chy·mo·ses
tar·dive
tare
tar·get
tar·ich·a·tox·in
Tar·nier sign
ta·ro
tar·ry
tars·ad·e·ni·tis
tar·sal
tar·sa·le
   pl tar·sa·li·a
tar·sal·gi·a
tar·sec·to·my
   pl tar·sec·to·mies
tar·si·tis
tar·so·chei·lo·plas·ty
tar·soc·la·sis
tar·so·ma·la·ci·a
tar·so·met·a·tar·sal
Tar·so·nem·i·dae
tar·so·pha·lan·ge·al
tar·so·phy·ma
   pl tar·so·phy·mas
   or tar·so·phy·ma·ta
tar·so·pla·si·a
tar·so·plas·ty
   pl tar·so·plas·ties
tar·sop·to·si·a
tar·sop·to·sis
   pl tar·sop·to·ses
tar·sor·rha·phy
   pl tar·sor·rha·phies
tar·sot·o·my
   pl tar·sot·o·mies
tar·sus
   pl tar·si
tar·tar

tar·tar·at·ed
   or tar·trat·ed
tar·tar·ic
tar·trate
tar·trat·ed
   or tar·tar·at·ed
tar·tra·zine
tar·tron·ic
Ta·ru·i dis·ease
Tash·kent ul·cer
taste
tat·too
Tau·ber test
tau·rine
tau·ro·cho·lan·o·poi·e·sis
tau·ro·cho·late
tau·ro·cho·lic
tau·ro·dont
tau·ryl
Taus·sig-Bing com·plex
Taus·sig-
   Bla·lock op·er·a·tion
tau·to·me·ni·al
tau·to·mer
tau·tom·er·al
tau·tom·er·ase
tau·to·mer·ic
tau·tom·er·ism
Ta·wa·ra node
tax·is
   pl tax·es
tax·o·di·um
tax·on
   pl tax·ons
   or tax·a
tax·o·nom·ic
   or tax·o·nom·i·cal
tax·o·nom·i·cal
   or tax·o·nom·ic
tax·o·nom·i·cal·ly
tax·on·o·mist
tax·on·o·my
   pl tax·on·o·mies
Tay cho·roid·i·tis
Tay-Sachs dis·ease
tea·ber·ry
Teal test
tear
tear·gas

teart
tease
tea·spoon
tea·spoon·ful
   pl tea·spoon·fuls
   or tea·spoons·ful
teat
teb·u·tate
tech·ne·ti·um
tech·ne·tron·ic
tech·nic
tech·ni·cal
tech·ni·cian
tecn·nique
tech·nol·o·gist
tech·nol·o·gy
   pl tech·nol·o·gies
tec·lo·zan
tec·no·cyte
   var of tek·no·cyte
tec·tal
tec·ti·form
tec·to·bul·bar
tec·to·ceph·a·ly
   pl tec·to·ceph·a·lies
tec·to·cer·e·bel·lar
tec·ton·ic
tec·to·ri·al
tec·to·ri·um
   pl tec·to·ri·a
tec·to·ru·bral
tec·to·spi·nal
tec·tum
   pl tec·ta
te·di·ous
teethe
Tee·van law
te·flu·rane
teg·men
   pl teg·mi·na
teg·men·tal
teg·men·to·ol·i·var·y
teg·men·tum
   pl teg·men·ta
   or teg·u·men·tum
teg·u·ment
   pl teg·u·men·ta
   or teg·men·tum
teg·u·men·tal

teg·u·men·ta·ry
Teich·mann crys·tals
tei·cho·ic
tei·chop·si·a
tek·no·cyte
te·la
   pl te·lae
tel·al·gi·a
tel·an·gi·ec·ta·si·a
   or tel·an·gi·ec·ta·sis
tel·an·gi·ec·ta·sis
   pl tel·an·gi·ec·ta·ses
   or tel·an·gi·ec·ta·si·a
tel·an·gi·ec·tat·ic
tel·an·gi·ec·to·des
tel·an·gi·o·ma
   pl tel·an·gi·o·mas
   or tel·an·gi·o·ma·ta
tel·an·gi·on
tel·an·gi·o·sis
   pl tel·an·gi·o·sis·es
   or tel·an·gi·o·ses
tel·an·gi·tis
tel·au·gic
tel·e·an·gi·ec·ta·sis
   pl tel·e·an·gi·ec·ta·ses
tel·e·car·di·og·ra·phy
tele·car·di·o·gram
tele·car·di·o·phone
tel·e·cep·tor
tel·e·ci·ne·si·a
tel·e·ci·ne·sis
tel·e·co·balt
tel·e·cu·rie
tel·e·den·drite
tel·e·den·dron
tel·e·di·a·stol·ic
tel·e·flu·or·os·co·py
te·leg·o·ny
   pl te·leg·o·nies
tel·e·ki·ne·sis
   pl tel·e·ki·ne·ses
tel·e·lec·tro·car·di·o·gram
tel·e·lec·tro·ther·a·peu·tics
te·lem·e·ter
tel·e·met·ric
tel·e·met·ri·cal·ly
te·lem·e·try
   pl te·lem·e·tries

tel·en·ce·phal·ic
tel·en·ceph·a·lon
   pl tel·en·ceph·a·la
tel·e·neu·rite
tel·e·neu·ron
te·le·o·log·ic
   or te·le·o·log·i·cal
te·le·o·log·i·cal
   or te·le·o·log·ic
te·le·ol·o·gy
   pl te·le·ol·o·gies
tel·e·o·mi·to·sis
tel·e·op·si·a
tel·e·or·gan·ic
te·le·o·roent·gen·o·gram
tel·e·o·ther·a·peu·tics
tel·e·path·ic
tel·e·path·i·cal·ly
te·lep·a·thist
te·lep·a·thy
   pl te·lep·a·thies
tel·e·ra·di·og·ra·phy
   pl tel·e·ra·di·og·ra·phies
tel·e·ra·di·um
tel·er·gy
   pl tel·er·gies
tel·e·roent·gen·o·gram
tel·e·roent·ge·nog·ra·phy
   pl tel·e·roent·ge·nog·ra·
     phies
tel·e·ster·e·o·roent·ge·nog·
   ra·phy
tel·es·the·si·a
tel·es·thet·ic
tel·e·sys·tol·ic
tel·e·ther·a·py
   pl tel·e·ther·a·pies
tel·lu·rate
tel·lu·ric
tel·lu·ri·um
tel·o·cen·tric
tel·o·coele
tel·o·den·dri·on
   pl tel·o·den·dri·a
tel·o·den·dron
tel·o·gen
tel·og·no·sis
tel·o·lec·i·thal
tel·o·lem·ma

tel·o·mer
tel·o·mere
te·lom·er·i·za·tion
te·lom·er·ize
tel·o·phase
tel·o·phrag·ma
   pl tel·o·phrag·ma·ta
Tel·o·spo·rid·i·a
tel·o·spo·ri·di·an
tel·o·syn·ap·sis
tem·per
tem·per·a·ment
tem·per·ance
tem·per·ate
tem·per·a·ture
tem·plate
tem·ple
tem·plet
   var of tem·plate
tem·po·la·bile
tem·po·ra
tem·po·ral
tem·po·ra·lis
tem·po·rary
tem·po·ri·za·tion
tem·po·rize
tem·po·ro·fron·tal
tem·po·ro·man·dib·u·lar
tem·po·ro·max·il·lar·y
tem·po·ro·oc·cip·i·tal
tem·po·ro·pa·ri·e·tal
tem·po·ro·pon·tine
tem·po·ro·sphe·noid
tem·po·sta·bile
tem·u·lence
tem·u·len·ti·a
te·na·cious
te·nac·i·ty
   pl te·nac·i·ties
te·nac·u·lum
   pl te·nac·u·lums
   or te·nac·u·la
ten·al·gi·a
ten·den·cy
   pl ten·den·cies
ten·der
ten·der·ness
ten·di·ni·tis
   or ten·don·i·tis

ten·di·no·plas·ty
pl ten·di·no·plas·ties
ten·di·no·su·ture
ten·di·nous
ten·do
pl ten·di·nes
ten·dol·y·sis
pl ten·dol·y·ses
ten·do·mu·cin
ten·do·mu·coid
ten·don
ten·don·i·tis
or ten·di·ni·tis
ten·do·plas·ty
pl ten·do·plas·ties
ten·do·syn·o·vi·tis
ten·do·vag·i·nal
ten·do·vag·i·ni·tis
te·neb·ric
Te·neb·ri·o
te·nec·to·my
pl te·nec·to·mies
te·nes·mic
te·nes·mus
te·ni·a
te·ni·a·cide
te·ni·ae co·li
te·ni·a·fuge
te·ni·a·sis
te·ni·form
te·ni·oid
te·ni·o·la
te·ni·o·pho·bi·a
ten·nis el·bow
te·no·de·sis
pl te·no·de·ses
ten·o·dyn·i·a
ten·o·fi·bril
te·nol·y·sis
pl te·nol·y·ses
te·nom·e·ter
te·no·my·o·plas·ty
pl te·no·my·o·plas·ties
te·no·my·ot·o·my
pl te·no·my·ot·o·mies
Ten·on cap·sule
ten·o·nec·to·my
pl ten·o·nec·to·mies
ten·o·ni·tis

ten·o·nom·e·ter
ten·on·to·dyn·i·a
ten·on·tog·ra·phy
ten·on·tol·o·gy
te·non·to·my·o·plas·ty
pl te·non·to·my·o·plas·ties
te·non·to·my·ot·o·my
pl te·non·to·my·ot·o·mies
te·non·to·the·ci·tis
ten·o·phyte
ten·o·plas·tic
ten·o·plas·ty
pl ten·o·plas·ties
ten·o·re·cep·tor
te·nor·rha·phy
pl te·nor·rha·phies
ten·o·si·tis
ten·os·to·sis
pl ten·os·to·si·es
or ten·os·to·se
ten·o·su·ture
ten·o·syn·o·vec·to·my
pl ten·o·syn·o·vec·to·mies
ten·o·syn·o·vi·al
ten·o·syn·o·vi·o·ma
pl ten·o·syn·o·vi·o·mas
or ten·o·syn·o·vi·o·ma·ta
te·no·syn·o·vi·tis
ten·o·tome
te·not·o·mist
te·not·o·mize
te·not·o·my
pl te·not·o·mies
ten·o·vag·i·ni·tis
ten·si·om·e·ter
ten·sion
ten·si·ty
ten·sive
ten·sor
ten·sure
ten·ta·cle
ten·ta·tive
tenth·me·ter
ten·tig·i·nous
ten·ti·go
ten·to·ri·al
ten·to·ri·um
pl ten·to·ri·a
ten·to·ri·um ce·re·bel·li

ten·u·ate
te·nu·i·ty
ten·u·ous
te·pa
teph·ro·my·e·li·tis
tep·id
te·por
ter in di·e
ter·ab·del·la
ter·a·mor·phous
ter·as
pl ter·a·ta
ter·at·ic
ter·a·tism
ter·a·to·blas·to·ma
pl ter·a·to·blas·to·mas
or ter·a·to·blas·to·ma·ta
ter·a·to·car·ci·no·ma
pl ter·a·to·car·ci·no·mas
or ter·a·to·car·ci·no·ma·ta
ter·a·to·gen
ter·a·to·gen·e·sis
pl ter·a·to·gen·e·ses
ter·a·to·gen·et·ic
or ter·a·to·gen·ic
ter·a·to·gen·ic
or ter·a·to·gen·et·ic
ter·a·tog·e·nous
ter·a·tog·e·ny
ter·a·toid
ter·a·to·log·ic
or ter·a·to·log·i·cal
ter·a·to·log·i·cal
or ter·a·to·log·ic
ter·a·tol·o·gist
ter·a·tol·o·gy
pl ter·a·tol·o·gies
ter·a·to·ma
pl ter·a·to·mas
or ter·a·to·ma·ta
ter·a·tom·a·tous
ter·a·to·pho·bi·a
ter·a·to·sis
pl ter·a·to·ses
ter·a·to·sper·mi·a
ter·bi·um
ter·chlor·eth·yl·ene
te·re
ter·e·bene

ter·e·bin·thi·nate
ter·e·bin·thine
ter·e·bin·thism
ter·e·bra·che·sis
   pl ter·e·bra·che·ses
ter·e·brat·ing
ter·e·bra·tion
teres
   pl ter·e·tes
term
ter·mi·nal
ter·mi·nal·i·za·tion
ter·mi·nal·ly
ter·mi·na·ti·o
   pl ter·mi·na·ti·o·nes
ter·mi·na·tion
ter·mi·na·ti·o·nes ner·vo·rum li·ber·ae
ter·mi·ni
ter·mi·nol·o·gy
   pl ter·mi·nol·o·gies
ter·mi·nus
   pl ter·mi·nus·es
   or ter·mi·ni
ter·na·ry
Ter·ni·dens
ter·o·di·line
ter·ox·a·lene
ter·pene
ter·pe·nic
ter·pe·nism
ter·pin
ter·pin·e·ol
ter·pi·nol
ter·ra
   pl ter·rae
Ter·ry meth·od
ter·tian
ter·ti·ar·ism
ter·ti·ar·y
   pl ter·ti·ar·ies
ter·ti·grav·i·da
ter·tip·a·ra
   pl ter·tip·a·ras
   or ter·tip·a·rae
ter·va·lence
Tes·chen dis·ease
Tes·la cur·rent
tes·sel·lat·ed

test
test-tube
tes·ta·ceous
tes·tal·gi·a
test·cross
tes·tec·to·my
tes·ti·cle
tes·tic·u·lar
tes·tis
   pl tes·tes
tes·ti·tis
tes·toid
tes·to·lac·tone
tes·tos·ter·one
tet·a·nal
te·ta·ni·a
te·tan·ic
te·tan·i·cal·ly
te·tan·i·form
tet·a·nig·e·nous
tet·a·nil·la
tet·a·nin
tet·a·nism
tet·a·ni·za·tion
tet·a·nize
tet·a·no·can·na·bin
tet·a·node
tet·a·noid
tet·a·no·ly·sin
tet·a·no·ly·sis
tet·a·nom·e·ter
tet·a·no·mo·tor
tet·a·no·pho·bi·a
tet·a·no·spas·min
tet·a·nus
tet·a·ny
   pl tet·a·nies
tet·ar·cone
   or tet·tar·to·cone
tet·ar·co·nid
   or te·tar·to·co·nid
te·tar·ta·no·pi·a
te·tar·ta·nop·si·a
te·tar·to·cone
   or tet·ar·cone
te·tar·to·co·nid
   or tet·ar·co·nid
tet·i·o·thal·ein
tet·mil

tet·ra·ba·sic
tet·ra·ba·sic·i·ty
   pl tet·ra·ba·sic·i·ties
tet·ra·ben·a·zine
tet·ra·bra·chi·us
tet·ra·bro·mo·phe·nol·phthal·e·in
tet·ra·caine
tet·ra·chei·rus
tet·ra·chlor·eth·ane
   or tet·ra·chlo·ro·eth·ane
tet·ra·chlo·ride
tet·ra·chlo·ro·eth·ane
   or tet·ra·chlor·eth·ane
tet·ra·chlo·ro·eth·yl·ene
tet·ra·chlo·ro·meth·ane
tet·ra·chrome
tet·ra·crot·ic
tet·ra·coc·cus
   pl tet·ra·coc·ci
tet·ra·cy·cline
tet·rad
tet·ra·dac·tyl
tet·ra·dac·ty·ly
te·trad·ic
tet·ra·eth·yl
tet·ra·eth·yl·am·mo·ni·um
tet·ra·eth·yl·py·ro·phos·phate
tet·ra·eth·yl·thi·u·ram
tet·ra·eth·yl·thi·u·ram di·sul·fide
tet·ra·gen·ic
te·trag·e·nous
tet·ra·go·num
tet·ra·hy·dric
tet·ra·hy·dro·can·nab·in·ol
tet·ra·hy·dro·fo·lic
tet·ra·hy·dro·zo·line
Tet·ra·hy·men·a
tet·ra·i·o·do·phe·nol·phthal·e·in
tet·ra·i·o·do·phthal·e·in
tet·ra·i·o·do·thy·ro·nine
te·tral·o·gy
   pl te·tral·o·gies
te·tral·o·gy of Fal·lot
tet·ra·mas·ti·a
tet·ra·mas·ti·gote

tet·ra·ma·zi·a
te·tram·e·lus
Te·tram·er·es
tet·ra·mer·ic
te·tram·er·ism
te·tram·er·ous
tet·ra·meth·yl·am·mo·ni·um
tet·ra·meth·yl·ene·di·a·mine
te·tram·i·sole
tet·ra·ni·trol
tet·ra·nop·si·a
tet·ra·nu·cle·o·tide
tet·ra·o·don·tox·in
   or tet·ro·do·tox·in
tet·ra·oph·thal·mus
tet·ra·o·tus
tet·ra·pa·re·sis
tet·ra·pep·tide
tet·ra·pho·co·me·li·a
tet·ra·ple·gi·a
tet·ra·ploid
tet·ra·ploid·y
tet·ra·pod
tet·ra·pus
tet·ra·pyr·ro·le
tet·ra·sac·cha·ride
te·tras·ce·lus
tet·ra·so·mic
tet·ra·so·my
tet·ras·ter
tet·ra·sti·chi·a·sis
tet·ra·thi·o·nate
tet·ra·tom·ic
tet·ra·vac·cine
tet·ra·va·lent
tet·ra·zole
tet·ra·zo·li·um
tet·relle
tet·ro·do·tox·in
   or tet·ra·o·don·tox·in
tet·ro·do·tox·ism
tet·ro·nal
tet·roph·thal·mus
tet·ro·qui·none
tet·rose
te·tro·tus
te·trox·ide

te·tryd·a·mine
tet·ter
Tex·as fe·ver
tex·is
tex·ti·form
tex·to·blas·tic
tex·tur·al
tex·ture
tex·tus
   pl tex·tus
T-group
thal·a·men·ce·phal·ic
thal·a·men·ceph·a·lon
   pl thal·a·men·ceph·a·la
tha·lam·ic
tha·lam·i·cal·ly
thal·a·mo·cele
   or thal·a·mo·coele
thal·a·mo·coele
   or thal·a·mo·cele
thal·a·mo·cor·ti·cal
thal·a·mo·ge·nic·u·late
thal·a·mo·len·tic·u·lar
thal·a·mo·mam·mil·lar·y
thal·a·mo·pa·ri·e·tal
thal·a·mo·per·fo·rate
thal·a·mo·teg·men·tal
thal·a·mot·o·my
   pl thal·a·mot·o·mies
thal·a·mus
   pl thal·a·mi
thal·as·sa·mi·a
   var of thal·as·se·mi·a
thal·as·se·mi·a
thal·as·se·mic
tha·las·so·pho·bi·a
tha·las·so·po·si·a
tha·las·so·ther·a·py
   pl tha·las·so·ther·a·pies
tha·lid·o·mide
thal·lei·o·quin
thal·i·um
Thal·loph·y·ta
thal·lo·phyte
thal·lo·phyt·ic
thal·lo·spore
thal·lo·tox·i·co·sis
   pl thal·lo·tox·i·co·ses

thal·lus
   pl thal·lus·es
   or thal·li
tha·mu·ri·a
than·a·to·bi·o·log·ic
than·a·to·gno·mon·ic
than·a·tog·ra·phy
than·a·toid
than·a·tol·o·gy
   pl than·a·tol·o·gies
than·a·to·ma·ni·a
than·a·to·phid·i·a
than·a·to·pho·bi·a
than·a·to·pho·ric
than·a·top·sy
   pl than·a·top·sies
than·a·tos
Thap·si·a
thas·sa·nae·mi·a
   var of thas·sa·ne·mi·a
thas·sa·ne·mi·a
thau·mat·ro·py
Thay·er-Doi·sy u·nit
the·ba·ic
the·ba·ine
the·be·si·an ves·sel
the·ca
   pl the·cae
the·cal
   or the·cate
the·cate
   or the·cal
the·ci·tis
thec·o·dont
the·co·ma
   pl the·co·mas
   or the·co·ma·ta
the·co·steg·no·sis
   pl the·co·steg·no·sis·es
   or the·co·steg·no·ses
the·e·lin
the·e·lol
Thei·ler vi·rus
Thei·le·ri·a
   pl Thei·le·ri·as
   or Thei·le·ri·ae
thei·le·ri·a·sis
the·ine
the·in·ism

Theis and Ben·e·dict
   meth·od
Theis meth·od
the·ism
the·lal·gi·a
the·lar·che
the·las·is
The·la·zi·a
thel·a·zi·a·sis
the·le·plas·ty
   pl the·le·plas·ties
the·ler·e·thism
the·li·o·ma
   pl the·li·o·mas
   or the·li·o·ma·ta
the·li·tis
the·li·um
   pl the·li·a
the·lon·cus
   pl the·lon·ci
the·lo·phleb·o·stem·ma
the·lor·rha·gi·a
the·lo·thism
thel·y·gen·ic
thel·y·go·ni·a
thel·y·to·ci·a
the·lyt·o·kous
the·lyt·o·ky
the·nar
then·yl·di·a·mine
then·yl·pyr·a·mine
The·o·bro·ma oil
the·o·bro·mine
the·o·ma·ni·a
the·o·pho·bi·a
the·o·phyl·line
the·o·ple·gi·a
the·o·ret·ic
   or the·o·ret·i·cal
the·o·ret·i·cal
   or the·o·ret·ic
the·o·ret·i·cal·ly
the·o·ry
   pl the·o·ries
the·o·ther·a·py
theque
ther·a·peu·sis
   pl ther·a·peu·ses

ther·a·peu·tic
   or ther·a·peu·ti·cal
ther·a·peu·ti·cal
   or ther·a·peu·tic
ther·a·peu·ti·cal·ly
ther·a·peu·tics
ther·a·peu·tist
ther·a·pi·a
ther·a·pi·a ster·i·li·sans
   mag·na
ther·a·pist
ther·a·py
   pl ther·a·pies
ther·en·ceph·a·lous
ther·i·ac
the·ri·a·ca
the·ri·a·ca an·drom·a·chi
the·ri·at·rics
Ther·i·di·i·dae
the·ri·od·ic
the·ri·o·gen·ol·o·gy
the·ri·o·ma
   pl the·ri·o·mas
   or the·ri·o·ma·ta
the·ri·o·mim·ic·ry
therm
ther·mae
therm·aes·the·si·a
   var of therm·es·the·si·a
therm·aes·the·si·om·e·ter
   var of therm·es·the·si·om·
   e·ter
therm·a·er·o·ther·a·py
ther·mal
therm·al·ge·si·a
ther·mal·gi·a
therm·an·aes·the·si·a
   var of therm·an·es·the·si·a
therm·an·al·ge·si·a
therm·an·es·the·si·a
ther·ma·to·log·ic
ther·ma·tol·o·gy
   pl ther·ma·tol·o·gies
ther·mel·om·e·ter
therm·es·the·si·a
therm·es·the·si·om·e·ter
therm·hyp·aes·the·si·a
   var of therm·hyp·as·
   the·si·a

therm·hy·per·aes·the·si·a
   var of therm·hy·per·es·the·
   si·a
therm·hy·per·es·the·si·a
therm·hyp·es·the·si·a
ther·mic
ther·mis·tor
ther·mo·an·aes·the·si·a
   var of ther·mo·an·es·
   the·si·a
ther·mo·an·al·ge·si·a
ther·mo·an·es·the·si·a
ther·mo·bi·ol·o·gy
ther·mo·cau·ter·y
   pl ther·mo·cau·ter·ies
ther·mo·chem·is·try
   pl ther·mo·chem·is·tries
ther·mo·chro·ism
ther·mo·co·ag·u·la·tion
ther·mo·cou·ple
ther·mo·cur·rent
ther·mo·dif·fu·sion
ther·mo·di·lu·tion
ther·mo·du·ric
ther·mo·dy·nam·ics
ther·mo·e·lec·tric
ther·mo·e·lec·tric·i·ty
ther·mo·ex·ci·to·ry
ther·mo·gen·e·sis
   pl ther·mo·gen·e·ses
ther·mo·gen·ic
ther·mog·e·nous
ther·mo·gram
ther·mo·graph
ther·mo·graph·ic
ther·mo·graph·i·cal·ly
ther·mog·ra·phy
   pl ther·mog·ra·phies
ther·mo·hyp·aes·the·si·a
   var of ther·mo·hyp·es·the·
   si·a
ther·mo·hy·per·aes·the·si·a
   var of ther·mo·hy·per·es·
   the·si·a
ther·mo·hy·per·al·ge·si·a
ther·mo·hy·per·es·the·si·a
ther·mo·hyp·es·the·si·a
ther·mo·in·hib·i·to·ry
ther·mo·la·bile

ther·mol·o·gy
ther·mol·y·sis
   pl ther·mol·y·ses
ther·mo·lyt·ic
ther·mo·mas·sage
ther·mom·e·ter
ther·mo·met·ric
ther·mom·e·try
   pl ther·mom·e·tries
ther·mo·neu·ro·sis
   pl ther·mo·neu·ro·ses
ther·moph·a·gy
   pl ther·moph·a·gies
ther·mo·phile
   or ther·moph·i·lous
   or ther·mo·phil·ic
ther·mo·phil·ic
   or ther·moph·i·lous
   or ther·mo·phile
ther·moph·i·lous
   or ther·mo·phile
   or ther·mo·phil·ic
ther·mo·pho·bi·a
ther·mo·phore
ther·mo·phy·lic
ther·mo·pile
ther·mo·plac·en·tog·ra·phy
ther·mo·plas·tic
ther·mo·ple·gi·a
ther·mo·pol·yp·ne·a
ther·mo·pol·yp·noe·a
   var of ther·mo·pol·yp·ne·a
ther·mo·re·cep·tor
ther·mo·reg·u·la·tion
ther·mo·reg·u·la·tor
ther·mo·reg·u·la·to·ry
ther·mo·scope
ther·mo·set
ther·mo·sta·bil·i·ty
ther·mo·sta·ble
ther·mo·stat
ther·mo·stat·i·cal·ly
ther·mo·ste·re·sis
   pl ther·mo·ste·re·ses
ther·mo·stro·muhr of Rein
ther·mo·sys·tal·tic
ther·mo·sys·tal·tism
ther·mo·tac·tic
ther·mo·tax·ic

ther·mo·tax·is
   pl ther·mo·tax·es
ther·mo·ther·a·py
   pl ther·mo·ther·a·pies
ther·mot·ics
ther·mo·to·nom·e·ter
ther·mo·tox·in
ther·mo·tra·che·ot·o·my
   pl ther·mo·tra·che·ot·o·mies
ther·mo·trop·ic
ther·mot·ro·pism
the·ro·morph
the·ro·mor·phi·a
the·ro·mor·phism
The·ro·pi·the·cus
the·sau·ris·mo·sis
the·sau·ro·sis
   pl the·sau·ro·sis·es
   or the·sau·ro·ses
the·sis
   pl the·ses
the·ta
the·tin
the·ve·tin
thi·a·ben·da·zole
thi·a·cet·a·zone
thi·am·a·zole
thi·a·min
   or thi·a·mine
thi·am·i·nase
thi·a·mine
   or thi·a·min
thi·am·i·prine
thi·am·phen·i·col
thi·am·y·lal
thi·az·e·sim
thi·a·zide
thi·a·zine
thi·a·zole
thi·a·zol·sul·fone
thick·wind·ed
Thie·mann dis·ease
Thie·mann-
   Fleisch·ner dis·ease
thi·e·mi·a
Thiersch graft
thi·eth·yl·per·a·zine
thigh

thigh·bone
thig·maes·the·si·a
   var of thig·mes·the·si·a
thig·man·aes·the·si·a
   var of thig·man·es·the·si·a
thig·man·es·the·si·a
thig·mes·the·si·a
thig·mo·tax·is
   pl thig·mo·tax·es
thig·mot·ro·pism
thi·hex·i·nol
thi·mer·o·sal
thin-lay·er chro·ma·tog·ra·phy
thi·o
thi·o·ac·e·tal
thi·o·al·de·hyde
thi·o·bac·te·ri·um
   pl thi·o·bac·te·ri·a
thi·o·bar·bi·tal
thi·o·bar·bit·u·rate
thi·o·bar·bi·tu·ric
thi·o·car·bam·ide
thi·o·car·ban·i·lide
thi·o·chrome
thi·oc·tic
thi·o·cy·a·nate
thi·o·cy·an·ic
thio·di·phe·nyl·am·ine
thi·o·glu·co·si·dase
thi·o·gua·nine
thi·ol
thi·ol·prive
thi·o·mer·sa·late
thi·o·ne·ine
thi·on·ic
thi·o·nin
thi·o·pen·tal
thi·o·pen·tone
thi·o·phene
thi·o·phile
thi·o·phil·ic
thi·o·pro·pa·zate
Thi·o·rho·da·ce·ae
Thi·o·rid·a·zine
thi·o·sa·lan
thi·o·sem·i·car·ba·zone
thi·o·sin·am·ine
thi·o·sul·fate

thi·o·sul·fur·ic
thi·o·tep·a
thi·o·thix·ene
thi·o·u·ra·cil
thi·o·u·re·a
thi·phen·a·mil
thi·ram
third-de·gree burn
thirst
Thi·ry fis·tu·la
thix·o·trop·ic
thix·ot·ro·pism
thix·ot·ro·py
  pl thix·ot·ro·pies
thlip·sen·ceph·a·lus
Tho·ma am·pul·la
Thom·as splint
Thom·as-
  La·vol·lay meth·od
Thom·sen dis·ease
Thom·so·ni·an·ism
thon·zyl·a·mine
tho·ra·cal·gi·a
tho·ra·cec·to·my
  pl tho·ra·cec·to·mies
tho·ra·cen·te·sis
  pl tho·ra·cen·te·ses
tho·rac·ic
tho·rac·i·co·lum·bar
tho·ra·co·ab·dom·i·nal
tho·ra·co·a·ceph·a·lus
tho·ra·co·a·cro·mi·al
tho·ra·co·ce·li·ot·o·my
tho·ra·co·ce·los·chi·sis
  pl tho·ra·co·ce·los·chi·i·es
  or tho·ra·co·ce·los·chi·ses
tho·ra·co·cen·te·sis
  pl tho·ra·co·cen·te·ses
tho·ra·co·coe·li·ot·o·my
  var of tho·ra·co·ce·li·ot·o·my
tho·ra·co·coe·los·chi·sis
  var of tho·ra·co·ce·los·chi·sis
tho·ra·co·cyl·lo·sis
  pl tho·ra·co·cyl·lo·sis·es
  or tho·ra·co·cyl·lo·se
tho·ra·co·cyr·to·sis
tho·ra·co·del·phus

tho·ra·co·did·y·mus
tho·ra·co·dyn·i·a
tho·ra·co·gas·tro·did·y·mus
tho·ra·co·gas·tros·chi·sis
  pl tho·ra·co·gas·tros·chi·sis·es
  or tho·ra·co·gas·tros·chi·ses
tho·ra·co·lap·a·rot·o·my
  pl tho·ra·co·lap·a·rot·o·mies
tho·ra·co·lum·bar
tho·ra·col·y·sis
  pl tho·ra·col·y·ses
tho·ra·com·e·lus
  pl tho·ra·com·e·li
tho·ra·com·e·ter
tho·ra·com·e·try
tho·ra·co·my·o·dyn·i·a
tho·ra·cop·a·gus
  pl tho·ra·cop·a·gus·es
  or tho·ra·cop·a·gi
tho·ra·co·par·a·ceph·a·lus
  pl tho·ra·co·par·a·ceph·a·li
tho·ra·co·par·a·si·tus
tho·ra·cop·a·thy
tho·ra·co·plas·ty
  pl tho·ra·co·plas·ties
tho·ra·co·pneu·mo·plas·ty
tho·ra·cos·chi·sis
  pl tho·ra·cos·chi·sis·es
  or tho·ra·cos·chi·ses
tho·ra·co·scope
tho·ra·co·scop·ic
tho·ra·cos·co·py
  pl tho·ra·cos·co·pies
tho·ra·co·ste·no·sis
tho·ra·cos·to·my
  pl tho·ra·cos·to·mies
tho·ra·cot·o·my
  pl tho·ra·cot·o·mies
tho·ra·del·phus
tho·rax
  pl tho·rax·es
  or tho·ra·ces
tho·ri·um
Thorn test
tho·ron
thor·ough·joint
thor·ough·pin

Thor·son-Bioerck-
  syn·drome
tho·zal·i·none
thread
thread·worm
thread·y
threat·en
threm·ma·tol·o·gy
thre·o·nine
thre·o·nyl
thre·ose
threp·sol·o·gy
  pl threp·sol·o·gies
thresh·old
thrill
thrix
thrix an·nu·la·ta
throat
throb
Throck·mor·ton re·flex
throe
throm·base
throm·bas·the·ni·a
throm·bec·to·my
  pl throm·bec·to·mies
throm·bin
throm·bin·o·gen
throm·bo·an·gi·i·tis
  pl throm·bo·an·gi·i·ti·des
throm·bo·an·gi·i·tis o·blit·
  er·ans
throm·bo·ar·ter·i·tis
throm·bo·as·the·ni·a
throm·bo·blast
throm·bo·cav·er·no·si·tis
throm·boc·la·sis
  pl throm·boc·la·ses
throm·bo·clas·tic
throm·bo·cyst
throm·bo·cys·tis
throm·bo·cyte
throm·bo·cy·thae·mi·a
  var of throm·bo·cy·the·
  mi·a
throm·bo·cy·the·mia
throm·bo·cyt·ic
throm·bo·cy·to·bar·in
throm·bo·cy·to·crit
throm·bo·cy·tol·y·sin

393

throm·bo·cy·tol·y·sis
throm·bo·cy·to·lyt·ic
throm·bo·cy·to·path·i·a
throm·bo·cy·to·path·ic
throm·bo·cy·to·top·a·thy
throm·bo·cy·to·pe·ni·a
throm·bo·cy·to·pe·nic
thrombo·cy·to·pher·e·sis
throm·bo·cy·to·poi·e·sis
  pl throm·bo·cy·to·poi·e·ses
throm·bo·cy·to·sis
  pl throm·bo·cy·to·ses
throm·bo·em·bo·lec·to·my
  pl throm·bo·em·bo·lec·to·mies
throm·bo·em·bol·ic
throm·bo·em·bo·lism
throm·bo·em·bo·li·za·tion
throm·bo·em·bo·lus
  pl throm·bo·em·bo·li
throm·bo·en·dar·ter·ec·to·my
  pl throm·bo·en·dar·ter·ec·to·mies
throm·bo·end·ar·ter·i·tis
throm·bo·en·do·car·di·tis
throm·bo·gen
throm·bo·gen·e·sis
throm·bo·gen·ic
throm·boid
throm·bo·ki·nase
throm·bo·lym·phan·gi·tis
  pl throm·bo·lym·phan·gi·ti·des
throm·bol·y·sis
  pl throm·bol·y·ses
throm·bo·lyt·ic
throm·bon
throm·bop·a·thy
  pl throm·bop·a·thies
throm·bo·pe·ni·a
throm·bo·pe·nic
throm·bo·phil·i·a
throm·bo·phle·bi·tis
  pl throm·bo·phle·bi·ti·des
throm·bo·plas·tic
throm·bo·plas·ti·cal·ly
throm·bo·plas·tid
throm·bo·plas·tin

throm·bo·plas·tin·o·gen
throm·bo·poi·e·sis
  pl throm·bo·poi·e·ses
throm·bo·poi·e·tic
throm·bose
throm·bo·sis
  pl throm·bo·ses
throm·bo·sta·sis
  pl throm·bo·sta·ses
throm·bo·sthe·nin
throm·bot·ic
thom·bo·zym
throm·bus
  pl throm·bi
throt·tle
throw·back
thrush
thryp·sis
Thu·ja
thu·jone
thu·li·um
thumb
thumb·nail
Thun·berg and Ahl·gren
  meth·od
thus
thy·la·ken·trin
thyme
thy·mec·to·mize
thy·mec·to·my
  pl thy·mec·to·mies
thy·mel·co·sis
thy·mer·ga·si·a
thy·mer·ga·sic
thy·mic
thy·mi·co·lym·phat·ic
thy·mi·dine
thy·mine
thy·mi·on
thy·mi·tis
thy·mo·cyte
thy·mo·gen·ic
thy·mo·hy·dro·qui·none
thy·mo·ke·sis
thy·mo·ki·net·ic
thy·mol
thy·mo·lep·tic
thy·mol·phthal·ein

thy·mo·ma
  pl thy·mo·mas
  or thy·mo·ma·ta
thy·mo·no·ic
thy·mo·nu·cle·ic
thy·mop·a·thy
  pl thy·mop·a·thies
thy·mo·pha·ryn·ge·al
thy·mo·priv·ic
thy·mo·pri·vous
thy·mo·sis
thy·mus
  pl thy·mus·es
  or thy·mi
thy·re·o·a·pla·si·a con·gen·i·ta
thy·re·o·gen·ic
thy·re·o·pri·val
thy·ro·ad·e·ni·tis
thy·ro·a·pla·si·a
thy·ro·ar·y·te·noid
thy·ro·cal·ci·to·nin
thy·ro·car·di·ac
thy·ro·cele
thy·ro·cer·vi·cal
thy·ro·chon·drot·o·my
  pl thy·ro·chon·drot·o·mies
thy·ro·cri·cot·o·my
  pl thy·ro·cri·cot·o·mies
thyro·ep·i·glot·tic
thy·ro·gen·ic
  or thy·rog·e·nous
thy·rog·e·nous
  or thy·ro·gen·ic
thy·ro·glob·u·lin
thy·ro·glos·sal
thy·ro·hy·al
thy·ro·hy·oid
  or thy·ro·hy·oi·de·an
thy·roid
thy·roi·hy·oi·de·an
  or thy·ro·hy·oid
thy·roi·dal
thy·roi·dec·to·mize
thy·roi·dec·to·my
  pl thy·roi·dec·to·mies
thy·roid·ism
thy·roid·i·tis
thy·roid·i·za·tion

394

thy·roi·dot·o·my
  pl thy·roi·dot·o·mies
thy·ro·i·o·dine
thy·roi·do·tox·in
thy·roid-
  stim·u·lat·ing hor·mone
thy·rol·y·sin
thy·ro·me·dan
thy·ro·meg·a·ly
thy·ro·mi·met·ic
thy·ron·cus
thy·ro·nine
thy·ro·nyl
thy·ro·par·a·thy·roi·dec·to·
  my
  pl thy·ro·par·a·thy·roi·dec·
    to·mies
thy·ro·pha·ryn·ge·al
thy·ro·pha·ryn·ge·us
thy·ro·pri·val
thy·ro·priv·ic
thy·ro·pro·te·in
thy·rop·to·sis
  pl thy·rop·to·sis·es
  or thy·rop·to·ses
thy·ro·sis
thy·ro·ther·a·py
thy·rot·o·my
  pl thy·rot·o·mies
thy·ro·tox·ic
thy·ro·tox·ic·i·ty
  pl thy·ro·tox·ic·i·ties
thy·ro·tox·i·co·sis
  pl thy·ro·tox·i·co·ses
thy·ro·tox·in
thy·ro·tro·phic
  or thy·ro·trop·ic
thy·ro·tro·phi·cal·ly
thy·ro·tro·phin
  or thy·ro·tro·pin
thy·ro·trop·ic
  or thy·ro·tro·phic
thy·ro·tro·pin
  or thy·ro·tro·phin
thy·rot·ro·pism
thy·rox·in
  or thy·rox·ine
thy·rox·ine
  or thy·rox·in

tib·i·a
  pl tib·i·as
  or tib·i·ae
tib·i·al
tib·i·al·gi·a
tib·i·a·lis
  pl tib·i·a·les
tib·io·fem·o·ral
tib·i·o·fib·u·la
  pl tib·i·o·fib·u·las
  or tib·i·o·fib·u·lae
tib·i·o·fib·u·lar
tib·i·o·tar·sal
ti·bro·fan
tic dou·lou·reux
tick
tick-borne
tic·po·lon·ga
tic·tol·o·gy
tid·al
tide
Tie·de·mann gland
Tiet·ze dis·ease
ti·ges·tol
tight·ness
ti·gog·e·nin
tig·o·nin
ti·groid
ti·grol·y·sis
  pl ti·grol·y·ses
Til·laux dis·ease
tilt
tim·ber
  or tim·bre
tim·bre
  or tim·ber
tim·o·thy
tin
tin·cal
tinc·tion
tinc·to·ri·al
tinc·to·ri·al·ly
tinc·tu·ra
tinc·ture
tine
tin·e·a
tin·e·a bar·bae
tin·e·a cap·i·tis
tin·e·a cor·po·ris

tin·e·a cru·ris
tin·e·a pe·dis
tin·e·a ver·si·co·lor
tin·e·al
Ti·nel sign
tin·gi·ble
tin·gle
tin·ni·tus
tin·tom·e·ter
tin·to·met·ric
tin·tom·e·try
  pl tin·tom·e·tries
Ti·pu·li·dae
ti·queur
tire
ti·sane
Tis·dall meth·od
Ti·se·li·us ap·pa·ra·tus
tis·sue
tis·su·lar
ti·ta·ni·um
ti·ter
tit·il·la·tion
ti·trant
ti·trate
ti·tra·tion
ti·tre
  var of ti·ter
ti·trim·e·ter
ti·tri·met·ric
ti·trim·e·try
tit·u·ba·tion
Tit·y·us
to·bac·co
  pl to·bac·cos
  or to·bac·coes
To·bey-Ay·er test
to·bra·my·cin
to·cam·phyl
to·co·al·gog·ra·phy
to·co·dy·na·mom·e·ter
  var of to·ko·dy·na·mom·e·
    ter
to·co·graph
  var of to·ko·graph
to·cog·ra·phy
  or to·kog·ra·phy
to·col·o·gist
  or to·kol·o·gist

to·col·o·gy
pl to·col·o·gies
or to·kol·o·gy
to·co·ma·ni·a
or to·ko·ma·ni·a
to·com·e·ter
var of to·kom·e·ter
to·com·e·try
var of to·kom·e·try
to·coph·er·ol
to·coph·er·so·lan
to·co·pho·bi·a
or to·ko·pho·bi·a
to·cus
or to·kus
Todd pa·ral·y·sis
toe
toe·drop
toe·nail
to·ga·vi·rus
toi·let
Toi·son so·lu·tion
To·ke·la·u ring·worm
to·ko·dy·na·mom·e·ter
to·ko·graph
to·kog·ra·phy
or to·cog·ra·phy
to·kol·o·gist
or to·col·o·gist
to·kol·o·gy
pl to·kol·o·gies
or to·col·o·gy
to·ko·ma·ni·a
or to·co·ma·ni·a
to·kom·e·ter
to·kom·e·try
to·ko·pho·bi·a
or to·co·pho·bi·a
to·kus
or to·cus
to·la·za·mide
to·laz·o·line
tol·bu·ta·mide
tol·er·ance
tol·er·ant
tol·er·ate
tol·er·a·tion
tol·er·o·gen

Tol·lens test
tol·naf·tate
to·lo·ni·um
tol·pyr·ra·mide
tol·u·ene
to·lu·ic
to·lu·i·dine
tol·u·ol
tol·u·yl·ene
tol·yl
to·ma·tin
tom·a·tine
to·men·tum
pl to·men·ta
Tomes fi·bers
Tom·ma·sel·li syn·drome
to·mo·gram
to·mo·graph
to·mo·graph·ic
to·mog·ra·phy
pl to·mog·ra·phies
to·mo·ma·ni·a
to·mo·to·ci·a
ton·al
to·na·pha·si·a
tone
tone-deaf
tone-deaf·ness
tongue
tongue-tie
ton·ic
ton·ic-clo·nic
to·nic·i·ty
pl to·nic·i·ties
To·ni-Fan·co·ni syn·drome
to·ni·tro·pho·bi·a
ton·ka
ton·o·clon·ic
to·no·fi·bril
to·no·fi·bril·la
pl to·no·fi·bril·lae
or to·no·fi·bril
to·no·gram
to·no·graph
to·nog·ra·phy
pl to·nog·ra·phies
to·nom·e·ter
to·no·met·ric

to·nom·e·try
pl to·nom·e·tries
to·no·plast
to·nos·cil·log·ra·phy
ton·o·scope
ton·sil
ton·sil·la
pl ton·sil·lae
ton·sil·lar
or ton·sil·lar·y
ton·sil·lar·y
or ton·sil·lar
ton·sil·lec·tome
ton·sil·lec·to·my
pl ton·sil·lec·to·mies
ton·sil·lit·ic
ton·sil·li·tis
ton·sil·lo·lith
ton·sil·lo·phar·yn·gi·tis
ton·sil·lo·tome
ton·sil·lot·o·my
pl ton·sil·lot·o·mies
ton·sil·lo·ty·phoid
ton·sil·sec·tor
ton·sure
to·nus
tooth
pl teeth
Tooth mus·cu·lar at·ro·
phy
tooth·ache
toothed
top·aes·the·si·a
var of top·es·the·si·a
top·ag·no·sis
pl top·ag·no·ses
to·pal·gi·a
to·pec·to·my
pl to·pec·to·mies
top·es·the·si·a
Töp·fer test
to·pha·ceous
to·phus
pl to·phi
top·ic
or top·i·cal
top·i·cal
or top·ic

top·i·cal·ly
To·pi·nard an·gle
top·o·al·gi·a
top·o·an·aes·the·si·a
   var of top·o·an·es·the·si·a
top·o·an·es·the·si·a
to·po·gen·e·sis
top·og·no·si·a
   or top·og·no·sis
top·og·no·sis
   pl top·og·no·sis·es
   or top·og·no·si·a
top·og·nos·tic
top·o·graph·ic
to·pog·ra·phy
   pl to·pog·ra·phies
to·pol·o·gy
   pl to·pol·o·gies
top·o·nar·co·sis
   pl top·o·nar·co·ses
top·o·neu·ro·sis
   pl top·o·neu·ro·ses
top·o·nym
to·pon·y·my
   pl to·pon·y·mies
top·o·pho·bi·a
top·o·phone
tor·cu·lar
tor·cu·lar He·roph·i·li
To·rek op·er·a·tion
to·ric
Tor·kild·sen pro·ce·dure
tor·mi·na
tor·mi·nal
tor·mi·nous
Torn·waldt dis·ease
to·rose
tor·pes·cence
tor·pid
tor·pid·i·ty
tor·por
tor·que
torr
tor·rec·fac·tion
tor·re·fy
Tor·ri·cel·lian vac·u·um
tor·si·oc·clu·sion
tor·si·om·e·ter

tor·sion
tor·sive
tor·si·ver·sion
tor·so
   pl tor·sos
   or tor·si
   or tor·soes
tor·soc·clu·sion
tort
tor·ti·col·lar
tor·ti·col·lis
tor·ti·pel·vis
tor·tu·os·i·ty
tor·tu·ous
Tor·u·la
   pl Tor·u·las
   or Tor·u·lae
tor·u·lar
tor·u·li tac·ti·les
tor·u·lo·ma
   pl tor·u·lo·mas
   or tor·u·lo·ma·ta
Tor·u·lop·sis
   pl Tor·u·lop·ses
tor·u·lo·sis
tor·u·lus
   pl tor·u·li
to·rus
   pl to·ri
tos·y·late
to·tal
to·ta·quine
To·ti op·er·a·tion
to·tip·o·tence
to·ti·po·ten·cy
   pl to·ti·po·ten·cies
to·tip·o·tent
to·ti·po·ten·tial
to·ti·po·ten·ti·al·i·ty
   pl to·ti·po·ten·ti·al·i·ties
touch
Tou·louse-
   Lau·trec dis·ease
tour de maî·tre
Tou·raine aph·tho·sis
Tou·rette dis·ease
Tour·nay sign
tour·ni·quet

Tou·ton cells
tow
Towne pro·jec·tion
Towne-
   Cham·ber·lain pro·jec·tion
Town·send op·er·a·tion
tox·ae·mi·a
   var of tox·e·mi·a
tox·ae·mic
   var of tox·e·mic
tox·al·bu·min
tox·al·bu·mose
tox·a·phene
Tox·as·ca·ris
tox·e·mi·a
tox·e·mic
tox·en·zyme
tox·ic
tox·i·cae·mi·a
   var of tox·i·ce·mi·a
tox·i·cant
tox·i·ce·mi·a
tox·i·cide
tox·ic·i·ty
   pl tox·ic·i·ties
tox·i·co·den·drol
Tox·i·co·den·dron
tox·i·co·der·ma
   pl tox·i·co·der·mas
   or tox·i·co·der·ma·ta
tox·i·co·der·ma·ti·tis
   pl tox·i·co·der·ma·ti·tis·es
   or tox·i·co·der·ma·ti·ti·des
tox·i·co·der·ma·to·sis
tox·i·co·gen·ic
tox·i·coid
tox·i·co·log·ic
   or tox·i·co·log·i·cal
tox·i·co·log·i·cal
   or tox·i·co·log·ic
tox·i·col·o·gist
tox·i·col·o·gy
   pl tox·i·col·o·gies
tox·i·co·ma·ni·a
tox·i·co·ma·ni·ac
tox·i·co·path·ic
tox·i·cop·a·thy

tox·i·co·pex·is
tox·i·co·phid·i·a
tox·i·co·pho·bi·a
tox·i·co·sis
   pl tox·i·co·ses
tox·i·der·ma·to·sis
   pl tox·i·der·ma·to·ses
tox·i·der·mi·tis
tox·if·er·ine
tox·if·er·ous
tox·i·gen·ic
tox·i·ge·nic·i·ty
   pl tox·i·ge·nic·i·ties
tox·ig·e·nous
tox·in
tox·in-an·ti·tox·in
tox·in·fec·tion
tox·ip·a·thy
tox·is·ter·ol
tox·i·ther·a·py
tox·i·tu·ber·cu·lide
Tox·o·car·a
tox·o·ca·ri·a·sis
tox·oid
tox·o·in·fec·tion
tox·o·lec·i·thin
tox·o·no·sis
tox·o·phil
tox·o·phil·ic
tox·o·phore
tox·o·phor·ic
   or tox·oph·o·rous
tox·oph·o·rous
   or tox·o·phor·ic
Tox·o·plas·ma
   pl Tox·o·plas·mas
   or Tox·o·plas·ma·ta
   or Tox·o·plas·ma
tox·o·plas·mat·ic
toxo·plas·mic
tox·o·plas·min
tox·o·plas·mo·sis
   pl tox·o·plas·mo·ses
Toyn·bee cor·pus·cle
tra·bec·u·la
   pl tra·bec·u·las
   or tra·bec·u·lae
tra·bec·u·lar
tra·bec·u·late

tra·bec·u·la·tion
trace
trac·er
tra·che·a
   pl tra·che·as
   or tra·che·ae
tra·che·a·ec·ta·sy
tra·che·al
tra·che·al·gi·a
tra·che·i·tis
tra·che·lag·ra
trach·e·lec·to·my
   pl trach·e·lec·to·mies
trach·e·le·ma·to·ma
   pl trach·e·le·ma·to·mas
   or trach·e·le·ma·to·ma·ta
tra·che·lism
trach·e·lis·mus
trach·e·li·tis
trach·e·lo·cyl·lo·sis
tra·che·lo·cys·ti·tis
trach·e·lo·dyn·i·a
trach·e·lo·ky·pho·sis
tra·che·lo·mas·toid
tra·che·lo·my·i·tis
trach·e·lo·par·a·si·tus
trach·e·lo·pex·i·a
tra·che·lo·pex·y
tra·che·lo·plas·ty
   pl tra·che·lo·plas·ties
tra·che·lor·rha·phy
   pl tra·che·lor·rha·phies
trach·e·lor·rhec·tes
trach·e·los·chi·sis
trach·e·lo·syr·in·gor·rha·
   phy
trach·e·lot·o·my
tra·che·o·a·er·o·cele
tra·che·o·blen·nor·rhe·a
tra·che·o·blen·nor·rhoe·a
   var of tra·che·o·blen·nor·
   rhe·a
tra·che·o·bron·chi·al
tra·che·o·bron·chi·tis
   pl tra·che·o·bron·chi·ti·des
tra·che·o·bron·chos·co·py
   pl tra·che·o·bron·chos·co·
   pies

tra·che·o·cele
tra·che·o·e·soph·a·ge·al
tra·che·o·fis·sure
tra·che·o·gram
tra·che·og·ra·phy
tra·che·o·la·ryn·ge·al
tra·che·o·lar·yn·got·o·my
tra·che·o·ma·la·ci·a
tra·che·o·path·i·a os·te·o·
   plas·ti·ca
tra·che·op·a·thy
tra·che·o·pha·ryn·ge·al
tra·che·oph·o·ny
   pl tra·che·oph·o·nies
tra·che·o·plas·ty
   pl tra·che·o·plas·ties
tra·che·o·py·o·sis
   pl tra·che·o·py·o·ses
tra·che·or·rha·gi·a
tra·che·or·rha·phy
tra·che·os·chi·sis
   pl tra·che·os·chi·sis·es
   or tra·che·os·chi·ses
tra·che·o·scop·ic
tra·che·os·co·py
   pl tra·che·os·co·pies
tra·che·o·ste·no·sis
   pl tra·che·o·ste·no·ses
tra·che·os·to·mize
tra·che·os·to·my
   pl tra·che·os·to·mies
tra·che·o·tome
tra·che·ot·o·mist
tra·che·ot·o·mize
tra·che·ot·o·my
   pl tra·che·ot·o·mies
tra·chi·el·co·sis
tra·chi·el·cus
tra·chi·tis
tra·cho·ma
tra·cho·ma·tous
tra·chy·chro·mat·ic
tra·chy·o·nych·i·a
tra·chy·pho·ni·a
trac·ing
tract
trac·tion
trac·tor

trac·tot·o·my
  pl trac·tot·o·mies
trac·tus
  pl trac·tus
Tra·cy meth·od
trade·mark
trag·a·canth
tra·gal
Tra·gi·a
tra·gi·cus
trag·o·mas·chal·i·a
trag·o·pho·ni·a
tra·goph·o·ny
tra·gus
  pl tra·gi
trail·er
train·a·ble
train·sick
train·sick·ness
trait
tram·a·dol
tra·maz·o·line
trance
tran·ex·am·ic
tran·quil·ize
tran·quil·iz·er
trans·ab·dom·i·nal
trans·ac·e·tyl·ase
trans·ac·e·tyl·a·tion
trans·ac·tion
trans·ac·y·lase
trans·ac·y·la·tion
trans·am·i·da·tion
trans·am·i·din·ase
trans·am·i·nase
trans·am·i·nate
trans·am·i·na·tion
trans·a·or·tic
trans·a·tri·al
trans·au·di·ent
trans·ax·i·al
trans·ax·o·nal
trans·ca·lent
trans·cal·lo·sal
trans·cav·i·tar·y
trans·con·dy·lar
trans·cor·ti·cal
trans·cor·tin
tran·scribe

tran·scrip·tion
trans·cu·ta·ne·al
  or trans·cu·ta·ne·ous
trans·cu·ta·ne·ous
  or trans·cu·ta·ne·al
trans·duce
trans·duc·er
trans·duc·tion
trans·du·o·de·nal
tran·sect
tran·sec·tion
trans·fer
trans·fer RNA
trans·fer·ase
trans·fer·ence
trans·fer·rin
trans·fix
trans·fix·ion
trans·fo·rate
trans·fo·ra·tion
trans·fo·ra·tor
trans·form
trans·for·ma·tion
trans·form·er
trans·fuse
trans·fu·sion
trans·fu·sion·al
trans·fu·sion·ist
trans·he·pat·ic
tran·sient
trans·il·i·ac
trans·il·lu·mi·na·ble
trans·il·lu·mi·nate
trans·il·lu·mi·na·tion
trans·il·lu·mi·na·tor
trans·isth·mi·an
tran·sis·tor
tran·si·tion·al
tran·si·to·ry
tran·si·to·zo·o·no·sis
trans·late
trans·la·tion
trans·lo·ca·tion
trans·lu·cen·cy
  pl trans·lu·cen·cies
trans·lu·cent
trans·lu·cid
trans·lu·mi·na·tion
trans·max·il·lar·y

trans·mem·brane
trans·meth·y·lase
trans·meth·yl·a·tion
trans·mi·gra·tion
trans·mis·si·bil·i·ty
  pl trans·mis·si·bil·i·ties
trans·mis·si·ble
trans·mis·sion
trans·mit
trans·mit·ta·ble
trans·mit·tance
trans·mit·ter
trans·mu·ral
trans·mu·ta·tion
trans·oc·u·lar
tran·so·nance
trans·or·bi·tal
trans·par·ent
trans·pep·ti·dase
trans·pep·ti·da·tion
trans·per·i·to·ne·al
trans·phos·pho·ryl·ase
trans·phos·phor·y·la·tion
tran·spir·a·ble
tran·spi·ra·tion
tran·spire
trans·pla·cen·tal
trans·plant
trans·plan·ta·tion
trans·pleu·ral
trans·port
trans·pose
trans·po·si·tion
trans·py·lo·ric
trans·ra·di·ant
trans·sa·cral
trans·seg·men·tal
trans·sep·tal
trans·sex·u·al
trans·sex·u·a·lism
trans·ten·to·ri·al
trans·tha·lam·ic
trans·tho·rac·ic
trans·tho·rac·i·cal·ly
trans·tra·che·al
trans·tym·pan·ic
tran·sub·stan·ti·ate
tran·sub·stan·ti·a·tion
tran·su·date

tran·su·da·tion
tran·su·da·to·ry
tran·sude
trans·u·ran·ic
trans·u·re·thral
trans·vag·i·nal
trans·ver·sa·lis
trans·verse
trans·ver·sec·to·my
 pl trans·ver·sec·to·mies
trans·ver·sion
trans·ver·sus
 pl trans·ver·si
trans·ves·i·cal
trans·ves·tism
trans·ves·tite
trans·ves·ti·tism
 var of trans·ves·tism
tran·yl·cy·pro·mine
tra·pe·zi·al
tra·pe·zi·form
tra·pe·zi·o·met·a·car·pal
tra·pe·zi·um
 pl tra·pe·zi·ums
 or tra·pe·zi·a
tra·pe·zi·us
trap·e·zoid
Trapp for·mu·la
Trau·be mem·brane
Trau·be-Her·ing curves
trau·ma
 pl trau·mas
 or trau·ma·ta
trau·mat·ic
trau·mat·i·cal·ly
trau·ma·tism
trau·ma·ti·za·tion
trau·ma·tize
trau·ma·tol·o·gy
 pl trau·ma·tol·o·gies
trau·ma·top·a·thy
trau·ma·top·ne·a
trau·ma·top·noe·a
 var of trau·ma·top·ne·a
trau·ma·to·sis
Traut·mann tri·an·gle
tra·vail
tray

Trea·cher Col·lins syn·
 drome
trea·cle
treat
treat·a·bil·i·ty
 pl treat·a·bil·i·ties
treat·a·ble
treat·ment
tre·foil
tre·ha·la
tre·ha·lase
tre·ha·lose
Treitz mus·cle
tre·ma
tre·mat·ic
Trem·a·to·da
trem·a·tode
trem·a·to·di·a·sis
 pl trem·a·to·di·a·ses
trem·ble
trem·bles
trem·el·loid
trem·el·lose
trem·e·tol
trem·o·gram
trem·o·graph
trem·o·la·bile
trem·o·lo
trem·o·pho·bi·a
trem·or
trem·o·sta·ble
trem·u·la·tion
tre·mu·lous
trem·u·lous·ly
trem·u·lous·ness
trench fe·ver
trench·foot
trench·mouth
Tren·de·len·burg po·si·tion
tre·pan
trep·a·na·tion
trep·a·nize
treph·i·na·tion
tre·phine
treph·o·cyte
treph·one
trep·i·dant
tre·pi·da·ti·o
trep·i·da·tion

trep·o·ne·ma
 pl trep·o·ne·mas
 or trep·o·ne·ma·ta
trep·o·ne·mal
Trep·o·ne·ma·ta·ce·ae
trep·o·ne·ma·to·sis
 pl trep·o·ne·ma·to·ses
trep·o·neme
trep·o·ne·mi·a·sis
 pl trep·o·ne·mi·a·ses
trep·o·ne·mi·ci·dal
trep·o·ne·min
tre·pop·ne·a
tre·pop·noe·a
 var of tre·pop·ne·a
trep·pe
Tre·sil·i·an sign
tre·sis
tre·tin·o·in
tri·ac·e·tate
tri·ac·e·tin
tri·ac·e·tyl·o·le·an·do·my·
 cin
tri·ad
tri·ad of Whip·ple
tri·age
tri·a·kai·dek·a·pho·bi·a
tri·al
tri·al·ist
tri·al·kyl·a·mine
tri·am·cin·o·lone
tri·am·py·zine
tri·am·ter·ene
tri·an·gle
tri·an·gu·lar
tri·an·gu·la·ris
 pl tri·an·gu·la·res
Tri·at·o·ma
tri·a·tom·ic
Tri·a·tom·i·dae
tri·a·tri·al
tri·ax·i·al
tri·a·zine
trib·ade
tri·bad·ic
trib·a·dism
trib·a·dy
 pl trib·a·dies
tri·ba·sic

tri·bas·i·lar
tribe
tri·bo·lu·mi·nes·cence
tri·bra·chi·us
tri·bro·mo·eth·a·nol
tri·bro·mo·meth·ane
tri·brom·sa·lan
tri·bu·tyr·in
tri·car·box·yl·ic
tri·cel·lu·lar
tri·ceph·a·lus
tri·ceps
   pl tri·ceps·es
   or tri·ceps
Tri·cer·com·o·nas
tri·cet·a·mide
trich·aes·the·si·a
   var of trich·es·the·si·a
trich·an·gi·ec·ta·si·a
trich·an·gi·ec·ta·sis
trich·a·tro·phi·a
trich·es·the·si·a
tri·chi·a·sis
tri·chi·na
   pl tri·chi·nas
   or tri·chi·nae
Trich·i·nel·la
   pl Trich·i·nel·lea
trich·i·nel·li·a·sis
   pl trich·i·nel·li·a·ses
trich·i·ni·a·sis
   pl trich·i·ni·a·ses
trich·i·ni·za·tion
trich·i·nize
tri·chi·no·scope
trich·i·no·sis
   pl trich·i·no·ses
trich·i·nous
trich·i·on
tri·chi·tis
tri·chlor·a·ce·tic
   or tri·chlo·ro·a·ce·tic
tri·chlor·eth·yl·ene
   or tri·chlo·ro·eth·yl·ene
tri·chlor·fon
tri·clo·ride
tri·clor·me·thi·a·zide
tri·clo·ro·ac·e·tal·de·hyde

tri·chlo·ro·a·ce·tic
   or tri·chlor·a·ce·tic
tri·chlo·ro·bu·tyl
tri·chlo·ro·eth·yl·ene
   or tri·chlor·eth·yl·ene
tri·chlo·ro·meth·ane
trich·o·aes·the·si·a
   var of trich·o·es·the·si·a
trich·o·an·aes·the·si·a
   var of trich·o·an·es·the·si·a
trich·o·an·es·the·si·a
trich·o·bac·te·ri·a
trich·o·be·zo·ar
Trich·o·bil·har·zi·a oc·el·
   la·ta
trich·o·car·di·a
trich·o·ceph·a·li·a·sis
   pl trich·o·ceph·a·li·a·ses
Trich·o·ceph·a·lus
trich·o·cla·si·a
tri·choc·la·sis
trich·o·clas·ma·ni·a
trich·o·cryp·to·sis
trich·o·cyst
Trich·o·dec·tes
Trich·o·der·ma
trich·o·ep·i·the·li·o·ma
   pl trich·o·ep·i·the·li·o·mas
   or trich·o·ep·i·the·li·o·ma·ta
trich·o·es·the·si·a
trich·o·es·the·si·om·e·ter
trich·o·gen
trich·o·gen·ic
   or tri·chog·e·nous
tri·chog·e·nous
   or trich·o·gen·ic
trich·o·glos·si·a
trich·o·hy·a·lin
trich·oid
trich·o·kryp·to·ma·ni·a
trich·o·lith
trich·o·lo·gi·a
tri·chol·o·gy
   pl tri·chol·o·gies
tri·cho·ma
trich·o·ma·de·sis
trich·o·ma·ni·a
trich·o·ma·tose
tri·cho·ma·to·sis

tri·chom·a·tous
trich·ome
trich·o·mic
trich·o·mo·na·ci·dal
trich·o·mo·na·cide
trich·o·mon·ad
tri·chom·o·nal
Trich·o·mon·as
trich·o·mo·ni·a·sis
   pl trich·o·mo·ni·a·ses
trich·o·mo·ni·cide
Trich·o·my·ce·tes
trich·o·my·co·sis
   pl trich·o·my·co·ses
tri·chon
trich·o·no·car·di·o·sis
trich·o·no·do·sis
   pl trich·o·no·do·ses·es
   or trich·o·no·do·ses
trich·o·no·sis
trich·o·path·ic
trich·o·path·o·pho·bi·a
tri·chop·a·thy
   pl tri·chop·a·thies
trich·o·pha·gi·a
tri·choph·a·gy
trich·o·pho·bi·a
trich·o·phyte
trich·o·phy·tid
trich·o·phy·tin
trich·o·phy·to·be·zo·ar
trich·o·phy·ton
   pl trich·o·phy·tons
   or trich·o·phy·ta
trich·o·phy·to·sis
trich·o·po·li·o·dys·tro·phy
trich·o·po·li·o·sis
trich·o·pti·lo·sis
   pl trich·o·pti·lo·ses
trich·o·rhi·no·pha·lan·ge·al
trich·or·rhe·a
trich·or·rhex·is
   pl trich·or·rhex·es
trich·or·rhex·o·ma·ni·a
trich·os·chi·sis
tri·chos·co·py
trich·o·sid·er·in
tri·cho·sis
   pl tri·cho·ses

Trich·o·spo·ron
trich·o·spo·ro·sis
    pl trich·o·spo·ro·sis·es
    or trich·o·spo·ro·ses
trich·o·sta·sis
    pl trich·o·sta·ses
trich·o·sta·sis spi·nu·lo·sa
trich·o·stron·gy·li·a·sis
trich·o·stron·gy·lo·sis
Trich·o·stron·gy·lus
trich·o·the·cin
trich·o·til·lo·ma·ni·a
trich·o·til·lo·man·ic
tri·chot·o·mous
tri·chot·o·my
    pl tri·chot·o·mies
tri·chro·ic
tri·chro·ism
tri·chro·mat
tri·chro·mat·ic
tri·chro·ma·tism
tri·chro·ma·top·si·a
tri·chrome
tri·chro·mic
trich·ter·brust
trich·u·ri·a·sis
    pl trich·u·ri·a·ses
Trich·u·ris
tri·cip·i·tal
tri·clo·bi·son·i·um
tri·clo·car·ban
tri·clo·fen·ol
tri·clo·fos
tri·corn
tri·cor·nute
tri·cre·sol
tri·crot·ic
tri·cro·tism
tri·cus·pid
tri·cus·pi·date
tri·cy·cla·mol
tri·dac·tyl
    or tri·dac·ty·lous
    or tri·dac·tyle
tri·dac·tyle
    or tri·dac·tyl
    or tri·dac·ty·lous
tri·dac·ty·lism

tri·dac·ty·lous
    or tri·dac·tyl
    or tri·dac·tyle
tri·dent
tri·den·tate
tri·der·mic
tri·der·mo·ma
    pl tri·der·mo·mas
    or tri·der·mo·ma·ta
tri·di·hex·eth·yl
trid·y·mite
trid·y·mus
tri·en·ceph·a·lus
tri·eth·a·nol·a·mine
tri·eth·i·o·dide
tri·eth·yl·a·mine
tri·eth·yl·ene·mel·a·mine
tri·eth·y·lene·thi·o·phos·
    phor·a·mide
tri·fa·cial
tri·fid
tri·flu·mi·date
tri·flu·o·per·a·zine
tri·flu·per·i·dol
tri·flu·pro·ma·zine
tri·flu·ro·meth·yl·thi·a·zide
tri·fo·cal
tri·fo·li·o·sis
    pl tri·fo·li·o·ses
Tri·fo·li·um
tri·fur·cate
tri·fur·ca·tion
tri·gas·tric
tri·gas·tri·cus
tri·gem·i·nal
tri·gem·i·no·tha·lam·ic
tri·gem·i·nus
    pl tri·gem·i·ni
tri·gem·i·ny
    pl tri·gem·i·nies
tri·gen·ic
tri·glyc·er·ide
tri·gon
    or tri·gone
tri·go·na fi·bro·sa cor·dis
tri·go·nal
tri·go·nal·ly
tri·gone
    or tri·gon

tri·gon·ec·to·my
Trig·o·nel·la
trig·o·nel·line
tri·go·nid
tri·go·ni·tis
trig·o·no·ce·phal·ic
    or trig·o·no·ceph·a·lous
trig·o·no·ceph·a·lous
    or trig·o·no·ce·phal·ic
trig·o·no·ceph·a·ly
    pl trig·o·no·ceph·a·lies
tri·go·num
    pl tri·go·nums
    or tri·go·na
tri·go·num ha·ben·u·lae
tri·hex·y·phen·i·dyl
tri·hy·brid
tri·hy·dric
tri·hy·drol
tri·hy·drox·y·ben·zo·ic
tri·hy·drox·y·pro·pane
tri·in·i·od·y·mus
tri·i·o·do·eth·i·on·ic
tri·i·o·do·meth·ane
tri·i·o·do·thy·ro·nine
tri·ke·to·cho·lan·ic
tri·ke·to·hy·drin·dene
tri·ke·to·pu·rine
tri·labe
tri·lam·i·nar
    or tri·lam·i·nate
tri·lam·i·nate
    or tri·lam·i·nar
tri·li·no·le·in
tri·lo·bate
tri·loc·u·la
    or tri·loc·u·late
tri·loc·u·lar
tri·loc·u·late
    or tri·loc·u·la
tril·o·gy
    pl tril·o·gies
tri·mal·le·o·lar
tri·man·u·al
tri·mas·ti·gate
tri·men·su·al
tri·mep·ra·zine
Trim·er·e·su·rus
tri·mes·ter

tri·meth·a·di·one
tri·meth·a·phan cam·syl·ate
tri·meth·i·din·i·um meth·o·sul·fate
tri·meth·o·benz·a·mide
tri·meth·o·prim
tri·meth·yl·a·ce·tic
tri·meth·yl·a·mine
tri·meth·yl·ene
tri·meth·yl·gly·cine
tri·meth·yl·xan·thine
tri·met·o·zine
tri·mip·ra·mine
tri·mor·phic
tri·mor·phism
tri·mor·phous
tri·mox·a·mine
tri·ni·tro·glyc·er·in
tri·ni·tro·phe·nol
tri·ni·tro·tol·u·ene
tri·no·mi·al
tri·nu·cle·ate
tri·nu·cle·o·tide
tri·o·ceph·a·lus
tri·o·le·in
tri·o·lism
tri·o·list
tri·oph·thal·mos
tri·o·pod·y·mus
tri·or·chid
tri·or·chi·dy
tri·or·chi·dism
tri·or·tho·cres·yl
tri·ose
tri·ose·phos·pho·ric
tri·o·tus
tri·ox·sa·len
tri·ox·ide
tri·ox·y·meth·yl·ene
tri·ox·y·pu·rine
tri·pal·mi·tin
trip·a·ra
 pl trip·a·ras
 or trip·a·rae
tri·par·tite
tri·pel·en·na·mine
tri·pep·tide
tri·pha·lan·gism

tri·pha·lan·gy
tri·phar·ma·con
tri·pha·sic
tri·phe·nyl·meth·ane
tri·phos·pha·tase
tri·phos·phate
tri·phos·pho·pyr·i·dine
tri·phos·pho·pyr·i·dine nu·cle·o·tide
tri·ple
tri·ple·gi·a
trip·let
tri·plex
trip·lo·blas·tic
trip·lo·co·ri·a
 var of trip·lo·ko·ri·a
trip·loid
trip·loi·dy
trip·lo·ko·ri·a
tri·plo·pi·a
tri·pod
tri·prol·i·dine
tri·pro·so·pus
trip·sis
Trip·te·ryg·i·um
tri·pus
tri·que·trous
tri·que·trum
 pl tri·que·tra
tri·ra·di·al
tri·ra·di·al·ly
tri·ra·di·ate
tri·ra·di·us
 pl tri·ra·di·us·es
 or tri·ra·di·i
tri·sac·cha·ride
tri·sect
tris·kai·dek·a·pho·bi·a
tris·mus
tri·so·mic
tri·so·mus
tri·so·my
 pl tri·so·mies
tri·splanch·nic
tri·ste·a·rin
tris·te·ma·ni·a
 or tris·ti·ma·ni·a
tri·stich·i·a
tris·ti·chi·a·sis

tris·ti·ma·ni·a
 or tris·te·ma·ni·a
tris·tis
tri·sul·cate
tri·sul·fate
tri·sul·fide
tri·ta·nope
trit·a·nop·i·a
tri·ter·pene
trit·i·ate
trit·i·a·tion
trit·i·ca·le
tri·ti·ce·o·glos·sus
tri·ti·ceous
tri·ti·ce·um
 pl tri·ti·ce·i
trit·i·co·nu·cle·ic
trit·i·cum
tri·ti·um
trit·o·cone
trit·o·co·nid
tri·ton
trit·o·pine
tri·tu·ber·cu·lar
trit·u·ra·ble
trit·u·rate
trit·u·ra·tion
trit·u·ra·tor
tri·va·lence
 or tri·va·len·cy
tri·va·len·cy
 pl tri·va·len·cies
 or tri·va·lence
tri·val·ent
tri·valve
tri·val·vu·lar
tro·car
tro·chan·ter
tro·chan·ter·ic
tro·chan·tin
 or tro·chan·tine
tro·chan·tine
 or tro·chan·tin
tro·chan·tin·i·an
tro·char
 var of tro·car
tro·che
tro·chis·ca·tion

tro·chis·cus
   pl tro·chis·ci
troch·le·a
   pl troch·le·ae
troch·le·ar
troch·le·ar·i·form
troch·le·ar·is
troch·o·car·di·a
troch·o·ce·pha·li·a
troch·o·ceph·a·lus
troch·o·ceph·a·ly
troch·o·gin·gly·mus
tro·choid
tro·choi·des
   pl tro·choi·des
troch·o·phore
troch·o·ri·zo·car·di·a
Trog·lo·tre·ma
Trog·lo·tre·mat·i·dae
Troi·sier sign
trol·a·mine
tro·land
tro·le·an·do·my·cin
trol·ni·trate
Trö·ltsch·cor·pus·cles
Trom·bic·u·la
trom·bic·u·li·a·sis
Trom·bic·u·li·dae
trom·bic·u·lo·sis
tro·meth·a·mine
Trom·mer test
Trom·ner sign
trom·o·ma·ni·a
tro·na
tro·pa·co·caine
tro·pae·o·lin
   var of tro·pe·o·lin
tro·pane
tro·pate
tro·pe·ine
tro·pe·o·lin
tro·pe·sis
troph·ec·to·derm
tro·phe·de·ma
   pl tro·phe·de·mas
   or tro·phe·de·ma·ta
tro·phe·ma
tro·phe·si·al

tro·phe·sic
troph·e·sy
   pl troph·e·sies
troph·ic
tro·phic·i·ty
troph·ism
troph·o·blast
troph·o·blas·tic
tro·pho·blas·to·ma
   pl tro·pho·blas·to·mas
   or tro·pho·blas·to·ma·ta
troph·o·chrome
troph·o·chro·mid·i·a
troph·o·cyte
troph·o·derm
troph·o·der·mal
troph·o·der·ma·to·neu·ro·sis
troph·o·dy·nam·ics
tro·pho·oe·de·ma
   pl tro·pho·oe·de·mas
   or tro·pho·oe·de·ma·ta
   var of tro·pho·e·de·ma
tro·phol·o·gy
   pl tro·phol·o·gies
troph·o·neu·ro·sis
   pl troph·o·neu·ro·ses
troph·o·neu·rot·ic
troph·o·no·sis
troph·o·nu·cle·us
   pl troph·o·nu·cle·us·es
   or troph·o·nu·cle·i
tro·phop·a·thy
   pl tro·phop·a·thies
troph·o·plasm
troph·o·plast
troph·o·spon·gi·a
troph·o·spon·gi·um
troph·o·tax·is
   troph·o·tax·es
troph·o·ther·a·py
troph·o·trop·ic
tro·phot·ro·pism
tro·pho·zo·ite
tro·pi·a
trop·ic ac·id
trop·i·cal
tro·pic·a·mide

tro·pin
tro·pine
tro·pism
tro·po·chrome
tro·po·col·la·gen
trop·o·lone
tro·pom·e·ter
tro·po·my·o·sin
tro·po·nin
tro·po·pause
tro·po·sphere
Trous·seau dis·ease
trox·i·done
troy
truem·mer·feld
Tru·e·ta shunt
trun·cal
trun·cate
trun·co·co·nal
trun·cus
   pl trun·ci
trun·cus ar·te·ri·o·sus
trunk
truss
tryp·a·fla·vine
try·pan blue
try·pan red
try·pan·o·ci·dal
try·pan·o·cide
try·pan·ol·y·sis
Try·pan·o·so·ma
   pl Try·pan·o·so·mas
   or Try·pan·o·so·ma·ta
try·pan·o·so·mal
Try·pan·o·so·mat·i·dae
try·pan·o·some
try·pan·o·so·mi·a·sis
   pl try·pan·o·so·mi·a·ses
try·pan·o·som·ic
try·pan·o·so·mi·cide
try·pan·o·so·mid
try·pan·o·so·mide
tryp·a·no·tox·yl
tryp·ar·sa·mide
tryp·sin
tryp·sin·i·za·tion
tryp·sin·o·gen
tryp·ta·mine

tryp·tase
tryp·tic
tryp·to·lyt·ic
tryp·to·phan
  or tryp·to·phane
tryp·to·pha·nae·mi·a
  var of try·to·pha·ne·mi·a
tryp·to·pha·nase
tryp·to·phane
  or tryp·to·phan
tryp·to·pha·ne·mi·a
tryp·to·phan·u·ri·a
tryp·to·phyl
Tscher·ning the·o·ry
tset·se
  pl tset·ses
  or tset·se
Tsu·chi·ya re·a·gent
Tsu·ga
tsu·tsu·ga·mu·shi
tu·a·mi·no·hep·tane
tu·ba
  pl tu·bae
tu·bage
tub·al
tube
tu·bec·to·my
  pl tu·bec·to·mies
tu·ber
  pl tu·bers
  or tu·ber·a
tu·ber ci·ne·re·um
tu·be·ral
tu·ber·cle
tu·ber·cled
tu·ber·cu·la co·ro·nae den·tis
tu·ber·cu·lar
tu·ber·cu·late
tu·ber·cu·la·tion
tu·ber·cu·lid
  or tu·ber·cu·lide
tu·ber·cu·lide
  or tu·ber·cu·lid
tu·ber·cu·lig·e·nous
tu·ber·cu·lin
tu·ber·cu·li·tis
tu·ber·cu·lo·cele

tu·ber·cu·lo·ci·dal
tu·ber·cu·lo·derm
  or tu·ber·cu·lo·der·ma
tu·ber·cu·lo·der·ma
  tu·ber·cu·lo·derm
tu·ber·cu·lo·fi·broid
tu·ber·cu·loid
tu·ber·cu·lo·ma
  pl tu·ber·cu·lo·mas
  or tu·ber·cu·lo·ma·ta
tu·ber·cu·lo·ma·ni·a
tu·ber·cu·lo·pho·bi·a
tu·ber·cu·lo·pro·te·in
tu·ber·cu·lose
tu·ber·cu·lo·sil·i·co·sis
tu·ber·cu·lo·sis
  pl tu·ber·cu·lo·ses
tu·ber·cu·lo·stat·ic
tu·ber·cu·lo·ste·ar·ic
tu·ber·cu·lot·ic
tu·ber·cu·lous
tu·ber·cu·lous·ly
tu·ber·cu·lum
  pl tu·ber·cu·la
tu·ber·cu·lum ci·ne·re·um
tu·ber·in
tu·ber·o·hy·po·phys·e·al
tu·ber·ose
  or tu·ber·ous
tu·ber·o·sis
tu·ber·os·i·tas
  pl tu·ber·os·i·ta·tes
tu·ber·os·i·ty
  pl tu·ber·os·i·ties
tu·ber·ous
  or tu·ber·ose
tu·bo·ab·dom·i·nal
tu·bo·ad·nex·o·pex·y
tu·bo·cu·ra·re
tu·bo·cu·ra·rine
tu·bo·lig·a·men·ta·ry
tu·bo·lig·a·men·tous
tub·o·o·var·i·an
tu·bo·o·var·i·ot·o·my
tu·bo·per·i·to·ne·al
tu·bo·plas·ty
tu·bo·tym·pan·ic
tu·bo·u·ter·ine

tu·bo·vag·i·nal
tu·bu·lar
tu·bule
tu·bu·lin
tu·bu·li·za·tion
tu·bu·lize
tu·bu·lo·ac·i·nous
tu·bu·lo·al·ve·o·lar
tu·bu·lo·cyst
tu·bu·lo·rac·e·mose
tu·bu·lor·rhex·is
tu·bu·lus
  pl tu·bu·li
tu·bus
  pl tu·bi
Tuf·fier in·fe·ri·or lig·a·ment
tu·la·re·mi·a
tu·la·re·mic
tulle gras
tu·me·fa·cient
tu·me·fac·tion
tu·me·fy
tu·men·ti·a
tu·mer·ic
tu·mes·cence
tu·mes·cent
tu·mid
tu·mid·i·ty
tum·my
  pl tum·mies
tu·mor
tu·mor·af·fin
tu·mor·al
tu·mor·i·ci·dal
tu·mor·i·gen·e·sis
  pl tu·mor·i·gen·e·ses
tu·mor·i·gen·ic
tu·mor·i·ge·nic·i·ty
  pl tu·mor·i·ge·nic·i·ties
tu·mor·let
tu·mor·ous
tu·mour
  var of tu·mor
tu·mul·tus
Tun·ga
tun·gi·a·sis
tung·sten

tu·nic
tu·ni·ca
   pl tu·ni·cae
tu·ni·ca al·bu·gi·ne·a
   pl tu·ni·cae al·bu·gi·ne·ae
tu·ni·cin
tun·ing fork
tun·nel
tu·ra·cin
tu·ra·nose
tur·bid
tur·bi·dim·e·ter
tur·bi·di·met·ric
tur·bi·di·met·ri·cal·ly
tur·bi·dim·e·try
   pl tur·bi·dim·e·tries
tur·bid·i·ty
   pl tur·bid·i·ties
tur·bi·nal
tur·bi·nate
tur·bi·nec·to·my
   pl tur·bi·nec·to·mies
tur·bi·no·tome
tur·bi·not·o·my
   pl tur·bi·not·o·mies
Türck bun·dle
tur·ges·cence
tur·ges·cent
tur·gid
tur·gid·i·ty
   pl tur·gid·i·ties
tur·gid·ness
tur·gor
tu·ris·ta
Türk cell
Tur·ling·ton bal·sam
tur·mer·ic
turn
Tur·ner syn·drome
turn·sick
tur·pen·tine
tur·ri·ceph·a·ly
   pl tur·ri·ceph·a·lies
tusk
tus·sal
tus·se·do
tus·sic·u·la·tion
Tus·si·la·go
tus·sis

tus·sive
tu·ta·men
Tut·hill meth·od
Tut·tle op·er·a·tion
twang
tween-brain
tweez·ers
twig
twin
twin-born
twinge
Twi·ning kink
twin·ning
twitch
ty·bam·ate
tyl·i·on
   pl tyl·i·a
ty·lo·ma
   pl ty·lo·mas
   or ty·lo·ma·ta
ty·lo·sin
ty·lo·sis
   pl ty·lo·ses
ty·lot·ic
ty·lox·a·pol
tym·pa·nal
tym·pa·nec·to·my
tym·pan·i·a
tym·pan·ic
tym·pa·nism
tym·pa·ni·tes
tym·pa·nit·ic
tym·pa·ni·tis
tym·pa·no·mas·toid
tym·pa·no·mas·toi·di·tis
   pl tym·pa·no·mas·toi·di·ti·
   des
tym·pa·no·plas·ty
   pl tym·pa·no·plas·ties
tym·pa·no·scle·ro·sis
tym·pa·no·sis
tym·pa·no·squa·mous
tym·pa·no·sta·pe·di·al
tym·pa·not·o·my
   pl tym·pa·not·o·mies
tym·pa·nous
tym·pa·num
   pl tym·pa·nums
   or tym·pa·na

tym·pa·ny
   pl tym·pa·nies
Tyn·dall phe·nom·e·non
Tyn·dal·li·za·tion
type
typh·lat·o·ny
typh·lec·ta·si·a
typh·lec·ta·sis
typh·lec·to·my
   pl typh·lec·to·mies
typh·len·ter·i·tis
typh·li·tis
typh·lo·cele
typh·lo·dic·li·di·tis
typh·lo·em·py·e·ma
   pl typh·lo·em·py·e·mas
   or typh·lo·em·py·e·ma·ta
typh·lo·en·ter·i·tis
typh·loid
typh·lo·lex·i·a
typh·lo·li·thi·a·sis
   pl typh·lo·li·thi·a·ses
typh·lo·meg·a·ly
   pl typh·lo·meg·a·lies
typh·lo·pto·sis
   pl typh·lo·pto·ses
typh·lo·sis
typh·lo·sole
typh·lo·spasm
typh·lo·ste·no·sis
typh·los·to·my
   pl typh·los·to·mies
typh·lot·o·my
ty·pho·bac·il·lo·sis of Lan·
   dou·zy
ty·pho·bac·ter·in
ty·phoid
ty·phoid·al
ty·pho·ma·lar·i·al
ty·pho·pneu·mo·ni·a
ty·phous
ty·phus
typ·i·cal
ty·po·scope
ty·pus de·gen·er·a·ti·vus
   am·ste·lo·da·men·sis
ty·ra·mine
tyr·an·nism
ty·rem·e·sis

406

ty·ro·ci·din
   or ty·ro·ci·dine
ty·ro·ci·dine
   or ty·ro·di·din
Ty·rode so·lu·tion
Ty·rog·e·nous
Ty·rog·ly·phus
ty·roid
ty·ro·ma
ty·ro·ma·to·sis

ty·ros·a·mine
ty·ro·si·nae·mi·a
   var of ty·ro·si·ne·mi·a
tyr·o·sin·ase
ty·ro·sine
ty·ro·si·ne·mi·a
ty·ro·si·no·sis
ty·ro·si·nu·ri·a
ty·ro·sis
ty·ro·syl

ty·ro·syl·u·ri·a
ty·ro·thri·cin
ty·ro·tox·ism
Ty·son glands
ty·vel·ose
Tyz·zer dis·ease
Tzanck test
tzet·ze
   var of tzet·se

U

u·ber·ous
u·ber·ty
   pl u·ber·ties
u·biq·ui·none
ud·der
Uf·fel·mann test
Uhl a·nom·a·ly
u·la
ul·cer
ul·cer·ate
ul·cer·a·tion
ul·cer·a·tive
ul·cer·o·gan·gre·nous
ul·cer·o·gen·ic
ul·cer·o·glan·du·lar
ul·cer·o·mem·bra·nous
ul·cer·ous
ul·cul
   pl ul·cera
ul·cus
   pl ul·ce·a
u·lec·to·my
ule·gy·ri·a
u·ler·y·the·ma
u·let·ic
u·lex·ine

u·li·tis
Ull·rich-
   Tur·ner syn·drome
ul·mus
ul·na
   pl ul·nas
   or ul·nae
ul·nad
ul·nar
ul·na·ris
ul·no·car·pal
ul·no·car·pe·us
ul·no·ra·di·al
u·loc·a·ce
u·lo·car·ci·no·ma
u·lo·der·ma·ti·tis
u·lo·glos·si·tis
u·loid
u·lon·cus
u·lor·rha·gi·a
u·lo·sis
   pl u·lo·sis·es
   or u·lo·ses
U·lo·so·ni·a par·vi·cor·nis
u·lot·ic
u·lot·o·my
   pl u·lot·o·mies

u·lot·ri·chous
ul·ti·mate
u·ti·mo·bran·chi·al
ul·ti·mo·gen·i·tar·y
ul·ti·mo·gen·i·ture
ul·ti·mum mor·i·ens
ul·tra·brach·y·ce·phal·ic
ul·tra·brach·y·cra·ni·al
ul·tra·cen·trif·u·gal
ul·tra·cen·tri·fu·ga·tion
ul·tra·cen·tri·fuge
ul·tra·dol·i·cho·cra·ni·al
ul·tra·fil·ter
ul·tra·fil·tra·tion
ul·tra·mi·cro·scope
ul·tra·mi·cro·scop·ic
   or ul·tra·mi·cro·scop·i·al
ul·tra·mi·cro·scop·i·cal
   or ul·tra·mi·cro·scop·ic
ul·tra·mi·cro·scop·i·cal·ly
ul·tra·mi·cros·co·py
   pl ul·tra·mi·cros·co·pies
ul·tra·mi·cro·tome
ul·tra·phag·o·cy·to·sis
ul·tra·red
ul·tra·son·ic
ul·tra·son·o·gram

ul·tra·so·nog·ra·phy
pl ul·tra·so·nog·ra·phies
ul·tra·son·o·scope
ul·tra·sound
ul·tra·struc·tur·al
ul·tra·struc·tur·al·ly
ul·tra·struc·ture
ul·tra·thin
ul·tra·vi·o·let
ul·u·la·tion
um·bel·li·fer
Um·bel·lif·er·ae
um·bel·lif·er·ous
um·ber
um·bi·lec·to·my
um·bil·i·cal
um·bil·i·cate
um·bil·i·ca·tion
um·bil·i·cus
pl um·bil·i·cus·es
or um·bil·i·ci
um·bo
pl um·bos
or um·bo·nes
um·bo·nate
um·bras·co·py
un·a·nes·the·tized
un·bal·ance
un·cal
un·ci·a
pl un·ci·ae
un·ci·form
un·ci·nal
Un·ci·nar·i·a
un·ci·na·ri·a·sis
pl un·ci·na·ri·a·ses
un·ci·nate
un·ci·na·tum
pl un·ci·na·tums
or un·ci·na·ta
un·ci·pi·si·for·mis
un·ci·press·ure
un·cir·cum·cised
un·com·pen·sat·ed
un·com·pli·cat·ed
un·con·di·tion·al
un·con·di·tion·ed
un·con·ju·gat·ed
un·con·scious

un·con·scious·ly
un·con·scious·ness
un·co·or·di·nat·ed
un·co·ver·te·bral
unc·tion
unc·tu·ous
unc·tu·ous·ly
un·cus
pl un·ci
un·dec·yl
un·dec·y·len·ate
un·dec·y·len·ic
un·de·fend·ed space of
    Pea·cock
un·der·a·chieve
un·der·a·chiev·er
un·der·arm
un·der·cut
un·der·de·vel·oped
un·der·de·vel·op·ment
un·der·lip
un·der·nour·ished
un·der·nu·tri·tion
un·der·sex·ed
un·der·shot
un·der·slung
un·der·toe
un·der·weight
Un·der·wood dis·ease
un·de·scend·ed
un·di·ag·nosed
un·dif·fer·en·ti·at·ed
un·di·gest·ed
un·dine
un·din·ism
un·do·ing
un·du·lant
un·du·late
un·du·la·tion
un·du·la·to·ry
un·en·cap·su·lat·ed
un·e·qual
un·e·rupt·ed
un·gual
or un·gui·nal
un·guent
un·guen·tum
Un·guic·u·la·ta
un·guic·u·late

un·gui·nal
or un·gual
un·guis
pl un·gues
un·gu·la
pl un·gu·lae
Un·gu·la·ta
un·gu·late
un·gu·li·grade
un·health·y
u·ni·al·gal
u·ni·ar·tic·u·lar
u·ni·ax·i·al
u·ni·ax·i·al·ly
u·ni·bas·al
u·ni·cam·er·al
u·ni·cam·er·al·ly
u·ni·cam·er·ate
u·ni·cel·lu·lar
u·ni·cel·lu·lar·i·ty
pl u·ni·cel·lu·lar·i·ties
u·ni·cen·tral
u·ni·cen·tric
u·ni·cor·nous
u·ni·cus·pid
or u·ni·cus·pi·date
u·ni·cus·pi·date
or u·ni·cus·pid
u·ni·di·rec·tion·al
u·ni·fac·to·ri·al
u·ni·fa·mil·i·al
u·ni·fi·lar
u·ni·fla·gel·late
u·ni·glan·du·lar
u·ni·grav·i·da
pl u·ni·grav·i·das
or u·ni·grav·i·dae
u·ni·lat·er·al
u·ni·lat·er·al·ly
u·ni·lo·bar
u·ni·loc·u·lar
u·ni·mo·lec·u·lar
un·im·paired
un·in·cis·ed
un·in·hib·i·ted
u·ni·nu·cle·ar
or u·ni·nu·cle·ate
u·ni·nu·cle·ate
or u·ni·nu·cle·ar

u·ni·nu·cle·at·ed
u·ni·oc·u·lar
un·ion
u·ni·o·val
  or u·ni·ov·u·lar
u·ni·ov·u·lar
  or u·ni·o·val
u·nip·a·ra
  pl u·nip·a·ras
  or u·nip·a·rae
u·ni·pa·ren·tal
u·ni·par·i·ens
u·nip·a·rous
u·ni·pen·nate
u·ni·po·lar
u·ni·po·lar·i·ty
  pl u·ni·po·lar·i·ties
u·ni·po·ten·cy
u·nip·o·tent
u·ni·po·ten·tial
u·ni·sep·tate
u·ni·sex·u·al
u·nit
u·ni·tar·y
u·ni·va·lent
u·ni·ver·sal
un·linked
un·load·ing
un·med·ul·lat·ed
un·mod·i·fied
un·my·e·li·nat·ed
Un·na bod·ies
Un·na-Thost syn·drome
un·of·fi·cial
un·or·ga·nized
un·paired
un·phys·i·o·log·ic
  or un·phys·i·o·log·i·cal
un·phys·i·o·log·i·cal
  or un·phys·i·o·log·ic
un·pig·ment·ed
un·re·ac·tive
un·re·al·i·ty
un·re·duced
un·re·spon·sive
un·rest
un·sat·u·rat·ed
un·sex
un·slaked

un·sound
un·sound·ness
un·spec·i·fied
un·sta·ble
un·stained
un·stri·at·ed
un·striped
un·treat·ed
un·u·nit·ed
un·vac·ci·nat·ed
Un·ver·richt dis·ease
un·well
up·per
up·set
up·take
u·ra·chal
u·ra·chus
u·ra·cil
u·ra·cra·si·a
u·ra·cra·ti·a
u·rae·mi·a
  var of u·re·mi·a
u·rae·mic
  var of u·re·mic
u·ra·gogue
u·ra·mil
u·ra·nal
u·ra·nal·y·sis
u·ra·nin
u·ran·i·nite
u·ra·nis·co·plas·ty
u·ra·nis·cor·rha·phy
u·ra·nis·cus
u·ra·nism
u·ra·ni·um
u·ra·no·col·o·bo·ma
u·ra·no·plas·tic
u·ra·no·plas·ty
  pl u·ra·no·plas·ties
u·ra·no·ple·gi·a
u·ra·nor·rha·phy
u·ra·nos·chi·sis
  pl u·ra·nos·chi·sis·es
  or u·ra·nos·chi·ses
u·ran·o·schism
u·ra·no·schis·ma
u·ra·no·staph·y·lo·plas·ty
  pl u·ra·no·staph·y·lo·plas·
   ties

u·ra·no·staph·y·lor·rha·phy
  pl u·ra·no·staph·y·lor·rha·
   phies
u·ra·no·staph·y·los·chi·sis
u·ra·nyl
u·ra·ro·ma
u·rar·thri·tis
u·rase
u·ra·sin
u·ra·tae·mi·a
  var of u·ra·te·mi·a
u·rate
u·ra·te·mi·a
u·rat·ic
u·ra·to·ma
u·ra·to·sis
u·ra·tu·ri·a
ur·ce·i·form
ur·ce·o·late
u·re·a
u·re·al
u·re·am·e·ter
u·re·am·e·try
  pl u·re·am·e·tries
u·re·a·poi·e·sis
u·re·ase
u·rec·chy·sis
u·re·de·ma
  pl u·re·de·mas
  or u·re·de·ma·ta
u·re·dep·a
u·re·he·pat·ic
u·re·ide
u·rel·co·sis
u·re·mi·a
u·re·mic
u·re·mi·gen·ic
u·re·om·e·ter
u·re·om·e·try
u·re·o·tel·ic
u·re·o·tel·ism
u·re·si·aes·the·si·a
  var of u·re·si·es·the·si·a
u·re·si·es·the·si·a
u·re·si·es·the·sis
u·re·sis
u·re·ter
u·re·ter·al
  or u·re·ter·ic

u·re·ter·al·gi·a
u·re·ter·ec·ta·si·a
  or u·re·ter·ec·ta·sis
u·re·ter·ec·ta·sis
  or u·re·ter·ec·ta·si·a
u·re·ter·ec·to·my
  pl u·re·ter·ec·to·mies
u·re·ter·ic
  or u·re·ter·al
u·re·ter·i·tis
u·re·ter·o·cele
u·re·ter·o·ce·lec·to·my
u·re·ter·o·co·los·to·my
  pl u·re·ter·o·co·los·to·mies
u·re·ter·o·cys·tic
u·re·ter·o·cys·to·scope
u·re·ter·o·cys·tos·to·my
  pl u·re·ter·o·cys·tos·to·mies
u·re·ter·o·di·al·y·sis
u·re·ter·o·en·ter·ic
u·re·ter·o·en·ter·os·to·my
  pl u·re·ter·o·en·ter·os·to·
   mies
u·re·ter·og·ra·phy
  pl u·re·ter·og·ra·phies
u·re·ter·o·hem·i·ne·phrec·
 to·my
u·re·ter·o·hy·dro·ne·phro·
 sis
  pl u·re·ter·o·hy·dro·ne·phro·
   ses
u·re·ter·o·il·e·al
u·re·ter·o·il·e·os·to·my
  pl u·re·ter·o·il·e·os·to·mies
u·re·ter·o·in·tes·ti·nal
u·re·ter·o·lith
u·re·ter·o·li·thi·a·sis
  pl ur·e·ter·o·li·thi·a·ses
u·re·ter·o·li·thot·o·my
  pl u·re·ter·o·li·thot·o·mies
u·re·ter·ol·y·sis
  pl u·re·ter·ol·y·ses
u·re·ter·o·meg·a·ly
u·re·ter·o·ne·o·cys·tos·to·
 my
  pl ur·e·ter·o·ne·o·cys·tos·to·
   mies

u·re·ter·o·ne·o·py·e·los·to·
 my
  pl u·re·ter·o·ne·o·py·e·los·
   to·mies
u·re·ter·o·ne·phrec·to·my
  pl u·re·ter·o·ne·phrec·to·
   mies
u·re·ter·op·a·thy
  pl u·re·ter·op·a·thies
u·re·ter·o·pel·vic
u·re·ter·o·pel·vi·o·plas·ty
u·re·ter·o·plas·ty
  pl u·re·ter·o·plas·ties
u·re·ter·o·py·el·i·tis
u·re·ter·o·py·e·log·ra·phy
  pl u·re·ter·o·py·e·log·ra·
   phies
u·re·ter·o·py·e·lo·ne·os·to·
 my
  pl u·re·ter·o·py·e·lo·ne·os·
   to·mies
u·re·ter·o·py·e·lo·ne·phri·
 tis
  pl u·re·ter·o·py·e·lo·ne·phri·
   ti·des
u·re·ter·o·py·e·lo·ne·phros·
 to·my
  pl u·re·ter·o·py·e·lo·ne·
   phros·to·mies
u·re·ter·o·py·e·lo·plas·ty
  pl u·re·ter·o·py·e·lo·plas·
   ties
u·re·ter·o·py·e·los·to·my
  pl u·re·ter·o·py·e·los·to·
   mies
u·re·ter·o·py·o·sis
u·re·ter·or·rha·gi·a
u·re·ter·or·rha·phy
  pl u·re·ter·or·rha·phies
u·re·ter·o·sig·moi·dos·to·
 my
  pl u·re·ter·o·sig·moi·dos·to·
   mies
u·re·ter·os·to·my
  pl u·re·ter·os·to·mies
u·re·ter·o·the·cal
u·re·ter·ot·o·my
  pl u·re·ter·ot·o·mies
u·re·ter·o·u·re·ter·al

u·re·ter·o·u·re·ter·os·to·my
u·re·ter·o·u·ter·ine
u·re·ter·o·vag·i·nal
u·re·ter·o·ves·i·cal
u·re·than
  or u·re·thane
u·re·thane
  or u·re·than
u·re·thra
  pl u·re·thras
  or u·re·thrae
u·re·thral
u·re·thral·gi·a
u·re·thra·tre·si·a
u·re·threc·to·my
  pl u·re·threc·to·mies
u·re·threm·phrax·is
u·re·thrism
u·re·thri·tis
  pl u·re·thri·ti·des
u·re·thro·bul·bar
u·re·thro·cele
u·re·thro·cu·ta·ne·ous
u·re·thro·cys·ti·tis
  pl u·re·thro·cys·ti·ti·des
u·re·thro·cys·to·cele
u·re·thro·dyn·i·a
u·re·thro·gram
u·re·thro·graph
u·re·throg·ra·phy
u·re·throm·e·ter
u·re·throm·e·try
u·re·thro·pe·nile
u·re·thro·per·i·ne·al
u·re·thro·per·i·ne·o·scro·tal
u·re·thro·phrax·is
u·re·thro·phy·ma
u·re·thro·plas·ty
  pl u·re·thro·plas·ties
u·re·thro·pros·tat·ic
u·re·thro·rec·tal
u·re·thror·rha·gi·a
u·re·thror·rha·phy
  pl u·re·thror·rha·phies
u·re·thror·rhe·a
u·re·thror·rhoe·a
  var of u·re·thror·rhe·a
u·re·thro·scope
u·re·thro·scop·ic

u·re·thros·co·py
  pl u·re·thros·co·pies
u·re·thro·spasm
u·re·thro·stax·is
u·re·thro·ste·no·sis
  pl u·re·thro·ste·no·ses
u·re·thros·to·my
  pl u·re·thros·to·mies
u·re·thro·tome
u·re·throt·o·my
  pl u·re·throt·o·mies
u·re·thro·tri·go·ni·tis
u·re·thro·vag·i·nal
u·re·thro·ves·i·cal
u·re·thro·ves·i·co·vag·i·nal
ur·gen·cy
  pl ur·gen·cies
Ur·gin·e·a
ur·hi·dro·sis
  pl ur·hi·dro·ses
u·ric
u·ric·ac·i·dae·mi·a
  var of u·ric·ac·i·de·mi·a
u·ric·ac·i·de·mi·a
u·ric·ac·i·du·ri·a
u·ri·cae·mi·a
  var of u·ri·ce·mi·a
u·ri·can·i·case
u·ri·case
u·ri·ce·mi·a
u·ri·col·y·sis
  pl u·ri·col·y·ses
u·ri·co·lyt·ic
u·ri·com·e·ter
u·ri·co·su·ri·a
u·ri·co·su·ric
u·ri·co·tel·ic
u·ri·co·tel·ism
u·ri·dine
u·ri·dro·sis
u·ri·dyl
u·ri·dyl·ic
u·ri·es·the·sis
u·ri·nal
u·ri·nal·y·sis
  pl u·ri·nal·y·ses
u·ri·nar·y
u·ri·nate
u·ri·na·tion

u·ri·na·tive
u·rine
u·ri·ne·mi·a
u·ri·nif·er·ous
u·ri·nif·ic
u·ri·nip·a·rous
u·ri·no·cry·os·co·py
u·ri·no·gen·i·tal
u·ri·nog·e·nous
u·ri·nol·o·gy
u·ri·no·ma
  pl u·ri·no·mas
  or u·ri·no·ma·ta
u·ri·nom·e·ter
u·ri·nom·e·try
  pl u·ri·nom·e·tries
u·ri·no·scop·ic
u·ri·nos·co·py
u·ri·nous
u·ri·po·si·a
u·ri·sol·vent
u·ri·tis
ur·ning
u·ro·ac·i·dim·e·ter
u·ro·an·the·lone
u·ro·az·o·tom·e·ter
u·ro·ben·zo·ic
u·ro·bi·lin
u·ro·bi·li·nae·mi·a
  var of u·ro·bi·li·ne·mi·a
u·ro·bi·li·ne·mi·a
u·ro·bi·li·nic·ter·us
u·ro·bi·lin·o·gen
u·ro·bi·lin·o·ge·nu·ri·a
u·ro·bi·li·noi·din
u·ro·bi·li·nu·ri·a
u·ro·can·ic
u·ro·cele
u·roch·e·ras
u·ro·che·si·a
u·ro·che·zi·a
u·ro·chlo·ral·ic
u·ro·chrome
u·ro·chro·mo·gen
u·ro·clep·si·a
u·ro·cris·i·a
u·ro·cri·sis
u·ro·cy·a·nin
u·ro·cy·an·o·gen

u·ro·cy·a·nose
u·ro·cy·a·no·sis
  pl u·ro·cy·a·no·ses
u·ro·cyst
u·ro·dac·um
  var of u·ro·de·um
u·ro·de·um
u·ro·dy·nam·ics
u·ro·dyn·i·a
u·roe·de·ma
  var of u·re·de·ma
u·ro·en·ter·one
u·ro·er·y·thrin
u·ro·fla·vin
u·ro·fus·cin
u·ro·fus·co·haem·a·tin
  var of u·ro·fus·co·hem·a·tin
u·ro·fus·co·hem·a·tin
u·ro·gas·trone
u·ro·gen·i·tal
u·rog·e·nous
u·ro·glau·cin
u·ro·gram
u·rog·ra·phy
  pl u·rog·ra·phies
u·ro·gra·vim·e·ter
u·ro·hae·ma·tin
  var of u·ro·he·ma·tin
u·ro·he·ma·tin
u·ro·haem·a·to·ne·phro·sis
  var of u·ro·hem·a·to·ne·
    phro·sis
u·ro·hem·a·to·ne·phro·sis
u·ro·haem·a·to·por·phy·rin
  var of u·ro·hem·a·to·por·
    phy·rin
u·ro·hem·a·to·por·phy·rin
u·ro·hy·per·ten·sin
u·ro·ki·nase
u·ro·ki·net·ic
u·ro·leu·kin·ic
u·ro·lite
u·ro·lith
u·ro·li·thi·a·sis
  pl u·ro·li·thi·a·ses
u·ro·lith·ic
u·ro·li·thot·o·my
u·ro·log·ic
  or u·ro·log·i·cal

u·ro·log·i·cal
  or u·ro·log·ic
u·rol·o·gist
u·rol·o·gy
  pl u·rol·o·gies
u·ro·lu·te·in
u·ro·man·cy
u·ro·man·ti·a
u·ro·mel·a·nin
u·rom·e·lus
u·rom·e·ter
u·ron·cus
u·ro·ne·phro·sis
u·ron·ic
u·ro·nol·o·gy
u·ron·on·com·e·try
u·ro·nos·co·py
  pl u·ro·nos·co·pies
u·rop·a·thy
  pl u·rop·a·thies
u·ro·pep·sin
u·ro·phan·ic
u·ro·phe·in
u·ro·pit·tin
u·ro·pla·ni·a
u·ro·poi·e·sis
  pl u·ro·poi·e·ses
u·ro·poi·et·ic
u·ro·por·phyr·i·a
u·ro·por·phy·rin
u·ro·por·phy·rin·o·gen
u·ro·psam·mus
u·ro·pyg·i·al
u·ro·rec·tal
u·ro·ro·se·in
u·ror·rha·gi·a
u·ror·rhe·a
u·ror·rho·din
u·ror·rho·din·o·gen
u·ro·ru·bin
u·ro·ru·bro·hem·a·tin
u·ro·sa·cin
u·ros·che·o·cele
u·ros·che·sis
  pl u·ros·che·ses
u·ro·scop·ic
u·ros·co·pist
u·ros·co·py
  pl u·ros·co·pies

u·ro·se·in
u·ro·sem·i·ol·o·gy
u·ro·sep·sin
u·ro·sep·sis
  pl u·ro·sep·ses
u·ro·spec·trin
u·ro·ste·a·lith
u·ro·the·li·al
u·ro·the·li·um
u·ro·tox·i·a
u·ro·tox·ic
u·ro·tox·ic·i·ty
  pl u·ro·tox·ic·i·ties
u·ro·tox·in
u·ro·tox·y
u·rou·re·ter
U·rov dis·ease
u·ro·xan·thin
ur·rho·din
ur·sol·ic
ur·sone
ur·ti·ca
ur·ti·cant
ur·ti·car·i·a
ur·ti·car·i·al
ur·ti·car·i·o·gen·ic
ur·ti·cate
ur·ti·ca·tion
u·ru·shi·ol
us·ne·in
us·nic
us·ti·lag·i·nism
Us·ti·la·go
us·tion
us·tu·la·tion
u·ta
u·ter·al·gi·a
u·ter·ine
u·ter·is·mus
u·ter·i·tis
u·ter·o·ab·dom·i·nal
u·ter·o·ad·nex·al
u·ter·o·cer·vi·cal
u·ter·o·col·ic
u·ter·o·en·ter·ic
u·ter·o·fix·a·tion
u·ter·o·ges·ta·tion
u·ter·og·ra·phy
  pl u·ter·og·ra·phies

u·ter·o·in·tes·ti·nal
u·ter·o·lith
u·ter·o·ma·ni·a
u·ter·om·e·ter
u·ter·o·o·var·i·an
u·ter·o·pa·ri·e·tal
u·ter·o·pel·vic
u·ter·o·pex·i·a
u·ter·o·pex·y
  pl u·ter·o·pex·ies
u·ter·o·pla·cen·tal
u·ter·o·plas·ty
  pl u·ter·o·plas·ties
u·ter·o·rec·tal
u·ter·o·sa·cral
u·ter·o·sal·pin·gog·ra·phy
  pl u·ter·o·sal·pin·gog·ra·
    phies
u·ter·o·scope
u·ter·ot·o·my
  pl u·ter·ot·o·mies
u·ter·o·ton·ic
u·ter·o·trac·tor
u·ter·o·tu·bal
u·ter·o·vag·i·nal
u·ter·o·ven·tral
u·ter·o·ves·i·cal
u·ter·us
  pl u·ter·us·es
  or u·ter·i
u·tri·cle
u·tric·u·lar
u·tric·u·li·tis
u·tric·u·lo·sac·cu·lar
u·tric·u·lus
  pl u·tric·u·li
u·va·ur·si
u·ve·a
u·ve·al
u·ve·it·ic
u·ve·i·tis
  pl u·ve·i·ti·des
u·ve·o·en·ceph·a·li·tis
u·ve·o·me·nin·go·en·ceph·
  a·li·tis
u·ve·o·neur·ax·i·tis
u·ve·o·pa·rot·id
u·ve·o·pa·rot·i·tis
u·ve·o·scle·ri·tis

u·vi·form
u·vi·o·fast
u·vi·om·e·ter
u·vi·o·re·sis·tant
u·vi·o·sen·si·tive
u·vu·la
  pl u·vu·las
  or u·vu·lae

u·vu·lap·to·sis
u·vu·lar
u·vu·lar·ly
u·vu·la·tome
  or u·vu·lo·tome
u·vu·lec·to·my
  pl u·vu·lec·to·mies
u·vu·li·tis

u·vu·lo·nod·u·lar
u·vu·lop·to·sis
  pl u·vu·lop·to·ses
u·vu·lo·tome
  or u·vu·la·tome
u·vu·lot·o·my
  pl u·vu·lot·o·mies

V

vac·cig·e·nous
vac·cin
vac·ci·na
vac·cin·a·ble
vac·ci·nal
vac·ci·nate
vac·ci·na·tion
vac·ci·na·tor
vac·cine
vac·ci·nee
vac·cin·i·a
vac·cin·i·al
vac·cin·i·form
vac·ci·ni·o·la
vac·ci·noid
vac·ci·no·pho·bi·a
vac·ci·no·style
vac·ci·no·ther·a·py
  pl vac·ci·no·ther·a·pies
vac·u·o·lar
vac·u·o·late
vac·u·o·la·tion
vac·u·ole
vac·u·o·li·za·tion
vac·u·ome
vac·u·um
  pl vac·u·ums
  or vac·u·a
va·gal

va·gi·na
  pl va·gi·nas
  or va·gi·nae
va·gi·na ten·di·nis
vag·i·nal
vag·i·na·lec·to·my
vag·i·na·li·tis
vag·i·nal·ly
va·gi·na·pex·y
  pl va·gi·na·pex·ies
vag·i·nate
vag·i·nec·to·my
  pl vag·i·nec·to·mies
vag·i·nic·o·line
vag·i·nif·er·ous
vag·i·nis·mus
vag·i·ni·tis
vag·i·no·ab·dom·i·nal
vag·i·no·cele
vag·i·no·dyn·i·a
vag·i·no·fix·a·tion
vag·i·no·la·bi·al
vag·i·no·my·co·sis
  pl vag·i·no·my·co·ses
vag·i·nop·a·thy
vag·i·no·per·i·ne·al
vag·i·no·per·i·ne·or·rha·
  phy

vag·i·no·per·i·ne·ot·o·my
  pl vag·i·no·per·i·ne·ot·o·
  mies
vag·i·no·per·i·to·ne·al
vag·i·no·plas·ty
  pl vag·i·no·plas·ties
vag·i·no·scope
vag·i·nos·co·py
  pl vag·i·nos·co·pies
vag·i·not·o·my
  pl vag·i·not·o·mies
vag·i·no·ves·i·cal
vag·i·tus
va·gi·tus u·ter·i·nus
va·go·ac·ces·so·ry
va·go·gram
va·go·hy·po·glos·sal
va·gol·y·sis
va·go·lyt·ic
va·go·mi·met·ic
va·go·pres·sor
va·got·o·mize
va·got·o·my
  pl va·got·o·mies
va·go·to·ni·a
  or va·go·to·ny
va·go·ton·ic
va·got·o·nin

413

va·go·to·ny
   pl va·go·to·nies
   or va·go·to·ni·a
va·go·trop·ic
va·go·va·gal
va·gus
   pl va·gi
va·gus·stoff
va·lence
va·len·cy
   pl va·len·cies
va·lent
Va·len·tin cor·pus·cles
val·er·ate
va·le·ri·an
va·le·ri·a·nate
va·le·ri·an·ic
va·le·ric ac·id
val·e·tham·ate
val·e·tu·di·nar·i·an
val·e·tu·di·nar·i·an·ism
val·gus
val·ine
val·i·ne·mi·a
val·in·o·my·cin
val·late
val·lec·u·la
   pl val·lec·u·lae
Val·leix points
Val·let mass
val·lum
   pl val·lums
   or val·la
val·noc·ta·mide
Val·sal·va ma·neu·ver
Val·su·a·ni dis·ease
val·va
   pl val·vae
valve
valve of Bau·hin
valve of Ger·lach
valve of Has·ner
valve of Hei·ster
valve of Hous·ton
valve of Kerch·ring
valve of The·be·si·us
valve of Vieus·sens
val·vi·form

val·vot·o·my
   pl val·vot·o·mies
val·vu·la
   pl val·vu·lae
val·vu·la co·li
val·vu·la con·ni·vens
   pl val·vu·lae con·ni·ven·tes
val·vu·la spi·ra·lis
   pl val·vu·lae spi·ra·les
val·vu·lar
val·vu·lec·to·my
val·vu·li·tis
val·vu·lo·plas·ty
   pl val·vu·lo·plas·ties
val·vu·lo·tome
val·vu·lot·o·my
   pl val·vu·lot·o·mies
val·yl
van·a·date
va·na·di·um
va·na·di·um·ism
van Bo·gaert leu·ko·en·
   ceph·a·li·tis
van Bo·gaert-Nys·sen
   dis·ease
van·co·my·cin
van Crev·eld-von Gierke
   dis·ease
van Deen test
Van de Graaff gen·er·a·
   tor
van den Bergh test
van der Hoeve syn·drome
van Ge·huch·ten cell
Van Gie·son stain
van Han·se·mann cells
van Hoorne ca·nal
Van Slyke and Cul·len
   test
Van Slyke and Kirk
   meth·od
Van Slyke and Neill
   method
Van Slyke and Pal·mer
   test
Van Slyke, Mac·Fad·yen,
   and Ham·il·ton nin·hy·
   drin test

Van Slyke meth·od
va·na·di·um
va·na·di·um·ism
van·co·my·cin
va·nil·la
va·nil·late
va·nil·lic
van·il·lin
van·nil·lism
van·il·lyl·man·del·ic
van't Hoff law
va·po·cau·ter·i·za·tion
va·por
va·po·res u·ter·i·ni
va·por·ish
va·por·i·za·tion
va·por·ize
va·por·iz·er
va·por·ther·a·py
   pl va·po·ther·a·pies
Va·quez dis·ease
var·i·a·bil·i·ty
   pl var·i·a·bil·i·ties
var·i·a·ble
var·i·ance
var·i·ant
var·i·a·tion
var·i·ca·tion
var·i·ce·al
var·i·cec·to·my
var·i·cel·la
var·i·cel·la·tion
var·i·cel·li·form
var·i·cel·loid
var·ic·i·form
var·i·co·bleph·a·ron
var·i·co·cele
var·i·co·ce·lec·to·my
   pl var·i·co·ce·lec·to·mies
var·i·cog·ra·phy
   pl var·i·cog·ra·phies
var·i·coid
var·i·com·pha·los
var·i·com·phal·lus
   pl var·i·com·pha·li
var·i·co·phle·bi·tis
   pl var·i·co·phle·bi·ti·des
var·i·cose

var·i·co·sis
   pl var·i·co·ses
var·i·cos·i·ty
   pl var·i·cos·i·ties
var·i·cot·o·my
   pl var·i·cot·o·mies
va·ric·u·la
   pl va·ric·u·las
   or va·ric·u·lae
var·i·e·gate
var·i·e·ty
var·i·form
va·ri·o·la
va·ri·o·la vac·cin·i·a
va·ri·o·lar
var·i·o·late
var·i·o·la·tion
var·i·ol·ic
var·i·ol·i·form
var·i·o·li·za·tion
va·ri·o·loid
va·ri·o·lous
va·ri·o·lo·vac·cine
va·ri·o·lo·vac·cin·i·a
var·ix
   pl var·i·ces
va·ro·li·an
var·us
vas
   pl va·sa
vas ab·er·rans
   pl va·sa ab·er·ran·ti·a
vas def·er·ens
   pl va·sa def·er·en·ti·a
va·sa brev·is
va·sa ef·fer·en·ti·a
va·sa va·so·rum
va·sal
vas·cu·lar
vas·cu·lar·i·ty
   pl vas·cu·lar·i·ties
vas·cu·lar·i·za·tion
vas·cu·lar·ize
vas·cu·la·ture
vas·cu·li·tis
   pl vas·cu·li·ti·des
vas·cu·lo·gen·e·sis
vas·cu·lop·a·thy

vas·cu·lum
   pl vas·cu·la
va·sec·to·mize
va·sec·to·my
   pl va·sec·to·mies
vas·i·cine
vas·i·fac·tion
vas·i·fac·tive
   or vas·o·fac·tive
vas·i·form
vas·i·for·ma·tion
vas·i·tis
va·so·ac·tive
va·so·ac·tiv·i·ty
   pl va·so·ac·tiv·i·ties
va·so·con·stric·tion
va·so·con·stric·tive
va·so·con·stric·tor
va·so·den·tin
va·so·den·tine
va·so·de·pres·sion
va·so·de·pres·sor
va·so·dil·a·ta·tion
va·so·di·la·tion
va·so·di·la·tive
va·so·di·la·tor
va·so·ep·i·did·y·mos·to·my
va·so·fac·tive
   or va·si·fac·tive
va·so·for·ma·tion
va·so·for·ma·tive
va·so·gan·gli·on
   pl va·so·gan·gli·ons
   or va·so·gan·gli·a
va·so·gen·ic
va·sog·ra·phy
   pl va·sog·ra·phies
va·so·hy·per·ton·ic
va·so·hy·po·ton·ic
va·so·in·hib·i·tor
va·so·in·hib·i·to·ry
va·so·li·ga·tion
va·so·mo·tion
va·so·mo·tor
va·so·mo·tric·i·ty
vas·o·neu·rop·a·thy
va·so·neu·ro·sis
   pl va·so·neu·ro·ses

va·so·or·chid·os·to·my
va·so·pa·ral·y·sis
va·so·pa·re·sis
va·so·pres·sin
va·so·pres·sor
va·so·punc·ture
va·so·re·flex
va·so·re·lax·a·tion
vas·or·rha·phy
vas·os·cil·la·tor
va·so·sec·tion
va·so·sen·sor·y
va·so·spasm
va·so·spas·tic
va·so·stim·u·lant
vas·os·to·my
va·so·to·cin
vas·ot·o·my
va·so·to·ni·a
va·so·ton·ic
va·so·to·nin
va·so·tribe
va·so·troph·ic
va·so·trop·ic
va·so·va·gal
va·so·vas·os·to·my
va·so·va·sot·o·my
va·so·ve·sic·u·lec·to·my
vas·tus
   pl vas·ti
vas·tus ex·ter·nus
vas·tus in·ter·me·di·us
vas·tus in·ter·nus
vas·tus lat·er·al·is
vas·tus me·di·al·is
Va·ter am·pul·la
Va·ter cor·pus·cle
Va·ter-Pa·ci·ni cor·pus·cle
vault
Veau op·er·a·tion
ve·cor·di·a
vec·tion
vec·tis
vec·tor
vec·tor·car·di·o·gram
vec·tor·car·di·o·graph
vec·tor·car·di·o·graph·ic

vec·tor·car·di·og·ra·phy
  pl vec·tor·car·di·og·ra·phies
vec·to·ri·al
Ved·der sign
veg·an
veg·a·nism
veg·e·ta·ble
veg·e·tal
veg·e·tar·i·an
veg·e·tar·i·an·ism
veg·e·ta·tion
veg·e·ta·tive
veg·e·to·an·i·mal
ve·hi·cle
veil
Veil·lo·nel·la
Veil·lon tube
vein
ve·la·men
  pl ve·lam·i·na
vel·a·men·tous
vel·a·men·tum
  pl vel·a·men·ta
ve·lar
ve·li·form
vel·li·cate
vel·li·ca·tion
vel·lus
ve·loc·i·ty
  pl ve·loc·i·ties
vel·o·pha·ryn·ge·al
Vel·peau ban·dage
ve·lum
  pl ve·la
ve·na
  pl ve·nae
ve·na ca·va
  pl ve·nae ca·vae
ve·na ca·val
ve·na co·mes
  pl ve·nae com·i·tes
ve·nae vor·ti·co·sae
ve·na·tion
ve·nec·ta·si·a
ve·nec·to·my
  pl ve·nec·to·mies
ven·e·nate
ven·e·na·tion
ven·e·nif·er·ous

ven·e·no·sa
ven·e·nous
ven·e·punc·ture
  or ven·i·punc·ture
ve·ne·re·al
ve·ne·re·o·log·i·cal
ve·ne·re·ol·o·gist
ve·ne·re·ol·o·gy
  pl ve·ne·re·ol·o·gies
ve·ne·re·o·pho·bi·a
ven·er·ol·o·gy
  pl ven·er·ol·o·gies
  var of ve·ne·re·ol·o·gy
ven·er·y
  pl ven·er·ies
ven·e·sec·tion
  or ven·i·sec·tion
ven·e·su·ture
  or ven·i·su·ture
ven·in
ven·i·punc·ture
  or ven·e·punc·ture
ven·i·sec·tion
  or ven·e·sec·tion
ven·i·su·ture
  or ven·e·su·ture
ve·noc·ly·sis
  pl ve·noc·ly·ses
ve·no·fi·bro·sis
  pl ve·no·fi·bro·ses
ve·no·gram
ve·no·graph·ic
ve·nog·ra·phy
  pl ve·nog·ra·phies
ven·om
ven·om·i·za·tion
ven·o·mo·sal·i·var·y
ve·no·mo·tor
ven·om·ous
ve·no·oc·clu·sive
ve·no·per·i·to·ne·os·to·my
  pl ve·no·per·i·to·ne·os·to·
  mies
ve·no·pres·sor
ve·no·scle·ro·sis
  pl ve·no·scle·ro·ses
ve·nose
ve·nos·i·ty
  pl ve·nos·i·ties

ve·nos·ta·sis
  pl ve·nos·ta·ses
ve·no·throm·bot·ic
ve·not·o·my
  pl ve·not·o·mies
ve·nous
ve·no·ve·nos·to·my
  pl ve·no·ve·nos·to·mies
vent
ven·ter
ven·ti·late
ven·ti·la·tion
ven·ti·lom·e·ter
ven·ti·lom·e·try
ven·trad
ven·tral
ven·tra·lis
ven·tri·cle
ven·tri·co·lum·na
  pl ven·tri·co·lum·nae
ven·tri·cor·nu
  pl ven·tri·cor·nu·a
ven·tri·cose
ven·tric·u·lar
ven·tric·u·lar·is
ven·tric·u·li·tis
ven·tric·u·lo·a·tri·al
ven·tric·u·lo·a·tri·os·to·my
ven·tric·u·lo·cis·ter·nos·to·
  my
  pl ven·tric·u·lo·cis·ter·nos·
  to·mies
ven·tric·u·lo·cor·dec·to·my
ven·tric·u·lo·gram
ven·tric·u·log·ra·phy
  pl ven·tric·u·log·ra·phies
ven·tric·u·lo·jug·u·lar
ven·tric·u·lo·mas·toi·dos·
  to·my
ven·tric·u·lom·e·try
ven·tric·u·lo·nec·tor
ven·tric·u·lo·per·i·to·ne·al
ven·tric·u·lo·pleu·ral
ven·tric·u·lo·punc·ture
ven·tric·u·lo·scope
ven·tric·u·los·co·py
  pl ven·tric·u·los·co·pies
ven·tric·u·los·to·my
  pl ven·tric·u·los·to·mies

ven·tric·u·lo·sub·a·rach·
    noid
ven·tric·u·lot·o·my
    pl ven·tric·u·lot·o·mies
ven·tric·u·lo·ve·nous
ven·tric·u·lus
    pl ven·tric·u·li
ven·tri·cum·bent
ven·tri·duct
ven·tri·duc·tion
ven·tri·lat·er·al
ven·tril·o·quism
ven·tri·me·sal
ven·trim·e·son
ven·tro·cys·tor·rha·phy
ven·tro·fix·a·tion
ven·tro·hys·ter·o·pex·y
    pl ven·tro·hys·ter·o·pex·ies
ven·tro·lat·er·al
ven·tro·lat·er·al·ly
ven·tro·me·di·al
ven·tro·me·di·al·ly
ven·trop·to·sis
ven·tros·co·py
    pl ven·tros·co·pies
ven·trose
ven·tros·i·ty
ven·tro·sus·pen·sion
ven·trot·o·my
ven·tro·ves·i·co·fix·a·tion
Ven·tu·ri waves
ven·tu·rim·e·ter
ven·u·la
    pl ven·u·lae
ven·u·lar
ven·ule
ve·nus
ver·a·ce·vine
ve·rat·ri·dine
ve·ra·trine
ve·rat·ro·sine
ve·ra·trum
ver·bal
ver·bal·ly
Ver·bas·cum
ver·big·er·a·tion
ver·bo·ma·ni·a
ver·di·gris
ver·do·glo·bin

ver·do·hae·min
    var of ver·do·he·min
ver·do·he·min
ver·do·nych·i·a
ver·do·per·ox·i·dase
verge
ver·gence
ver·gens
ver·ge·ture
Ver·hoeff stain
ver·mi·ci·dal
ver·mi·cide
ver·mic·u·lar
ver·mic·u·late
ver·mic·u·la·tion
ver·mi·cule
ver·mic·u·lose
ver·mic·u·lous
ver·mic·u·lus
    pl ver·mic·u·li
ver·mi·form
ver·mi·fu·gal
ver·mi·fuge
ver·mi·lin·gual
ver·mil·ion
ver·mil·ion·ec·to·my
    pl ver·mil·ion·ec·to·mies
ver·min
    pl ver·min
ver·mi·na·tion
ver·mi·no·sis
    pl ver·mi·no·ses
ver·mi·nous
ver·mi·nous·ly
ver·mi·pho·bi·a
ver·mis
    pl ver·mes
ver·mix
ver·nal
Ver·net syn·drome
Ver·neuil neu·ro·ma
ver·ni·er
ver·nine
ver·nix
ver·nix ca·se·o·sa
Ver·no·ni·a
Ver·o·cay bod·ies
ve·ro·di·gen

ver·ru·ca
    pl ver·ru·cae
ver·ru·ca a·cu·mi·na·ta
ver·ru·ca plan·tar·is
ver·ru·ca se·ni·lis
ver·ru·ca vul·gar·is
ver·ru·ci·form
ver·ru·coid
ver·ru·cose
ver·ru·co·sis
    pl ver·ru·co·ses
ver·ru·cous
ver·ru·ga
ver·ru·ga per·u·a·na
ver·si·col·or
ver·sion
ver·te·bra
    pl ver·te·bras
    or ver·te·brae
ver·te·bra·dym·i·a
ver·te·bral
ver·te·bral·ly
ver·te·bra·ri·um
ver·te·brar·te·ri·al
Ver·te·bra·ta
ver·te·brate
ver·te·brec·to·my
    pl ver·te·brec·to·mies
ver·te·bro·bas·i·lar
ver·te·bro·con·dral
ver·te·bro·cos·tal
ver·te·bro·di·dym·i·a
ver·te·bro·sa·cral
ver·te·bro·ster·nal
ver·tex
    pl ver·tex·es
    or ver·ti·ces
ver·ti·cal
ver·ti·ca·lis
ver·ti·cal·ly
ver·ti·cil
ver·ti·cil·late
ver·tig·i·nous
ver·ti·go
    pl ver·ti·gos
    or ver·tig·i·nes
    or ver·ti·goes
ver·tig·ra·phy
ver·u·mon·ta·ni·tis

ver·u·mon·ta·num
ve·sa·li·a·num
Ve·sa·li·us bone
ve·sa·ni·a
ve·sa·nic
ve·si·ca
  pl ve·si·cae
ves·i·cal
ves·i·cant
ves·i·cate
ves·i·ca·tion
ves·i·ca·to·ry
  pl ves·i·ca·to·ries
ves·i·cle
ves·i·co·ab·dom·i·nal
ves·i·co·bul·lous
ves·i·co·cele
ves·i·co·cer·vi·cal
ves·i·coc·ly·sis
ves·i·co·en·ter·ic
ves·i·co·fix·a·tion
ves·i·co·in·tes·ti·nal
ves·i·co·pros·tat·ic
ves·i·co·pu·bic
ves·i·co·pu·den·dal
ves·i·co·pus·tu·lar
ves·i·co·pus·tule
ves·i·co·rec·tal
ves·i·co·rec·to·vag·i·nal
ves·i·co·sig·moid
ves·i·co·sig·moi·dos·to·my
ves·i·co·spi·nal
ves·i·cos·to·my
ves·i·cot·o·my
  pl ves·i·cot·o·mies
ves·i·co·um·bil·i·cal
ves·i·co·u·re·ter·al
ves·i·co·u·re·thral
ves·i·co·u·re·thro·vag·i·nal
ves·i·co·u·ter·ine
ves·i·co·u·ter·o·vag·i·nal
ves·i·co·vag·i·nal
ve·sic·u·la
  pl ve·sic·u·las
  or ve·sic·u·lae
ve·sic·u·lar
ve·sic·u·late
ve·sic·u·la·tion

ve·sic·u·lec·to·my
  pl ve·sic·u·lec·to·mies
ve·sic·u·li·form
ve·sic·u·li·tis
ve·sic·u·lo·bron·chi·al
ve·sic·u·lo·bul·lous
ve·sic·u·lo·cav·ern·ous
ve·sic·u·lo·gram
ve·sic·u·log·ra·phy
  pl ve·sic·u·log·ra·phies
ve·sic·u·lo·pap·u·lar
ve·sic·u·lo·pus·tu·lar
ve·sic·u·lot·o·my
  pl ve·sic·u·lot·o·mies
ve·sic·u·lo·tym·pan·ic
ves·sel
ves·tib·u·lar
ves·ti·bule
ves·tib·u·lo·cer·e·bel·lar
ves·tib·u·lo·coch·le·ar
ves·tib·u·lo·oc·u·lar
ves·tib·u·lo·plas·ty
ves·tib·u·lo·spi·nal
ves·tib·u·lot·o·my
  pl ves·tib·u·lo·to·mies
ves·tib·u·lo·u·re·thral
ves·tib·u·lum
  pl ves·tib·u·la
ves·tige
ves·tig·i·al
ves·ti·gi·al·ly
ves·tig·i·um
  pl ves·tig·i·a
ve·ta
vet·er·i·nar·i·an
vet·er·i·nar·y
  pl vet·er·i·nar·ies
vi·a
  pl vi·as
  or vi·ae
vi·a·bil·i·ty
  pl vi·a·bil·i·ties
vi·a·ble
vi·a·bly
vi·al
vi·bes·ate
vi·bex
  pl vi·bi·ces
vi·brate

vi·bra·tile
vi·bra·tion
vi·bra·tor
vi·bra·to·ry
Vib·ri·o
vib·ri·o·ci·dal
vi·bri·on
vib·ri·o·sis
  pl vib·ri·o·ses
vi·bris·sa
  pl vi·bris·sae
vi·bro·car·di·o·gram
vi·bro·car·di·og·ra·phy
vi·bro·mas·sage
vi·bro·ther·a·peu·tics
vi·bur·num
vi·car·i·ous
vice
vic·i·a·nose
vi·cious
Vicq d'A·zyr tract
vid·e·og·no·sis
Vid·i·an ar·ter·y
Vie·us·sens an·sa
vig·il
vig·il·am·bu·lism
vig·i·lance
vig·or
Vil·la·ret syn·drome
vil·li
vil·lik·i·nin
vil·li·tis
vil·lo·ma
vil·lose
vil·lo·si·tis
vil·los·i·ty
  pl vil·los·i·ties
vil·lous
vil·lous·ly
vil·lus
  pl vil·li
vil·lus·ec·to·my
  pl vil·lus·ec·to·mies
vin·bar·bi·tal
vin·blas·tine
Vin·ca
vin·ca·leu·ko·blas·tine
Vin·cent an·gi·na
vin·cris·tine

418

vin·cu·lum
   pl vin·cu·lums
   or vin·cu·la
Vine·berg op·er·a·tion
vin·e·gar
Vine·land scale
vin·gly·ci·nate
vi·nic
vin·leu·ro·sine
vin·ro·si·dine
Vin·son-
   Plum·mer syn·drome
vi·nous
vi·nyl
vi·nyl et·her
vi·nyl·ben·zene
vi·nyl·ene
vi·nyl·i·dene
vi·o·la·ceous
vi·o·la·quer·ci·trin
vi·o·la·tion
vi·o·my·cin
vi·os·ter·ol
vi·per
Vi·per·i·dae
vi·rae·mi·a
   var of vi·re·mi·a
vi·ral
Vir·chow law
Vir·chow-Rob·in spa·ces
vi·re·mi·a
vi·re·mic
vir·gin
vir·gin·al
vir·gin·i·ty
   pl vir·gin·i·ties
vir·gin·i·um
vir·i·ci·dal
vir·i·cide
vir·i·dans strep·to·coc·ci
vir·i·din
vi·rid·o·ful·vin
vir·ile
vir·i·les·cence
vir·i·les·cent
vir·i·lism
vi·ril·i·ty
   pl vi·ril·i·ties
vir·i·li·za·tion

vir·i·lize
vi·ri·on
vi·rip·o·tent
vi·ro·cyte
vi·ro·log·ic
   or vi·ro·log·i·cal
vi·ro·log·i·cal
   or vi·ro·log·ic
vi·ro·log·i·cal·ly
vi·rol·o·gist
vi·rol·o·gy
   pl vi·rol·o·gies
vi·ro·pex·is
vi·ro·sis
   pl vi·ro·ses
vir·tu·al
vi·ru·ci·dal
vi·ru·cide
vi·ru·ci·din
vir·u·lence
   or vir·u·len·cy
vir·u·len·cy
   pl vir·u·len·cies
   or vir·u·lence
vir·u·lent
vir·u·lent·ly
vir·u·lif·er·ous
vir·u·ri·a
vi·rus
vi·rus·cyte
vir·u·stat·ic
vis
   pl vi·res
vis a ter·go
   pl vi·res a ter·go
vis·am·min
vis·cer·a
vis·cer·ad
vis·cer·al
vis·cer·al·gi·a
vis·cer·o·car·di·ac
vis·cer·o·cep·tor
vis·cer·o·gen·ic
vis·cer·o·in·hib·i·to·ry
vis·cer·o·meg·a·ly
   pl vis·cer·o·meg·a·lies
vis·cer·o·mo·tor
vis·cer·o·pa·ri·e·tal
vis·cer·o·per·i·to·ne·al

vis·cer·o·pleu·ral
vis·cer·op·to·sis
   pl vis·cer·op·to·ses
vis·cer·op·tot·ic
vis·cer·o·sen·sor·y
vis·cer·o·skel·e·tal
vis·cer·o·so·mat·ic
vis·cer·o·tome
vis·cer·ot·o·my
vis·cer·o·to·ni·a
vis·cer·o·ton·ic
vis·cer·o·troph·ic
vis·cer·o·trop·ic
vis·cer·ot·ro·pism
vis·cid
vis·cid·i·ty
   pl vis·cid·i·ties
vis·com·e·ter
vis·co·liz·er
vis·com·e·try
   pl vis·com·e·tries
vis·co·sim·e·ter
vis·co·sim·e·try
   pl vis·co·sim·e·tries
vis·cos·i·ty
   pl vis·cos·i·ties
vis·cous
vis·cus
   pl vis·cer·a
vis·i·bil·i·ty
vis·i·ble
vi·sion
vis·na
vi·su·al
vis·u·al·i·za·tion
vi·su·al·ize
vi·su·al·iz·er
vis·u·o·au·di·tor·y
vis·u·og·no·sis
   pl vis·u·og·no·ses
vis·u·o·mo·tor
vis·u·o·psy·chic
vis·u·o·sen·so·ry
vi·sus
vi·tal
vi·tal·ism
vi·tal·ist
vi·tal·is·tic

vi·tal·i·ty
  pl vi·tal·i·ties
vi·tal·ize
vi·ta·lom·e·ter
vi·tals
vi·ta·mer
vi·ta·min
vi·ta·min·i·za·tion
vi·ta·min·ize
vi·ta·min·ol·o·gy
  pl vi·ta·min·ol·o·gies
vi·tel·lin
vi·tel·line
vi·tel·lo·gen·e·sis
  pl vi·tel·lo·gen·e·ses
vi·tel·lo·in·tes·tin·al
vi·tel·lo·lu·te·in
vi·tel·lo·mes·en·ter·ic
vi·tel·lo·ru·bin
vi·tel·lus
  pl vi·tel·li
vi·ti·a·tion
vit·i·lig·i·nes
vit·i·lig·i·nous
vit·i·li·go
vit·i·li·goi·de·a
vi·trec·to·my
vit·re·in
vit·re·o·den·tin
vit·re·o·den·tine
vit·re·ous
vi·tres·cence
vi·tres·cent
vit·re·um
vit·ric
vi·tri·na
vit·ri·ol
vit·ri·ol·ic
vit·ro·pres·sion
vit·rum
vi·var·i·um
  pl vi·var·i·ums
  or vi·var·i·a
vi·vax ma·lar·i·a
viv·i·di·al·y·sis
vi·vi·dif·fu·sion
vi·vi·fi·ca·tion
vi·vi·par·i·ty
  pl vi·vi·par·i·ties

vi·vip·a·rous
vi·vi·sect
viv·i·sec·tion
viv·i·sec·tion·al
viv·i·sec·tion·ist
viv·i·sec·tor
Vlem·inckx so·lu·tion
vo·cal
vo·ca·lis
Vo·ges-
  Pros·kau·er re·ac·tion
Vogt point
Vogt-Ko·ya·na·gi-
  Ha·ra·da syn·drome
voice
void
Voille·mier point
vo·la
vo·lar
vo·la·ris
vol·a·tile
vol·a·til·i·za·tion
vol·a·til·ize
vol·az·o·cine
vole
vo·le·mic
Vol·hard and Fahr test
Vol·hard-Har·vey meth·od
Vol·hyn·i·a fe·ver
vo·li·tion
vo·li·tion·al
Volk·mann ca·nal
vol·ley
  pl vol·leys
  or vol·lies
Voll·mer patch test
vol·sel·lum
  pl vol·sel·la
volt
volt·age
vol·ta·ic
vol·ta·ism
volt-am·me·ter
volt·am·pere
Vol·ter·ra meth·od
volt·me·ter
vol·ume
vol·ume·nom·e·ter
vol·u·met·ric

vol·u·mom·e·ter
vol·un·tar·y
vo·lute
vol·u·tin
vol·vox
vol·vu·lo·sis
vol·vu·lus
vo·mer
vo·mer·ine
vom·er·o·bas·i·lar
vom·er·o·na·sal
vom·i·ca
  pl vom·i·cae
vom·it
vom·it·ing
vom·i·tive
vom·i·to ne·gro
vom·i·to·ry
vom·i·tu·ri·tion
vom·i·tus
von Al·dor test
von den Vel·den meth·od
von Ec·o·no·mo dis·ease
von Gier·ke dis·ease
von Grae·fe sign
von Hip·pel-
  Lin·dau dis·ease
von Jaksch a·ne·mi·a
von Jaksch-Pol·lak test
von Kós·sa stain
von Noor·den treat·ment
von Pir·quet test
von Reck·ling·hau·sen
  dis·ease
von Stein test
von Wil·le·brand dis·ease
vo·ra·cious
Vo·ro·noff op·er·a·tion
vor·tex
  pl vor·tex·es
  or vor·ti·ces
vor·ti·ces pi·lo·rum
vor·ti·cose
Vos·si·us ring
vox
  pl vo·ces
vo·yeur
vo·yeur·ism

vo·yeur·is·tic
Vro·lik dis·ease
vu·e·rom·e·ter
vul·can·i·za·tion
vul·can·ize
vul·gar·is
vul·ner·a·bil·i·ty
  pl vul·ner·a·bil·i·ties
vul·ner·a·ble
vul·ner·ar·y
  pl vul·ner·ar·ies

vul·nus
  pl vul·ner·a
Vul·pi·an at·ro·phy
Vul·pi·an-Hei·den·han-
  Sher·ring·ton phe·nom·
  e·non
vul·sel·lum
  pl vul·sel·la
vul·va
  pl vul·vae
vul·vae a·cu·tum ul·cus

vul·val
vul·var
vul·vec·to·my
  pl vul·vec·to·mies
vul·vis·mus
vul·vi·tis
vul·vo·cru·ral
vul·vo·u·ter·ine
vul·vo·vag·i·nal
vul·vo·vag·i·ni·tis

W

Wa·chen·stein-Zak
  meth·od
Wa·da test
wad·ding
wad·dle
wa·fer
Wag·ner cor·pus·cles
Wag·ner-Jau·regg
  treat·ment
Wag·staffe frac·ture
Wahl sign
waist
waist·line
wake·ful·ness
Wal·den·ström syn·drome
Wal·dey·er ep·i·the·li·um
Wal·dey·er ton·sil·lar ring
Wal·dey·er zo·nal lay·er
Walk·er-
  Rei·sin·ger meth·od
Wal·lace-
  Dia·mond meth·od
Wal·len·berg syn·drome
Wal·le·ri·an de·gen·er·a·
  tion
wall·eye
Wal·thard in·clu·sions

Wal·ther gan·gli·on
Wal·ton op·er·a·tion
Wang test
Wan·gen·steen ap·pa·ra·
  tus
war·bles
War·burg ap·pa·ra·tus
ward
Ward tri·an·gle
War·dell meth·od
War·drop dis·ease
war·fa·rin
warm-blood·ed
warm-blood·ed·ness
War·ner hand
War·ren in·ci·sion
wart
War·ten·berg dis·ease
War·thin sign
War·thin-
  Fin·kel·dey gi·ant cells
War·thin-Star·ry meth·od
wart·y
Was·ser·mann an·ti·body
Was·ser·mann-fast
waste

wa·ter pick
  or wa·ter tooth·
    pick
wa·ter tooth·pick
  or wa·ter pick
wa·ter·borne
Wa·ter·house-
  Fri·der·ich·sen syn·
  drome
Wa·ters pro·jec·tion
wa·ter·shed
Wat·son meth·od
Wat·son-Crick mo·del
Wat·son-Schwartz test
watt
watt·age
watt·me·ter
Waugh-Rud·dick test
wave
wave·length
wean
wean·ling
wea·sand
web
We·ber cor·pus·cle
Web·er dis·ease
Web·er-Chris·tian dis·ease

We·ber-Fech·ner law
Web·ster op·er·a·tion
Wechs·ler-Belle·vue in·tel·li·gence scale
We·den·sky fa·cil·i·ta·tion
weep·ing
We·ge·ner gran·u·lo·ma·to·sis
Weg·ner dis·ease
Weich·sel·baum coc·cus
Wei·del re·ac·tion
Wei·gert law
Wei·gert-Mey·er law
weight
weight·less·ness
Weil dis·ease
Weil test
Weil-Fe·lix re·ac·tion
Wein·back meth·od
Wein·grow heel re·flex
Weir op·er·a·tion
Weis·bach an·gle
Weis·mann the·o·ry
Weiss sign
Weisz test
Welch ba·cil·lus
well-born
well-bred
Wells fa·ci·es
Wells-Sten·ger test
Welt·mer·ism
wen
Wen·cke·bach phe·nom·e·non
Werd·nig-Hoff·mann at·ro·phy
Werl·hof dis·ease
Wer·ne·kink com·mis·sure
Wer·ner dis·ease
Wer·ner-His dis·ease
Wer·ni·cke a·pha·si·a
Wer·ni·cke-Mann pa·ral·y·sis
Werth tu·mor
Wert·heim op·er·a·tion
Wert·heim-Schau·ta op·er·a·tion
West syn·drome

Wes·ter·gren meth·od
West·phal dis·ease
West·phal-Pilcz re·flex
West·phal-Strüm·pell pseu·do·scle·ro·sis
wet-nurse
Wet·zel grid
We·ver-Bray ef·fect
Weyl test
Whar·ton duct, jel·ly
wheal
wheel·chair
Wheel·house op·er·a·tion
wheeze
whelp
whey
whip·lash
Whip·ple op·er·a·tion
whip·worm
whis·per
White meth·od
white·comb
white·head
white·pox
Whit·field oint·ment
whit·low
whoop·ing cough
whorl
Whytt dis·ease
Wick·ham stri·ae
wick·ing
Wi·dal re·ac·tion
Wig·and ma·neu·ver
Wil·bur and Ad·dis meth·od
Wild·bolz re·ac·tion
Wil·der test
Wil·der·muth au·ri·cle, ear
Wil·hel·mi meth·od
Wilks syn·drome
Wil·lems meth·od
Wil·li-Pra·der syn·drome
Wil·liam·son sign
Wil·lis ar·ter·y, cir·cle, cords
Wilms tu·mor
Wil·son dis·ease

Wil·son-Mik·i·ty syn·drome
Wim·ber·ger line
Win·ckel dis·ease
wind·age
Win·daus dig·i·to·nin test
wind·bro·ken
wind·burn
wind·chill
wind·gall
wind·kes·sel
win·dow
wind·pipe
wind·puff
wind·suck·ing
Win·i·war·ter op·er·a·tion
Wins·low fo·ra·men
Win·ter·bot·tom sign
win·ter·green
Win·ter·nitz phe·nom·e·non
Win·trich sign
Win·trobe-Lands·berg meth·od
Win·trobe meth·od
wir·ing
Wir·sung ca·nal
wish ful·fill·ment
wish·ful think·ing
Wis·kott-Al·drich syn·drome
Wis·tar rat
Wib·teb·sky sub·stance
with·draw·al
with·ers
Witt·maak-Ek·bom syn·drome
Wit·zel op·er·a·tion
wit·zel·sucht
wob·bles
Wohl·fahr·ti·a mag·nif·i·ca
Wohl·ge·muth meth·od
Woil·lez dis·ease
Wolff law
Wolff-Eis·ner test
Wolff·i·an bod·y, duct
Wolff-Park·in·son-White syn·drome
wolf·jaw

Wöl·fler op·er·a·tion
wolf·ram
Wol·fring glands
wolfs·bane
Wol·hyn·i·a fe·ver
Wol·las·ton doub·let
Wol·man dis·ease
Wolt·man-
  Ker·no·han syn·drome
womb
Wong meth·od
Wood light
Wool·ner tu·ber·cle,
  point, tip

wool·sort·er dis·ease
word-as·so·ci·a·tion test
word sal·ad
work-up
  or work·up
worm
Wor·mi·an bone
worm·seed
Woulff bot·tle
wound
Wre·den op·er·a·tion
Wre·den-Stone
  op·er·a·tion
Wright stain

wrin·kle
Wris·berg car·ti·lage,
  nerve
wrist
wrist·drop
writ·er's cramp
wry·head
wry·neck
Wu·cher at·ro·phy
Wu·cher·er·i·a ban·crof·ti
wu·cher·e·ri·a·sis
Wun·der·lich curve
Wundt tet·a·nus
Wy·lie op·er·a·tion

X

Xan·thate
xan·thel·as·ma
  pl xan·the·las·mas
  or xan·the·las·ma·ta
xan·the·las·moi·de·a
xan·them·a·tin
xan·the·mi·a
xan·thene
xan·thic
xan·thine
xan·thi·nol ni·a·cin·ate
xan·thi·nu·ri·a
xan·thi·u·ri·a
xan·tho·chroi·a
xan·tho·chro·mat·ic
xan·tho·chro·mi·a
xan·tho·chro·mic
xan·thoch·ro·ous
xan·tho·cy·a·no·pi·a
xan·tho·cy·a·nop·si·a
xan·tho·cyte
xan·tho·der·ma

xan·tho·fi·bro·ma the·co·
  cel·lu·lar·e
xan·tho·gran·u·lo·ma
  pl xan·tho·gran·u·lo·mas
  or xan·tho·gran·u·lo·ma·ta
xan·tho·gran·u·lo·ma·to·
  sis
xan·tho·ky·an·o·py
xan·tho·ma
  pl xan·tho·mas
  or xan·tho·ma·ta
xan·tho·ma·to·sis
  pl xan·tho·ma·to·ses
xan·thom·a·tous
xan·thone
xan·tho·phane
xan·tho·phore
xan·tho·phose
xan·tho·phyll
xan·tho·pi·a
xan·tho·pro·te·ic
xan·tho·pro·te·in
xan·thop·si·a

xan·thop·sin
xan·thop·sy·dra·ci·a
xan·thop·ter·in
xan·tho·rham·nin
xan·thor·rhe·a
xan·thor·rhoe·a
  var of xan·thor·rhe·a
xan·tho·sine
xan·tho·sis
  pl xan·tho·ses
xan·thous
xan·thox·y·lum
xan·thu·re·nic
xan·thy·drol
xan·thyl·ic
xe·nic
xe·ni·cal·ly
xe·no·bi·ol·o·gy
xen·o·di·ag·no·sis
  pl xen·o·di·ag·no·ses
xen·o·di·ag·nos·tic
xen·o·gen·e·ic
xen·o·gen·e·sis

xen·o·gen·ic
xen·og·e·nous
xen·o·graft
xe·nol·o·gy
xen·o·me·ni·a
xe·non
xen·o·par·a·site
xen·o·pho·bi·a
xen·o·pho·ni·a
xen·oph·thal·mi·a
xen·o·plas·tic
xen·o·plas·ty
Xen·op·syl·la
Xen·o·pus
xe·ran·sis
xe·ran·tic
xe·ra·si·a
xe·ro·chei·li·a
xe·ro·der·ma
xe·ro·der·mos·te·o·sis
xe·rog·ra·phy
xe·ro·ma
xe·ro·me·ni·a
xe·ro·myc·te·ri·a
xe·ron·o·sus

xe·ro·pha·gi·a
  or xe·roph·a·gy
  pl xe·roph·a·gies
xe·roph·a·gy
  pl xe·roph·a·gies
  or xe·ro·pha·gi·a
xe·roph·thal·mi·a
xe·roph·thal·mic
xe·ro·ra·di·og·ra·phy
  pl xe·ro·ra·di·og·ra·phies
xe·ro·sis
  pl xe·ro·ses
xe·ro·sto·mi·a
xe·ro·tes
xe·ro·tic
xe·ro·to·ci·a
xe·ro·trip·sis
xiph·i·ster·nal
xiph·i·ster·num
  pl xiph·i·ster·na
xiph·o·cos·tal
xi·phod·y·mus
xiph·o·dyn·i·a
xi·phoid
  or xi·phoi·dal

xi·phoi·dal
  or xi·phoid
xiph·oid·i·tis
xi·phop·a·gus
xiph·o·um·bil·i·cal
X-ir·ra·di·ate
X-ir·ra·di·a·tion
X-ra·di·a·tion
X-ray
xy·lam·i·dine
xy·lan
xy·lem
xy·lene
xy·le·nol
xy·li·dine pon·ceau
X-linked
xy·lo·ke·tose
xy·lol
xy·lo·me·taz·o·line
xy·lo·pho·bi·a
xy·lose
xy·lo·ther·a·py
xy·lu·lose
xy·lyl
xy·ro·spasm
xys·ma
xys·ter

Y

Yaw
yaw·ey
yawn
yaws
yeast
yel·low
Ye·men ul·cer
yer·ba
yilt
  var of gilt
yo·ghurt
  or yo·gurt

yo·gurt
  or yo·ghurt
yo·him·bé
  or yo·him·bi
yo·him·bi
  or yo·him·bé
yo·him·bine
yoke
yolk
yolk sac
yolk stalk

Yo·shi·da tu·mor
Young·burg and Fo·lin
  meth·od
y·per·ite
yp·sil·i·form
yt·ter·bi·um
yt·tri·um
Yu·ge syn·drome
Y·von co·ef·fi·cient
Y·von test

424

Z

ze·a·tin
ze·a·xan·thin
zed·o·ar·y
Zee·man ef·fec
ze·in
Zeis glands
Zel·ler test
Zen·ker flu·id
ze·o·lite
ze·o·scope
ze·ro
  pl ze·ros
  or ze·roes
Zie·hem-
  Op·pen·heim dis·ease
Ziehl-Neel·sen stain
Ziems·sen point
Zieve syn·drome
Zim·mer·lin type
Zim·mer·mann re·ac·tion,
  test
zinc
zinc·if·er·ous
zinc·ite
zin·coid
zin·gi·ber
Zinn lig·a·ment
Zins·ser-Eng·man-Cole
  syn·drome
zir·co·ni·um
zo·ac·an·tho·sis
  pl zo·ac·an·tho·ses
zo·an·thro·py
  pl zo·an·thro·pies
zo·et·ic
zo·e·trope
  or zo·o·trope
zo·ic
zo·la·mine
zo·ler·tine
Zol·lin·ger-
  El·li·son syn·drome
Zöll·ner lines
zo·na
  pl zo·nas
  or zo·nae
zo·na pel·lu·ci·da
  pl zo·nae pel·lu·ci·dae

zo·naes·the·si·a
  var of zo·nes·the·si·a
zo·nal
zo·nar·y
zon·ate
zo·nes·the·si·a
zo·nif·u·gal
zon·ing
zo·nip·e·tal
zo·nu·la
  pl zo·nu·las
  or zo·nu·lae
zo·nu·lar
zo·nule
z·onu·le of Zinn
zo·nu·li·tis
zo·nu·lol·y·sis
zo·nu·lot·o·my
zo·nu·ly·sis
  pl zo·nu·ly·ses
zo·o·bi·ol·o·gy
zo·o·chem·is·try
zo·o·der·mic
zo·o·dy·nam·ics
zo·o·e·ras·ti·a
zo·o·ge·ne·ous
  or zo·og·e·nous
zo·o·gen·ic
zo·og·e·nous
  or zo·o·ge·ne·ous
zo·og·e·ny
zo·o·ge·o·graph·ic
  or zo·o·ge·o·graph·i·cal
zo·o·ge·o·graph·i
  or zo·o·ge·o·graph·ic
zo·o·ge·og·ra·phy
  pl zo·o·ge·og·ra·phies
zo·o·gle·a
zo·o·gloe·a
  var of zo·o·gle·a
zo·og·o·ny
  pl zo·og·o·nies
zo·o·graft·ing
zo·og·ra·phy
  pl zo·og·ra·phies
zo·oid
zo·o·lag·ni·a
zo·ol·o·gist
zo·ol·o·gy

Zo·o·mas·ti·gi·ni·a
zo·on·o·my
  pl zo·on·o·mies
zo·o·no·sis
  pl zo·o·no·ses
zo·o·not·ic
zo·o·par·a·site
zo·o·par·a·sit·ic
zo·o·pa·thol·o·gy
  pl zo·o·pa·thol·o·gies
zo·oph·a·gous
zo·o·phile
zo·o·phil·i·a
  or zo·oph·i·lism
zo·o·phil·ic
zo·oph·i·l·sm
  or zo·o·phil·i·a
zo·oph·i·list
zo·oph·i·lous
zo·o·pho·bi·a
zo·o·phyte
zo·o·plank·ton
zo·o·plas·tic
zo·o·plas·ty
  pl zo·o·plas·ties
zo·op·si·a
zo·o·spore
zo·os·ter·ol
zo·o·tech·nics
zo·o·ther·a·peu·tics
zo·o·ther·a·py
  pl zo·o·ther·a·pies
zo·ot·o·my
zo·o·to·xin
zo·o·trope
  or zo·e·trope
zo·o·troph·ic
zos·ter
zos·ter·i·form
zos·ter·oid
Z-plas·ty
zuck·er·guss
Zuck·er·kan·dl bod·ies
zuck·ung
Zwem·er test
zwit·ter·i·on
zy·gal
zyg·a·poph·y·se·al

zy·ga·poph·y·sis
  pl zy·ga·poph·y·ses
zyg·i·on
  pl zyg·i·ons
  or zyg·i·a
zy·goc·i·ty
  pl zy·goc·i·ties
zy·go·dac·ty·ly
  pl zy·go·dac·ty·lies
zy·go·ma
  pl zy·go·mas
  or zy·go·ma·ta
zy·go·mat·ic
zy·go·mat·i·co·au·ric·u·la·
  ris
  pl zy·go·mat·i·co·au·ric·u·
    la·res
zy·go·mat·i·co·fa·cial
zy·go·mat·i·co·max·il·lar·y
zy·go·mat·i·co·or·bit·al
zy·go·mat·i·co·tem·por·al
zy·go·mat·i·cus
zy·go·max·il·lar·e
zy·go·max·il·lar·y

zy·go·my·ce·tes
zy·go·my·ce·tous
zy·gon
zy·go·ne·ma
zy·go·sis
  pl zy·go·ses
zy·gos·i·ty
  pl zy·gos·i·ties
zy·go·sperm
zy·go·spore
zy·go·style
zy·gote
zy·go·tene
zy·got·ic
zy·mase
zyme
zy·mic
zy·mo·gen
zy·mo·gen·ic
zy·mog·e·nous
zy·mo·gram
zy·mo·hex·ase
zy·mo·hy·drol·y·sis
  pl zy·mo·hy·drol·y·ses

zy·moid
zy·mo·log·ic
zy·mol·o·gy
  pl zy·mol·o·gies
zy·mol·y·sis
  pl zy·mol·y·ses
zy·mo·lyte
zy·mo·lyt·ic
zy·mom·e·ter
zy·mo·nem·a·to·sis
zy·mo·phore
zy·mo·pho·ric
zy·mo·plas·tic
zy·mo·pro·te·in
zy·mo·san
zy·mo·scope
zy·mose
zy·mo·sis
  pl zy·mo·ses
zy·mos·ter·ol
zy·mos·then·ic
zy·mot·ic
zy·mot·i·cal·ly
zy·mur·gy

APPENDIX 1 Abreviations

A

a   accommodation; acetum; acid; acidity; actin; activity; allergist; allergy; alpha; ampere; anode; answer; ante; anterior; aqua; area; argon; artery; asymmetric; asymmetry; atria
A   absorbance
Å   angstrom unit
A_2 aortic second sound
AA   achievement age; Alcoholics Anonymous
AAF   ascorbic acid factor
AAL   anterior axillary line
A & P   anterior and posterior; auscultation and percussion
A & W   alive and well
ab   abort; abortion; about
AB   add to blind; Bachelor of Arts
ABC   atomic, biological, and chemical
abd   abdomen; abdominal
abdom   abdomen; abdominal
abort   abortion
abs   absent; absolute
ABS   acute brain syndrome
abt   about
ac   acute
Ac   actinium; acetyl
Ac   air conduction; anodic closure; axiocervical; alternating current
acc   acceleration; according
ACE   adrenocortical extract
acG   accelerator globulin (Factor V)
ACG   apex cardiogram
ACh   acetylcholine
ACHE   acetylcholinesterase
AcPase   acid phosphatase
ACS   antireticular cytotoxic serum
act   active
ACTH   adrenocorticotrophic hormone
A disk   anisotropic disk
Ad   anisotropic disk

AD   average deviation; right ear (auris dextra)
ADC   Aid to Dependent Children; anodic duration contraction; axiodistocervical
add   adduction; adductor
ADH   antidiuretic hormone
adj   adjunct
ADL   activities of daily living
adm   administration; administrator; admission; admit
ADP   adenosine diphosphate
ADPase   adenosine diphosphatase
ae   of age, aged (aet, aetat)
AF   audio frequency; auricular fibrillation
AFB   acid-fast bacillus
Ag   silver (argentum)
AGA   accelerated growth area
A/g ratio   albumin-globulin ratio
agglut   agglutination
agt   agent
ah   hypermetropic astigmatism
AHF   antihemolytic factor; antihemophilic factor
AHG   antihemophilic globulin; antihuman globulin
AI   aortic insufficiency; artificial insemination
AID   artificial insemination by donor
AIH   artificial insemination by husband
AJ   ankle jerk
AK   above knee
Al   aluminum
alb   albumin
alc   alcohol
ALG   antilymphocyte globulin; antilymphocytic globulin
alk   alkaline
als   amyotrophic lateral sclerosis; antilymphocyte serum; antilymphocytic serum

427

alt   alternate; altitude
alv   alveolar
am   ametropia; meter-angle, myopic astigmatism; ammeter; ampere-meter; amplitude modulation
AM   Master of Arts
Am   americium
AMA   against medical advice
amb   ambulance; ambulatory
AMI   acute myocardial infarction
AML   acute myoblastic leukemia
amp   amperage; ampere; ampule; amputation
AMP   adenosine monophosphate
AMPase   adenosine monophosphatase
amt   amount
An   anisometropia; anodal; anode
ANA   American Nurses Association
anal   analysis; analytic; analyze
anat   anatomic; anatomical; anatomy
anh   anhydrous
ans   answer
ANS   anterior nasal spine; autonomic nervous system
A-P   anteroposterior
A & P   auscultation and percussion
ap   apothecaries
AP   action potential; alkaline phosphatase; anterior pituitary; aortic pressure
APC   virus adenovirus; aspirin, phenacetin, and caffeine
A-P & Lat   anteroposterior and lateral
APF   animal protein factor (vitamin B_{12})
app   appendix
appl   applied
approx   approximate; approximately
appt   appointment
AQ   accomplishment quotient; achievement quotient
AQRS   mean manifest electrical axis of the QRS complex
Ar   argon
AR   alarm reaction
ARD   acute respiratory disease
as   astigmatism

As   arsenic
AS   left ear (auris sinistra); aortic stenosis; arteriosclerosis
ASA   aspirin (acetylsalicylic acid)
ASAP   as soon as possible
ASCVD   arteriosclerotic cardiovascular disease
ASHD   arteriosclerotic heart disease
ASLO   antistreptolysin-O
assn   association
Asst   assistant
Ast   astigmatism
as tol   as tolerated
at   airtight
At   astatine
AT   achievement test; mean manifest magnitude of repolarization of the myocardium
ATCC   American Type Culture Collection
atm   atmosphere; atmospheric
ATN   acute tubular necrosis
ATP   adenosine triphosphate
ATPase   adenosine triphosphatase
ATS   equine antitetanus serum
at vol   atomic volume
at wt   atomic weight
Au   gold (aurem)
au   angstrom unit; antitoxin unit
aux   auxiliary
av   average
Av   avoirdupois weight
AV   auriculoventricular; arteriovenous; atrioventricular
ax   axis
Az   nitrogen (azote)
AZT   Aschheim-Zondek test

B

b   balnium; barometric; bath; Baumé scale; behavior; Benoist scale; born; brother
B   boron; bacillus; boils at; buccal
Ba   barium
BA   bronchial asthma; buccoaxial
bact   bacteria; bacterial; bacteriological; bacteriology; bacterium

BaE or BAE barium enema
bal balance
BAL British Anti-Lewisite (dimer-
     caprol)
B & O belladonna and opium
bar barometer; barometric
baso basophil
BBB bundle branch block
BBT basal body temperature
BCG Bacillus Calmette-Guérin
     (tuberculosis vaccine); ballis-
     tocardiogram; bromcresyl
     green
BE barium enema; below elbow
Be beryllium
Bé Baumé
bev billion electron volts
BFP biological false-positive reac-
     tion
BH bill of health
BHC benzene hexachloride
BHL biological half-life
Bi bismuth
bili bilirubin
biol biologic; biological; biologist;
     biology
BJ biceps jerk
Bk berkelium
BK below knee
bld blood
BM Bachelor of Medicine; basal
     metabolism; bowel movement
BMR basal metabolic rate
BNA Basle Nomina Anatomica
BO body odor
BOD biochemical oxygen demand;
     biological oxygen demand
bot botanical; botany; bottle
BP blood pressure; British Pharma-
     copoeia
bp boiling point
Br bromine
BRP bathroom privileges
BS blood sugar; bowel sounds;
     breath sounds
BSA body surface area; bovine se-
     rum albumin
BSR blood sedimentation rate

BST blood serological test
BT bedtime; brain tumor
BTU British thermal unit
BUN blood urea nitrogen
BW blood Wassermann; body
     weight
Bx biopsy

C

c centum; deciduous canine; calorie;
   cathode; cervical; clonus; closure;
   cobalt; cocaine; coefficient; con-
   tact; coulomb
C canine of second dentition; chest,
   carbon; Celcius; centigrade; com-
   plement; closure; cylinder; con-
   traction
Ca calcium; cancer; carcinoma; car-
    diac
CA chronological age; cardiac arrest
CAC cardiac accelerator center
CAD coronary artery disease
CAI confused artificial insemination
cal small calorie
Cal large calorie
canc canceled
cap capacity; capsule
CAR conditioned avoidance re-
     sponse
CAT children's apperception test
cath cathartic; catheter
cav cavity
Cb columbium
CB Bachelor of Surgery (Chirurgiae
    Baccalaureus)
CBC complete blood count
CBD closed bladder drainage; com-
     mon bile duct
CBF cerebral blood flow
CBG corticosteroid-binding globulin
CBR chemical, bacteriological, and
     radiological
CBS chronic brain syndrome
CBW chemical and biological war-
     fare
cc cubic centimeter

CC   chief complaint; commission certified; critical condition; current complaint
CCA   chick cell agglutination; chimpanzee corzya agent
CCI   chronic coronary insufficiency
CCK   cholecystokinin
Ccr   creatinine clearance
CCT   chocolate-coated tablet
CCTe cathodal closure tetanus
CCU   coronary care unit
cd   candela
Cd   cadmium
CD   communicable disease; constant drainage; contagious disease; convulsive disorder; curative dose
CDC   calculated date of confinement; Center for Disease Control
Ce   cerium
CE   cardiac enlargement
Cel   Celsius
cen   central
Ceph floc cephalin flocculation
CER   conditioned emotional response; conditioned escape response
cert certificate, certified
cerv cervical
CES   central excitatory state
cf   compare (confer)
Cf   californium
CF   chest and left leg; complement fixation; cystic fibrosis
CFT   complement fixation test
CG   center of gravity; chorionic gonadotropin
cgs   centimeter gram-second
ch   child, chronic
ChB   Bachelor of Surgery (Chirurgiae Baccalaureus)
CHD   childhood disease; congenital heart disease; coronary heart disease
ChE   cholinesterase
chem chemical; chemist; chemistry
CHF   congestive heart failure
chg   change

chl   chloroform
CHINA chronic infectious neuropathic agent
CHO   carbohydrate
chol cholesterol
chr   chronic
Ci   curie
CI   chemotherapeutic index; color index
CICU coronary intensive care unit
CID   cytomegalic inclusion disease
CIE   counterimmunoelectrophoresis
cir   circular
circ circulation
cl   centiliter; clavicle; clinic; closure
Cl   chloride; chlorine
CL   chest and left arm; corpus luteum; critical list
clin clinical
CLL   chronic lymphocytic leukemia
CLO   cod liver oil
CLSH corpus luteum–stimulating hormone
cm   centimeter
Cm   curium
CM   Master of Surgery (Chirurgiae Magister); circular muscle
cmm   cubic millimeter
CMR   cerebral metabolic rate
CMV   cytomegalovirus
CNS   central nervous system
Co   cobalt, coenzyme
CO   carbon monoxide; cardiac output
c/o   complains of
coag coagulate; coagulation
coag time coagulation time
COC   cathodal opening contraction
COCl cathodal opening clonus
COD   chemical oxygen demand
coeff or coef coefficient
COH   carbohydrate
col   colony; color
coll collect; collection; colloidal; collyrium
comp comparative; compare; composition; compound
compl completed; complications
conc concentrated; concentration

cond   condition
cond ref   conditioned reflex
cond resp   conditioned response
conf   conference
cong   congenital
const   constant
cont   containing; contents; continue; continued
conv   convalescent
coord   coordination
COPD   chronic obstructive pulmonary disease
COPE   chronic obstructive pulmonary emphysema
cor   corrected
CoR   congo red
cort   cortex; cortical
CP   capillary pressure; cerebral palsy; chemically pure; compare; constant pressure; cor pulmonale
CPC   chronic passive congestion
cpd   compound
CPD   cephalopelvic disproportion
CPE   cytopathogenic effects
CPI   constitutional psychopathic inferiority
CPK   creatine phosphokinase
cpm   cycles per minute
CPM   counts per minute
cps   cycles per second
CPZ   chlorpromazine
Cr   chromium; creatinine
CR   cardiorespiratory; chest and right arm; clot retraction; conditioned reflex; conditioned response
CRD   chronic respiratory disease
CRF   corticotropin-releasing factor
crit   critical
CRM   cross-reacting material
CRO   cathode-ray oscilloscope
CrP   creatine phosphate
CRP   C-reactive protein
CRS   Chinese restaurant syndrome
CRT   cathode-ray tube; complex reaction time
cryst   crystalline; crystallized

cs   cesarean section; case; conditioned stimulus; consciousness; corticosteroid; current strength
Cs   cesium
CSF   cerebrospinal fluid
CSM   cerebrospinal meningitis
CSR   corrected sedimentation rate
CST   convulsive shock therapy
CT   circulation time; coated tablet; corrective therapist
CTa   catamenia (menstruation)
CTC   chlortetracycline
ctr   center
CTR   cardiothoracic ratio
CTU   centigrade thermal unit
cu   cubic
Cu   copper
CU   clinical unit
CUC   chronic ulcerative colitis
cult   culture
cur   curative; current
CV   cardiovascular
CVA   cardiovascular accident; costovertebral angle; cerebrovascular accident
CVD   cardiovascular disease
CVP   central venous pressure
CVR   cardiovascular renal; cardiovascular respiratory; cerebrovascular resistance
CVS   clean voided specimen
CW   crutch walking
cwt   hundredweight
Cx   cervix
Cy   cyanogen
Cyl   cylinder; cylindrical lens
cytol   cytological; cytology

D

d   date; dead; deceased; deciduous; degree; density; developed; deviation; dexter; diameter; died; diopter; disease; divorced; distal; give (da); let it be given (detur); dorsal; dose; duration
d   dextrorotary
D   deuterium

da   daughter, day
DA   delayed action; developmental age; dopamine
DAH   disordered action of the heart
D & C   dilatation and curettage
DAT   delayed action tablet; differential aptitude test
dB   decibel
dbl   double
DBP   diastolic blood pressure
DBT   dry bulb temperature
DC   Dental Corps; diagnostic center; direct current; distocervical; Doctor of Chiropractic
DCc   double concave
DCR   direct critical response
DDS   Doctor of Dental Science; Doctor of Dental Surgery
DDT   dichlorodiphenyltrichloroethane
dec   decreased; decompose
decd deceased; dead
def   defecation; deficient; definite
deg   degeneration; degree
del   delusion
dent dental; dentist; dentistry
depr depression
derm dermatology
detn detention
devel development
dg   decigram
DHHS Department of Health and Human Services
DHO   deuterium hydrogen oxide
DI   deterioration index; diabetes insipidus
dia   diameter; diathermy
diab diabetic
diag diagnosis; diagnostic; diagonal; diagram
diam diameter
diath diathermy
diff difference; differential blood count
dil   dilute
dilat dilatation
dim   diminished
DIP   distal interphalangeal
diph diphtheria

dis   disabled; disease
disc discontinue; discontinued
disch discharge; discharged
disp dispensary
dissd dissolved
div   divide; division; divorced
DJD   degenerative joint disease
dkg   dekagram
dkl   dekaliter
dkm   dekameter
dl   deciliter
DL   danger list
DLE   disseminated lupus erythematosus
dm   decimeter
DM   diabetes mellitus; diastolic murmur
DMD   Doctor of Dental Medicine (dentariae medicinae doctor)
DMF   decayed, missing, and filled teeth
DMSA dimercaptosuccinic acid
DMSO dimethylsulfoxide
DMT   dimethyltryptamine
DNA   deoxyribonucleic acid
DNB   dinitrobenzene
DO   diamine oxidase; Doctor of Optometry; Doctor of Osteopathy
DOA   dead on arrival
DOB   date of birth
doc   document
DOE   dyspnea on exertion
dom   domestic; dominant
DOPA dihydroxyphenylalanine
dos   dosage
doz   dozen
DP   deep pulse; diphosgene; Doctor of Podiatry; Doctor of Pharmacy
DPA   diphenylamine
DPH   Department of Public Health; Doctor of Public Health
DPN   diphosphopyridine nucleotide
DPT   diphtheria-pertussis-tetanus (vaccines)
DQ   deterioration quotient; developmental quotient
dr   dram; dressing
Dr   doctor
DR   delivery room

DS dead air space; dilute strength; dioptric strength
DSC Doctor of Surgical Chiropody
DSD dry sterile dressing
DT delirium tremens; distance test; duration of tetany
DTMA desoxycorticosterone trimethylacetate
DTN diphtheria toxin normal
DTPA diethylene triamine pentaacetic acid
DTR deep tendon reflex
DU diagnosis undetermined
dup duplicate
DV dilute volume
DVM Doctor of Veterinary Medicine
DW distilled water
dwt pennyweight
Dx diagnosis
Dy dysprosium

E

e electron
E einstein; emmetropia; enema; enzyme; experimenter; eye
ea each
EA educational age
EBV Epstein-Barr virus
ECF extracellular fluid
ECG electrocardiogram
ECS electroconvulsive shock
ECT electroconvulsive therapy
ED effective dose; erythema dose
ED$_{50}$ median effective dose
EDC expected date of confinement
EDN electrodessication
EDR effective direct radiation; electrodermal response
EDTA ethylenediaminetetraacetic acid
EENT eye, ear, nose, and throat
eg for example (exempli gratia)
Eh standard oxidation-reduction potential

EHBF estimated hepatic blood flow; extrahepatic blood flow
EHL effective half-life
EJ elbow jerk
EKG electrocardiogram; electrocardiograph
EKY electrokymogram
elec electric; electrical; electricity
elix elixir
EM electron microscope
emb embryo; embryology
EMC encephalomyocarditis
EMF electromotive force; erythrocyte maturation factor
EMG electromyogram; electromyography
EMIC emergency maternity and infant care
emul emulsion
enl enlarged
ENT ear, nose, and throat
EOA examination, opinion, and advice
EOG electrooculogram; electrooculograph
EOM extraocular movement
eos eosinophil
epil epilepsy; epileptic
epith epithelial; epithelium
eq equal; equivalent
EQ educational quotient
Er erbium
ER emergency room; endoplasmic reticulum; equivalent roentgen; extended release
ERBF effective renal blood flow
ERG electroretinogram
ERPF effective renal plasma flow
ERV expiratory reserve volume
Es Einsteinium
ESF erythropoietic-stimulating factor
esp especial; especially
ESP extrasensory perception
ESR electron spin resonance; erythrocyte sedimentation rate
EST electroshock therapy

ET   educational therapy
et al   and elsewhere (et alibi); and others (et alii)
etc   and so forth (et cetera)
et seq   and the following one (et sequens); and the following ones (et sequentes or et sequentia)
Eu   europium
eV   electron volt
ex   examined; example; exercise
exam   examination
exc   except; exception
exp   experiment; experimental; expired
expt   experiment
exptl   experimental
ext   external; extract; extremity

F

f   failure; family; farad; father; female; feminine; fibrous; focal length; foot; function; son (filius); brother (frater)
F   fluorine; Fahrenheit; formula; fellow
FA   fatty acid; filterable agent; first aid; folic acid
FACP   Fellow, American College of Physicians
FACS   Fellow, American College of Surgeons
FAD   flavin adenine dinucleotide
fah or Fahr   Fahrenheit
fam   family
FAMA   Fellow, American Medical Association
fb   finger-breadth
FB   foreign body
FBS   fasting blood sugar
FD   fan douche; fatal dose; focal distance
FDA   Food and Drug Administration
Fe   iron
fem   female; feminine; femur
ff   following

FF   fat free; filtration fraction; force fluid
FFA   free fatty acid
FFT   flicker fusion threshold
FH   family history
FHS   fetal heart sounds
FHT   fetal heart tone
fib   fibrillation
fig   figure
fl   fluid
fl dr   fluid dram
FL   focal length
fl oz   fluid ounce
Fm   fermium
FMD   foot and mouth disease
FMN or FM   flavin mononucleotide
fp   freezing point; foot-pound
fpm   feet per minute
fps   feet per second
fr   from
FR   flocculation reaction
Fr   francium
FRC   functional residual capacity
freq   frequency
FRF   follicle-stimulating hormone releasing factor
fsd   focus-to-skin distance
FSF   fibrin-stabilizing factor
FSH   follicle-stimulating hormone
ft   feet; foot
FUO   fever of undetermined origin
Fx   fracture

G

g   gauge; gender; gingival; glucose; grain; gram; gravity
G   gonidial (colony); gravitational constant
Ga   gallium
GA   gastric analysis
GABA   gamma aminobutyric acid
gal   galactose; gallon
galv   galvanic; galvanism; galvanized
gang or gangl   ganglion; ganglionic
G-A-S   general adaptation syndrome
GB   gallbladder; sarin (code name)

GBS   gallbladder series
GC   *Gonococcus*
Gd   gadolinium
Ge   germanium
GE   gastroenterology
gen   general; genus
GFR   glomerular filtration rate
GH   growth hormone
GHRF   growth hormone–releasing factor
gl   gland; glands
GI   gastrointestinal; globin insulin; growth-inhibiting
GL   greatest length
GLC   gas-liquid chromatography
gm   gram
GM and S   General Medicine and Surgery
GMP   guanosine monophosphate
GOE   gas, oxygen, and ether (anesthesia)
GOR   general operating room
GOT   glutamic-oxaloacetic transaminase
gp   group
GP   general paralysis; general paresis; general practitioner
GPT   glutamic-pyruvic transaminase
GpTH   group therapy
gr   gamma roentgen; grain; gravity
grad   gradient; graduated
GRAS   generally recognized as safe
grav   gravid; gravity
GSH   glutathione (reduced form)
GSSG   glutathione (oxidized form)
GSW   gunshot wound
GU   genitourinary
guid   guidance
GV   gentian violet
GYN   gynecologic; gynecological; gynecologist; gynecology

H

h   height; hour; horizontal; hundred; Planck constant
H   henry; heroin; hydrogen; hypermetropia; hypodermic

HA   headache
HAA   hepatitis-associated antigen
HAD   hospital administration
Hb   hemoglobin
HB   heart block
HBP   high blood pressure
HC   home care; hydrocortisone
HCG   human chorionic gonadotropin
HCT   hematocrit
HCVD   hypersensitive cardiovascular disease
HD   Hansen disease; hearing distance
HDLW   distance at which a watch is heard with left ear
HDRW   distance at which a watch is heard with right ear
He   helium
HE virus   human enteric virus
HEENT   head, eye, ear, nose, and throat
hemi   hemiplegia
Hf   hafnium
HF   Hageman factor (factor XII)
hg   hectogram; hemoglobin; hyperglycemic factor (hectogram)
Hg   mercury (hydrargyrum)
hgb   hemoglobin
HGF   hyperglycemic factor (hyperglycemic-glycogenolytic factor)
HGH   human growth hormone
HH   heard of hearing
HHb   reduced hemoglobin
HI   hemagglutination inhibition
HIC   heart information center
HID   headache, insomnia, and depression
HIF   Health Information Foundation
hl   hectoliter
HL   half-life
HM   hand movements
HMC   heroin, morphine, and cocaine
HMD   hyaline membrane disease
HMG   human menopausal gonadotropin
HMO   heart minute output
HN   head nurse

Ho   holmium
HOP   high oxygen pressure
hor   horizontal
hosp   hospital
Hp   haptoglobin
HP   high potency; high pressure; hot pack; hot pad; hydrostatic pressure
hpf   high power field
HPG   human pituitary gonadotropin
HPI   history of present illness
HPN   hypertension
hr   hour
HR   heart rate
HRH   hypothalamic-releasing factors
HS   heart sounds; house surgeon
HSA   human serum albumin
HSV   herpes simplex virus
ht   height
HT   hydrotherapy; hypodermic tablet
HV   hyperventilation
HVD   hypertensive vascular disease
HVL   half-value layer
Hx   history; hypoxanthine
Hy   hypermetropia
hyd   hydrautics; hydrostatics
hyg   hygiene
hyp   hyperresonance; hypertrophy
hys   hysteria
Hz   hertz

I

i   incisor (deciduous); insoluble; optically inactive
I   incisor (permanent); iodine; internal medicine
IA   impedance angle; intraarterial
IAA   indoleacetic acid
IAFI   infantile amaurotic familial idiocy
I & D   incision and drainage
I & O   intake and output
ibid   in the same place (ibidem)
IB   inclusion body
IC   inspiratory capacity; inspiratory center; intensive care; intercostal; interstitial cell; intracerebral; intracutaneous
ICF   intracellular fluid
ICN   International Council of Nurses
ICPMM   incisors, canines, premolars, and molars
ICT   inflammation of connective tissue; insulin coma therapy
ICU   intensive care unit
id   same (idem)
ID   dentification; inside diameter; intradermal
ie   that is (id est)
IE   immunizing unit (immunitäts Einheit)
IF   interstitial fluid
Ig   immunoglobulin
IH   infectious hepatitis
IHSA   iodinated human serum albumin
IHSS   idiopathic hypertrophic subaortic stenosis
IL   illinium
IM   intramuscular; intramuscularly
immunol   immunology
imp   important; impression
in   inch
In   indium
inc   incomplete; inconclusive; increase
incl   including; inclusive
incr   increase; increased; increment
incur   incurable
ind   independent
IND   investigational new drug
indic   indication; indicative
inf   infant; infantile; infected; infection; inferior; infusion; infirmary
infl   influence
ing   inguinal
INH   isoniazid
INI   intranuclear inclusion
inj   injection; injury
INPRONS   information processing in the central nervous system
ins   insurance
insol   insoluble
insp   inspiration

inst institute
instr instructor
int intermittent; intern; internal
inv inversion
invol involuntary
IO intraocular
IOP intraocular pressure
IP International Pharmacopoeia; interphalangeal; intraperitoneal
IPH interphalangeal
IPPB intermittent positive pressure breathing
IPPR intermittent positive pressure respiration
IPSP inhibitory postsynaptic potential
IQ intelligence quotient
Ir iridium
IR infrared; internal resistance
IRI immunoreactive insulin
is island
IS intercostal space
ISC interstitial cell
ISF interstitial fluid
isom isometric
ISP distance between iliac spines
IST insulin shock therapy
ITP idiopathic thrombocytopenic purpura
ITT insulin tolerance test
IU immunizing unit; international unit
IUD intrauterine contraceptive device
IV intravenous; intravenously; intraventricular
IVC inferior vena cava
IVCD intraventricular conduction delay
IVD intervertebral disc
IVP intravenous pyelogram
IVT intravenous transfusion
IZS insulin zinc suspension

J

J joint; joule
JAI juvenile amaurotic idiocy

jct junction
JJ jaw jerk
JNA Jena Nomina Anatomica
JND just noticeable difference
jour journal
jt or jnt joint
juv juvenile

K

K absolute zero; constant; kelvin; potassium (kalium)
ka cathode (kathode)
kc kilocycle
KC cathodal closing
kcal kilocalorie
KCC cathodal closing contraction
kCi kilocurie
kcps kilocycle per second
KCT cathodal closing tetanus
KD cathodal duration
KDT cathodal duration tetanus
keV kiloelectron volt
kg kilogram
kg-cal kilogram-calorie
kHz kilohertz
KI Krönig's isthmus
KJ knee jerk
KK knee kick
kl kiloliter
km kilometer
kMc kilomegacycle
kMcps kilomegacycles per second
KOC cathodal opening contraction
Kr krypton
KS ketosteroid
KUB kidney, ureter, and bladder
kV kilovolt
KW kilowatt
kW-hr kilowatt hour

L

L Latin; left; lethal; lewisite; licensed; light; liter; lower; lumen
La lanthanum

437

LA   left angle; left atrium; left auricle
lab   laboratory
lab proc   laboratory procedure
lac   laceration
LAD   lactic acid dehydrogenase
L & A   light and accommodation (pupil reaction)
L & B   left and below
L & W   living and well
lap   laparotomy
LAP   leukocyte alkaline phosphatase
laryngol   laryngologist; laryngology
lat   lateral; latitude
LATS   long-acting thyroid stimulator
lb   pound
LB   low back
LBD   left border dullness
LBH   length, breadth, and height
LBP   low back pain; low blood pressure
LCCS   low cervical cesarean section
LCM   left costal margin; lymphocytic choriomeningitis
LD   lethal dose
LDH   lactate dehydrogenase; lactic dehydrogenase
LE   left eye; lower extremity; lupus erythematosus
LES   local excitatory state
Leu   leucine
LF   limit of flocculation; low frequency
LGV   lymphogranuloma venereum
LH   left hand; luteinizing hormone
LHRH   luteinizing hormone–releasing hormone
Li   lithium
LIF   left iliac fossa
lig   ligament
lin   linear
liq   liquid; liquor
LKS   liver, kidney, and spleen
LLBCD   left lower border of cardiac dullness
LLE   lower left extremity
LLL   left lower lobe (lung)
LLQ   left lower quadrant (abdomen)
lm   lumen

LM   longitudinal muscle
LMD   local medical doctor
LMP   last menstrual period
LNMP   last normal menstrual period
LOA   leave of absence
loc cit   in the place cited (loco citato)
log   logarithm
LOM   limitation of motion
LOP   leave on pass
LP   latent period; low pressure; lumbar puncture
lpf   lower power field
LPF   leukocytosis-promoting factor
LPN   licensed practical nurse
LQ   lower quadrant
Lr   lawrencium
LR   latency relaxation
LRF   liver residue factor
LS   lumbosacral
LSB   left sternal border
LSD   lysergic acid diethylamide
LSK   liver, spleen, and kidneys
lt   left; light
LTB   laryngeal-tracheal bronchitis
ltd   limited
LTH   luteotropic hormone
Lu   lutetium
LUE   left upper extremity
LUL   left upper lobe (lung)
LUQ   left upper quadrant (abdomen)
lv   leave
LV   left ventricle
LVH   left ventricular hypertrophy
LVN   licensed vocational nurse
lymph   lymphocyte

M

m   macerate; male; malignant; married; masculine; mass; mature; mean; melts at; memory; chin (mentum); noon (meridies); metabolite; meter; minute; molar; molecular weight; morphine; mother; murmur; muscle; dullness (mutitas); myopia
M   *Micrococcus*

mA   milliampere
MA   menstrual age; mental age; mentum anterior
MABP   mean arterial blood pressure
mac   macerate
MAC   maximum allowable concentration
MAF   minimum audible field
mag   magnification; large (magnus)
MAO   monoamine oxidase
MAOI   monoamine oxidase inhibitor
MAP   minimum audible pressure
masc   masculine
MAT   manual arts therapist
max   maximum
MBC   maximum breathing capacity
MBP   mean blood pressure
Mc   megacycle
MCAT   Medical College Admissions Test
MCB   membranous cytoplasmic bodies
MCD   mean corpuscular diameter
mcg   microgram
mch   millicurie hour
MCH   mean corpuscular hemoglobin
MCHC   mean corpuscular hemoglobin concentration
mCi   millicurie
MCi   megacurie
MCL   midclavicular line
MCV   mean corpuscular volume
md   median
MD   medical department; Doctor of Medicine; mentally deficient; mitral disease; muscular dystrophy
MDH   malic dehydrogenase
MDR   minimum daily requirement
MDS   Master of Dental surgery
Me   methyl
ME   medical examiner; middle ear
meas   measure; measurement
MeB   methylene blue
med   medial; median; medical; medicinal; medicine; medium
MED   minimal effective dose; minimum erythema dose
MEF   maximal expiratory flow

meg   megacycle
mem   member
memb   membrane
MEP   mean effective pressure; motor end plate
mEq   milliequivalent
Met   methionine
MFD   minimum fatal dose
MFG   modified heat degraded gelatin
MFT   muscle function test
mg   milligram
Mg   magnesium
MH   marital history; menstrual history; mental health
MHB   maximum hospital benefit
MHD   minimum hemolytic dose
mHg   millimeters of mercury
MHz   megahertz
MI   mitral insufficiency; myocardial infarction
mid   middle
MID   minimum infective dose
min   minimal; minimum; minute
MIO   minimal identifiable odor
misc   miscellaneous
MIT   monoiodothyrosine
mit insuf   mitral insufficiency
mixt   mixture
mks   meter-kilogram-second
ml   midline; milliliter
MLD   minimum lethal dose
mm   millimeter
mM   millimole
MM   mucous membrane
MMPI   Minnesota Multiphasic Personality Inventory
MMT   manual muscle test
Mn   manganese
mo   month
Mo   molybdenum
MO   mineral oil
mod   moderate
mol   molecular; molecule
MON   milk of magnesia
mon or mono   monocyte; mononucleosis
morph   morphological; morphology
mOsm   milliosmol

mp melting point
MP metacarpophalangeal (wrist);
    metatarsophalangeal (ankle);
    mentum posterior; mesiopulpal
MPC maximum permissible concen-
    tration
MPH Master of Public Health
MPI Multiphasic Personality Inven-
    tory
MPN most probable number
mr milliroentgen
MR mentally retarded; metabolic
    rate; methyl red
mrd millirutherford
MRD minimum reacting dose
mrhm milliroentgen per hour at one
    meter
MRL medical record librarian
mRNA messenger RNA
MRU minimal reproductive units
MS Master of Science; Master of
    Surgery; mitral stenosis; mor-
    phine sulfate; multiple sclerosis
msec millisecond
MSG monosodium glutamate
MSH melanocyte-stimulating hor-
    mone
MSL midsternal line
MSN Master of Science in Nursing
MSRPP multidimensional scale for
    rating psychiatric patients
MST mean survival time
MSW Master of Social Welfare;
    Master of Social Work
MT medical technologist; medical
    technology; metatarsal
MTT mean transit time
MTX methotrexate
musc muscle
mv millivolt
Mv mendelvium
MVV maximum voluntary ventila-
    tion
MW molecular weight
my myopia
myco mycobacterium
myelo myelocyte

N

N   nasal; nerve; neurology; neuter;
    neutron dosage unit; nitrogen;
    nonmalignant; normal; number
Na sodium
NA Nomina Anatomica; numerical
    aperture; nurse's aide
NAD nicotinamide-adenine dinu-
    cleotide; no appreciable dis-
    ease
NADP nicotinamide-adenine dinu-
    cleotide phosphate
NAMH National Association for
    Mental Health
N & T nose and throat
N & V nausea and vomiting
nat native; natural
Nb niobium
NB newborn; note well (nota bene)
NBM nothing by mouth
nc nanocurie
Nd neodymium
ND neutral density
Ne neon
NE not enlarged
neg negative
neurol neurological; neurology
NF National Formulary
ng nanogram
NG nasogastric; no good
Ni nickel
nl nanoliter; is not permitted (non
    licet)
nm nanometer
NM neuromuscular; nitrogen mus-
    tard
NMI no middle initial
NMN nicotinamide mononucleotide
NMR nuclear magnetic resonance
nn nerves
NND new and nonofficial drugs
NNR new and nonofficial remedies
no number
No nobelium
NO nitric oxide
NOP not otherwise provided for
norm normal
NOS not otherwise specified

Np   neptunium

np   neuropsychiatric; neuropsychiatry; nucleoplasmic; nucleoprotein; nursing procedure

NPO   nothing by mouth (non per os)

NPT   normal pressure and temperature

nr   near

NR   neutral red; no refill; normal range

NS   nervous system; neurosurgery; normal saline; normal serum

NSFTD   normal spontaneous full-term delivery

NSR   normal sinus rhythm

NSU   nonspecific urethritis

NT   no test

NTP   normal temperature and pressure

nuc   nucleated

nucl   nucleus

Nv   naked vision

NYD   not yet diagnosed

O

O   occiput; oculus (eye); oral; orally; oxygen

O_2 cap   oxygen capacity

O_2 sat   oxygen saturation

OA   occiput anterior; old age; osteoarthritis

O & C   onset and course

OASP   organic acid soluble phosphorus

ob   he died (obiit); obstetrical; obstetrician; obstetrics

OBG or OB-GYN   obstetrician-gynecologist; obstetrics-gynecology

obs   observed, observer; observation

obstet   obstetrical; obstetrics

OC   oxygen consumed

occas   occasionally

occup   occupation; occupational

OD   Doctor of Optometry, occupational disease; optical density;

outside diameter; overdose; right eye (oculus dexter)

OF   occipital-frontal

OFC   occipitofrontal circumference

off   official

OHD   organic heart disease

OHI   ocular hypertension indicator

oint   ointment

OJ   orange juice

ol   oleum

OM   otitis media

ONP   operating nursing procedure

OOB   out of bed

OOLR   ophthalmology, otology, laryngology, and rhinology

OP   occiput posterior; operation; osmotic pressure; other than psychotic; outpatient

OPC   outpatient clinic

op cit   in the work cited (opere citato)

OPD   outpatient department; outpatient dispensary

oph or ophth   ophthalmic; ophthalmologic; ophthalmologist; ophthalmology; ophthalmoscope; ophthalmoscopy

opt   optical; optician; optics; optional

OR   operating room

O-R   oxidation-reduction

ord   orderly

org   organic

orig   origin; original

Os   osmium; left eye (oculus sinister)

OT   objective test; occupational therapy

OTC   over-the-counter; oxytetracycline

oz   ounce

P

P   parental; part; percentile; pharmacopeia; phosphorus; pint; plasma; pole; population; position; positive; posterior; postpartum; presbyopia; premolar; pressure; psychiatry; pulse; pupil

p   radiant flux

P_2 pulmonic second heart sound

Pa   protactinium

PA   paralysis agitans; pernicious anemia; posteroanterior; posteroanterior projection; psychoanalyst; pulmonary artery

PABA   para-aminobenzoic acid

PAC   phenacetin, aspirin, and caffeine

PAD   phenacetin, aspirin, and deoxyephedrine

palp   palpable

P & A   percussion and auscultation

P & N   psychiatry and neurology

pap   papilla

PAP   primary atypical pneumonia

PAR   postanesthetic recovery

PARU   postanesthetic recovery unit

PAS   para-aminosalicylic acid

PASA   para-aminosalicylic acid

pat   patent

path   pathological; pathologist; pathology

Pb   lead (plumbum); presbyopia

PB   pressure breathing

PBI   protein-bound iodine

PC   phosphocreatine; present complaint

PCG   phonocardiogram

pCi   picocurie

PCT   plasmacrit test

PCV   packed cell volume

pD   prism diopter; pupillary distance

PD   interpupillary distance; Doctor of Pharmacy; papilla diameter; paralyzing dose; pediatrics

PDA   patent ductus arteriosus

PDB   paradichlorobenzene

PDC   private diagnostic clinic

pdr   powder

Pe   pressure on expiration

PE   physical examination; probable error; pulmonary embolism

PEG   pneumoencephalogram; pneumoencephalography

penic   penicillin

PEP   phosphoenolpyruvate

per   period; periodic; person

perf   perforated; perforation

perm   permanent

perp   perpendicular

pers   personal

pg   picogram

PG   postgraduate; prostaglandin

pga   pteroylglutamic acid

PGR   psychogalvanic response

ph   phenyl

pH   hydrogen ion concentration

PH   pharmacopoeia; past history; previous history; public health

PHA   phytohemagglutinin

pharm   pharmaceutical; pharmacist; pharmacy

Phc   pharmaceutical chemist

PhD   Doctor of Philosophy

PHK cells   postmortem human kidney cells

phys   physical; physician

physiol   physiological; physiologist; physiology

PI   present illness; proactive inhibition; protamine insulin

PID   pelvic inflammatory disease

PIE   pulmonary infiltration with eosinophilia

PIF   prolactin inhibitory factor

PIP   proximal interphalangeal

PITR   plasma iron turnover rate

pk   dissociation constant; ionization constant

PK   psychokinesis

pKU   phenylketonuria

pl   place; plate

PL   light perception

Pm   promethium

PM   physical medicine; after noon (post meridiem); postmortem; presystolic murmur

PM & R   physical medicine and rehabilitation

PMA test   primary mental abilities test

PMB   polymorphonuclear basophilic (leukocytes)

PMD   private medical doctor

442

PME   polymorphonuclear eosinophil-
      ic (leukocytes)
PMH   past medical history
PMI   past medical illness; point of
      maximum impulse; point of
      maximum intensity; previous
      medical illness
PMN   polymorphonuclear neutro-
      philic (leukocytes)
PMP   previous menstrual period
PMS   postmenopausal syndrome;
      pregnant mare's serum
PN   peripheral nerve; practical
      nurse; psychiatry neurology;
      psychoneurotic
PNC   penicillin
PND   paroxysmal nocturnal dyspnea;
      postnasal drip
PNH   paroxysmal nocturnal hemo-
      globinuria
PNPR positive-negative pressure
      respiration
PNS   peripheral nervous system
pnx   pneumothorax
Po   polonium
PO   phone order; postoperative
POA   primary optic atrophy
poly polymorphonuclear leukocyte
pop   population
poplit popliteal
pos   position; positive
post posterior; postmortem
post-op postoperative
pot   potential; potion
PP   near point (punctum proximum);
      postpartum; postprandial
PPC   progressive patient care
PPCF plasma prothrombin conver-
      sion factor
PPD   purified protein derivative
PPF   pellagra preventive factor
ppg   picopicogram
PPLO pleuropneumonia-like organ-
      ism (mycoplasma)
ppm   parts per million
ppt   precipitate
Pr   praseodymium; presbyopia; pro-
      pyl; prism

PR   percentile rank; pressoreceptor;
      proctologist
PRA   plasma renin activity
prac practice
pract practical
PRD   partial reaction of degeneration
PRE   progressive resistive exercise
pref preference
preg pregnant
prelim preliminary
pre-op preoperative
prep prepare, preparation
prev preventive; prevention; previous
prin principal
priv private
proc procedure; proceedings; pro-
      cess
Proct proctologist; proctology
prod product; production
prog prognosis
proj project
pros prostate
prosth prosthesis
prot protein
prox proximal
Ps   prescription
PS   plastic surgery; pulmonary ste-
      nosis; serum from a pregnant
      woman
psAn psychoanalysis; psychoanalyst;
      psychoanalytic; psychoanalyti-
      cal
PSE   point of subjective equality
PSF   prolactin-stimulating factor
psi   pounds per square inch
PSL   potassium, sodium chloride;
      sodium lactate
PSMA progressive spinal muscular
      atrophy
P sol partly soluble
psych or psychol psychology
pt   part, patient, pint, point
Pt   platinum
PT   physical therapy
PTA   plasma thromboplastin anteced-
      ent; prior to admission
PTC   phenylthiocarbamide; plasma
      thromboplastin component
PTF   plasma thromboplastin factor

PTH parathyroid hormone
PTT partial thromboplastin time
PTU propylthiouracil
Pu plutonium
PU pregnancy urine
pub public; published; publisher
pulm pulmonary
PUO pyrexia of undetermined origin
PV plasma volume
pva polyvinyl alcohol
PVC premature ventricular contraction
PVD peripheral vascular disease
PVM pneumonia virus of mice
PVP polyvinylpyrrolidone
pvt private
Px past history; physical examination; pneumothorax; prognosis
Pyr pyridine
PZI protamine zinc insulin

Q

Q electric quantity; quantity; quartile
QNS quantity not sufficient
QRS segment of electrocardiograph
qt quart
qual qualitative; quality
quant quantitative; quantity
quar quarter; quarterly
qv which see (quod vide)

R

R radioactive mineral; rectal; regression coefficient; resistance; resistant; respiration; response; review; right; roentgen; roentgenologist; roentgenology
Ra radium
RA rheumatoid arthritis; right atrium; right auricle
rac racemic
rad radical; radius
RAIU radioactive iodine uptake
R & D research and development

R & R rate and rhythm (or pulse)
RAS reticular-activating system
Rb rubidium
RBC red blood cells; red blood count
RBD right border of dullness
RBE relative biological effectiveness
RBF renal blood flow
RC red cell; respiration ceased; respiratory center
RCM right costal margin
RCO aliphatic acyl radical
RCT Rorschach Content Test
rd rutherford
RD reaction of degeneration; retinal detachment
RdA reading age
RdQ reading quotient
RDS respiratory distress syndrome
Re rhenium
RE reticuloendothelium; right eye
readm readmission
rec record; recreation; recurrent
recond recondition
reconstr reconstruction
recryst recrystallize
rect rectified
ref reference
reg region; registered; regular
regen regenerate; regeneration
reg umb umbilical region
rehab or rehabil rehabilitation
rel relative
REL rate of energy loss
rem dosage of ionizing radiation equivalent in effect to one roentgen of X-ray or gamma-ray dosage (roentgen equivalent man)
REM rapid eye movement
rep repeat; report
REP retrograde pyelogram
res research; reserve; residence; resident
RES reticuloendothelial system
resp respiration; respiratory; responsible
ret retired

retic   reticulocyte

rev   reverse; review; revolution

RF   rheumatic fever; rheumatoid factor

RFR   refraction

RGE   relative gas expansion

rh   rhonchi

Rh   Rhesus (blood factor); rhodium

RH   relative humidity; right hand

RHC   respirations have ceased

RHD   relative hepatic dullness; rheumatic heart disease

rheum   rheumatic; rheumatism

RHF   right heart failure

Rhin   rhinologist; rhinology

RI   refractive index; respiratory illness; retroactive inhibition

RICM   right intercostal margin

RIF   right iliac fossa

RISA   radioactive iodinated serum albumin

rl   fine rales

Rl   medium rales

RL   coarse rales; reduction level

RLE   right lower extremity

RLF   retrolental fibroplasia

RLL   right lower lobe (lung)

RLQ   right lower quadrant (abdomen)

RLR   right lateral rectus

RM   respiratory movement

RML   right mediolateral; right middle lobe

Rn   radon

RN   registered nurse

RNA   ribonucleic acid

RNase or RNAase   ribonuclease

Rnt   roentgenologist; roentgenologist; roentgenology

RO   routine order

R/O   rule out

ROM   range of motion

rot   rotation

RPF   relaxed pelvic floor; renal plasma flow

rpm   revolutions per minute

rps   renal pressure substance; revolutions per second

rpt   report

RPT   registered physical therapist

RQ   recovery quotient; respiratory quotient

RR   radiation response; recovery room

RR & E   round, regular, and equal (eye pupils)

RS   reinforcing stimulus; review of symptoms

rt   right

RT   radiotherapy; reaction time; reading test; recreational therapy; registered technician

Ru   ruthenium

RU   Roentgen unit

RUE   right upper extremity

RUL   right upper lobe (lung)

rupt   rupture

RUQ   right upper quadrant (abdomen)

RV   residual volume; retroversion; right ventricle

RVH   right ventricular hypertrophy

Rx   prescription; therapy; treatment

S

s   left (sinister); half (semis); second

S   sacral; scruple; second; section; sensation; sign; single; singular; son; stimulus; subject; sulfur; surgeon; spherical; spherical lens

Sa   samarium

SA   surface area; sinoatrial

SAD   sugar, acetone, and diacetic acid

SAH   subarachnoid hemorrhage

sanit   sanitary; sanitation

sapon   saponification

sat   satelite; saturated

sat sol   saturated solution

Sb   antimony (stibium); strabismus

SB   Bachelor of Science (Scientiae Baccalaureus); Stanford-Binet (intelligence test)

sc   science; scientific; subcutaneously

Sc   scandium; scapula

SCAT sheep cell agglutination test
SCB strictly confined to bed
sci science; scientific
SCU special care unit
SCV smooth; capsulated; virulent
SD skin dose; standard deviation
SDA specific dynamic action; succinic dehydrogenase
sds sounds
Se selenium
SE saline enema; sanitary engineer; standard error
sec second; secondary; section
SEC soft elastic capsules
sed sedimentation
SED skin erythemal dose
sed rate sedimentation rate (erythrocyte)
sem semen; seminal
sem ves seminal vesicle
sep separate; separated; separation
ser serial; series; service
serv services
SF spinal fluid
SFC spinal fluid count
SFW slow-filling wave
sg specific gravity
SGOT serum glutamic oxaloacetic transaminase
SGPT serum glutamic pyruvic transaminase
sh short; shoulder
SH serum hepatitis; social history; somatotrophic hormone
Si silicon
SI saturation index; soluble insulin (Systemes International d'Unités)
SIADH syndrome of inappropriate antidiuretic hormone
sib sibling
SIC surgical intensive care
SID sudden infant death
SIG sigmoidoscopy
sing singular
SK streptokinase
sl slightly
SL small lymphocyte
SLDH serum lactate dehydrogenase

SLE Saint Louis encephalitis; systemic lupus erythematosus
sm small
Sm samarium
SM Master of Science (scientiae magister); streptomycin
SMR somnolent metabolic rate; submucous resection
Sn tin (stannum)
SN student nurse
SNDO Standard Nomenclature of Diseases and Operations
SNM Society of Nuclear Medicine
SNS sympathetic nervous system
SOB shortness of breath
soc social
sol soluble; solution
soln solution
S-O-R stimulus-organism-response
sp species; specific; spinal
SP sacrum to pubis
S/P status post
SPCA serum prothrombin conversion accelerator; Society for the Prevention of Cruelty to Animals
spec special, specific, specimen
sp fl spinal fluid
sp gr specific gravity
spir spiral
spon spontaneous
sq square
SQ subcutaneous
Sr strontium
SR sedimentation rate; sigma reaction; sinus rhythm; stomach rumble; systems review
SRN state registered nurse
sRNA soluble RNA; transfer RNA
SRS slow reacting substance
SS saline soak; soapsuds; sterile solution
SSD source skin distance
SSE soap solution enema
sss layer on layer (stratum super stratum)
st stimulus

ST sedimentation time; slight trace; standardized test; surface tensions; survival time
sta station
Staph *Staphylococcus*
std standard
STD skin test dose; standard test dose
STH somatotrophic hormone
STP standard temperature and pressure; standard temperature and pulse
STREP *Streptococcus*
struct structure
STS serum test for syphilis
STU skin test unit
SU sensation unit
subsp subspecies
sup superior; supination; above (supra)
supp suppository
surg surgeon; surgery; surgical
sv single vibrations
SV simian virus; sinus venosus; stroke volume
SVC superior vena cava
SWR serum Wassermann reaction
Sx symptoms
sym symmetrical
syst system; systolic

T

T temperature; temporal; tension; thoracic; time; topical; total; trace; transverse
T_3 triiodothyronine
T_4 thyroxine
Ta tantalum
TA toxin-antitoxin; transaldolase; tuberculin alkaline
tab tablet
TAB typhoid, parathyphoid A, and parathyphoid B (vaccine)
TAH total abdominal hysterectomy
TAM toxoid-antitoxin mixture

T & A tonsillectomy and adenoidectomy; tonsillitis and adenoiditis; tonsils and adenoids
TAT tetanus antitoxin; Thematic Apperception Test; toxin-antitoxin
Tb terbium
TB thymol blue; tubercle bacillus; tuberculosis
TBG thyroxine-binding globin
TBLC term birth, living child
TBPA thyroxine-binding proalbumin
tbsp tablespoon
Tc technetium
TC tetracycline; tissue culture
TCA trichloroaectic acid
TCP tricresyl phosphate
TD thyphoid dysentery
Te tellurium; tetanus
TE trial and error
tech technical
TED threshold erythema dose
temp temperature; temporal; temporary
TEPA triethylenephosphoramide
TEPP tetraethyl pyrophosphate
term terminal
tert tertiary
TF tactile fremitus; tuberculin filtrate; tuning fork
TG type genus
TGA thyroglobin antibodies
TGE transmissible gastroenteritis; tryptone glucose extract
TGT thromboplastin generation test
Th thoracic; thorax; thorium
TH thyroid hormone
THC tetrahydrocannabinol
Ti titanium
TI transverse diameter between ischia; tricuspid insufficiency
TIA transient ischemic attack
tinct tincture
TJ triceps jerk
Tl thallium
TL terminal lumen; tubal ligation
TLC tender loving care; thin-layer chromatography; total lung capacity

Tm   thulium
TM   transport mechanism
TMV   tobacco mosaic virus
Tn   normal intraocular tension
TNT   trinitrotoluene
TO   target organ; telephone order; oral temperature
TP   total protein; tuberculin precipitation
TPC   thromboplastic plasma component
TPN   triphospopyridine nucleotide
TPP   thiamine pyrophosphate
TPR   temperature, pulse, and respiration; total peripheral resistance
tr   tincture; trace; traction; tremor
TR   rectal temperature; therapeutic radiology; tuberculin R; turbidity reducing
trans   transaction; transverse
TRF   thyrotropin-releasing factor
trg   training
TRH   thyrotropin-releasing hormone
TRI   total response index
tRNA   transfer RNA
TS   terminal sensation; test solution; thoracic surgery; tricuspid stenosis; triple strength; tubular sound
TSD   target skin distance
TSH   thyroid-stimulating hormone
TSI   thyroid-stimulating immunoglobulin
tsp   teaspoon
TT   transit time; tuberculin tested
TTH   thyrotrophic hormone
TU   toxic unit; transmission unit
tus   a cough (tussis)
TV   tetrazolium violet; tidal volume; total volume; tuberculin volutin

U

U   unit; uranium; urology
U & C   urethral and cervical
UBA   undenatured bacterial antigen
UBI   ultraviolet blood irradiation
UCHD   usual childhood diseases

UCL   urea clearance test
UCR   unconditioned response
USC   unconditioned stimulus
UCV   uncontrolled variable
UD   urethral discharge; uridine diphosphate
UDC   usual diseases of childhood
UFA   unesterified fatty acid
UGI   upper gastrointestinal
UHF   ultrahigh frequency
UIBC   unsaturated iron binding capacity
umb   umbilical; umbilicus
UP   uteropelvic
UQ   upper quadrant (abdomen)
UR   unconditioned response
URI   upper respiratory infection
urol   urological; urologist; urology
US   unconditioned stimulus
USD   United States Dispensatory
USP   United States Pharmacopoeia
UTI   urinary tract infection
UTP   uridine triphosphate
UV   ultraviolet; uterovesical

V

V   valve; vanadium; vein; vertex; see (vide); virulence; vision; volt; volume
va   volt-ampere
VA   visual acuity
vac   vacuum
vacc   vaccination
vag   vaginal
V & T   volume and tension (of pulse)
var   variation; variety
VAR   visual-aural range
vasc   vascular
VAT   ventricular activation time
VC   color vision; vital capacity
VCC   vasoconstrictor center
VCG   vector cardiogram
VCS   vasoconstrictor substance
VD   veneral disease
VDA   visual discriminatory acuity
VDC   vasodilator center

448

VDG   veneral disease-gonorrhea
VDH   valvular disease of the heart
VDM   vasodepressor material
VDRL   Venereal Disease Research
       Laboratory
VDS   vasodilator substance; venereal
       disease-syphilis
VE   vesicular exanthema
vel   velocity
Vet   veteran; veterinary
VF   visual field; vocal fremitus
VG   ventricular gallop; very good
VH   Veterans Hospital
VHF   very high frequency
VI   volume index
VIC   vasoinhibitory center
VIG   vaccinia immune globulin
VL   vision—left
VLF   very low frequency
VM   vasomotor; vestibular mem-
       brane; voltmeter
VO   verbal order
vol   volar; volume; volumetric; vol-
       untary; volunteer
VP   vapor pressure; venous pressure
VPB   ventricular premature beat
vps   vibrations per second
VR   variable ratio; vision—right; vo-
       cal resonance
VRI   virus respiratory infection
VS   vesicular sound; vesicular sto-
       matitis; Veterinary Surgeon; vi-
       tal signs; volumetric solution
VU   volume unit
VV   vulva and vagina
VW   vessel wall

W

W   tungsten; water; watt; weight;
       wide; width

WAIS   Wechsler Adult Intelligence
       Scale
Wass   Wassermann test
WB   whole blood
WBC   white blood count; white
       blood cell
WC   wheelchair
WD   well developed; wet dressing
wk   week
WL   waiting list; wavelength
WN   well nourished
WO   written order; water-in-oil
WP   wet pack
WR   Wassermann reaction
ws   water soluble
wt   weight

X

X   Keinböck unit of x-ray dosage
Xe   xenon

Y

Y   young; yttrium
Yb   ytterbium
yd   yard
y/o   years old
yr   year
ys   yellow spot (on retina)

Z

z   atomic number
Z   contraction (Zuckung); zero; zone
Zn   zinc
zool   zoological; zoology
ZPG   zero population growth
Zr   zirconium

APPENDIX 2 Units of measurement

2-1. Conversion factors

Conversion rules: To convert units of one system into the other, multiply the number of units in the first column by the equivalent factor in the second column.

WEIGHT

Unit	Equivalent
1 milligram	0.015432 grain
1 gram	15.432 grains
1 gram	0.25720 apothecaries' dram
1 gram	0.03527 avoirdupois ounce
1 gram	0.03215 apothecaries' or troy ounce
1 kilogram	35.274 avoirdupois ounces
1 kilogram	32.151 apothecaries' or troy ounces
1 kilogram	2.2046 avoirdupois pounds
1 grain	64.7989 milligrams
1 grain	0.0648 gram
1 apothecaries' dram	3.8879 grams
1 avoirdupois ounce	28.3495 grams
1 apothecaries' or troy ounce	31.1035 grams
1 avoirdupois pound	453.5924 grams

CAPACITY (FLUID OR LIQUID)

Unit	Equivalent
1 milliliter	16.23 minims
1 milliliter	0.2705 fluid dram
1 milliliter	0.0338 fluid ounce
1 liter	33.8148 fluid ounces
1 liter	2.1134 pints
1 liter	1.0567 quart
1 liter	0.2642 gallon
1 fluid dram	3.697 milliliters
1 fluid ounce	29.573 milliliters
1 pint	473.166 milliliters
1 quart	946.332 milliliters
1 gallon	3.785 liters

VOLUME (AIR OR GAS)

Unit	Equivalent
1 cubic centimeter	0.06102 cubic inch
1 cubic meter	35.314 cubic feet
1 cubic meter	1.3079 cubic yard
1 cubic inch	16.3872 cubic centimeters
1 cubic foot	0.02832 cubic meter

MISCELLANEOUS CONVERSION FACTORS
Pressure

To obtain	Multiply	By
lb/sq in	atmospheres	14.696
lb/sq in	in of water	0.03609

From Mosby's medical & nursing dictionary, St. Louis, 1983, The C.V. Mosby Co.

To obtain	Multiply	By
lb/sq in	ft of water	0.4335
lb/sq in	in of mercury	0.4912
lb/sq in	kg/sq meter	0.00142
lb/sq in	kg/sq cm	14.22
lb/sq in	cm of mercury	0.1934
lb/sq ft	atmospheres	2116.2
lb/sq ft	in of water	5.1981
lb/sq ft	ft of water	62.378
lb/sq ft	in of mercury	70.727
lb/sq ft	cm of mercury	27.845
lb/sq ft	kg/sq meter	0.20482
lb/cu in	gm/ml	0.03613
lb/cu ft	lb/cu in	1728.0
lb/cu ft	gm/ml	62.428
lb/US gal	gm/ml	8.345
in of water	in of mercury	13.60
in of water	cm of mercury	5.3524
ft of water	atmospheres	33.93
ft of water	lb/sq in	2.311
ft of water	kg/sq meter	0.00328
ft of water	in of mercury	1.133
ft of water	cm of mercury	0.4460
atmospheres	ft of water	0.02947
atmospheres	in of mercury	0.03342
atmospheres	kg/sq cm	0.9678
bars	atmospheres	1.0133
in of mercury	atmospheres	29.921
in of mercury	lb/sq in	2.036
mm of mercury	atmospheres	760.0
gm/ml	lb/cu in	27.68
gm/sq cm	lb/sq in	70.31
gm/sq cm	kg/sq meter	0.1
kg/sq meter	in of water	25.38
kg/sq meter	in of mercury	345.32
kg/sq meter	cm of mercury	135.95
kg/sq meter	atmospheres	10332.0
kg/sq cm	atmospheres	1.0332

Flow rate

To obtain	Multiply	By
cu ft/hr	cc/min	0.00212
cu ft/hr	L/min	2.12
L/min	cu ft/hr	0.472

Parts per million

Conversion of parts per million (ppm) to percent: 1 ppm = 0.0001%, 10 ppm = 0.001%, 100 ppm = 0.01%, 1000 ppm = 0.1%, and 10,000 ppm = 1%.

2-2. Metric doses and apothecary equivalents

LIQUID MEASURE

Metric	Approximate apothecary equivalents
Milliliters	
1000	1 quart
750	1½ pints
500	1 pint
250	8 fluid ounces
200	7 fluid ounces
100	3½ fluid ounces
50	1¾ fluid ounces
30	1 fluid ounce
15	4 fluid drams
10	2½ fluid drams
8	2 fluid drams
5	1¼ fluid drams
4	1 fluid dram
3	45 minims
2	30 minims
1	15 minims
0.75	12 minims
0.6	10 minims
0.5	8 minims
0.3	5 minims
0.25	4 minims
0.2	3 minims
0.1	1½ minims
0.06	1 minim
0.05	¾ minim
0.03	½ minim

WEIGHT

Metric	Approximate apothecary equivalents
Grams	Grains
.0002	1/300
.0003	1/200
.0004	1/150
.0005	1/120
.0006	1/100
.001	1/60
.002	1/30
.005	1/12
.010	1/6
.015	1/4
.025	3/8
.030	1/2
.050	3/4
.060	1
.100	1½
.120	2
.200	3
.300	5
.500	7½
.600	10
1	15
2	30
4	60

2-3. Units of length, volume, and weight

Arabic numbers are used with weights and measures, as 10 gm or 3 ml. Portions of weights and measures are usually expressed decimally. For practical purposes, 1 cc is equivalent to 1 ml and 1 drop (gtt) of water is equivalent to 1 minim (m).

LINEAR MEASURE

1 inch = 2.54 centimeters
40 rods = 1 furlong
8 furlongs = 1 statute mile

12 inches = 1 foot
3 feet = 1 yard
5.5 yards = 1 rod

1 statute mile = 5280 feet
3 statute miles = 1 statute league

UNITS OF LENGTH

Millimeters	Centimeters	Inches	Feet	Yards	Meters
1 mm = 1.0	0.1	0.03937	0.00328	0.0011	0.001
1 cm = 10.0	1.0	0.3937	0.03281	0.0109	0.01
1 in = 25.4	2.54	1.0	0.0833	0.0278	0.0254
1 ft = 304.8	30.48	12.0	1.0	0.333	0.3048
1 yd = 914.40	91.44	36.0	3.0	1.0	0.9144
1 m = 1000.0	100.0	39.37	3.2808	1.0936	1.0

1 μ = 1 mu = 1 micrometer = 0.001 millimeter. 1 mm = 1000 μ.
1 Km = 1 kilometer = 1000 meters = 0.6215 mile.
1 mile = 5280 feet = 1.609 kilometers.

VOLUME CONVERSIONS

Metric

Milliliters	Minims	Fluid drams	Fluid ounces	Pints
1	16.2	.27	.0333	.0021
.0616	1	1/60	1/480	1/7680
3.697	60	1	1/8	1/128
29.58	480	8	1	1/16
473.2	7680	128	16	1

Apothecary

Liters	Gallons	Quarts	Fluid ounces	Pints
1	.2642	1.057	33.824	2.114
3.785	1	4	128	8
.946	1/4	1	32	2
.473	1/8	1/2	16	1
.0296	1/128	1/32	1	1/16

APPROXIMATE* HOUSEHOLD MEASUREMENT EQUIVALENTS (VOLUME)

		1 tsp =	5 ml
	1 tbsp =	3 tsp =	15 ml
	1 fl oz =	2 tbsp = 6 tsp =	30 ml
1 cup =	8 fl oz		= 240 ml
1 pt = 2 cups =	16 fl oz		= 480 ml
1 qt = 2 pt = 4 cups =	32 fl oz		= 960 ml
1 gal = 4 qt = 8 pt = 16 cups =	128 fl oz		= 3840 ml

*Household measures are not precise. For instance, 1 household tsp will hold from 3 ml to 5 ml of liquid. Therefore do not substitute household equivalents for prescribed medication.

WEIGHT CONVERSIONS (METRIC AND APOTHECARY)

Grams	Milligrams	Grains	Drams	Ounces	Pounds
1	1000	15.4	.2577	.0322	.00268
.001	1	.0154	.00026	.0000322	.00000268
.0648	64.8	1	1/60	1/480	1/5760
3.888	3888	60	1	1/8	1/96
31.1	31104	480	8	1	1/12
373.25	373248	5760	96	12	1

WEIGHT CONVERSIONS (METRIC AND AVOIRDUPOIS)

Grams	Kilograms	Ounces	Pounds
1	.001	.0353	.0022
1000	1	35.3	2.2
28.35	.02835	1	1/16
454.5	.4545	16	1

TROY WEIGHT (USED FOR WEIGHING GOLD, SILVER, AND JEWELS)

24 grains = 1 pennyweight
20 pennyweights = 1 ounce
12 ounces = 1 pound

MISCELLANEOUS WEIGHTS AND MEASURES

Apothecaries' weight

20 grains = 1 scruple

3 scruples = 1 dram

Avoirdupois weight

27.343 grains = 1 dram
2000 pounds = 1 short ton
1 oz troy = 480 grains
1 lb troy = 5760 grains

16 drams = 1 ounce
100 pounds = 1 hundredweight
2240 pounds = 1 long ton
1 oz avoirdupois = 437.5 grains
1 lb avoirdupois = 7000 grains

Circular measure

60 seconds = 1 minute
90 degrees = 1 quadrant

60 minutes = 1 degree
4 quadrants = 360 degrees = circle

Cubic measure

1728 cubic inches = 1 cubic foot
2150.42 cubic inches = 1 standard bushel
1 cubic foot = about four-fifths of a bushel

27 cubic feet = 1 cubic yard
268.8 cubic inches = 1 dry gallon (US)
128 cubic feet = 1 cord (wood)

Dry measure

2 pints = 1 quart

8 quarts = 1 peck

4 pecks = 1 bushel

Liquid measure

1000 milliliters = 1 liter
4 gills = 1 pint

31.5 gallons = 1 barrel (US)

2 barrels = 1 hogshead (US)

Barrels and hogsheads vary in size. One US gallon is equal to 0.8327 British gallon; therefore, 1 British gallon is equal to 1.201 US gallons. 1 liter is equal to 1.0567 quarts.

2-4. Temperature

To convert Centigrade or Celsius degrees to Fahrenheit degrees: multiply the number of Centigrade degrees by ⅘ and add 32 to the result. *To convert* *Fahrenheit degrees to Centigrade degrees:* Subtract 32 from the number of Fahrenheit degrees and multiply the difference by ⁵⁄₉.

FAHRENHEIT AND CELSIUS EQUIVALENTS: BODY TEMPERATURE RANGE

F°	C°	F°	C°	F°	C°	F°	C°
94.0	34.44	97.6	36.44	101.2	38.44	104.8	40.44
94.2	34.56	97.8	36.56	101.4	38.56	105.0	40.56
94.4	34.67	98.0	36.67	101.6	38.67	105.2	40.67
94.6	34.78	98.2	36.78	101.8	38.78	05.4	40.78
94.8	34.89	98.4	36.89	102.0	38.89	105.6	40.89
95.0	35.00	98.6	37.00	102.2	39.00	105.8	41.00
95.2	35.11	98.8	37.11	102.4	39.11	106.0	41.11
95.4	35.22	99.0	37.22	102.6	39.22	106.2	41.22
95.6	35.33	99.2	37.33	102.8	39.33	106.4	41.33
95.8	35.44	99.4	37.44	103.0	39.44	106.6	41.44
96.0	35.56	99.6	37.56	103.2	39.56	106.8	41.56
96.2	35.67	99.8	37.67	103.4	39.67	107.0	41.67
96.4	35.78	100.0	37.78	103.6	39.78	107.2	41.78
96.6	35.89	100.2	37.89	103.8	39.89	107.4	41.89
96.8	36.00	100.4	38.00	104.0	40.00	107.6	42.00
97.0	36.11	100.6	38.11	104.2	40.11	107.8	42.11
97.2	36.22	100.8	38.22	104.4	40.22	108.0	42.22
97.4	36.33	101.0	38.33	104.6	40.33		

FAHRENHEIT AND CELSIUS EQUIVALENTS

F°	C°	F°	C°	F°	C°	F°	C°
−40	−40.0	−30	−34.44	−20	−28.89	−10	−23.33
−39	−39.44	−29	−33.89	−19	−28.33	−9	−22.78
−38	−38.89	−28	−33.33	−18	−27.78	−8	−22.22
−37	−38.33	−27	−32.78	−17	−27.22	−7	−21.67
−36	−37.78	−26	−32.22	−16	−26.67	−6	−21.11
−35	−37.22	−25	−31.67	−15	−26.11	−5	−20.56
−34	−36.67	−24	−31.11	−14	−25.56	−4	−20.0
−33	−36.11	−23	−30.56	−13	−25.0	−3	−19.44
−32	−35.56	−22	−30.0	−12	−24.44	−2	−18.89
−31	−35.0	−21	−29.44	−11	−23.89	−1	−18.33

Continued.

F°	C°	F°	C°	F°	C°	F°	C°
0	−17.78	45	7.22	90	32.22	135	57.22
1	−17.22	46	7.78	91	32.78	136	57.78
2	−16.67	47	8.33	92	33.33	137	58.33
3	−16.11	48	8.89	93	33.89	138	58.89
4	−15.56	49	9.44	94	34.44	139	59.44
5	−15.0	50	10.0	95	35.0	140	60.0
6	−14.44	51	10.56	96	35.56	141	60.56
7	−13.89	52	11.11	97	36.11	142	61.11
8	−13.33	53	11.67	98	36.67	143	61.67
9	−12.78	54	12.22	99	37.22	144	62.22
10	−12.22	55	12.78	100	37.78	145	62.78
11	−11.67	56	13.33	101	38.33	146	63.33
12	−11.11	57	13.89	102	38.89	147	63.89
13	−10.56	58	14.44	103	39.44	148	64.44
14	−10.0	59	15.0	104	40.0	149	65.0
15	−9.44	60	15.56	105	40.56	150	65.56
16	−8.89	61	16.11	106	41.11	151	66.11
17	−8.33	62	16.67	107	41.67	152	66.67
18	−7.78	63	17.22	108	42.22	153	67.22
19	−7.22	64	17.78	109	42.78	154	67.78
20	−6.67	65	18.33	110	43.33	155	68.33
21	−6.11	66	18.89	111	43.89	156	68.89
22	−5.56	67	19.44	112	44.44	157	69.44
23	−5.0	68	20.0	113	45.0	158	70.0
24	−4.44	69	20.56	114	45.56	159	70.56
25	−3.89	70	21.11	115	46.11	160	71.11
26	−3.33	71	21.67	116	46.67	161	71.67
27	−2.78	72	22.22	117	47.22	162	72.22
28	−2.22	73	22.78	118	47.78	163	72.78
29	−1.67	74	23.33	119	48.33	164	73.33
30	−1.11	75	23.89	120	48.89	165	73.89
31	−0.56	76	24.44	121	49.44	166	74.44
32	0.0	77	25.0	122	50.0	167	75.0
33	0.56	78	25.56	123	50.56	168	75.56
34	1.11	79	26.11	124	51.11	169	76.11
35	1.67	80	26.67	125	51.67	170	76.67
36	2.22	81	27.22	126	52.22	171	77.22
37	2.78	82	27.78	127	52.78	172	77.78
38	3.33	83	28.33	128	53.33	173	78.33
39	3.89	84	28.89	129	53.89	174	78.89
40	4.44	85	29.44	130	54.44	175	79.44
41	5.0	86	30.0	131	55.0	176	80.0
42	5.56	87	30.56	132	55.56	177	80.56
43	6.11	88	31.11	133	56.11	178	81.11
44	6.67	89	31.67	134	56.67	179	81.67

F°	C°	F°	C°	F°	C°	F°	C°
180	82.22	189	87.22	197	91.67	205	96.11
181	82.78	190	87.78	198	92.22	206	96.67
182	83.33	191	88.33	199	92.78	207	97.22
183	83.89	192	88.89	200	93.33	208	97.78
184	84.44	193	89.44	201	93.89	209	98.33
185	85.0	194	90.0	202	94.44	210	98.89
186	85.56	195	90.56	203	95.0	211	99.44
187	86.11	196	91.11	204	95.56	212	100.0
188	86.67						

2-5. Physical elements*

Element	Symbol	Valence	Atomic number	Atomic weight†
Actinium	Ac	3	89	(227.0278)
Aluminum	Al	3	13	26.98154
Americium	Am	3,4,5,6	95	(243.0614)
Antimony	Sb	3,5	51	121.75
Argon	Ar	0	18	39.948
Arsenic	As	3,5	33	74.9216
Astatine	At	1,3,5,7	85	(209.987)
Barium	Ba	2	56	137.34
Berkelium	Bk	3,4	97	(247.0703)
Beryllium	Be	2	4	9.01218
Bismuth	Bi	3,5	83	208.9804
Boron	B	3	5	10.81
Bromine	Br	1,3,5,7	35	79.904
Cadmium	Cd	2	48	112.40
Calcium	Ca	2	20	40.08
Californium	Cf	3	98	(251.0796)
Carbon	C	2,4	6	12.011
Cerium	Ce	3,4	58	140.12
Cesium	Cs	1	55	132.9054
Chlorine	Cl	1,3,5,7	17	35.453
Chromium	Cr	2,3,6	24	51.996
Cobalt	Co	2,3	27	58.9332
Columbium	See:	Niobium		
Copper	Cu	1,2	29	63.546

*The 103 chemical elements known at present are included in this table. Some of those recently discovered have been obtained only as unstable isotopes.

†Based on Carbon-12. Figures enclosed in parentheses represent the mass number of the most stable isotope.   *Continued.*

Physical elements—cont'd

Element	Symbol	Valance	Atomic number	Atomic weight†
Curium	Cm	3	96	(247.0704)
Dysprosium	Dy	3	66	162.50
Einsteinium	Es		99	(254.0881)
Erbium	Er	3	68	167.26
Europium	Eu	2,3	63	151.96
Fermium	Fm		100	(257.0951)
Fluorine	F	1	9	18.9984
Francium	Fr	1	87	(223.0198)
Gadolinium	Gd	3	64	157.25
Gallium	Ga	2,3	31	69.72
Germanium	Ge	4	32	72.59
Glucinum	See:	Beryllium		
Gold	Au	1,3	79	196.9665
Hafnium	Hf	4	72	178.49
Helium	He	0	2	4.0026
Holmium	Ho	3	67	164.9304
Hydrogen	H	1	1	1.0079
Indium	In	3	49	114.82
Iodine	I	1,3,5,7	53	126.9045
Iridium	Ir	3,4	77	192.22
Iron	Fe	2,3	26	55.847
Krypton	Kr	0	36	83.30
Lanthanum	La	3	57	138.9055
Lawrencium	Lw		103	(256.0986)
Lead	Pb	2,4	82	207.2
Lithium	Li	1	3	6.941
Lutetium	Lu	3	71	174.97
Magnesium	Mg	2	12	24.305
Manganese	Mn	2,3,4,6,7	25	54.938
Mendelevium	Md		101	(257.0956)
Mercury	Hg	1,2	80	200.59
Molybdenum	Mo	3,4,6	42	95.94
Neodymium	Nd	3	60	144.24
Neon	Ne	0	10	20.179
Neptunium	Np	4,5,6	93	237.0482
Nickel	Ni	2,3	28	58.70
Niobium	Nb	3,5	41	92.9064
Nitrogen	N	3,5	7	14.0067
Nobelium	No		102	(255.0933)
Osmium	Os	2,3,4,8	76	190.2
Oxygen	O	2	8	15.9994
Palladium	Pd	2,4,6	46	106.4
Phosphorus	P	3,5	15	30.98376

Element	Symbol	Valance	Atomic number	Atomic weight†
Platinum	Pt	2,4	78	195.09
Plutonium	Pu	3,4,5,6	94	(244.0642)
Polonium	Po	2,4	84	(208.9824)
Potassium	K	1	19	39.098
Praseodymium	Pr	3	59	140.9077
Promethium	Pm	3	61	(144.9128)
Protactinium	Pa		91	(231.0359)
Radium	Ra	2	88	(226.0254)
Radon	Rn	0	86	(222.0176)
Rhenium	Re		75	186.207
Rhodium	Rh	3	45	102.9055
Rubidium	Rb	1	37	85.4678
Ruthenium	Ru	3,4,6,8	44	101.07
Samarium	Sm	2,3	62	150.4
Scandium	Sc	3	21	44.9559
Selenium	Se	2,4,6	34	78.96
Silicon	Si	4	14	28.086
Silver	Ag	1	47	107.868
Sodium	Na	1	11	22.98977
Strontium	Sr	2	38	87.62
Sulfur	S	2,4,6	16	32.06
Tantalum	Ta	5	73	180.9479
Technetium	Tc	6,7	43	96.9062
Tellurium	Te	2,4,6	52	127.60
Terbium	Tb	3	65	158.9254
Thallium	Tl	1,3	81	204.37
Thorium	Th	4	90	232.0381
Thulium	Tm	3	69	168.9342
Tin	Sn	2,4	50	118.69
Titanium	Ti	3,4	22	47.90
Tungsten	W	6	74	183.85
Uranium	U	4,6	92	238.029
Vanadium	V	3,5	23	50.9414
Xenon	Xe	0	54	131.30
Ytterbium	Yb	2,3	70	173.04
Yttrium	Y	3	39	88.9059
Zinc	Zn	2	30	65.38
Zirconium	Zr	4	40	91.22

APPENDIX 3   Prefixes and Suffixes

The ability to break down medical terms into separate components or to recognize a complete word depends on the mastery of the combining forms (a stem or root with an "o" attached), roots or stems that appear in medical terms, and prefixes and suffixes that alter or modify meaning and usage of a term.

3-1. Prefixes

Prefixes, the most frequently used elements in the formation of Greek and Latin words, consist of one or more syllables (prepositions or adverbs) placed before words or roots to show various kinds of relationships. They are never used independently, but when added before verbs, adjectives, or nouns, they modify the meaning. Most prefixes are a part of words in ordinary speech and do not refer specifically to medical or scientific terminology, but many occur frequently in medical terminology.

Prefixes

Prefix	Translation of Greek or Latin	Examples
a-, an-	Without, lack of	Apathy (lack of feeling) Apnea (without breath) Aphasia (without speech) Anemia (lack of blood)
ab-	Away from	Abductor (leading away from) Aboral (away from mouth)
ad-	To, toward, near to	Adductor (leading toward) Adhesion (sticking to) Adnexia (structures joined to) Adrenal (near the kidney)
ambi-	Both	Ambidextrous (ability to use hands equally) Ambilateral (both sides)
amphi-	About, on both sides, both	Amphibious (living on both land and in water)
ampho-	Both	Amphogenic (producing offspring of both sexes)

From Austrin, M.G.: Young's learning medical terminology step by step: textbook and workbook, ed. 5, St. Louis, 1983, The C.V. Mosby Co.

Prefixes—cont'd

Prefix	Translation of Greek or Latin	Examples
ana-	Up, back, again, excessive	Anatomy (a cutting up) Anagenesis (reproduction of tissue) Anasarca (severe edema)
ante-	Before, in front of	Antecubital (in front of elbow) Anteflexion (bending forward)
anti-	Against, opposed to, reversed	Antiperistalsis (reversed peristalsis) Antisepsis (against infection)
ap-, apo-	From, separation	Apolepsis (stopping of a function) Apochromatic (free from distortion of shape or color)
bi-	Twice, double	Biarticulate (double joint) Bifocal (two foci) Bifurcation (two branches)
cata-	Down, under, lower, against	Catabolism (breaking down) Catalepsy (diminished movement)
circum-	Around, about	Circumflex (winding about) Circumference (surrounding) Circumarticular (around joint)
com-, con-	With, together	Commissure (sending or coming together) Conductor (leading together) Concentric (having a common center) Concrescence (growing together)
contra-	Against, opposite	Contralateral (opposite side) Contraception (prevention of conception) Contraindicated (not indicated)
de-	Away from	Dehydrate (remove water) Dedentition (removal of teeth) Decompensation (failure of compensation)
dia-	Between, through, apart, across, completely	Diaphragm (wall across) Diapedesis (ooze through) Diagnosis (complete knowledge)

Continued.

Prefix	Translation of Greek or Latin	Examples
dis-	Reversal, apart from, separation	Disinfection (apart from infection) Disarticulation (separation at a joint) Dissect (cut apart)
e-, ex-	Out, away from	Enucleate (remove from) Eviscerate (take out viscera or bowels) Exostosis (outgrowth of bone)
ec-	Out from	Ectopic (out of place) Eccentric (away from center) Ectasia (stretching out or dilation)
ecto-	On outer side, situated on	Ectoderm (outer skin) Ectoretina (outer layer of retina)
em-, en-	In	Empyema (pus in) Encephalon (in the brain)
endo-	Within	Endocardium (within heart) Endometrium (within uterus)
epi-	Upon, on	Epidural (upon dura) Epidermis (on skin)
exo-	Upon, on, outside, on outer side, outer layer	Exogenous (originating outside) Exocolitis (inflammation of outer coat of colon)
extra-	Outside	Extracellular (outside cell) Extrapleural (outside pleura)
hyper-	Excessive, over, above	Hyperemia (excessive blood) Hypertrophy (overgrowth) Hyperplasia (excessive formation)
hypo-	Under, below, deficient	Hypotension (low blood pressure) Hypothyroidism (deficiency or underfunction of thyroid)
im-, in-	In, into	Immersion (act of dipping in) Infiltration (act of filtering in) Injection (act of forcing fluid into)
im-, in-	Not	Immature (not mature) Involuntary (not voluntary) Inability (not able)

Prefix	Translation of Greek or Latin	Examples
infra-	Below	Infraorbital (below eye) Infraclavicular (below clavicle or collar bone)
inter-	Between	Intercostal (between ribs) Intervene (come between)
intra-	Within	Intracerebral (within cerebrum) Intraocular (within eye) Intraventricular (within ventricles)
intro-	Into, within	Introversion (turning inward) Introduce (lead into)
meta-	Beyond, after, change	Metamorphosis (change of form) Metastasis (beyond original position) Metacarpal (beyond wrist)
opistho-	Behind, backward	Opisthotic (behind ears) Opisthognathous (beyond jaws)
para-	Beside, beyond, near to	Paracardiac (beside the heart) Paraurethral (near the urethra)
per-	Through, excessive	Permeate (pass through) Perforate (bore through) Peracute (excessively acute)
peri-	Around	Periosteum (around bone) Periatrial (around atrium) Peribronchial (around bronchus)
post-	After, behind	Postoperative (after operation) Postpartum (after childbirth) Postocular (behind eye)
pre-, pro-	Before, in front of	Premaxillary (in front of maxilla) Preoral (in front of mouth) Prognosis (foreknowledge) Projection (throw forward)
re-	Back, again, contrary	Reflex (bend back) Revert (turn again to) Regurgitation (backward flowing, contrary to normal)

Continued.

Prefixes—cont'd

Prefix	Translation of Greek or Latin	Examples
retro-	Backward, located behind	Retrocervical (located behind cervix) Retrograde (going backward) Retrolingual (behind tongue)
sub-	Under	Subcutaneous (under skin) Subarachnoid (under arachnoid) Subungual (under nail)
super-	Above, upper, excessive	Supercilia (upper brows) Supernumerary (excessive number) Supermedial (above middle)
supra-	Above, upon	Suprarenal (above kidney) Suprasternal (above sternum) Suprascapular (on upper part of scapula)
sym-, syn-	Together, with	Symphysis (growing together) Synapsis (joining together) Synarthrosis (articulation of joints together)
trans-	Across, through, beyond	Transection (cut across) Transduodenal (through duodenum) Transmit (sent beyond)
ultra-	Beyond, in excess	Ultraviolet (beyond violet end of spectrum) Ultraligation (ligation of vessel beyond point of origin) Ultrasonic (sound waves beyond the upper frequency of hearing by human ear)

3-2. Suffixes

Suffixes are the one or more syllables or elements added to the root or stem of a word (the part that indicates the essential meaning) to alter the meaning or indicate the intended part of speech.

To make a word pronounceable, the last letter or letters of the root to which the suffix is attached may be changed. The last vowel may be changed to an "*o*" or an "*o*" may be inserted if it is not already present before a suffix beginning with a consonant, as in cardiology. The final vowel in the root may be dropped before a suffix beginning with a vowel, as in neuritis.

Most suffixes are in common use in English, but some are peculiar to medical science. The suffixes most commonly used to indicate disease are *itis*, meaning inflammation; *oma*, meaning tumor; and *osis*, meaning a condition, usually morbid. The suffixes listed occur often in medical terminology, but they are also in use in ordinary language. These suffixes apply to Greek and Latin words.

Suffixes

Suffix	Use	Examples
-ize, -ate	Add to nouns or adjectives to make verbs expressing to use, to act like, to subject to, make into	Visualize (able to see) Impersonate (act like) Hypnotize (put into state of hypnosis)
-ist, -or, -er	Add to verbs to make nouns expressing agent or person concerned or instrument	Anesthetist (one who practices the science of anesthesia) Dissector (instrument that dissects or person who dissects) Donor (one who donates)
-ent	Add to verbs to make adjectives or nouns of agency	Recipient (one who receives) Concurrent (happening at the same time)
-sia, -y, -tion	Add to verbs to make nouns expressing action, process, or condition	Anesthesia (process or condition of not feeling) Therapy (treatment) Inhalation (act of inhaling)
-ia, -ity	Add to adjectives or nouns to make nouns expressing quality or condition	Septicemia (poisoning of blood) Disparity (inequality) Acidity (condition of excess acid) Neuralgia (pain in nerves)
-ma (mata), -men (-mina), -ment, -ure	Add to verbs to make nouns expressing result of action or object of action	Trauma (injury) Foramina (openings) Ligament (tough fibrous band holding bone or viscera together) Fissure (groove)

Continued.

Suffixes—cont'd

Suffix	Use	Examples
-ium, -olus, -olum, -culus, -culum, -cule, -cle, -ellum	Add to nouns to make diminutive nouns	Bacterium (one-cell organism) Alveolus (air sac) Follicle (little bag) Cerebellum (little brain) Molecule (little mass) Ossicle (little bone)
-ible, -ile	Add to verbs to make adjectives expressing ability or capacity	Contractile (ability to contract) Edible (capable of being eaten) Flexible (capable of being bent)
-al, -c, -ious, -tic	Add to nouns to make adjectives expressing relationship, concern, or pertaining to	Neural (referring to nerve) Neoplastic (referring to neoplasm) Cardiac (referring to the heart) Delirious (suffering from delirium)
-id	Add to verbs or nouns to make adjectives expressing state or condition	Flaccid (state of being weak or lax) Fluid (state of being liquid)
-tic	Add to a verb to make an adjective showing relationship	Caustic (referring to burn) Acoustic (referring to sound or hearing)
-oid, -form	Add to nouns to make adjectives expressing resemblance	Polypoid (resembling polyp) Plexiform (resembling a plexus) Fusiform (resembling a fusion) Epidermoid (resembling epidermis)
-ous	Add to nouns to make adjectives expressing material	Ferrous (composed of iron) Serous (composed of serum) Mucinous (composed of mucin)

APPENDIX 4 Common abbreviations used in writing prescriptions

Abbreviation	Derivation	Meaning
āā	ana	of each
a.c.	ante cibum	before meals
ad	ad	to, up to
ad lib.	ad libitum	freely as desired
aq.	aqua	water
aq. dest.	aqua destillata	distilled water
b.i.d.	bis in die	two times a day
b.i.n.	bis in noctis	two times a night
c.	cum	with
caps.	capsula	capsule
comp.	compositus	compound
dil.	dilutus	dilute
elix.	elixir	elixir
ext.	extractum	extract
fld.	fluidus	fluid
Ft.	fiat	make
g.	gramme	gram
gr.	granum	grain
gtt.	gutta	a drop
h.	hora	hour
h.s.	hora somni	hour of sleep (bedtime)
M.	misce	mix
m.	minimum	a minim
mist.	mistura	mixture
non rep.	non repetatur	not to be repeated
noct.	nocte	in the night
O	octarius	pint
ol.	oleum	oil
o.d.	omni die	every day
o.h.	omni hora	every hour
o.m.	omni mane	every morning
o.n.	omni nocte	every night
os	os	mouth
oz.	uncia	ounce
p.c.	post cibum	after meals
per	per	through or by
pil.	pilula	pill
p.r.n.	pro re nata	when required
q.h.	quaque hora	every hour

From Bergerson, B.S.: Pharmacology in nursing, ed. 14, St. Louis, 1979, The C.V. Mosby Co. *Continued.*

Common abbreviations used in writing prescriptions—cont'd

Abbreviation	Derivation	Meaning
q. 2h.		every two hours
q. 3h.		every three hours
q. 4h.		every four hours
q.i.d.	quater in die	four times a day
q.s.	quantum sufficit	as much as is required
℞	recipe	take thou
s	sine	without
Sig. or S.	signa	write on label
s.o.s.	si opus sit	if necessary
sp.	spiritus	spirits
ss	semis	a half
stat.	statim	immediately
syr.	syrupus	syrup
t.i.d.	ter in die	three times a day
t.i.n.	ter in nocte	three times a night
tr. or tinct.	tinctura	tincture
ung.	unguentum	ointment
vin.	vini	wine